Dermatologic, Cosmeceutic, and Cosmetic Development

Dermatologic, Cosmeceutic, and Cosmetic Development

Therapeutic and Novel Approaches

Edited by

Kenneth A. Walters
An-eX Analytical Services Ltd.
Cardiff, United Kingdom

Michael S. Roberts
School of Medicine, University of Queensland
Princess Alexandra Hospital
Buranda, Australia

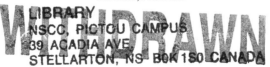
informa
healthcare

New York   London

Informa Healthcare USA, Inc.
52 Vanderbilt Avenue
New York, NY 10017

International Standard Book Number-10: 0-8493-7589-4 (hb : alk. paper)
International Standard Book Number-13: 978-0-8493-7589-7 (hb : alk. paper)

Library of Congress Cataloging-in-Publication Data

Dermatologic, Cosmeceutic, and Cosmetic Development: Therapeutic and Novel Approaches / edited by Kenneth A. Walters, Michael S. Roberts.
     p. ; cm.
  Includes bibliographical references and index.
  ISBN-13: 978-0-8493-7589-7 (hb : alk. paper)
  ISBN-10: 0-8493-7589-4 (hb : alk. paper)
  1. Skin—Diseases—Chemotherapy. 2. Dermatopharmacology. 3.
Cosmetics—Side effects. I. Walters, Kenneth A., 1949- II. Roberts, Michael S., 1949-
  [DNLM: 1. Skin Diseases—drug therapy. 2. Administration, Cutaneous.
3. Cosmetics—adverse effects. 4. Cosmetics—pharmacokinetics. 5.
Dermatologic Agents—adverse effects. 6. Dermatologie
Agents—pharmacokinetics. 7. Skin Absorption. WR 650 D4355 2007]
  RL801.D473 2007
  616.5'061—dc22   2007031863

**For Corporate Sales and Reprint Permissions call 212-520-2700 or write to:
Sales Department, 52 Vanderbilt, 16th floor, New York, NY 10017.**

**Visit the Informa Web site at
www.informa.com**

**and the Informa Healthcare Web site at
www.informahealthcare.com**

Preface

Skin disorders can be both physically and psychologically traumatic for the patient. Reactions can range from the extreme discomfort of infantile eczema to the painful embarrassment of teenage acne to the midlife desire to reduce facial wrinkles and hyperpigmentation. Researchers and clinicians within the pharmaceutical and cosmetic industries strive to find those treatments that will successfully alleviate the distressing symptoms. Basic researchers are continually searching for causative factors, be they immunologically, genetically, or environmentally mediated. As this research continues, it is safe to say that there have been many recent, significant advances in our understanding of the development and morphology of normal skin, and this has led to a more reliable ability to deliver therapeutic compounds to selected targeted areas both within the skin and systemically.

This book provides an overview of the current pharmaceutical and cosmeceutical practices in the management of both major and minor skin disorders. It is divided into eight parts. The first section is concerned with specific factors affecting efficacy of topical therapy and includes an overview of the range of skin disorders, drugs used to manage these disorders, sites where an effect is sought, and how percutaneous absorption is affected by age, skin site, race, and skin disease or damage. This section also considers delivery to the systemic circulation, appendages, and nails. The second section discusses pharmaceutical therapy from the viewpoint of topical absorption and covers treatment of the major skin diseases and injuries such as wounds and burns, with particular emphasis on novel approaches.

The third section introduces the underlying principles defining cosmeceuticals and goes on to examine their applications, sources, and formulations. The skin absorption and use of specific cosmeceuticals are then considered, covering both cosmeceutical and cosmetic agents such as hair dyes, sunscreens, oils, hydroxyacids, moisturizers, and insect repellents. The next section includes an evaluation of the evidence base for cosmeceuticals, their appropriate use, and the safety and toxicity issues.

The final portion of the book is concerned with improving therapeutic outcomes. The various methods used to improve drug transport into and across the skin, including more accurate dosing regimens, chemical penetration enhancers, physical enhancement, and the use of microneedles and high impact powder, or biolistic, delivery.

This book has been written for scientists interested in dermatological therapy and those concerned with the marketing of pharmaceutical and cosmeceutical products; in addition, it will prove useful to students and those involved in research and development in the pharmaceutical and cosmetic industries.

We have been fortunate to obtain the agreement of many internationally recognized experts in the field of dermal pharmaceutics and cosmeceuticals to provide coverage of their specific fields of expertise. To all of our authors we extend our sincere thanks for their unreserved efforts and time.

Kenneth A. Walters
Michael S. Roberts

Contents

Part V: Safety Considerations

Part VI: Skin Assessment

Part VII: Improving Therapeutic Outcomes Using Chemical Techniques

Part VIII: Improving Therapeutic Outcomes Using Physical Techniques

Contributors

Chris Anderson Department of Dermatology, Linköping University, Linköping, Sweden

Jorge Arrese Department of Dermatopathology, University Hospital of Liège, Liège, Belgium

Heather A. E. Benson School of Pharmacy, Curtin University of Technology, Perth, Western Australia, Australia

James Birchall Welsh School of Pharmacy, Cardiff University, Cardiff, U.K.

Michael Bonner School of Pharmacy, University of Bradford, Bradford, West Yorkshire, U.K.

Marcel Borgers Barrier Therapeutics NV, Geel, Belgium, and Department of Molecular Cell Biology, Maastricht University, Maastricht, Netherlands

Joke Bouwstra Leiden/Amsterdam Center for Drug Research, Leiden, the Netherlands

Keith R. Brain An-eX Analytical Services Ltd. and Cardiff University, Cardiff, U.K.

Robert L. Bronaugh Office of Cosmetics and Colors, Food and Drug Administration, College Park, Maryland, U.S.A.

Daniel A. W. Bucks Dow Pharmaceutical Sciences, Inc., Petaluma and Department of Dermatology, School of Medicine, University of California, San Francisco, San Francisco, California, U.S.A.

Christine F. Carson Department of Microbiology and Immunology, School of Biomedical, Biomolecular, and Chemical Sciences, Faculty of Life and Physical Sciences, The University of Western Australia, Crawley, Western Australia, Australia

Geert Cauwenbergh Barrier Therapeutics Inc., Princeton, New Jersey, U.S.A.

Thomas C. K. Chan ArQule Inc., Woburn, Massachusetts, U.S.A.

Susan Ciotti Pfizer Global Research and Development, Ann Arbor, Michigan, U.S.A.

Robert A. Coburn Therex LLC, Buffalo, New York, U.S.A.

Sheree E. Cross Therapeutics Research Unit, School of Medicine, University of Queensland, Princess Alexandra Hospital, Woolloongabba, Queensland, Australia

Grazyna Cynkowska Psivida Inc., Watertown, Massachusetts, U.S.A.

Tadeusz Cynkowski Psivida Inc., Watertown, Massachusetts, U.S.A.

Maxim Darvin Universitätsklinikum Charité, Klinik für Dermatologie, Venerologie und Allergologie, Berlin, Germany

Liévin Daugimont Unité de Pharmacie Galénique, Université Catholique de Louvain, Avenue Emmanuel Mounier, 73 UCL, Brussels, Belgium

Adrian F. Davis Limeway Consultancy, Dorking, Surrey, U.K.

Apostolos G. Doukas Wellman Center for Photomedicine, Massachusetts General Hospital, Boston, Massachusetts, U.S.A.

William E. Dressler Shelton, Connecticut, U.S.A.

Joseph A. Dunn Therex LLC, Buffalo, New York, U.S.A.

Anthony C. Dweck Dweck Data, Salisbury, Wiltshire, U.K.

Richard T. Evans Therex LLC, Buffalo, New York, U.S.A.

Françoise Falson Faculté de Pharmacie, Université de Lyon, Lyon, France

Des Fernandes The Renaissance Body Science Institute, Cape Town, South Africa

Joachim W. Fluhr Skin Physiology Laboratory, Department of Dermatology, Friedrich Schiller University of Jena, Jena and Bioskin, Berlin, Germany

Claudine Piérard-Franchimont Department of Dermatopathology, University Hospital of Liège, Liège, Belgium

Carlos Galzote Johnson & Johnson, Asia Pacific Skin Testing Center, Parañaque City, Metro Manila, Philippines

Robert J. Genco Therex LLC, Buffalo, New York, U.S.A.

Raman Govindarajan Johnson & Johnson Singapore Research Center, Singapore

Jeffrey E. Grice Therapeutics Research Unit, School of Medicine, University of Queensland, Princess Alexandra Hospital, Woolloongabba, Queensland, Australia

Kate A. Hammer Department of Microbiology and Immunology, School of Biomedical, Biomolecular, and Chemical Sciences, Faculty of Life and Physical Sciences, The University of Western Australia, Crawley, Western Australia, Australia

Greg G. Hillebrand Procter & Gamble, Cincinnati, Ohio, U.S.A.

Xiaoying Hui University of California, San Francisco, San Francisco, California, U.S.A.

Amit Jain Department of Chemical Engineering, University of California, Santa Barbara, Santa Barbara, California, U.S.A.

Narayanasamy Kanikkannan Tyco Healthcare Mallinckrodt, Webster Groves, Missouri, U.S.A.

Pankaj Karande Department of Chemical Engineering, University of California, Santa Barbara, California, U.S.A.

Gerald B. Kasting James L. Winkle College of Pharmacy, University of Cincinnati Academic Health Center, Cincinnati, Ohio, U.S.A.

Mark A. F. Kendall Australian Institute for Bioengineering and Nanotechnology (AIBN), The University of Queensland, Brisbane, Queensland, Australia

Neil Kitson Department of Dermatology and Skin Science, University of British Columbia, Vancouver, British Columbia, Canada

Juergen Lademann Universitätsklinikum Charité, Klinik für Dermatologie, Venerologie und Allergologie, Berlin, Germany

Chong Jin Loy Johnson & Johnson Asia Pacific, Singapore Research Center, Singapore

Guang Wei Lu Pfizer Global Research and Development, Ann Arbor, Michigan, U.S.A.

Howard I. Maibach University of California, San Francisco, San Francisco, California, U.S.A.

Paul John Matts Procter & Gamble Beauty, Egham, Surrey, U.K.

Lars E. Meyer Universitätsklinikum Charité, Klinik für Dermatologie, Venerologie und Allergologie, Berlin, Germany

Matthew A. Miller James L. Winkle College of Pharmacy, University of Cincinnati Academic Health Center, Cincinnati, Ohio, U.S.A.

Maria Miteva Skin Physiology Laboratory, Department of Dermatology, Friedrich Schiller University of Jena, Jena, Germany

Samir Mitragotri Department of Chemical Engineering, University of California, Santa Barbara, Santa Barbara, California, U.S.A.

Jesper B. Nielsen Institute of Public Health, University of Southern Denmark, Odense C, Denmark

Johannes M. Nitsche Department of Chemical Engineering, State University of New York at Buffalo, Buffalo, New York, U.S.A.

Sumit Paliwal Department of Chemical Engineering, University of California, Santa Barbara, Santa Barbara, California, U.S.A.

Gérald E. Piérard Department of Dermatopathology, University Hospital of Liège, Liège, Belgium

Fabrice Pirot Faculté de Pharmacie, Université de Lyon, Lyon, France

Véronique Préat Unité de Pharmacie Galénique, Université Catholique de Louvain, Avenue Emmanuel Mounier, 73 UCL, Brussels, Belgium

Pascale Quatresooz Department of Dermatopathology, University Hospital of Liège, Liège, Belgium

Anthony Vincent Rawlings AVR Consulting Ltd., Northwich, Cheshire, U.K.

Jürgen Reichling Department of Biology, Institut of Pharmacy and Molecular Biotechnology, University of Heidelberg, Heidelberg, Germany

Michael S. Roberts School of Medicine, University of Queensland, Princess Alexandra Hospital, Woolloongabba, Queensland, Australia

Mantu Sarkar University of Queensland, Princess Alexandra Hospital, Woolloongabba, Queensland, Australia

Ulrich F. Schäfer Biopharmaceutics and Pharmaceutical Technology, Saarbruecken, Saarland University, Germany

Sonja Schmitt Department of Biology, Institut of Pharmacy and Molecular Biotechnology, University of Heidelberg, Heidelberg, Germany

Jürgen Schneele Department of Biology, Institut of Pharmacy and Molecular Biotechnology, University of Heidelberg, Heidelberg, Germany

Jagdish Singh Department of Pharmaceutical Sciences, College of Pharmacy, North Dakota State University, Fargo, North Dakota, U.S.A.

Michael Suero Johnson & Johnson, Asia Pacific Skin Testing Center, Parañaque City, Metro Manila, Philippines

Satyanarayana Valiveti Pfizer Global Research and Development, Ann Arbor, Michigan, U.S.A.

Gaëlle Vandermeulen Unité de Pharmacie Galénique , Université Catholique de Louvain, Avenue Emmanuel Mounier, 73 UCL, Brussels, Belgium

Valérie Vroome Barrier Therapeutics NV, Geel, Belgium

Kenneth A. Walters An-eX Analytical Services Ltd., Cardiff, U.K.

Michael W. Whitehouse University of Queensland, Princess Alexandra Hospital, Woolloongabba, Queensland, Australia

R. Randall Wickett James L. Winkle College of Pharmacy, University of Cincinnati, Cincinnati, Ohio, U.S.A.

Johann W. Wiechers JW Solutions, Gouda, Netherlands

Adrian C. Williams Reading School of Pharmacy, University of Reading, Reading, U.K.

Introduction

Skin Structure, Pharmaceuticals, Cosmetics, and the Efficacy of Topically Applied Agents

Michael S. Roberts

School of Medicine, University of Queensland, Princess Alexandra Hospital, Woolloongabba, Queensland, Australia

Kenneth A. Walters

An-eX Analytical Services Ltd., Cardiff, U.K.

INTRODUCTION

The structure of human skin is a formidable barrier to determining the efficacy of topically applied compounds. Much emphasis is placed on the efficacy of topically applied therapeutic agents and developing appropriate formulations (pharmaceuticals) to facilitate their delivery. Because the structure of the skin, especially the stratum corneum, in relation to its role in percutaneous absorption has been discussed in Chapter 1 in the companion volume (1), this aspect is not being considered here. The emphasis in this chapter is on introducing key concepts in dermatological and cosmetic development, which are dealt with in greater detail in the other chapters of this book.

STRUCTURE AND THE SKIN IN RELATION TO SKIN FUNCTION

Figure 1 shows an overview of the skin in terms of the functions it performs. Protection, homeostatic, and sensing are both integrated and overlapping (2). Many products are applied to the skin to modify skin function. However, classifying them as a cosmetic or as a pharmaceutical is often difficult. Products applied to the skin to provide color or smell can be argued to not directly affect skin function. In contrast, all moisturizing cosmetic products applied to the skin do affect skin function. Both stratum corneum hydration and the rate of its turnover by desquamation can be affected when an occlusive product is applied to the skin. Further, a number of localized events follow perturbation in stratum corneum function by interventions such as delipidization, stratum corneum stripping, and surfactant applications (2). These events are discussed in Chapter 5 of the companion volume (1).

COSMETICS, COSMECEUTICALS, AND PHARMACEUTICALS

In previous decades, skin conditions, such as male-pattern baldness, dandruff, skin aging, and wrinkles, were managed using cosmetics (3). In general, *cosmetics* are asserted not to have any therapeutic effects and have been defined by the U.S. Federal Food, Drug, and Cosmetic Act (FD&C) as "an article intended to be applied to the human body…for cleansing, beautifying, promoting attractiveness, or altering the appearance without affecting the body's structure or function." In contrast, a *drug* is defined by FD&C (2) as "an article intended for use in the diagnosis, cure,

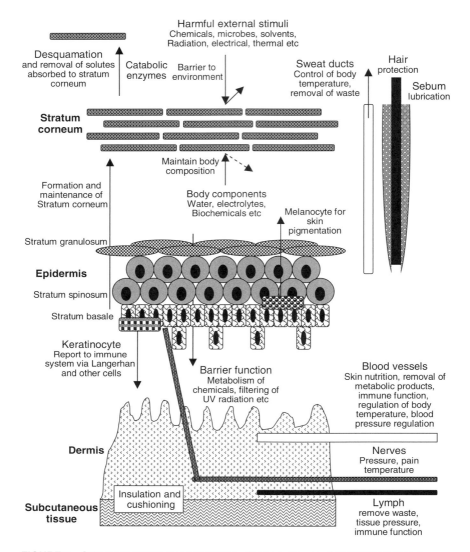

FIGURE 1   Skin components and functions performed. *Source*: Adapted from Ref. 2.

mitigation, treatment or prevention of disease, (or) intended to affect the structure or any function of the body." Thus, the conundrum, if a topical product modifies the skin, is it a cosmetic or is it a drug? What is a side effect? Hence, a deodorant is a cosmetic, whereas an antiperspirant is a drug; a shampoo is a cosmetic, whereas an antidandruff shampoo is a drug and so on. Hence, it is the purpose of the product rather than what is in it that defines its category. At this time, as is evident for very effective ingredients, such as the antiseptic tea tree oil, it is not what the products or ingredients do to the skin but rather what is stated on the label to be the intended use of the product. In general, cosmetic products should contain generally regarded

TABLE 1 The Continuum of Dermatological Knowledge

Dermatology	Cosmetic physician	Beauty therapist
Infections	Preventative antiseptics	Hygiene
Ichthyosis	Xerosis	Dry skin
Photodermatoses	Prevention of photoaging	Prevention of sunburn
Premature aging	Photoaging	Wrinkles
Pigmentary disorders	Melasma, actinic lentigines	Desire for bleaching
Acne	Hyperseborrhea	Oily skin
Scalp psoriasis	Seborrheic dermatitis	Dandruff
Hyperhidrosis	Hyperhidrosis	Sweating
Rosacea	Erythrosis	Red skin
Adipose tissue diseases	Adipose dystrophy	Cellulite
Alopecia	Male-pattern alopecia	Hair loss
Allergic dermatitis	Irritant dermatitis	Sensitive skin
Hypertrichosis	Idiopathic hirsutism	Socially excessive facial hair

Source: From Ref. 5.

as safe ingredients as defined by the U.S. Food Drug Administration (FDA) (i.e., not contain harmful substances). The European Commission's Scientific Committee on Consumer Products (SCCP) follows directives that state "a cosmetic product shall mean any substance or preparation intended to be placed in contact with the various parts of the human body (epidermis, hair system, nails, lips and external genital organs) or with the teeth and the mucous membranes of the oral cavity with a view exclusively or mainly to cleaning them, perfuming them, changing their appearance and/or correcting body odours and/or protecting them or keeping them in good condition" (2) and that a cosmetic product "must not cause damage to human health when applied under normal or reasonably foreseeable conditions of use" (4).

Wallach (5) has pointed out that the definition of a skin disease is not straightforward. Although a number of dermatoses, such as malignancies, autoimmune diseases, and severe adverse drug reactions, can be considered as diseases, there are a number that are not but may benefit from a cosmetic or other intervention. These include conditions such as greasy hair, oily skin, wrinkles, and sensitive skin. In reality, as shown in Table 1, there is a continuum of dermatological knowledge, and no clear demarcation exists between the categories requiring intervention by a dermatologist, cosmetic physician, and a beauty therapist. He points out that a drug or pharmaceutical is intended to prevent or treat a disease and that its efficacy must be proven by a double-blind, random, controlled trial. However, safety is a major consideration for such agents. In contrast, a cosmetic is intended to improve the appearance of the skin. Here, efficacy is whether it provides "beauty," and this may include acting as a camouflage for a disfiguration. In contrast, safety considerations need to carefully evaluated, recognizing that, in the past, systemic toxicity has resulted from cosmetic use. An example is hexachlorophene-containing cosmetic products, which were responsible for the death of 36 babies in France in 1972 (6).

Cosmeceuticals were originally proposed for drugs with efficacy in topical conditions, such as topical minoxidil and retinoic acid (3). A 2007 Medline search of this term reveal only 14 articles using this term since 2005. Hence, topical products are generally considered either cosmetics or pharmaceuticals. As Wallach (5) points out the key areas of overlap between these agents are in hygiene/prevention of infection, moisturizers, sunscreens, aging skin, acne, scaly scalp conditions, hyperhidrosis, and rosacea. Chapters 2 and 3 emphasize traditional pharmaceutical approaches whereas Chapter 4 emphasizes application of cosmeceutic principles.

PHARMACEUTICALS

The formulation of cosmetics and pharmaceuticals is critical not only to their efficacy but also to patient acceptance. As discussed in the companion volume, formulation can be used to maximize penetration and efficacy (1). A number of the technologies used in cosmetic formulations have been summarized by Morganti et al. (7). They classify these as closed system, open system, and polymeric reservoir. The first two of these systems are summarized in Tables 2 and 3. A key strategy in each of these systems is to leave a residue that is undetectable to the eye and neither tacky nor greasy. A number of strategies that facilitate penetration by affecting the stratum corneum integrity may also be used, and these are summarized in Figure 2. The processes associated with each strategy and examples in practice are discussed more fully in Chapters 30–36. Cosmetic product stability is also important and should be on two levels: the product and its ingredient. Product stability normally entails an assessment of the physical characteristics (e.g., rheology, evaporation rate) of the system, whereas ingredient stability is usually concerned with minimal degradation during various storage conditions. Many cosmetic products now contain either solid lipid nanoparticles or nanostructured lipid carriers. The cosmetic benefits

TABLE 2   Closed Systems

	Liposomes	Cyclodextrins	Microcapsules	Submicrocapsules
Average size	40–300 nm	Variable; 3-D structure	50–500 nm	0.1–1.0 nm
Wall composition	Phospholipid, POE, alkyl ethers, fatty acids, ceramides, or polyglycerol ethers	Oligosaccharide matrix consisting of 6, 7, or 8 glucopyranose units	Gelatin, polyvinyl alcohol, ethyl cellulose, urethane	Gelatin, alginate, albumin, carrageenan
Mode of action	Release occurs when the vesicle wall is disrupted while in contact with the SC	Release occurs when the complex is disrupted while in contact with the SC	Release occurs when the shell is disrupted by shear, abrasion, or pressure or by permeability	Release occurs when the matrix is disrupted by shear, abrasion, or pressure or by permeability
Other	May be unilamellar (single layer membrane) or multilamellar	Host complex can accommodate single molecule of active component. Cds are also hygroscopic	Composition of shell can function as membrane to control release	Matrix can be coated or uncoated; release or nonrelease can be designed

Abbreviations: POE, polyoxyethylene; SC, stratum corneum; Cds, cyclodextrins.
Source: From Ref. 7.

TABLE 3 Open Systems

	Microsponge	Polymeric liquid reservoir
Average size	5–300 nm	Variable
Composition	Polymeric: usually cross-linked, substituted acrylate	Polyester or polyurethane polymers: cross-linked or linear
Mode of action	Release occurs via several different "triggers": applied physical pressure, skin temperature, solvent for entrapped active, perspiration, and evaporation	Diffusion of active into the epidermis by partitioning mechanism: degree of skin penetration is dependent on geometry and molecular weight of polymer
Other	Porous and weblike systems: function through sorption-desorption mechanism	Co-compatibility of the polymer with actives and excipients is related to the relative polarity of the polymer

Source: From Ref. 7.

of these lipid ingredients are reported to be enhanced chemical stability of active components, formation of a film, controlled occlusion, skin hydration, enhanced skin bioavailability, and physical stability (8). Other products include a water-dissolvable cellulose film for a localized antiwrinkle effect (9). Packaging can be crucial, as evidenced by the better compliance when a "luxury jar" was used (10). Ultimately, more research is needed in this area—especially in relation to the "metamorphosis" of the vehicle after application to the skin (11). Here, the initial organization and composition of the product is altered with the evaporation of ingredients and friction associated with the product application.

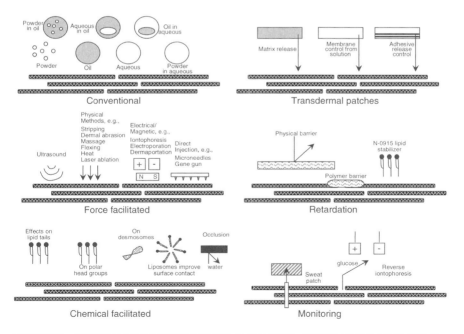

FIGURE 2 Strategies for altering percutaneous absorption. *Source*: Updated from Ref. 2.

EFFICACY

There are now many biophysical methods available to measure efficacy of products applied to treat local skin conditions. In assessing skin hydration, transepidermal water loss (TEWL) remains one of the most widely used because TEWL correlates directly with skin barrier dysfunction. Other measures, as discussed in Chapter 7, rely on measuring skin relief by using the electrical properties of the skin, such as conductance and capacitance. More advanced techniques include near infrared multispectral imaging, nuclear magnetic resonance spectroscopy, and optical coherence tomography. Laser Doppler flowmetry is used to measure local skin blood flow.

TESTING OF DERMATOLOGICS, COSMETICS, AND THEIR SAFETY EVALUATION

The United States distinguishes cosmetics and dermatologics through congressional legislature. In general, cosmetics beautify, cleanse, or promote attractiveness. When they go beyond this action, affecting the structure or function of the body, they become a drug. In relation to dermatologics, the FDA issued a white paper on critical paths on March 16, 2004 for the development of new medical products (12). A key focus in this white paper is updating the tools currently used to assess the safety and efficacy of new medical products. These tools need to be characterized by well-defined procedures, validation, standardized training, reproducibility, predictability, and clinical relevance. The FDA advocates a "maximal-use" study in the patient population of interest for topical products and an emphasis on systemic safety. This involves representing the largest anticipated usage/exposure that is consistent with the clinical trials and anticipated indication/labeling. Three categories of drugs are of interest: 505(b)(1)—classical new drug, 505(b)(2)—new formulation/form, and 505(j)—generic drug applications. In all cases, validation is the key to acceptance. In addition, as discussed in the accompanying volume (2), there is a range of safety tests required for topical products. Issues to be considered may include acute (single-patch) and cumulative (repeated-patch) irritation, use of neat or diluted material, open or occlusive, risk-benefit, type of irritation, and the selection of negative and positive controls for appropriately sensitive individuals.

In the European setting, SCCP provides guidance for the testing of cosmetic ingredients and their safety evaluation. The sixth revision of their guidance notes was adopted by the SCCP during the 10th plenary meeting in December 19, 2006 (4). SCCP points out that although cosmetic products have used a variety of ingredients derived from plants, animals, and mineral sources for thousands of years, a number of synthetic and semisynthetic ingredients have been added in recent times. Further, cosmetic products are now widely and extensively used. Although there are rare associations with serious health hazards, there is a need for a long-term safety assessment and monitoring of cosmetic ingredient chemical structures, toxicity profiles, and exposure patterns. Accordingly, the safety requirements for cosmetic products are becoming more similar to those imposed on drugs being applied for therapeutic purposes. The main difference in requirements between these two groups appears to be in relation to proof of efficacy.

Safety evaluation of cosmetic ingredients relies on data obtained from in vivo animal studies, in vitro test, quantitative structure-activity relationships, clinical studies, epidemiological studies, and reported adverse incidents. There is now an

TABLE 4 SSCP Safety Evaluation of Cosmetic Requirements

Chemical and physical specifications of cosmetic ingredients
  Chemical identity
  Physical form molecular weight
  Characterization and purity of the chemical
  Characterization of the impurities or accompanying contaminants
  Solubility
  Partition coefficient (log P_{ow})
  Additional relevant physical and chemical specifications
Relevant toxicity studies on cosmetic ingredients
  Acute toxicity
  Irritation and corrosivity
  Skin sensitization
  Dermal/percutaneous absorption
  Repeated dose toxicity
  Mutagenicity, genotoxicity, and carcinogenicity
  Reproductive toxicity
  Toxicokinetic studies
  Photoinduced toxicity
  Human data
Toxicological requirements for inclusion of a substance in one of the annexes to Dir. 76/768/EEC
  (which are evaluated by the SCCP)
    General toxicological requirements
    Annex II
    Annex III
    Annex IV
    Annex VI
    Annex VII
    Requirements for partial evaluations
Basic requirements for cosmetic ingredients (which are evaluated by individual safety assessors)
  General toxicological requirements
  Identification of mineral, animal, botanical, and biotechnological ingredients
  Fragrance materials
  Potential endocrine disruptors
  Animal-derived ingredients, including BSE issues
  CMR ingredients
  Nanoparticles
General principles for the calculation of the MoS and lifetime cancer risk for a cosmetic ingredient
  Introduction: definitions
  MoS
  Dermal absorption issues in the calculation of the SED
  MoS for children
  TTC
  Lifetime cancer risk

Abbreviations: BSE, bovine spongiform encephalopathy; CMR, carcinogenic, mutagenic, toxic to reproduction; MoS, margin of safety; SCCP, Scientific Committee on Consumer Products; SED, systemic exposure dosage; TTC, threshold of toxicological concern.
Source: From Ref. 4.

increasing emphasis on non-animal–based safety evaluations as per their Dir. 2003/15/EC2. SCCP relies on a risk assessment procedure consisting of the following (4): (i) hazard identification, (ii) dose-response assessment, (iii) exposure assessment, and (iv) risk characterization. In the case of a threshold effect, the margin of safety (MoS) is calculated according to the following formula: MoS = no observable effect level (NOAEL)/SED, where SED represents the systemic exposure dosage. For nonthreshold effects (e.g., nonthreshold carcinogenic effect), the lifetime risk usually

TABLE 5   SCCP Safety Evaluation of Finished Cosmetic Products

Categories of cosmetic products and exposure levels in use
Guidelines for the safety evaluation of finished cosmetic products
   Toxicological profile of the ingredients
   Stability and physical and chemical characteristics of the finished cosmetic product
   Evaluation of the safety of the finished product
Guidelines on microbiological quality of the finished cosmetic product
   Quantitative and qualitative limits
   Challenge testing
   Good manufacturing practice

Abbreviation: SCCP, Scientific Committee on Consumer Products.
Source: From Ref. 4.

is determined through the use of a dose descriptor. The SCCP also emphasizes the need to assess the safety profile of cosmetic ingredients (defined in Table 4) and their products (defined in Table 5).

In addition to experimental data, SCCP seeks (i) any report on epidemiological and/or observational experiences, (ii) description of all available ecological, and environmental effects of the respective substance/compound/preparation, (iii) all relevant published literature, (iv) a description of the bibliographical methods used, (v) any useful finding to the applicant's best ability, and (vi) any "gray material" available elsewhere. Table 5 shows SCCP guidelines for cosmetic product evaluations.

In general, the MoS used to extrapolate from test animals to sensitive human subpopulations must be at least 100 and is defined as a factor 10 for the extrapolation from animal to man and another factor 10 taking into account the interindividual variations within the human population (Fig. 3). According to Organisation for Economic Co-operation and Development Guideline 428 (Skin Absorption: In Vitro Method), normally, 1–5 mg/cm^2 for a solid and up to 10 μL/cm^2 for liquids should be used in in vitro tests to have an application that mimics human exposure (4). Exposure values used for various products are shown in Table 6.

As a result of such deliberations, the SCCP provides opinions on various products. One recent opinion, adopted in March 21, 2007, is on the UV filter homosalate (13). This opinion concluded, "Based on the information provided, the SCCP is of the opinion that the use of homosalate at a maximum concentration of 10%w/w in cosmetic sunscreen does not pose a risk to the health of the consumer. Use of homo-

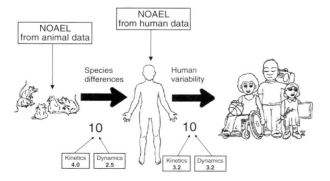

FIGURE 3 Approach to assessment of safety margin using animal and human studies. *Source*: From Ref. 4.

TABLE 6 Daily Consumer Exposure Values

Product type	Amount of substance applied (g)	Retention factor	Daily exposure calculated (g/day)
Shampoo	10.46	0.01	0.11
Face cream	1.54	1.0	1.54
Body lotion	7.82	1.0	7.82
Deodorant			
Stick	1.51	1.0	1.51
Spray	6.54	1.0	6.54
Lipstick, lip salve	0.057	1.0	0.057
Toothpaste (adult)	2.75	0.05	0.138

Source: From Ref. 4.

salate in other types of cosmetic products at concentrations up to 10.0% also does not pose a risk to the health of the consumer."

IS IT A SUCCESSFUL PRODUCT?

There are a number of necessary prerequisites for a topical dermatological or cosmetic product, including meeting technical, user acceptance, health care provider acceptance, regulatory approval, and adequate financial return considerations. At the end of the day, user acceptance and an adequate financial return may be the main determinants for product success. However, without a product, these conditions are rather irrelevant.

CONCLUSION

The success of both cosmetic and pharmaceutical products depends on an appropriate integration of skin structure and function aspects with the nature of the formulation (pharmaceuticals), its efficacy as defined by the goal of the product (cosmetic or pharmaceutical), and its safety. The function of the skin and especially the morphology of the stratum corneum are dependent on whether the barrier has been modified by hydration or by a perturbation, with consequences for the lipid assembly of the intercellular stratum corneum lipids (2). As Morganti et al. (7) point out, "To be really effective, each product should contain the right active principles in the right dose to be transported by the right carrier onto the selected skin area. These active principles have to be released by the carrier on the skin and remain there for the time needed to fulfil their function." The question remains, will cosmetic products ever become more, that is, will any of these products be commonly referred to in the future as "cosmeceuticals"? Ultimately, however, the efficacy and toxicity of a topically applied agent will depend on the intrinsic activity of any active ingredient, its interaction with the formulation, and how its ingredients affect the skin.

REFERENCES

1. Roberts MS, Walters KA. The relationship between structure and barrier function of skin. In: Roberts MS, Walters KA, eds. Dermal Absorption and Toxicity Assessment. Marcel Dekker, 1998; 91:1–42.

2. Roberts MS, Walters KA. Human skin morphology and dermal absorption. In: Roberts MS, Walters KA, eds. Dermal Absorption and Toxicity Assessment, 2nd edition. New York: Informa Healthcare, 2008; 1–13.
3. Lavrijsen AP, Vermeer BJ. Cosmetics and drugs. Is there a need for a third group: cosmeceutics? Br J Dermatol 1991; 124:503–504.
4. The SCCP's Notes of Guidance for the Testing of Cosmetic Ingredients and Their Safety Evaluation. 6th rev., European Commission, 2006. (http://ec.europa.eu/health/ph_risk/committees/04_sccp/docs/sccp_o_03j.pdf).
5. Wallach D. The field of cosmetic dermatology: the need for a patient-centred approach. J Cosmet Dermatol 2002 Oct; 1(3):137–141.
6. Editorial. Hexachlorophene today. Lancet 1982; 1:87–88.
7. Morganti P, Ruocco E, Wolf R, Ruocco V. Percutaneous absorption and delivery systems. Clin Dermatol 2001 Jul–Aug; 19(4):489–501.
8. Muller RH, Petersen RD, Hommoss A, Pardeike J. Nanostructured lipid carriers (NLC) in cosmetic dermal products. Adv Drug Deliv Rev 2007; (59):522–530.
9. Legendre JY, Schnitzler I, Li QY, et al. Formulation, characterization, and efficacy of an adenosine-containing dissolvable film for a localized anti-wrinkle effect. J Cosmet Sci 2007 Mar–Apr; 58(2):147–155.
10. Lodén M, Buraczewska I, Halvarsson K. Facial anti-wrinkle cream: influence of product presentation on effectiveness: a randomized and controlled study. Skin Res Technol 2007 May; 13(2):189–194.
11. Zhang J, Smith EW, Surber C. Galenical principles in skin protection. Curr Probl Dermatol 2007; 34:11–18.
12. Innovation or Stagnation: Challenge and Opportunity on the Critical Path to New Medical Products. U.S. Food and Drug Administration, Rockville, MD, 2006. (www.fda.gov/oc/initiatives/criticalpath/whitepaper.html). Accessed July 2007.
13. SCCP. Opinion on Homosalate. European Commission, 2006. (http://ec.europa.eu/health/ph_risk/committees/04_sccp/docs/sccp_o_097.pdf). Accessed July 2007.

2 Drugs Used for Skin Diseases

Neil Kitson

Department of Dermatology and Skin Science, University of British Columbia, Vancouver, British Columbia, Canada

INTRODUCTION

The origin of treatments for skin disease does not lie in science. Although modern methods of drug and vehicle creation and development, as well as increased understanding of the mechanisms of disease, are playing important roles in modern medicine, the reality of therapeutic life "in the trenches" has its origin in the medical apprenticeship tradition, in which methods based on experience are handed down from generation to generation of practitioners. Many of these methods, needless to say, have not been subjected to the laborious and expensive testing required for adequate statistical validation; nevertheless, it is certain that not all are useless. These methods are considered in this chapter to provide nonclinical professionals some insight into the practice of dermatology. In addition, the reality of patients is also considered because it is undoubtedly true that the patient's perception of treatment will markedly affect its success. The confirmation of this can be found in the placebo effect. Effective doctors will choose treatments in appropriate cases in such a way as to manipulate the placebo effect for the patient's maximal therapeutic advantage, and some insight into these aspects of clinical behavior will help those inventing new treatments.

THE "ART" OF DERMATOLOGICAL PRACTICE
Diagnosis
History

A brief excursion into the history of dermatological diagnosis is helpful in understanding the apparently arcane language used by clinicians in describing and treating skin disease. As with many branches of science and medicine, real understanding was preceded by various attempts at classification. Holubar (1) pointed out that Linnaeus provided a classification of human diseases in the 18th century, as did de Sauvages, and, subsequently, Plenck in Hungary published the first classification of skin diseases. Plenck, in turn, influenced the Englishman Robert Willan and his colleague Thomas Bateman, who provided the first clinically relevant classification, which has gone on to serve as the basis for current nomenclature. The primary basis for classification was the appearance (usually called morphology) of the individual lesion. Although formed from careful clinical observation, this classification essentially ignored the mechanism of the underlying pathology and was subsequently extended by Hebra, so that similar pathological processes were grouped together (e.g., inflammation, neoplasm).

In general, this approach to classification persists to the present day; clinical diagnosis is still very much based on the morphology of individual lesions, together with the distribution and time course. Experienced clinicians can frequently make diagnoses rapidly on the basis of pattern recognition, and to a novice, this process can appear very intuitive. It is, however, very similar to experienced garage mechanics making diagnoses based on evidence that is no more than "listening to the engine." An exception to this is the immunocompromised patient, in which classical morphology is often disrupted.

A further consideration is the nature of the diagnosis itself. The work of the 18th-century clinician Thomas Sydenham established the concept of disease independent of the sufferer. This idea, now taken for granted, was a revolution in medicine and remains essential to current medical practice, although the underlying mechanism of the disease may not be known. This raises the question of when a disease can be considered to be an individual entity and when it is a part of a spectrum of similar disorders that share an underlying mechanism but which may vary in expression because of many other factors. To the outsider, discussions among clinicians as to whether individually recognized diseases are, in fact, separate entities may come dangerously close to sophistry. Nevertheless, it has been repeatedly demonstrated that careful clinical observation may indeed delineate different disorders, and a striking example of this is the classification of the genetic blistering diseases, many of which have now been shown to have individual molecular mechanisms (2–4). In many other common and uncommon diseases (e.g., irritant contact dermatitis and the inherited scaling disorders known as the "ichthyoses"), the mechanisms are still not always clear, but the practice of careful clinical observation and classification has undeniable merit, particularly in relation to correlation with treatment and communication among clinicians. However, the danger of sophistry is always with us and should be guarded against.

Current Practice

The teaching of dermatological diagnosis continues to be based primarily on the morphology of individual lesions, together with their distribution and time course. In addition, there are simple bedside examinations that will assist in individual cases. An example is diascopy, in which a glass slide is pressed firmly against a lesion to compress the local blood vessels, and this is of particular value with pathology located deeper in the skin. Other simple procedures such as magnification, illumination with the so-called Wood's light ("black light," radiation at about 365 nm) is helpful in some disorders (e.g., differentiating among and between and bacterial infections), but its use is determined by diagnostic categories provided by the original examination based on morphology and distribution.

In practice, skin biopsy is frequently an invaluable aid to diagnosis. As Hebra foresaw, the information available from appropriate microscopic examination has provided great insight to the clinical diagnosis. This is particularly so in immunosuppressed patients. In such cases, the clinical appearances of common disorders may be so altered as to be unrecognizable, and the pathology becomes essential to diagnosis. Fortunately, small suitable samples of the skin can be taken for pathological examination without undue distress or cosmetic damage.

Jargon

Because of this history, names of many diagnoses are quite old, may commonly be derived from Latin and Greek, and may seem to those trained in the physical sciences to be at best arcane, and at worst, deliberately obscure. A similar lack of clarity for outsiders occurs when syndromes are linked to names (e.g., Netherton's syndrome), a practice that conveys absolutely nothing about the disorder unless this is already known. More rational systems have been suggested. Williams and

Elias (5) proposed that various epidermal disorders having a bewildering variety of names could be called collectively "disorders of cornification" and be given individual numbers (e.g., DOC9). This has not caught on, and it is unlikely the old Latin names for certain disorders or the eponymous syndromes are likely to disappear soon. Medical culture tends to resist sudden changes in direction and has (as do other branches of knowledge) an inherent respect for its own history. This is not all bad. However, simplifications in terminology will continue to occur, particularly as the biological basis for disease is better understood. Nevertheless, scientists trained in pharmacology and toxicology who have regular contact with dermatologists will continue to encounter these names and descriptive practices.

Lesions

The official morphological terms for individual lesions were proposed about the time of Willan and Bateman, originally in Latin, and these have now been anglicized and adapted similarly in other languages. Although the official definitions of these terms are somewhat arbitrary, and academic discussions of distinctions among them may leave outsiders temporarily stunned, there is general agreement on their qualitative meanings (Table 1). The real value of such terms is in forcing careful observation and subsequent description. It is said of those beginning to learn dermatology that they frequently look but do not see. A second important benefit is in assisting clinical communication and may be equally important in communication between clinicians and pharmaceutical scientists, an obvious example being the development of clinical criteria for trials of therapeutic agents. In preparing a protocol for clinical trials to avoid error or omission that will prove costly, it is essential to involve a dermatologist.

Adjectives

These can be derived from names for lesions (e.g., *macular* from macule) or may occasionally be ascribed to the nature of the disorder (e.g., *eczematous* from eczema). The latter category conveys less meaning to outsiders, and presupposes the correct diagnosis. A third category relates to the geographic distribution (e.g., annular, arciform, grouped, scattered, and so on). The usefulness of these descriptions is mainly in diagnosis.

Colors

These again are mainly useful in diagnosis, and occasionally certain color descriptions are associated with particular disorders. Psoriasis is frequently described

TABLE 1 Dermatological Jargon

Term	Meaning
Macule	Flat area <1 cm, color different from surrounding skin
Patch	Same as that of macule but >1 cm in diameter
Papule	Raised area <1 cm in diameter
Plaque	Raised area >1 cm in diameter
Vesicle	Blister <1 cm in diameter
Bulla	Blister >1 cm in diameter
Atrophy	Loss of substance in one or more parts of the skin (e.g., epidermis, dermis, etc.)
Erosion	Area in which epidermis is lost
Ulcer	Area in which dermis is lost
Pustule	Pus-filled cavity
Nodule	Palpable lump that extends deep to usual skin surface

as being "salmon pink," but certainly there is color variation among the different forms of psoriasis as, in fact, there is among salmon. Similarly, variations in skin color among different racial groups also modify the perceived color of various skin disorders (an obvious example being erythema in black patients), and considerable experience is required to appreciate these differences. Nevertheless, the terms are intended to convey a perception of color that is shared among experienced clinicians but is neither readily quantified nor communicated to those outside the field unless they themselves obtain sufficient clinical exposure. Thus, color description is most useful for diagnosis and communication about diagnosis.

Summary
Dermatological diagnosis is based on a clinical tradition of careful visual observation that has produced its own classification and language. Knowledge of this tradition will help scientists to communicate with clinicians and better understand the basis for some clinical decisions.

Nature of Dermatological Disorders
Wet Versus Dry
This concept influences many routine clinical decisions. The distinction is essentially between those lesions that look and feel wet because of processes, particularly inflammation, that disturb the permeability barrier and allow accumulation of serum, blood, and/or inflammatory cells and those in which there is an intact barrier such that the lesion feels dry. In general, the former involve acute inflammation, whereas the latter are more chronic in nature. Topical applications for "wet" lesions contain far more water, so that this eventually evaporates without further contributing to the "discomfort" or messiness of the original. This venerable practice is frequently used without active agents as in the so-called tap water compresses or wet-to-dry dressings. In these situations, an absorbent cloth is made wet with an aqueous solution at a comfortable temperature, applied to the skin, and allowed to dry to a significant extent. This provides a soothing sensation and allows easy removal of unpleasant, unsightly, or uncomfortable debris that accumulates with acute inflammation. An additional advantage is removal of a focus for infection or colonization by bacteria. Commonly used aqueous solutions may contain salts (e.g., Burrow's solution containing aluminum acetate), but these have not been shown to have significant advantages over plain water.

For lesions considered "dry," typically those that are scaly and thickened (e.g., chronic eczema, plaque-type psoriasis, some congenital scaling disorders), a more hydrophobic application is desired. Traditional teaching is that this helps to "hydrate" or "lubricate" the skin, but the precise meanings of these terms are unclear. It is undeniable, however, that such hydrophobic applications (e.g., hydrophilic petrolatum), with or without active agents, are in themselves therapeutic in many "dry" disorders and will be selected by experienced clinicians over others in these circumstances.

Hair-Bearing Versus "Glabrous" Skin
The presence of terminal hairs, as found in the scalp or axilla, also changes the choice of vehicle. This is usually quite simple in that the more aqueous preparations are well tolerated in hairy areas, and the more hydrophobic preparations are not.

Irritability

In general, the more inflammatory disorders are more easily "irritated." In practical terms, this means production of erythema and discomfort of a "stinging" nature. In some cases, particularly psoriasis, this can lead to an exacerbation of the underlying pathology. As described above, clinicians will generally try to use more aqueous solutions rather than hydrophobic applications, but the addition of alcohol as a means of solubilizing active agents will tend to increase such irritation. Thus, inflammatory psoriasis of the scalp involves a wet lesion in a hairy area, but the use of alcoholic lotions containing corticosteroids is sufficiently troublesome as to produce very poor compliance. Thus, the nature of the vehicle may dictate the choice of the formulation used as much as the selection of the active agent.

Patient Perceptions

Placebo Effect

As discussed recently by Pearce (6), therapeutic effects may be obtained for subjective complaints (such as itch or pain) or in objective measurement such as exercise tolerance. Unfortunately, there have been few studies of the placebo effect in dermatological treatment, particularly in topical treatments, but there can be little doubt that it exists. Many placebo-controlled studies in the literature (7–10) concentrate (not surprisingly) on the differences between placebo and active treatment groups. The statistical significance of the placebo effect alone is usually ignored.

Experienced clinicians will frequently sense the patient's preference for types of treatment, or this may be overtly stated. Alternatively, certain forms of treatment may be resisted. Not surprisingly, clinical decisions consistent with patient preferences are likely to be more successful, whether because of the placebo effect, improved compliance, or other factors. A corollary of this approach is that the treatment works best when it "makes sense" to the patient. This may sometimes merely involve taking the time to give an explanation in plain words or may involve playing to the patient's preconceptions. An obvious example is the use of intralesional corticosteroids (i.e., direct injection of a steroid suspension into the skin) in situations where a "superpotent" topical steroid would probably be equally effective with less pain. Patients may either have "faith" in "the needle" or, alternatively, have lost faith in creams and ointments because the appearances of these are much the same and may have frequently been given in the past.

Amounts to Dispense

There are clinical rules of thumb for deciding on amounts to dispense based on frequency of application and body surface area to be covered (11). Other factors may be even more important. Clinical experience suggests the use of a topical preparation is directly related to the size of the container. Thus, for conditions such as chronic eczema in which the application of the vehicle is as important in many cases as the active agent, dispensing small amounts of cream or ointment will result in inadequate use. Conversely, when it is desirable to use only small amounts of application, such as the superpotent topical steroids, the use of small containers will promote more miserly use.

Similarly, it is often true that the use of a topical preparation is inversely related to its cost. Thus, the use of large containers of economical preparations will promote liberal use and vice versa. In day-to-day clinical practice, these factors are as important to therapeutic outcome as the extent of body surface area to be treated.

Compliance

Failure to comply costs untold amounts of money to the health care system. Although explanations of dermatological diseases and their treatment can be very time consuming, patient's prejudices and misconceptions can interfere with effective use of established treatment. Clinical experience suggests that in the current climate, authoritarian "directive" medicine does not work for most patients, and lack of adequate time for discussion with patients is a frequent cause of treatment failure (12–14).

DERMATOLOGICAL THERAPY
Dressings
"Old" Dressings

These have been more important in the past than they are now. Many chronic skin disorders such as psoriasis and pemphigus were disabling and sometimes lethal, and given the opportunity, patients spent extensive periods in hospitals. In that setting, complex routines were evolved for bandaging and dressing wounds, and these were combined often with existing topical applications such as tars, astringents (salt solutions designed to precipitate protein and, therefore, reduce oozing and crusting), or powders designed to absorb water. With the development of newer forms of treatment, particularly anti-inflammatory drugs and various forms of phototherapy, such complex inpatient regimens are less commonly used. In fact, many large hospitals have very few dedicated dermatology beds, and most patients are treated as outpatients. Residual forms of these treatments are generally found in psoriasis units where extensive topical applications are done by staff rather than the patients, but the overnight stay and associated bed are no longer necessary.

"New" Dressings

Newer forms of dressings, beyond the scope of this article, are designed to promote wound healing. Others promote penetration of active molecules through the permeability barrier of the skin. These generally work through the phenomenon of "occlusion," which means covering normal or diseased skin with a vapor-impermeable dressing. This is best known through the use of plastic wraps (e.g., Saran wrap) to cover corticosteroid ointments (15), a technique pioneered by Sulzberger and Witten (16). The mechanism of increased penetration is not clear, but the benefit has been established after the work of Vickers (17) and may be related to the so-called reservoir effect. In dermatological therapeutics, an ointment may be chosen in preference to a cream or lotion for the same purpose, that is, to improve penetration of the active ingredient (see below). Occlusive dressings are also an integral component of many "transdermal" preparations, but these are not relevant to dermatological therapy.

Vehicle

Because of improvements in therapy, clinicians have not needed as wide a knowledge of topical formulation as previously. Indeed, many restrict themselves to formulations available off the shelf, and their knowledge of formulation techniques and the associated physical chemistry is rudimentary. In practice, preparations are divided into lotions, creams, ointments, and gels with excursions into other formulations, such as powders and pastes, made only occasionally and usually in the setting of intensive treatment such as psoriasis day care. Selections are generally made on clinical criteria as discussed above, and in this light, it can be seen that there are still some unfilled needs in formulations. Examples include an aqueous corticosteroid lotion that does not contain ethanol and therefore does not sting and a corticosteroid ointment for hand dermatitis that does not result in a persistent greasy feel. In the future, some means for the delivery of large therapeutic molecules that is practical, cost-effective, and painless must also be found. It is doubtful that such technology will be based on passive diffusion as is the case for current dermatological or transdermal formulations.

Compounding

This, of course, has been a significant part of the traditional "art" of dermatological practice. More recently, there have been two developments discouraging this practice. One is the evolution of more effective topical medications (such as the imidazoles and allylamines for fungal infections), and the second is the requirement by all major drug regulatory agencies such as the U.S. Food and Drug Agency, Health Protection Branch, Canada, and others for new pharmaceutical agents to be shown to have efficacy and safety. In addition to these, there is a corresponding decrease in interest among pharmacists in acquiring the skills and resources to perform extemporaneous compounding, or if they do, their increased costs are passed on to the patients. Finally, such increased costs may not be covered by third-party insurers. Although there are many expressions of frustration on the part of the medical profession with this state of affairs, it is an open question as to whether dermatological practice is impaired in any way by being restricted to "off-the-shelf" products provided by pharmaceutical and proprietary manufacturers. It can certainly be said that there is a lack of convincing evidence that this is the case.

A more serious problem is the persistence of old habits of compounding to involve more complex newer topical preparations. As discussed by Krochmal and Patel (18), there are a myriad of potential problems that may be encountered either when new ingredients are added to an existing formulation or when existing formulations are mixed together. These include interactions of the active agents and interactions of the vehicles with each other or the added agents. The results range from the development of a completely useless formulation to, at best, one in which there is absolutely no evidence for efficacy. Examples are the reduction in corticosteroid efficacy in compounds containing tar (19,20) and the oxidation and photodegradation that occurs when tretinoin is used in extemporaneously compounded medication. Although the dangers of irrational compounding seem obvious to most practitioners and pharmaceutical scientists, the practice nevertheless persists and may require another generation to be eradicated. Excuses generally offered by practitioners include the requirement of individual patients to have "tailored" topical preparations and that there are requirements for preparations that are not manufactured. In our opinion, there is absolutely no evidence to support such an approach. It should also be pointed out that "extemporaneous compounding," by definition, is the preparation of any therapeutic material from initial ingredients. The mixing of two or more proprietary or pharmaceutical topical preparations is not extemporaneous compounding and is not part of any curriculum in medicine or pharmacy.

Drugs

It is obviously not possible to review comprehensively the drugs used in dermatology. The reader is referred to other chapters in this volume and to the most complete and continuing source of information, the *Skin Therapy Letter* (21).

The Future—Needs and Possibilities

This is obviously a matter of opinion. In our view, the focus should not merely be on the development of new molecules but also on the means to deliver both the newer classes of drugs and older drugs with less toxicity.

Old Drugs in New Vehicles

It is possible that formulation of systemic drugs such as methotrexate in new ways might allow some form of "targeting" that would direct the drug away from the liver, the site of a major limiting toxicity. This would obviously not affect the other significant issue, long-term immunosuppression, but may still offer a significant therapeutic advantage. Similarly, improvement in topical formulations may allow the use of drugs in situations where now only systemic delivery is effective yet the toxicity is unacceptable (Table 2). An obvious example is lamellar ichthyosis, which responds well to systemic retinoids but cannot be treated with these because of potential long-term systemic toxicity. An improved formulation might significantly increase topical delivery, therapeutic effects might be obtained, and long-term side effects might be made acceptable.

TABLE 2 Systemic Agents Commonly Used in Dermatology

Corticosteroids
Prednisone
Methylprednisolone
Antibiotics
Tetracyclines
Erythromycin
Antifungals
Griseofulvin
Imidazoles
Terbinafine
Cytotoxic/immunomodulatory drugs
Azathioprine
Cyclophosphamide
Methotrexate
Cyclosporine
Thalidomide
Hydroxychloroquine
Dapsone
Retinoids
13-*cis* retinoic acid
Acitretin
Photosensitizers
Psoralens
Agents for "photodynamic therapy"
"Biologics"

Source: From Ref. 22.

New Drugs in New Vehicles

Newer classes of compounds are being developed for therapeutic use, obvious examples being antisense drugs and genetic material for gene therapy. These have many potential applications, but a limiting technical problem is satisfactory delivery. Despite some published claims to the contrary (23,24), we believe that there is no convincing evidence that large molecules can penetrate the skin by means of passive diffusion. This implies that either some new form of topical delivery that is both safe and practical or a delivery vehicle for systemic use must be developed. Both these approaches hold promise for both improved treatment of common problems and effective treatment of diseases for which there is now no adequate therapy.

SUMMARY

Treatments for skin disease have a long history that precedes "scientific" medicine. Some of these, e.g., tars, although in widespread clinical use, have uncertain clinical value over placebo. Others, e.g., anthralin, have been clearly shown to be of use. Further developments in these fields will probably consist of refining and delivering more effective forms of the drugs or, alternatively, drugs of equal effectiveness but reduced toxicity. New classes of compounds show great promise for dermatology, but the challenge will be to find practical means of delivery. Although skin disease is rarely lethal, it is frequently disabling, and the constant challenge is to reduce the disability without causing harm through treatment. Although there is no substitute for concerned and competent clinicians, such clinicians must have at their disposal therapy that is both effective and safe.

REFERENCES

1. Holubar K. The rise of Western dermatology. The London, Paris, and Vienna schools and their influence on the development of the dermatologic alphabet. Int J Dermatol 1989 Sep; 28(7):471–474.
2. Korge BP, Krieg T. The molecular basis for inherited bullous diseases. J Mol Med 1996; 74(2):59–70.
3. Fuchs E. Keratins and the skin. Annu Rev Cell Dev Biol 1995; 11:123–153.
4. Kirtschig G, Wojnarowska F. Autoimmune blistering diseases: an up-date of diagnostic methods and investigations. Clin Exp Dermatol 1994; 19:97–112.
5. Williams ML, Elias PM. From basket weave to barrier. Unifying concepts for the pathogenesis of the disorders of cornification. Arch Dermatol 1993 May; 129:626–629.
6. Pearce JMS. The placebo enigma. Q J Med 1995; 88:215–220.
7. Sherwood PA. The use of topical anesthesia in removal of port-wine stains in children. J Pediatr 1993 May; 122:S36–S40.
8. Kragballe K. Vitamin D3 and skin diseases. Arch Dermatol Res 1992; 284(Suppl. 1):S30–S36.
9. Kragbelle K. Treatment of psoriasis with calcipotriol and other vitamin D analogues. J Am Acad Dermatol 1992; 27:1001–1008.
10. Meinardi MM, de Rie MA. Oral cyclosporin A in the treatment of psoriasis: an overview of studies performed in The Netherlands. Br J Dermatol 1990; 122:27–31.
11. Ramsay B, Lawrence CM. Measurement of involved surface area in patients with psoriasis. Br J Dermatol 1991; 124:565–570.
12. Bigby M, Gadenne AS. Understanding and evaluating clinical trials. J Am Acad Dermatol 1996:34:555–590.
13. Draelos ZK. Patient compliance: enhancing clinical abilities and strategies. J Am Acad Dermatol 1995; 32:S42–S48.
14. Witkowski JA. Compliance: the dermatologic patient. Int J Dermatol 1988; 27:608–611.
15. Sneddon IB. Clinical use of topical cortisteroids. Drugs 1976; 11:193–199.

16. Sulzberger MB, Witten VH. Thin plastic films in topical dermatologic therapy. Arch Dermatol 1961; 84:1027–1028.
17. Vickers CFH. Existence of reservoir in stratum corneum: experimental proof. Arch Dermatol 1963; 88:20–23.
18. Krochmal L, Patel B. Topical product design and extemporaneous compounding in dermatology. Adv Dermatol 1992; 7:231–252.
19. Lester RS. Corticosteroids. Clin Dermatol 1989; 7:80–97.
20. Krochmal L, Wang JC, Patel B, et al. Topical corticosteroid compounding: effects on physicochemical stability and skin penetration rate. J Am Acad Dermatol 1989; 21:979–984.
21. www.SkinTherapyLetter.com.
22. Pirzada S, Tomi Z, Gulliver W. A review of biologic treatments for psoriasis with emphasis on infliximab. Skin Ther Lett 2007; 12(3):1–4.
23. Yarosh D, Bucana C, Cox P, Alas L, Kibitel J, Kripke M. Localization of liposomes containing a DNA repair enzyme in murine skin. J Invest Dermatol 1994; 103:461–468.
24. Short SM, Rubas W, Paasch BD, Mrsny RJ. Transport of biologically active interferon-gamma across human skin in vitro. Pharm Res 1995; 12:1140–1145.

3 Treatment of Dermatitis

Chris Anderson

Department of Dermatology, Linköping University, Linköping, Sweden

INTRODUCTION

The term "dermatitis" is deeply entrenched in the nosological history of diseases of the skin. As a term, it describes the organ as the skin and indicates that there is a component of inflammation. Even patients have a broad concept of what the skin might look like in this condition and actually use the term in a relatively correct context, to the extent that they can communicate about a condition that up to a quarter of those seeking advice for a dermatological condition may have (Table 1). The more useful and correct term when attempting an overview of the conditions we are to address in this chapter is "eczema". In practice, however, the terms eczema and dermatitis can be considered synonymous. Therapeutic principles relevant to eczema have considerable generalized relevance to other inflammatory conditions in dermatology.

Eczema, the Synonym for Dermatitis

Eczema is an inflammatory condition of the skin, the cause of which can be exogenous, endogenous, or a combination of both (Table 2). Eczema can be identified clinically by its main symptom, itch, and by the cardinal morphological components of erythema (redness), papules (a palpable component), and vesicles (small blisters). If this constellation of components exists in a dermatological condition, then a differential diagnosis of eczema can be entertained. What causes confusion

TABLE 1 Group Name, Common Dermatoses Assigned to Groups, and Indication of the Proportion (%) of Cases in Groups at Two Dermatological Clinics at the Assigned Antipodeal Ends of the World (Linköping, Sweden and Liverpool, Australia).

Group[a]	Examples of dermatoses	% of new visits
Special dermatology	Genodermatoses, blistering dermatoses, scleroderma, collagenoses, vasculitis, sarcoidosis, panniculitis, necrobiosis	10–15
Eczema/allergy	Atopic eczema, contact eczema, other forms of eczema, photodermatoses, urticaria	20–25
Psoriasis	Psoriasis, pustulosis palmoplantaris, pityriasis rosea, pityriasis lichenoides, parapsoriasis, lichen ruben	15
Infections	Viral bacterial and fungal infections	5
Acne	Acne, rosacea, hydradenitis suppurativa	5
Tumor	Benign and malignant skin tumors, metastatic malignoma	30–40
Ulcers	Venous and arterial leg ulcers, lymphedema, decubitus ulcers, thrombophlebitis	5
Other	Pruritus, excoriation, elastosis, hair and nail disease, hyperhidrosis, parasitosis, etc.	10–5

[a]In dermatology, there are more than 600 diagnoses, according to the International Statistical Classification of Diseases and Related Health Problems, 10th Revision. Diagnoses were grouped to give an overview of the dermatological conditions for which patients are referred.

TABLE 2   Clinical Signs, Symptoms, and Histology of Eczema

Eczema: Inflammatory condition of the skin
Pathogenesis: Exogenous, endogenous, or a combination
Symptom: Itch

Clinical signs		
Primary	Secondary	Secondary
Erythema	Infiltration	Erosion
Papules	Desquamation	Excoriation
Vesicles		Infection
		Lichenification

Histology		
Epidermis	Dermis	
Spongiosis	Lymphocytes	
Acanthosis	Vascular dilatation	
Parakeratosis		
Lymphocytes		
	Acute–subacute–chronic[a]	

[a]While the differentiation of different types of eczema is usually not possible on histology, the spectrum of features, chiefly in the epidermis, can indicate whether the condition is acute, subacute, or chronic.

diagnostically in individual cases is the range of secondary features caused by the eczematous rash progressing from its primary components. Thus, the pronounced itch can lead to scratch marks and excoriations, the vesicles can rupture to leave erosions (weeping areas), crusts, and even secondary bacterial infection from the skin's commensal organisms or by pathogens taking advantage of an opportune route past the skin's normal barrier against microbial invasion.

Histological examination after biopsy reveals inflammation in both the dermis and the epidermis, with the earliest changes in the epidermis in the form of separation of the keratinocytes in the stratum spinosum (spongiosis) and a subsequent dermal inflammatory cell infiltrate. The epidermis (apart from on the palms and soles) is only 0.1 mm thick. The skin barrier function resides in the stratum corneum, only a fraction of a tenth of a millimeter thick. The dermal stroma contains all the necessary components for amplification and modification of the cellular response. While the differentiation of different types of eczema is not usually possible on histology, the spectrum of features, chiefly those seen in the epidermis, can indicate whether the condition is acute, subacute, or chronic.

Examples of Exogenous and Endogenous Types of Eczema
As seen in Table 2, the very definition of eczema demands consideration of causative factors (i.e., exogenous/endogenous) and the acceptance that the individual patient's situation at a particular time may be a point on a spectrum of possibilities.

Contact Eczema
Contact eczema can be considered the flagship of the patho-etiologic approach to eczema, illustrating exogenous causes because it is per se an exogenous eczema. Contact eczema is of two basic types: allergic contact eczema (a type IV, delayed, cell-mediated immune response according to Gell and Coombs) and irritant contact eczema (which can be considered to be due to activation of the skin's innate response system) chiefly centered initially on the direct effects of xenobiotics on keratinocytes (1). Irritant contact dermatitis has a number of clinical subsets in presentation and

morphology. In type IV allergy, a sensitization process, usually involving a more pronounced initial exposure to the allergen, is required. In irritant contact eczema, no such previous exposure is necessary; different skin types, however, react to variable degrees. Often, the two types of contact eczema coexist; this is interpreted to imply that an initial irritant eczema causes increased percutaneous penetration of a xenobiotic, which increases the available dose to the immune system and thus the likelihood of sensitization. In broad terms, in both allergic and irritant contact eczema, the occurrence and variability in grade are due to variable irritant capacity of the xenobiotic, variable propensity of the individual to react, and the general inflammatory environment at the time. The allergenicity and irritancy of xenobiotics is, to some extent, predictable based on structural activity relationships. There is no known hereditary basis for individual propensity to develop contact allergy, although some individuals clearly have a propensity to develop multiple contact allergies. Atopics are clearly predisposed to irritant contact eczema as are, to a lesser extent, individuals with pale skin and those with constitutionally dry skin, which actually constitutes a hereditary component.

Atopic Eczema

The classic example of an eczema in which the endogenous component is of great relevance is atopic eczema. The phenotype of atopy is identified by a history of childhood eczema (mostly flexural eczema), current flexural eczema, hay fever, and a tendency to develop type I allergic reactions, e.g., to dog or cat hair or to latex. As many as 25% of individuals in such countries as Sweden and Australia can be classified as having atopic phenotypes (2). There is also a tendency to dry skin in the atopic phenotype, most often clinically expressed as wintertime chapping of the dorsal side of the hands, the lips, and even generalized dry skin, which can lead to irritant contact eczema. Because of the possible occurrence of type I allergy in this patient group, it becomes necessary to be able to separate an eczematous component from an urticarial component. Urticaria is characterized by itchy, raised, red and white, papular or round, annular or gyrate lesions on the skin that arise quickly, itch intensively, and subside without leaving any trace within several to 24 hours. Because new lesions can arise on new areas of skin, the condition can continue for days, but the individual lesions will resolve within 24 hours, with no scaling or redness left at the individual site. Classically, urticaria can be associated with angioedema (swelling of the mucous membranes, face, hands, or other areas), asthma, and anaphylaxis—a constellation of symptoms demanding their own investigation and treatment. Treatment for urticarial components of a clinical picture is based on antihistamines, which, however, will have no effect on eczema. The genetic basis for the known hereditary features of the atopic diathesis remains unclear, although there are a number of candidate genes under investigation on the immunological side (3). Recently, a loss-of-function gene for the keratinocyte protein filaggrin has been demonstrated, which seems to explain the origin of the epidermal barrier dysfunction in atopy (4). Other skin barrier dysfunctions that are also operative and explanative for the mix of immunological and barrier dysfunction remain to be elucidated.

Pathogenetic Studies in Eczema

In the pathogenetic study of eczema, there is a long tradition of the use of models for contact eczema. The provocation is delineated (known doses under known methods of application of dinitrochlorobenzene, oxazolone, croton oil, sodium lauryl sulfate, for example), and the material is available for a broad range of observations on the chronology and the biology of the reactions.

Studies in these models identify possible targets of therapy for the condition studied. Table 3 illustrates the cells identified in the dermal cellular infiltrate in an experimental model in a range of reactions caused by agents applied topically or injected into the skin (which is equivalent to the access through a damaged skin barrier). The counts are based on simple morphology in the upper dermis but illustrate the cells participating and the variability at different time points after provocation. In this guinea pig model, the basophil granulocyte and the lymphocyte typified the allergic contact reaction, the lymphocyte and, at higher concentrations, the neutrophil granulocyte typified the irritant eczema, and urticarial responses demonstrated a decrease in granulated mast cells (5).

At this level, one can guess that antihistamines will be without effect in nonurticarial reactions and that a broad range of anti-inflammatory mechanisms aiming at both lymphocyte and granulocyte mechanisms may be available in contact reactions. Another therapeutic lesson from studies shows the time course of a contact reaction after application of agents topically in an experimental model. The contact eczematous reactions are inherently self-limiting. In a therapeutic situation in which an exogenous cause is predominant, identification and removal of the offending agent is of primary importance. Indeed, the most robust of therapies will fail if the offending agent is not identified and removed.

Experimental models offer a range of opportunities to investigate therapeutic strategies but only within contact reactions and immediate hypersensitivity reaction. Sadly, we lack models of other aspects of the eczema spectrum and much of

TABLE 3 Models of Eczema Pathogenesis. Mean Cell Response in Various Reaction Types Three and 24 Hours After Testing

Agent	n	Cell response (total cells)	Monocytes	Mast cells	% of cell response		
					Basophils	Eosinophils	Neutrophils
3 hrs after test							
Ovalbumin[a]	13	4	Loss[b]	Loss	2	21	77
DMSO 100%[c]	10	11	54	Loss	20	12	15
Oxazolone[d]	5	8	78	3	7	15	1
24 hrs after test							
Ovalbumin[a]	13	12	55	Loss	17	21	7
DMSO 100%	10	13	67	1	21	10	2
Oxazolone[d]	52	21	65	1	30	4	1
Croton oil[e]	53	12	85	3	9	3	2
SLS 2%[f]	10	4	83	4	8	4	0
DMSO 12%[f]	10	9	82	4	9	2	4

Note: Eczema pathogenesis can be studied in models, e.g., study of dermal inflammatory cell infiltrate in a guinea pig contact reaction model.
[a]Ovalbumin (10 μg) injected intradermally in sensitized animals causes an immediate allergic reaction (atopy patch test model).
[b]Loss indicates a lesser amount of cells found in the dermal reaction than that found in the same animals normal skin.
[c]DMSO (100%) causes a nonimmunological immediate contact reaction in unsensitized animals.
[d]Oxazolone (0.2%) applied epicutaneously to sensitized animals elicits a delayed allergic reaction type (type IV reaction).
[e]Croton oil produces a toxic reaction in unsensitized animals (irritant reaction).
[f]Repetitive application of 2% SLS or 12% DMSO causes an irritant reaction in unsensitized animals.
Abbreviations: DMSO, dimethyl sulfoxide; SLS, sodium lauryl sulfate.

our knowledge has been built up empirically. Central in the clinical situation is the relief of itch, which, in turn, is a good parameter for effect on other aspects of inflammation. SCORAD is an example of a structured clinical scoring system (6).

THE PATIENT WITH ECZEMA

In health surveys on populations, "Do you suffer from skin allergy?" is the question most likely to be answered with "yes." Exact figures for the prevalence of eczema are not known. As can be seen in Table 1, "allergy" including eczema constitutes a significant proportion of the dermatological clientele. The proportion remains the same over the age groups, but the spectrum of eczema types and patient situations is diverse. It is important that patient care is holistic and not merely a question of prescription of pharmaceuticals.

Classification of Eczema

The definition of eczema in Table 2 is based on occurrence of symptoms and signs, the histological features that reflect a chronology, and the knowledge that endogenous and exogenous factors can have dominating or variable roles. The terminology used to delineate eczema diagnoses is sometimes confusing, reflecting classical presentations, anatomical distributions, empirical knowledge of clinical entities, and even purely descriptive terms. In a clinical situation, a number of other factors need to be considered to clarify the terminology, steer investigation, and then give appropriate therapy. For instance, delineation of a contact urticarial mechanism is important. In Table 4, diagnoses are presented in the order in which they are treated in this chapter, with annotations that may have significance for the above factors.

The Investigation of Eczema

As in all clinical situations, taking a history including a family and social history followed by an examination of the morphology and the distribution of the rash will be the basis for a correct diagnosis. An important issue, especially in cases not responding to therapy is the consideration of adverse reaction to current or previous therapy. Contact allergy to prescribed topical drugs is common and even more

TABLE 4 Eczema Classification

Contact dermatitis	Allergic (Photoallergic)	Irritant (Phototoxic)
Atopic		
Seborrheic		
Venous/gravitational eczema		
Lichen simplex chronicus (neurodermatitis)		
Asteatotic eczema		
Discoid (nummular)		
Pityriasis alba (pityriasis sicca)		
Intertriginous eczema		
Hand eczema	Pompholyx	Hyperkeratotic hand eczema
Infective/microbial eczema		
Generalized eczema		

Note: The progression in the list will be used to discuss therapy for main eczema scenarios, specific eczema types, and more complex eczema scenarios. The list is not all-inclusive.

common to over-the-counter, traditional, or alternative medicine preparations. This can complicate both diagnosis and further treatment. Similarly, a role for light in causality of eczema needs to be considered either in the form of photoallergy or phototoxicity ("phototoxicity" is the term used in preference to the more logical "photoirritancy"). Classical photodermatoses such as polymorphic light eruption need to be differentiated from eczematous conditions.

Epicutaneous Patch Test

The epicutaneous (patch) test is the classic test initiated by Jadassohn more than 100 years ago (7). It remains the definitive test for confirming contact allergy despite attempts to use blood testing, which is mostly based on lymphocyte transformation test to confirm the presence or absence of contact allergy. More than 3000 agents are reported to cause contact allergy. Common contact allergens are, however, a much smaller group. Typically, chronic eczema is investigated by use of a "standard patch test series" aimed at detecting possible allergy for the 30 most common contact allergens. Specific patch test series can be conducted according to the patient's occupation or exposure. Preferably, commercially produced pharmaceutical-grade patch testing material is used. It is, however, sometimes necessary to use the patient's products, which are then prepared in concentrations and in vehicles previously shown by the collective experience of patch testing technique to be acceptable—sufficiently strong to detect allergy but sufficiently weak not to induce allergy. The classic epicutaneous patch test involves application of small amounts of allergen in a chamber applied under occlusion to the skin of the back for 48 hours. Assessment of the test is performed after a further 24 hours and in a second reading 5 to 10 days after the first reading because the delay in the reaction might be increased after this period. Morphological criteria for positivity must be maintained. After morphological positivity is established, the question of relevance needs to be assessed—is the patient exposed to the positively testing allergen and can it explain the presenting symptoms? Relevance can be of present importance or of previous importance. The ultimate aim of patch testing is to localize relevant allergens that can be subsequently removed in their entirety (often down to the last molecule) from the patient's environment.

No specific test is available for testing of irritant capacity for agents suspected of being involved in an irritant contact dermatitis. There is, however, a large body of evidence about potential for irritancy and grade of irritancy, which is helpful.

Individual (Patient) Variability Is Marked

In testing of atopic individuals, especially infants with atopy, a test called the atopy patch test has been developed. This type of testing needs different approaches to classic epicutaneous patch testing and is, at present, best performed in the hands of experts with special interest in the area.

Contact Urticaria Testing

Contact urticaria gives lesions of urticaria, which are similar to idiopathic urticaria but have the history of appearing shortly after topical exposure for an agent. Classic examples of agents that cause contact urticaria are cat and dog hair and latex. There is a long list of potential contact urticaria agents. When the situation is less clear, topical application of small amounts of the suspected agent for short periods, with short follow-up for 20 minutes, is the basis for protocols used. Contact urticaria, of allergic or nonallergic mechanism, can occur after application of the agent to intact skin but can also be demonstrable when the agent is applied to damaged skin, such as eczematous skin. The urticarial component of the patient's symptoms will then be separate from the patient's eczema. In these situations, antihistamines may be of use, although they are classically not used in eczematous lesions. Again, avoidance of the agent is of prime importance.

Chronicity
Clinically, patients present, of course, without any guarantees of isolated etiologies. The patient with an isolated allergy to an epoxy that is acquired, for instance, during industrial exposure may well solve her or his problem merely by avoiding the allergen. Allergies to substances that are more ubiquitous present greater problems, and particular allergens, such as nickel, are known to be associated with chronicity, which persists despite attempts to remove the allergen. This phenomenon is seen with a broad range of irritants and allergens, and the concept of "post-occupational eczema" describes part of the problem in chronicity. An important point for chronicity is that early investigation and intervention is vital.

Endogenous Factors
The most common complicating factor to the contact eczema scenario is that of endogenous predisposition. The best example of this is the case of atopic eczema, an eczema with exogenous components but with a pronounced and multifaceted endogenous background, explaining the coexistence of irritant contact eczema mechanisms and a tendency to develop type I allergy according to Gell and Coombs. All this is important background information to therapeutic strategies in dermatitis/eczema.

THERAPY FORMS

Both the patient and the treating doctor want therapy to be effective and convenient to administer. There is a general tendency away from complicated, often messy ex tempore preparations, but these are sometimes necessary and effective (almost every ex tempore preparation can be said to represent a business opportunity in product development). Physical therapy forms can be less convenient and may necessitate visits to the doctor's office or to an outpatient apartment but are effective. Systemic therapy is usually considered to be somewhat of a "step," the patient being dubious and the treating doctor often being conservative because of the risk of potential side effects with almost all therapies. Comprehensive reviews of dermatological therapy are available in main dermatological textbooks (8, 9), national guidelines (10), and national formularies. Local tradition, even down to a hospital level, and marketing have influences.

Bathing and Soaks
Use of baths and soaks fulfills (at least) three functions: The patient often experiences relief from itch, the cardinal symptom of eczema. Although such relief may be short-lived, it is valued. Bathing can have astringent properties on skin, which is exudative. An exudative, or crusted, surface will have a bacterial proliferation, usually *Staphylococcus aureus*. Removing or reducing the inoculum size is an important feature of allowing the skin's natural antibacterial capacity to operate.

Water

Water is effective for bathing eczematous lesions. It should not be warmer than tepid to avoid leaching of valuable skin lipids from both normal and damaged skin. Water does not need to be sterile. Previous tradition of using sodium chloride, one tablespoon in one L of water, is of uncertain efficacy compared with ordinary water.

Aluminium Acetate

Burow's solution consists of 13% aluminium acetate. Diluted 1:20 or 1:40, it can be used for rinsing or on compresses used as soaks for 10 to 20 minutes. Aluminium acetate solutions containing up to 10% additional ethanol can increase astringent properties.

Potassium Permanganate

Potassium permanganate is a classic dermatological treatment agent with antiseptic and fungicidal activity based on its oxidizing capacity. In a 0.1% solution, it can be applied on a cotton stick to the fissure, blister, or eroded area. Diluted approximately 1:10, it can be used in soaks for 10 to 15 minutes. Whole-body potassium permanganate baths in similar strength are useful in widespread eczema, often having quick and marked effects on the patient's symptoms. Continued for too long, potassium permanganate can dry the skin. Some patients have poor tolerance.

Emollients

Use of moisturizing creams is an important base plate in both prevention and treatment of all eczema types. An important feature is the consistency of the preparation. Patients with dry skin often appreciate ointments, whereas a patient with normal skin often finds them too occlusive and greasy. Creams are generally used if the skin is normal or if there are exudating areas on the skin. Lotions containing increased water content can be more acceptable if there is a high degree of exudation. Evaporation of the product's water from the skin can ease itching.

Patients will have a wide variety of opinion about creams, which partly explains the plethora of different alternatives available both over the counter and by prescription. It is important to avoid creams containing potential allergens. Natural agents are common causes of contact allergy as indeed are perfumes and even preservatives. In the production of high-quality emollients, potential allergens and irritants should be excluded all the way back to raw material supply.

Emollients can prevent eczema, especially irritant contact eczema, by bolstering skin barrier function, which, in turn, prevents derangement of water content in the viable layers of the epidermis, which is the site of irritation of eczema. In the postinflammatory phase of acute dermatitis, scaliness can be alleviated by use of emollients. In chronic dermatitis, the scaling may be more pronounced, and use of emollients becomes more important. The concept of the "barrier cream" is not generally accepted in academic circles. Some emollients, however, do have important preventive properties used before wet work, and the use of creams before dirty work may ease the subsequent cleaning of the can, which will reduce subsequent damage from soaps and detergents.

Topical Corticosteroids

Topical corticosteroids are certainly the mainstay of dermatological treatment of inflammatory conditions. The discovery of the hydrocortisone molecule in 1952 revolutionized the possibilities of treating not only eczema but also many other inflammatory dermatoses (11). Corticosteroids function via membrane receptors by inducing suppression of inflammatory cytokines and inhibiting function of T cells and a range of other inflammatory cells (12). The production of arachidonic acid is affected as well as the function of vascular and connective tissues. Modification of the original steroid molecule, which consists of four ring structures and side chains, have led to a range of corticosteroids with differing specificity of action, potency, and range of side effects. Available steroids can be classified according to their ring structure. The potency of a steroid is based on its effect on biological mechanisms. The most common classification method is the assessment of vasoconstriction in human subjects because the ability to produce pallor correlates with the potency of the steroid in terms of both innate strength and vehicle efficacy (13,14). The most commonly used clinical classification of potency is the four-point scale of mild, moderate, potent, and very potent (Table 5). This is expressed numerically as groups I–IV in ascending order of potency. Side effects, especially after long-term use, include atrophy of the skin, occurrence of telangiectasia, and, particularly in the elderly, skin purpura. Secondary infection can be a problem, particularly folliculitis and a special form of dermatitis called perioral dermatitis, which became common quite quickly after the introduction of potent steroids. Use of appropriate strengths for different localizations on the body alleviates some of the side effect problems. For instance, the face should only be treated with weak steroids, and intertriginous areas (groin and axilla) should only be treated with weak or moderate-strength steroids. Intermittent dosage schedules can also be used and are of particular importance in chronic conditions and for the safe use of strong steroids.

Calcineurin Antagonists

Calcineurin antagonists induce T-cell suppression (15). Pimecrolimus and tacrolimus were originally used as oral medication in transplantation management. Both agents have been developed for topical use as a corticosteroid alternatives particularly for atopic dermatitis (16,17). Both have been shown to have efficacy in atopic dermatitis even a range of other eczemas and inflammatory conditions. Side effects of the nature of subjective skin symptoms such as burning occur in a proportion of

TABLE 5 Classification of Steroids According to Strength[a]

Mild (group I)
   Hydrocortisone
   Hydrocortisone acetate
   Desonide
Moderate (group II)
   Hydrocortisone butyrate
   Clobetasone butyrate
   Triamcinolone acetonide
Potent (group III)
   Betamethasone diproprionate
   Betamethasone valerate
   Fluticasone propionate
   Mometasone
   Triamcinolone acetonide
   Methylprednisolone aceponate
Very potent (group IV)
   Clobetasone propionate

[a]Changing concentration can alter strength, as can vehicle modification.

patients. Discussion continues about the appropriate place for these agents, based particularly on the known side effects of oral immunosuppressive medications in the transplant situation, where skin cancer and secondary infection are known to be more common. Studies and follow-up of use are being conducted to clarify the situation. Use of these agents will, therefore, need to be the subject to appropriate information and control mechanisms for patients or their parents. Concurrent use of therapeutic light or climatic light should be avoided. Eczematous conditions can very often be extremely disruptive and distressing, and it is important that these agents find their correct place in the therapeutic arsenal (18).

Antiseptics and Antibiotics for Secondary Infection
Astringents, especially potassium permanganate, have good antibacterial activity and are often adequate to handle mild secondary infections. Use of antiseptic solutions containing triclosan or chlorhexidine is part of therapeutic tradition in some parts of the world, although there are environmental and irritancy issues that are under discussion. Use of topical antibiotics is not favored. In the first instance, sensitization can often occur to topically applied antibiotics, e.g., neomycin. Common skin pathogens can also develop resistance to antibiotics that are used extensively in the topical situation. This is of great general concern because it has consequences for the usefulness of antibiotics in more serious situations of systemic infection. Restrictions on the topical use of antibiotics mean that systemic antibiotic therapy can be necessary for widespread secondary infections and, of course, for erysipelas or other serious skin infections. The focus is definitely on *S. aureus*, which is commonly cultured from damaged skin and for which super antigen capacities are suspected in the pathogenesis of eczematous lesions.

Chlorhexidine
Chlorhexidine solution (0.5 mg/mL) can be used for bathing secondarily infected skin areas. It can also be used in a preventive way to keep bacteria counts low in normal skin areas subject to repeated infections.

Mupirosin
This antibiotic is not known for the above problems of sensitization and development of resistance. It is applied daily for 7 to 10 days. A nasal preparation for the treatment of carrier status is also available.

Hydrogen Peroxide Cream
Another agent not known to cause resistance in bacteria is hydrogen peroxide, which can be stabilized in a cream base for topical application at a concentration of 1%.

Ex Tempore Preparations
Dermatological tradition is steeped in the art of the ex tempore preparations. Although preparations with historic names such as Kligman's ointment or Lindgren's starka have their place, use of pharmaceutical-grade preparations is becoming more common. Situations where use of ex tempore preparations is indicated will be taken up under the discussion of specific conditions.

Physical Therapy as an Adjunct to Topical Therapy
Wet Dressings
The wet dressing is a classic dermatological maneuver that not only heightens the efficacy of an applied topical pharmaceutical agent but also causes relief by physical means. It is commonly used for troublesome eczematous areas and even in generalized eczema. The topical agent to be used, whether group 1 steroids or stronger steroids, is applied to the wet skin, after which wet clothing or towels are used to cover most of the body. An extra blanket may be required to maintain warmth, and the use of warm water will also facilitate temperature holding. A period of 15 to 60 minutes is used for the wet dressing; then, the skin is dried, and an additional layer of moisturizer applied. The operative mechanism is occlusion, but even the evaporative effect, which produces skin cooling, can have a beneficial effect on itch and inflammation.

Occlusion
Occlusion by any means changes the function of the skin including decreased epidermal cell turnover and dendritic cell function and will often result in decreased itch. An additional benefit is that the patient is unable to reach the area of skin that may have been the site of a lichen simplex chronicus (neurodermatitis), thus preventing the mechanism of itch and scratch that perpetuates the inflammation at the site. Application of a topical agent under the occlusion will increase penetration. A steroid becomes more effective than its original grade would indicate. Occlusion can be left in place for several days, and some dressings, for instance, ointment-treated gauze dressings on the limbs can be left in place for up to a week.

Phototherapy
Natural sunlight can have a very positive effect on skin conditions such as psoriasis and eczema. The development of use of artificial UV light in dermatology (19) took pace in the 1950s and was used in large scale in the Scandinavian countries in the 1960s and 1970s, where it was shown that large numbers of patients could be given the therapy effectively in outpatient departments. Originally, broadband UVB (wavelength 292–320 nm) was used. The use of photochemotherapy (psoralen + UVA = PUVA) was shown to have great effect on psoriasis and even eczema. Side effects, however, in the form of skin atrophy, hyperpigmentation, and even skin cancer were more frequent with PUVA than with UVB. The discovery of the efficacy of narrowband UVB, where the 311-nm wavelength is prioritized, gave effects approaching those of PUVA. UVA therapy in higher doses than are available in natural sunlight was also shown to be effective. Combinations of UVA and UVB are also attractive particularly in the area of eczema. UV can be administered selectively to regions such as the hands, avoiding unnecessary treatment of otherwise normal areas of skin.

In regard to eczema, whole-body broadband UVB or whole-body narrowband UVB are the most common treatment forms being administered three to four times a week in increasing dosage for periods of six to eight weeks. Addition of UVA can be used especially in atopic eczema. The benefit of UV treatment for the patient needs to be weighed against potential risks. In all but those patients with a strong personal or family history of skin cancer, this cost-benefit analysis is usually favorable. Limits are placed on the number of lifetime treatments of PUVA. There is a suggestion of a limit for narrowband UVB but no consensus as yet. Other positive features of phototherapy is that there is a nonspecific positive effect on itch and the treatment reaches all parts of the body and is thus almost a systemic treatment. UV can be also used to normalize the function of a healed eczema.

Grenz Ray

Grenz rays, also known as Bucky rays, are very soft X rays (20). They can be administered in an office environment from machines that do not demand special safety standards (as with standard X-ray machines). Therapy is administered once a week for a period of 6 weeks, and the indications include localized areas of lichen simplex chronicus and hyperkeratotic hand eczema. Grenz ray treatment is only available at specific institutions that have chosen to adopt the therapy.

Systemic Therapy

Apart from use of oral antibiotics, systemic therapy for eczematous conditions is relatively uncommon and reserved for the more serious and chronic situations. Often, patients will have extensive eczema, but severe eczema of the hands even in the presence of perfect skin on the rest of the body may motivate consideration of systemic therapy.

Corticosteroids

Systemic corticosteroid therapy is the main line of systemic therapy (8). It is most clearly indicated for symptomatic relief when the cause of the eczema is known and the duration of the eczema can be expected to be limited. Prednisolone, in doses of 25 to 50 mg/day and administered as a single dose in the mornings, is the most common regime. After three to four days, the dose can be reduced during two weeks. Chronic use of corticosteroids systemically should be avoided because of the risks of long-term therapy.

Classical Immunosuppressive Agents

The most common immunosuppressive agents used are azathioprine (21), methotrexate (22), and cyclosporine (23). The antimetabolite azatioprine can be used as a steroid-sparing agent or in its own right in doses of 1 to 2 mg/kg/day. Methotrexate is a less commonly used agent for eczema, but familiarity with the agent is increasing because of therapy for psoriasis, rheumatoid arthritis, and other rheumatological conditions. It is administered in a divided dose once a week. Cyclosporine is a potent agent in the treatment of eczema such as contact eczema or atopic eczema, but short-term vigilance in administration to avoid renal and blood pressure side effects is needed, and therapy in the longer term is not optimal. A number of less commonly used agents can also be included in the list of possible immunosuppressive agents such as thioguanine, mycophenalate, and 6-mercaptopurine.

Retinoids

Synthetic derivatives of vitamin A have effects on cell differentiation, cell growth, and immune response. In the field of hyperkeratotic eczema of the hands (and feet), the use of retinoids can be considered. Side effects of dry skin and chapped lips always occur. Newer retinoids are being developed, which may increase the positive response rate in hand eczema. Retinoids can also be used to heighten response to phototherapy, which is more often used for psoriasis than for eczema.

Biologics

Biologics are a class of systemic drugs that are designed to perform specific functions in the pathogenetic processes of diseases (23–25). In dermatology, psoriasis is the forerunner to other dermatoses including eczema. The currently available biologics for dermatological (mostly psoriasis) use target tumor necrosis factor α or lymphocyte function. Little is established at the moment about the role of the available biologics for eczematous conditions, but it is to be expected that applications will be found.

TWO MAIN ECZEMA TREATMENT SCENARIOS

To exemplify treatment situations, contact eczema and atopic eczema can be used to illustrate two basic approaches to general aspects of management: management of the first presentation of a patient with eczema and the ongoing management situation that chronic eczema demands. Treatment of other eczema forms can then be then seen against this background.

Scenario 1: Contact Eczema

In this eczema group, exogenous causes predominate. Hereditary issues will be of less importance, with the exception of the establishment of an atopic diathesis, which is known to predispose to irritant contact eczema. The time course for nonurticarial reactions to exogenous agents will be delayed from several hours to several days, making detective work as to causality more difficult for patients. Exposure in the workplace, in the home environment, and in hobbies and sports needs to be considered and very often tested for. Eczema is an inflammation typified classically by rubor (redness), calor (warmth), dolor (pain), tumor (swelling), and functio laesa (loss of function). An inflamed organ, whether skin, bone, or any other organ, will need to be rested. This may involve sick leave for the patient or modification of duties at the workplace and at home. General supportive measures need to be facilitated, and irritative factors need to be avoided. The avoidance of irritation demands education of the patient and will involve decreasing exposure to water, personal cleansing items such as soap, detergents, shampoos, and any other irritating factors for the patient's skin (Table 6).

First Presentation

Patients may present with an acute dermatitis with severe itch, redness, swelling, weeping, and even blister formation. Even if the provoking factor is obvious and a spontaneous resolution of lesions can be expected provided the provoking agent is avoided, symptomatic relief will still be required, and a biphasic recovery period (return to normal appearance followed by return to normal function) will need to be planned for. Another presentation form is a more gradual onset of itch, erythema, and dryness over weeks or months. Symptomatic and supportive treatment is again required pending investigation.

Mild to Moderate Eczema

Normal treatment will involve use of a group III (potent) steroid applied thinly, twice daily for a period of two to three weeks. Instruction should be given to reduce frequency of application after that time introducing treatment-free days and a gradual cessation of therapy for the next two to three weeks. Table 7 shows the amounts

TABLE 6 Protecting a Fraction of a Tenth of a Millimeter (Thickness of the Stratum Corneum Everywhere Except the Palms and Soles)

Irritant	Comment
Water	Lessen exposure to water, and use lower temperature.
Soaps and shampoos	Avoid or use cream based soap substitutes without tensides
Summer	Sweating should be avoided through use of behaviors and ventilated clothing.
Winter	Dry, cold weather indoors and out exacerbates eczema. Use appropriate clothing, extra emollients, and humidifiers. Avoid indoor warmth.
Food preparation	Wet foodstuffs and juice from foodstuffs are irritants as well as potential urticants and allergens
Textiles with sharp fibers	Cotton and silk have soft fibers. Wool and synthetics irritate skin mechanically.
Animal fur	Hair and fur are irritants and cause allergy
Dirt and dust	For sensitive skin, dirt and dust are a diminutive form of sand blasting; thus, avoid them.
Cosmetics	Can be irritants—even the expensive ones. Try to totally avoid for several weeks.
Workplace	Follow appropriate guidelines for prevention in individual workplaces. Chiefly, there is a question of hand dermatitis; wet work is the worst!

Note: Avoidance of irritants is a vital aspect of the management of eczema. Most irritant factors act by a cumulative insult mechanism. Because damage may arise first after many, sometimes hundreds, of individual exposures, the road back to fully functional skin demands determined and disciplined avoidance of irritants.

necessary to treat—a 15-g tube is in, most situations, not a basis for an adequate trial of therapy. The face and the skin fold areas are usually not treated with stronger steroids. Group I (mild) should be used, and these can be applied more frequently. Fissured or eroded skin is not a contraindication to use of steroids. Emollients should be introduced at the same time as steroids are commenced. The patient may need to try several emollients to find the preparation that is preferred (and will therefore be used). Areas of exudative (weeping) dermatitis can be treated with bathing. Potassium permanganate is a useful agent, and this is painted on with a cotton stick or during bathing. Aluminium sulfate bathing can be more convenient for the patient.

Severe Eczema

A contact eczema that appears as severe may well be secondarily infected. Pronounced weeping with crust formation can indicate secondary infection especially

TABLE 7 Intermittent Protocol for Group IV (and Group III) Topical Corticosteroids.

Induction phase
  Corticosteroid applied twice daily for 4 days (emollients);
    3 corticosteroid-free days
  Corticosteroid applied twice daily for 2 days;
    2 corticosteroid-free days
  Corticosteroid twice a day
  Corticosteroid free day
  Corticosteroid twice a day
Maintenance phase
  One or two applications per day, 2 days a week, e.g. Monday and Thursday. On other days, use emollients.

if a yellowish hue in the lesion is seen. Given the use restrictions for local antibiotics, systemic antibiotics usually directed at *S. aureus* are often necessary in a 7- to 10-day course. Whole-body potassium permanganate baths are helpful. In severe eczema, a course of systemic corticosteroids can be motivated. Prednisolone in a dose of 30 mg/day that is reduced over two to three weeks is appropriate, provided there are no contraindications. Such courses should not be repeated often, and every effort should be made to avoid continual use. Wet dressings can be helpful.

Ongoing Management

Despite the tendency of contact eczema to be self-limiting, chronicity is often seen because of undiscovered or inadequately avoided allergens, failure in avoidance of irritants (or a too marked constitutional susceptibility to everyday irritants), a strong endogenous component (often but not solely atopy), or the little understood phenomenon of chronicity. This is particularly likely to occur in irritant contact eczema, but nickel allergy is notorious for its association with chronic hand eczema. Emollients are always important as well as discipline in preventive measures. Coaching and encouragement are important to increase compliance. Topical steroids remain important but need to be used intermittently to avoid risk for tachyphylaxis (loss of function due to receptor saturation) and other side effects (26). Intermittent use of corticosteroids utilizes the steroid reservoir, which builds up in the stratum corneum. Two general approaches to intermittent therapy can be delineated, both of which have acceptable long-term safety. A strong steroid can be used twice a day, 2–3 days in a row, twice a month without an undue risk for long-term side effects. An alternative method is seen in Table 7, where the aim is to establish treatment only twice a week. This works best with group IV steroids, but the regime can also be used for group III steroids. Systemic steroids for exacerbations can be used, but long-term, low-dose steroids should be avoided. Immunosuppressants such as azothioprine and cyclosporine can be used for severe cases. Use of biologics has not yet found a place, but this is an area to keep an eye on. Typically, patients in these tough situations think, "Am I prepared to take the risk of side effects with the systemic agents being suggested?" For the treating physician (at least this one), the question is, "Should I have been more aggressive in treatment earlier in the course of the illness?" There is, at present, little guidance from the literature about these matters.

Scenario 2: Atopic Eczema

Atopic eczema is characterized by a predisposition to eczema based on allergic mechanisms chiefly of type I allergy nature and susceptibility to irritant eczema based on faulty stratum corneum barrier function. Atopic patients can also develop contact allergy, although this seems to be less common in mild atopics. Atopics are exposed to many pharmaceutical preparations, and the contact allergy–risk of these agents [for instance, corticosteroids (27)] and of the excipients in emollients increases. Severe atopics can have multiple contact allergies. There are three main types presentation for atopic eczema:

1. The infantile variant, which affects large areas of the body, mostly the extensor areas, e.g., cheek, lateral arms and legs, lateral torso
2. The flexural eczema stage, which affects the knee and the elbow creases
3. Adult atopics who have a preponderance of lesions on the face and upper torso, a feature that is attributed to *Pityrosporum ovale* colonization

A fourth presentation pattern, most obvious in cold, dry climates is that of irritant contact eczema of the hands, which is markedly overrepresented in atopics. Other classical patterns of presentations for atopics in adult life are dry periorbital eczema and exacerbation of eczema during pregnancy.

All grades of atopy will be seen, and the clinical situation will follow a chronic remitting course of varying intensity. Care of atopic eczema includes due attention to the other manifestations of atopy (asthma and rhinoconjunctivitis). Type I allergic reactions to a broad range of substances including foods can also be a problem. In general terms, the younger the patient, the more that food allergy will be a problem (for children younger than two years old, comanagement between pediatric allergists and dermatologists is to be recommended). Irritant factors as itemized for contact dermatitis need to be avoided. Additionally, atopics are typically irritated by fibers other than soft cotton fibers and by clothing, which accentuates sweating.

First Presentation
In western societies, an atopic diathesis is present in 20% to 25% of the population. Presentation can occur in early childhood or later in life. It is likely that at the time of presentation symptoms may be mild. Although the need for effective therapy, as in contact eczema, can apply, and, indeed, the same approach can be used, treatment of atopic dermatitis can, with advantage, be viewed as a stepwise model in which a base plate of maintenance therapy is built up and other therapies added as necessary. Who is an atopic? A "yes" answer to the question, "Did you have eczema as a child?," has been validated as a reliable tag for an atopic. A personal and family history of atopic symptoms and the appearance of keratosis pilaris on the extensor skin are helpful indicators. In fact, the visage of an atopic is often easily recognizable.

The base plate of therapy for atopic eczema is care of skin that has a constitutionally defective barrier function. Emollients are important as is avoidance of the irritant factors itemized for irritant contact eczema. Indeed, presentation with irritant contact eczema of the hands or periorbitally is a common presentation for "historic atopics" (no adult history of eczema but an almost forgotten history of flexural eczema as a child). Atopics need also to avoid noncotton fabric close to the skin and tight sweat-promoting clothing. Allergies to dog and cat hair and to latex are very likely to occur, and these exposures should be avoided both for secondary and primary prevention. The supposition should be that correct preventive management can markedly inhibit exacerbations of eczema in atopics.

Mild to Moderate Eczema
Mild forms of atopic eczema may need no more than emollients and group I topical steroids in addition to the preventive base plate. The patient needs to become aware of the importance of prevention and the necessity for adequate therapy of other atopic manifestations (asthma and rhinoconjunctivitis).

More pronounced eczema will need the addition of group III steroids but often only for a number of days (depending on how long the eczema has been undertreated). Opinion among dermatologists varies as to the place of group II steroids—patients often find managing a range of steroid strengths to be difficult. Intermittent or interval treatment with a potent steroid is increasingly favored. Atopics will often have isolated areas of more difficult eczema. Usually, this is a question of "lichenification" caused by intense scratching. The "itch–scratch cycle" gives an indurated patch of eczema that is similar to lichen simplex chronicus (also known as neurodermatitis). This mechanism demands a potent steroid and a longer period of treatment—classically six weeks, the length of time needed for the itch to be subdued to lose the complex reflex mechanism that maintains the itch–scratch habit. Occlusion is the simplest way of helping the steroids work. Intralesional steroids can also be of use. Calcineurin antagonists (tacrolimus and pimecrolimus) can be considered in mild to moderate eczema, but the prescriber needs to keep abreast of recommended treatment regimes and cautions. In particular, contemporaneous exposure to sunlight should be avoided. At present, the half-life for the disappearance of immunological effects of relevance to sunlight exposure is not established. Head and neck localization can indicate that therapy directed at *P. ovale* (*M. furfur*) can be indicated. Some, possibly as many as half of atopics, have a type I allergy for this commensal. Medicated shampoos (e.g., ketaconazole) can reduce colonization. Iconazole preparations with or without hydrocortisone can have good effect. Again, an empirical approach is needed—trial therapy in head and neck localization and assessment of outcome. Eczema of the eyelids is common in atopics. Care should be taken with corticosteroids in the periorbital area, but with group I steroids, margins of safety are high in the short term (1–2 weeks).

Severe Eczema

Severe atopic eczema is often secondarily infected (impetiginized). The secondary infection can be localized or generalized. Fever and systemic malaise indicate infection beyond the skin (erysipelas or other cause) and should be investigated and treated accordingly. Two additions on the therapy staircase to cope with secondary infection are whole-body potassium permanganate baths and systemic antibiotics aiming at *S. aureus*. Bacterial culture should be performed (*Streptococcus pyogenes* is another possible cause). If the lesions are less widespread, bathing, mupirocin, and hydrogen peroxide cream can be used. Fucidic acid topically and in combination with hydrocortisone has been effective, but the development of resistance to topically applied fucidic acid is a problem that affects use. Exacerbations of atopic eczema can be sufficiently severe to warrant systemic steroids—under cover of antibiotics if secondary infection is present. Doses can be in the range 20–25 mg of prednisolone, and the dose reduction phase needs to be extended at lower levels (5–10 mg/day) to enable the reestablishment of other supportive therapy and prevent rebound. In cases not responding to therapy, frequent reviews of basic treatment principles (down to the level of type of soap, water temperature, presence of any external stresses) are necessary. Patients (and parents), family, friends, and the workplace need continuing coaching and support. Rehabilitation in the workplace may be needed.

Ongoing Management

Like green (or brown) eyes, the atopic diathesis will not change. The manifestations may, however, keep a low profile for long periods—longer if preventive strategies are followed. There are, however, patients with a chronic remitting course and exacerbations that come frequently and are severe, and in these cases, systemic therapy can be considered. The mildest systemic intervention is the use of phototherapy. Broadband UVB, narrowband UVB, and a combination with extra UVA can be very effective (Figure 1). Children can also be treated from the age at which they can be instructed and reassured about the actual process of standing in the light box (with the mother or father outside). Phototherapy is a useful way of giving a break from reliance on topical steroids. In Scandinavia, the long winter can

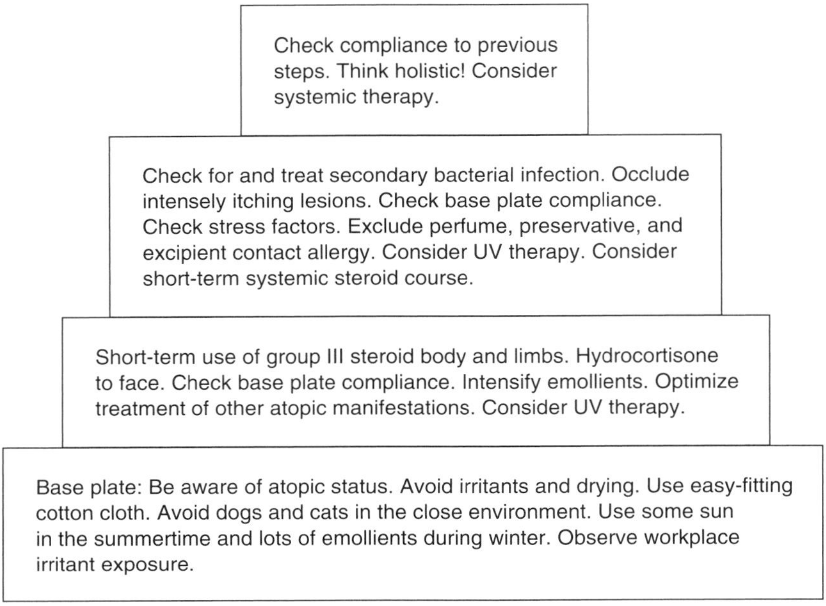

Check compliance to previous steps. Think holistic! Consider systemic therapy.

Check for and treat secondary bacterial infection. Occlude intensely itching lesions. Check base plate compliance. Check stress factors. Exclude perfume, preservative, and excipient contact allergy. Consider UV therapy. Consider short-term systemic steroid course.

Short-term use of group III steroid body and limbs. Hydrocortisone to face. Check base plate compliance. Intensify emollients. Optimize treatment of other atopic manifestations. Consider UV therapy.

Base plate: Be aware of atopic status. Avoid irritants and drying. Use easy-fitting cotton cloth. Avoid dogs and cats in the close environment. Use some sun in the summertime and lots of emollients during winter. Observe workplace irritant exposure.

FIGURE 1   Therapeutic steps for atopic eczema.

be broken by six weeks of phototherapy. It needs to be remembered that natural sunlight is not always easy to access just because the climate is inherently sunny — many parts of Sydney are a long way from the beach! Light in a box can often be administered with less sweatiness and warmth (not good for atopics) than a visit to a local pool or the beach. Cumulative dose in formal phototherapy is documented, and the educational and placebo effect of visiting the dermatological nursing staff is considerable.

Light is not universally effective. Two systemic immunomodulating drugs are most often used. Azathioprine can have a long-term effect at relatively low doses for six to 12 months. Cyclosporine has a more immediate effect and is often, if effective, continued for one to two years. Both have potential side effects, the most common being gastrointestinal symptoms and bone-marrow depression for azathioprine and elevated blood pressure and depressed renal function for cyclosporine. There are well-functioning monitoring regimes for a correct management of these agents, and patients in a situation warranting their trial should be informed and encouraged (but not pressured into) treatment. Some patients have a seriously disruptive eczema, and their physicians are seriously challenged in their ability to manage them. To say that we are grateful for all contributions is an understatement—and the contributions are needed across the therapeutic board, from soap substitutes to biologics specifically targeting eczema mechanisms.

SPECIFIC ECZEMA TYPES AND TREATMENT MODIFICATIONS

The therapeutic approaches and the agents used in the above two scenarios are adaptable to other forms of eczema. In the following sections, relevant additional modalities will be mentioned after a brief sketch of the actual conditions.

Seborrheic Eczema

This common eczema is named because of its manifestation in areas of more pronounced sebaceous gland activity (scalp, face, sternum, and intertriginous areas). The condition is constitutional and of variable expression, depending on systemic well-being and local factors in the skin. A role for *Malassezia furfur* is postulated, although the mechanism is unclear (possibly not via type I allergy as in atopics). Empirically, agents that suppress the growth of the organism help atopic eczema. Examples are shampoos containing ketoconazole, selenium sulfide, zinc pyrithione, and other agents that are used two to three times a week. Other agents are applied as creams before shampooing. Examples range from classical agents such as sulfur, tar, and propylene glycol to specific agents such as imidazoles. Inflammation can be pronounced, and intermittent use of corticosteroids is often required, most commonly in the scalp, where group III steroids in a solution, gel, or mousse can be safely and conveniently used. On the face, combination, preparations of group I steroids and imidazoles are popular and safe. In the flexural areas, stronger steroids should be avoided because of the risk for atrophy, but intermittent use of a group II steroid can be used. Sunlight can improve seborrheic eczema, but in some cases, sunlight seems an aggravating factor. Systemic therapy is seldom required. One situation is an attempt to reduce *M. furfur* by oral anti-yeast therapy. Another situation is the therapy-resistant adult with a general heightening of sebaceous gland activity for whom retinoids, as for acne, can be tried to reduce sebaceous gland size.

Venous and Gravitational Eczema

Eczema of the legs is common in situations of venous hypertension. This occurs after deep vein thrombosis and in the presence of varicosities, particularly deeper venous insufficiency. Valves in the veins are damaged, leading to poor venous return and pooling of blood in the lower limbs. This results in poor capillary function at a tissue level and a relative oxygen and nutrient deficiency in the dermis and epidermis. The result, dermatologically, is eczema, which is typified by itch and the classic morphology of eczema, with additional hemosiderin staining caused by (gravitational) leakage of red blood cells. The causal treatment of this eczema form is operative (after appropriate investigation). The main therapeutic measure awaiting operation is pressure bandage support and gravitational relief of swelling by raising the legs above the level of the heart at periods throughout the day. Symptomatic treatment of eczema can be used, aiming for relief of itch using a group III steroid. Often, one or two applications a week will suffice. An emollient is also often required. Venous eczema can be seen together with venous ulcers. The eczema seen around the ulcer can be treated as above. Vigilance is needed as to the possible complication of contact allergy to therapeutic agents. Leg ulcer treatment often attracts a plethora of different topical therapies. For some unclear reason, the lower limb, especially in the presence of ulceration, is an ideal site for sensitization. It is important to keep topical treatments simple and (from a contact allergy point of view) safe. Patch testing is often necessary.

Lichen Simplex Chronicus

In some countries, the term neurodermatitis is a synonym for this condition, which is based on a complex reflex itch–scratch mechanism. The original cause of the first episode of itch becomes irrelevant, and therapy is directed at relief of itch and prevention of scratch. The eczema form can appear in its own right or as a part of another eczema or dermatosis. Group III steroids and occlusion (by several means) are the mainstays of therapy and need to be kept in place for five to six weeks (i.e., longer than for standard eczema). In the long term, emollients and the use of occlusion (without necessarily corticosteroids) can be useful. It is likely that some individuals are predisposed, and it seems as though stress may have a part in the pathogenesis.

Asteatotic Eczema

Dry skin is an objective sign; asteatos means lack of lipid. Itch is subjective. When dry skin itches, it becomes an eczema terminologically. Asteatotic eczema is most common in the elderly, in younger people with a constitutional general dryness, and in unwell individuals, e.g. individuals who have been admitted to hospital for a period. The stratum corneum dries out like mud at the bottom of a summer-dry water bed in a hexagonal splitting pattern. The tissue at the base of the cracks is the focus for the itch-producing inflammation. Avoidance of irritants and use of emollients and topical steroids are usually helpful. Continued preventive management is necessary.

Discoid Eczema

This eczema-giving lesions on the trunk and extremities has a descriptive name. A synonym is nummular (coin-shaped) eczema. A disk-shaped lesion on a patient who obviously has atopic eczema does not warrant a change in the diagnosis. Rather, the term is used to convey the appearance of a separate group of eczema patients for whom dry skin may be the predisposing factor. The acute lesions can be treated with group III steroids, emollients, and attention to irritant factors. Phototherapy can facilitate a return of the skin to normal function.

Pityriasis Alba (Pityriasis Sicca)

The common presentation of this eczema is in the early summer after the patient has noted pale patches on the extremities and torso. It is usually not symptomatic, but occasionally, areas of slight erythema can be seen within the white (=alba) patches. This is "status post" eczema from the previous winter and is extremely common in countries with long winters. Low-grade, dry (=sicca), usually asymptomatic eczema during the winter goes unobserved by the patient until the summer sun pigments the normal skin but not the healed eczema patches, which display a postinflammational hypopigmentation due to abnormalities in melanocytes. Quite often, the skin has a degree of keratosis pilaris, the follicular dryness that can indicate an atopic diathesis. The acute lesions can be treated with mild steroids, emollients, and attention to irritant factors. As the summer progresses, pigmentation will return. Changes need to be made for the coming winter in regard to irritant exposure (water and soap essentially).

Intertriginous Eczema

Two folds of skin abutting on each other create an occluded environment that predisposes to barrier abnormality (through increased hydration) and a relative immunosuppression (through surface effects and dendritic and other cell effects). Bacterial, yeast, and even dermatophyte infections can become more common. Localization of rash to skin fold areas is common in psoriasis and seborrheic eczema. Eczema in these areas can occur in isolation. In addition to eczema treatments as previously outlined, attention to drying of moisture in skin folds is required by use of powders, either bland talcum or imidazole powders. Classic treatments in inter-trigo include painting with Gentian violet, a messy but effective anti-yeast agent that can additionally act as a representative for a group of dyes previously used in dermatological therapies.

MORE COMPLEX ECZEMA SCENARIOS

Fortunately, most patients with eczema can expect good relief from their condition even if they may need to continually observe preventive measures. There are, how-ever, complex treatment scenarios at the difficult end of the eczema spectrum.

Hand Eczema

Hand eczema is common. In Sweden, the 1-year prevalence of hand eczema in some degree is 10% (28). In warmer climates with shorter and less dry winters, the preva-lence of irritant hand eczema is patently less, but in all countries, hand eczema can have devastating effects on an individual's life. In many cases, we are at a loss on how to manage the chronic, unremitting course of the disease. Terminology for hand der-matoses across the world is not entirely uniform, but there are some general rules.

The first general rule is that in more than 90% of dermatoses of the hands, the cause will be eczema, psoriasis, or a dermatophyte infection. The remaining per-centage may be caused by dozens of alternative diagnoses.

Among eczemas of the hands, the causality may be atopic dermatitis per se, allergic contact dermatitis, irritant contact dermatitis (atopics are predisposed to ir-ritant dermatitis of the hands without other concurrent atopic skin manifestations), or a number of hand eczema types whose delineation needs to be discussed.

Pompholyx is a variant of hand eczema involving episodic vesicular lesions of the hands and feet. Dyshydrotic eczema is a term favored by some—the name reflect-ing an original theory that abnormal sweating was involved. In the Scandinavian tra-dition, the term vesicular hand eczema is more commonly used—the argument being that it is descriptively correct. Whatever way the discussion is conducted—vesicles indicate activity, being the macroscopic manifestation of the histological spongiosis, the histological hallmark of eczema. On the hands and feet, because the epidermis is thicker, intact vesicles are seen more often and for longer periods than at other skin sites.

Hyperkeratotic hand eczema is a descriptive term that is much clearer in its usage. Irritant mechanisms are more pronounced than specific allergy, and chronic-ity is common. Endogenous factors including, but not exclusively, atopy are sus-pected, and this is undoubtedly true if one accepts that the occurrence of chronicity itself reflects a constitutional expression. Ongoing management has been covered in the two main scenarios—typical for eczema located to the hands is that the patient's livelihood as well as discomfort and quality of life are at stake.

Infective or Microbial Eczema

The terms infective eczema or microbial eczema are not synonymous with secondarily infected eczema. An atopic eczema or a hand eczema that becomes impetiginized ex-acerbates. In microbial eczema, the eczematous process itself speeds up and spreads. Often, one area of eczema shows obvious infection, after which distant skin sites de-velop eczema. These distant sites need not necessarily be positive in culture. An old tradition of Scandinavian dermatology differentiated between dry and wet types of discoid eczema. In the wet type, the bacterial culture was often positive and accompanied by a tendency to spread or "generalize." Typically, this occurs in middle-aged or older men, and quite often, the initial lesions are on the legs. Sometimes, a point of trauma becomes infected, and this is the initial event. Treatment with antibiotics in these patients is not merely a question of getting rid of the secondary infection; it can actually be a form of pathogenetic intervention. These eczema forms are difficult to treat and often persist for years. The prognosis is better with early treatment.

Generalized Eczema

Generalization of eczema can sometimes be quite dramatic. One of the situations in which this occurs is in infective eczema. The tendency of the body to react generally has been termed an id reaction. Another term used is status eczematicus. Exact mechanisms are unknown. Patients in this situation are therapeutic challenges. A very specific form of widespread eczema is erythroderma ("red man syndrome"). Erythroderma, a serious condition with risks for sepsis and cardiac failure, can have various causes, four of which are psoriasis, drug reactions, seborrheic eczema, and atopic eczema. Treatment is complex, often involving prolonged hospitalization.

FUTURE ISSUES

Our framework for the treatment of eczema is empirical. Improvements in our knowledge base are necessary in many areas. Understanding of innate reactivity in the skin especially the role of the dermis in orchestrating reactivity is an important issue. The benefits that the rheumatological diseases and psoriasis have gained from biologics needs to happen for eczema patients. A better understanding of chronicity mechanisms would give therapeutic clues. At the moment, our knowledge that early treatment improves prognosis needs to better permeate health care delivery. It is best to prevent the problem. Identifying susceptible phenotypes, working out relevant preventive strategies, and then implementing them efficiently have great potential for improvement at a population level. When eczema has become established, specific treatments for allergy or therapy directed at reversing chronicity mechanisms are needed. Increased innovation in basic research, better topical and systemic agents, and improved clinical use of the therapeutic agents we have available will also help this large and long-suffering patient group.

REFERENCES

1. Elias P, Wood L, Feingold K. Epidermal pathogenesis of inflammatory dermatoses. Am J Contact Dermat 1999; 10:119–126.
2. Williams H, Robertson C, Stewart A, et al. Worldwide variation in the prevalence of symptoms of atopic eczema in the International Study of Asthma and Allergies in Childhood. J Allergy Clin Immunol 1999; 103:125–138.
3. Novak N, Bieber T, Allam J-P. Recent highlights in the pathophysiology of atopic eczema. Int Arch Allergy Immunol 2005; 136(2):191–197.
4. Palmer C, Irvine A, Terron-Kwiatkowski A, et al. Common loss-of-function variants of the epidermal barrier protein filaggrin are a major predisposing factor for atopic dermatitis. Nat Genet 2006; 38, 441–446.
5. Sjögren F, Anderson C. The spectrum of inflammatory cell response to dimethyl sulfoxide. Contact Dermatitis 2000;42(4):216–221.

6. Taieb A, Ring J, Stalder JF, Labreze L, Oranje AP, Kunz B. Clinical validation and guidelines for the SCORAD index: consensus report of the European Task Force on Atopic Dermatitis. Dermatitis 1997; 195(1):10–19.
7. Devos S, Van Der Valk. Epicutaneous patch testing. Eur J Dermatol 2002; 12. 506–513.
8. Burns T, Breathnach S, Cox N, Griffiths C., eds. Rook's Textbook of Dermatology. 7th ed. Vol. 2. Oxford: Blackwell Science.
9. Freedberg IM, Eisen AZ, Wolff K, Austen KF, Goldsmith LA, Katz SI. Fitzpatrick's Dermatology in General Medicine. 6th ed. Vol. 2. New York: McGraw-Hill.
10. Therapeutic Guidelines: Dermatology. Version 2. Melbourne: Therapeutic Guidelines Limited, 2004.
11. Carson-Jurica MA, Schrader WT, O'Malley BW.Z. Endocr Rev 1990; 11:201–220.
12. Gehring U. The structure of glucocorticoid receptors. J Steroid Biochem Mol Biol 1993; 45:183–190.
13. Marks R, Pongsehirum D, Saylan T. A method for the assay of topical corticosteroids. Br J Dermatol 1973; 88:69–74.
14. McKenzie AW, Stoughton RB. Method for comparing percutaneous absorption of steroids. Arch Dermatol 1962; 86:608–610.
15. Kapturczak MH, Meier-Kriesche HU, Kaplan B. Pharmacology of calcineurin antagonists. Transplant Proc 2004; 36(2 Suppl.): 25S–32S.
16. Kapp A, Papp K, Bingham A, et al. Long-term management of atopic dermatitis in infants with topical pimecrolimus, a non-steroid anti-inflammatory drug: flare reduction in eczema with Elidel (infants) multicenter investigator study group. J Allergy Clin Immunol 2002; 110:277–284.
17. Kang S, Lucky AW, Pariser D, et al. Long-term safety and efficacy of tacrolimus ointment for the treatment of atopic dermatitis in children. J Am Acad Dermatol 2001; 44: S58–S64.
18. Garside R, Stein K, Castelnuovo E, et al. The effectiveness and cost-effectiveness of pimecrolimus and tacrolimus for atopic eczema: a systematic review and economic evaluation. Health Technol Assess 2005; 9:1–230.
19. Larko O. Phototherapy of eczema. Photodermatol Photoimmunol Photomed 1996; 12:91–94.
20. Lindelof B, Wrangsjo K, Liden S. A double blind study of Grenz ray therapy in chronic hand eczema. Br J Dermatol 1987; 117:77–80.
21. Meggit SJ, Reynolds N J. Azathioprine for atopic dermatitis. Clin Exp Dermatol 2001; 26(5):369–375.
22. Weatherhead S, Wahie S, Reynolds N, Meggit S. An open label dose-ranging study of methotrexate for moderate to severe adult atopic eczema. Br J Dermatol 2007; 156:346–351.
23. Granlund H, Erkko P, Reitamo S. Long-term follow up of eczema patients treated with cyclosporine. Acta Derm Venereol 1998; 78:40–43.
24. Connell L, McInnes I. New cytokine targets in inflammatory rheumatic diseases. Best Pract Res Clin Rheumatol 2006; 20:865–278.
25. Gottlieb A. Tumor necrosis factor blockade: mechanisms of action. J Invest Dermatol Symp Proc 2007; 12(1):1–4.
26. du Vivier A. Tachyphylaxis to topically applied steroids. Arch Dermatol 1976; 112: 1245–1248.
27. Burden AD, Beck MH. Contact hypersensitivity to topical corticosteroids. Br J Dermatol 1992; 127: 497–500.
28. Meding B, Jarvholm B. Hand eczema in Swedish adults—changes in prevalence between 1983 and 1996. J Invest Dermatol 2002; 118, 719–723.

4 Evolution of Cosmeceuticals and Their Application to Skin Disorders, Including Aging and Blemishes

Des Fernandes
The Renaissance Body Science Institute, Cape Town, South Africa

INTRODUCTION

From time immemorial, people have tried to maintain healthy skin or to treat skin problems with such topical applications as mud, urine, animal products, oils, plants, or plant extracts and resins, and others. All of these were virtually ineffective except mud applications, which did have the advantage of providing UV protection. Generally, cosmetics developed into applications of colored substances on the skin to disguise the problems beneath. Over time, simple creams came into use and with them a burgeoning industry that today makes a fortune selling creams, gels, and other topical products largely produced from inexpensive ingredients such as simple fats or oils and emulsifiers or gelling agents, with colors and added perfumes to disguise the natural smell. The industry was built on selling "hope in a jar" because the most that these products could do was to create a surface barrier or oil that would inhibit the natural loss of water through the epidermis and thereby alleviate dry skin. Mesmerizing advertisements to promote the latest magical ingredient promising eternal youth and beautiful skin were the only effective ingredients in the whole package. There has never been a shortage of gullible buyers, and so the cosmetics industry eventually became an industry driven by seductive titles and fanciful packages containing ineffective serums or creams laden with inviting colors and perfumes.

Fortunately, we now live in a new age where scientific research has shown us that real science can be included in the cosmetic pot and make positive changes to skin. The creams containing these active, scientifically proven ingredients are called cosmeceuticals, and they have now become the key driver in the cosmetic industry. The cosmeceutical market in the first world was valued at about U.S. $20 billion in 2005 and may top U.S. $30 billion by 2010 as more and more men and women try to make a difference in their aging skin.

THE ORIGIN OF THE CONCEPT OF COSMECEUTICALS

The cosmetics industry entered a transition phase in the last quarter of the 20th century when Albert Kligman, a U.S. dermatologist, coined the term cosmeceuticals to describe a new form of cosmetic based on essential micronutrients to gently nurture and rehabilitate photoaged skin. As introduced in Chapter 1, cosmeceuticals are not simply a traditional cosmetic but a skin care system that includes active ingredients that create physiological changes in skin cells to make skin appear younger and healthier. Topical medications had helped us to understand that the epidermis was not a total barrier, and one could influence the state of the skin by applying various medications, such as cortisone and antibiotics. The next step that led to the concept of cosmeceuticals was the realization that wrinkles, pigmentation blemishes, and other signs of photoaging are not simple "conditions" of normal skin and a natural effect of getting older but are in fact varying degrees of a serious skin disease. They are merely the earliest signs of actinic skin damage that eventually leads to the development of solar keratoses and skin cancer. The recognition of wrinkles and pigmentary blemishes as a disease is a major philosophical and physiological step that many clinicians have great difficulty in taking. Photoaged skin is diseased skin and needs to be treated with appropriate products. Treatment of the early signs of sun damage is quite clearly preventive medicine, and so one really needs "medicines" to deal with the problem. This is where cosmeceuticals come into the picture. We need active cosmetics that have a therapeutic effect on the skin. The word cosmeceutical conveys the meaning of *cosme*tics that have a pharma*ceutical* effect in the same way topical medicines do, and this word introduced a revolution in skin care.

Cosmeceuticals have become a household word, and it also one of the most misleading words in the cosmetic industry, which has seized on the term and realized another successful marketing myth. Clearly, to claim that a product is a cosmeceutical, it has to fulfill three important conditions:

1. It has to include scientifically proven active ingredients at concentrations that have physiological effects and make observable improvements of human skin. The effects would be

    · reduction of fine lines and wrinkles,
    · thickening of the epidermis,
    · increased, normal collagen network,
    · improved elastin deposition,
    · restoration of natural moisturizing factors,
    · normalization of skin color and removal of pigmentation blemishes, or
    · normalization of sebum secretion.

2. A cosmeceutical should be formulated to give optimum penetration of the active ingredients. A product with adequate concentrations of effective ingredients will not work as a cosmeceutical if the formula does not ensure good penetration of those ingredients into the area where they are needed. In some cases, transdermal penetration has to be enhanced to position the active molecule where it is most needed.

3. A cosmeceutical should not expose the client to any deleterious consequences, although one has to realize that because effective concentrations of active ingredients are used, the possibility of transient skin reactions does increase. This is in keeping with the Gauss distribution curve. Inevitably, some people may develop skin irritation, whereas most get good changes or even superb changes to their skin. For that reason, cosmeceuticals should only be administered by trained skin care therapists who can advise clients on the proper way to use them, and ideally cosmeceuticals should not be sold over-the-counter in department stores and others.

This chapter only deals with agents that are considered cosmeceutical. Most physicians interpret cosmeceuticals as glycolic acid and other α-hydroxy acids (AHAs), but, in fact, they have rather small cosmeceutical effects on skin cell physiology. Glycolic acid has minimal effects on skin cell metabolism and acts mainly as an abrasive-type agent that works mainly on the stratum corneum and sheds the superficial corneocytes. Its effects on collagen formation are related to its peeling properties, and if glycolic acid is supplied as glycolates at a more physiological pH (about 4.5–6.5), there is minimal observable impact on the skin. The main impact of AHAs on skin is as a peeling agent and not as a cosmeceutical. Very largely, AHAs are impostors in the field of cosmeceuticals, although they do have observable effects on photoaging. There are far more worthy cosmeceutical ingredients than AHA when treating photoaging.

THE SIGNS OF PHOTOAGING

Tanned skin is so common that people fail to recognize that it is the first sign of photo-aging. Tanning occurs because DNA has been damaged by UV light, and this induces the release of nitrous oxide, which initiates the production of melanin. The horny layer is thickened, and this may make the surface of the skin feel rough. Most photo-damage occurs before the age of 20, and young patients are often shocked to hear that they already manifest the earliest signs of photodamage. The signs of photoaging are attributable to damage to each of the four important cells in the epidermis and dermis and to the blood vessels and structural proteins in between the cells. In the epider-mis, these are the (1) keratinocytes, (2) melanocytes, and (3) Langerhans cells, and in the dermis, (1) fibroblasts, (2) collagen and elastin, (3) water-retaining substances between the cells, and (4) blood vessels.

Changes in the Epidermis

The keratinocytes and keratinocyte stem cells may produce clones of abnormal cells of varying size, pycnotic nuclei with abnormal DNA, and an irregular growth pattern. They contain more melanin granules, and this the first easily detectable sign of photo-aging. Irregular clumps of pigmentation are observed instead of the normal even dis-tribution of melanin. UV irradiation promotes the release of active substances from the keratinocyte that promote the production of melanin in the melanocytes. Altered kera-tinization of the dermis results in a thickened rough skin, which leads to an impaired barrier (stratum corneum) and, subsequently, dry skin. With progressive sun damage, the basement membrane and the rete pegs are affected, and the epidermis becomes thin and atrophic with flattened rete pegs. There is a loss of the fine fibers anchoring the epidermis to the basement membrane and dermis. DNA damage, if unrepaired, leads to actinic keratoses and may progress to basal and squamous cell carcinomas.

Langerhans cells are responsible for immune functions of the skin and would normally detect cells that have undergone DNA damage and mutation. However, Langerhans cells are also susceptible to UV irradiation, and as a result, these aber-rations are not detected and clones of abnormal keratinocytes and melanocytes may proliferate (1). Irradiated Langerhans cells have fewer Birbeck granules and lose their dendrites, and when they are impaired, the following clinical conditions may occur:

- Solar keratoses develop in irradiated skin and may progress into skin cancer.
- Skin allergies become more common.
- Patients are more prone to skin infections.

Melanocytes are responsible for melanin production, and abnormalities result in the following:

- Tanned skin in the short term. The DNA of melanocytes may mutate to pro-duce much more melanin than normal. Each melanocyte supplies melanin to its melanocyte unit of about 36 to 40 keratinocytes and sometimes to fibroblasts. These melanocytes slowly form a clone of hyperactive cells. Although the change may only be detectable initially with the Woods light, later on, this will manifest as typical mottled aged skin, but, if you catch this early on and treat it properly, then you can avoid it.

· Irregular pigmentation blotches may develop and coalesce into melasma. In some people, particularly in darker skinned people, ugly pigmentation blemishes may occur on the main sun-exposed areas of the face, which are particularly resistant to treatment. This poses one of the most difficult problems that we have to deal with among Asian people and creates a special value for cosmeceuticals.

· Although exposure to sunlight seems to play an important part in the development of melanoma, the exact causes are still unknown.

Changes in the Dermis

Fibroblasts produce less matrix substances of the dermis, which promote the manifestation of wrinkles. The delicate skin of the lower eyelid may be the first area to show damage. Wrinkles may be because of a loss of the anchoring fibrils below the basement membrane (2). These are composed of type VII collagen, and they are destroyed by matrix metalloproteinase 2. Normal structural collagen of the dermis is also destroyed by light. Collagen mRNA is down-regulated, and with increased metalloproteinases, this results in a net loss of collagen, which is also damaged by UV light (3).

Elastin, by contrast, is formed in greater quantities, but the elastin fibers become thickened instead of forming a healthy fine mesh to support the skin. Elastin fibers are fractured by UV light, and they roll up into little balls that can be seen quite easily on the neck skin in even only moderately sun-damaged people. As a result of defective action of elastin and diminished support from collagen, the skin starts to sag. In addition, there is less glycosaminoglycans and other water-retaining molecules in the skin, and so the skin becomes dry. Solar irradiation damages the collagen support around blood vessels and causes dilation of these vessels. Poor circulation shows up as a sallow, poorly nourished skin.

UNDERSTANDING THE MECHANISMS THAT PRODUCE PHOTOAGED SKIN

We have to understand the mechanism of solar damage in order to mount a scientific attack on photoaging. The simple acceptance of photoaging as a condition endured by aging people is incorrect because clinicians will then follow irrational marketing advice and, in ignorance, suggest "cosmeceutical" products containing AHAs, such as glycolic acid, instead of recommending a focused cosmeceutical product. We have to know how light, particularly UV light, damages skin. Light consists of a spectrum of photons, which are "packets" of energy that vary according to the wavelength. Essentially, light enters into the skin and certain wavelengths of light (photons) can damage the skin by either interacting on the molecular level with chromophores to changing their chemical structure or on the subatomic level by creating free radicals. Most people believe that the damage is done by UV light only, but in fact, even green, blue, and violet light can damage cells. Few people are aware that even "soft" green light can damage keratinocytes sufficiently to stimulate melanocytes to make more melanin! Because the production of melanin is only induced by damage to the keratinocytes' DNA, every "beautiful" tan is in fact evidence of photodamage.

Skin Chromophores

On the molecular level, a photon's energy can be absorbed into the molecule, which is then altered. In some cases, this interaction causes heat (e.g., when light interacts with melanin) or light (photoluminescence) or the chemical nature of the molecule may be altered. This is the change that interests us most, and the prime example of this is vitamin A. When vitamin A molecules (particularly retinyl palmitate) absorb the energy of photons in the range of about 334 nm, the increased energy changes the structure of the molecule, and vitamin A activity is lost. As a result, a localized deficiency of vitamin A and other photosensitive molecules develops after exposure to sunlight.

The chromophores for UVB are melanin, DNA, urocanic acid, vitamin E, advanced glycation end products and 7-dehydrocholesterol. Melanin does not, in general, pose a problem because it absorbs energy and will only create heat and absorbs any free radicals as well as chelating heavy metals.

DNA absorbs UVB at about 260 nm, and this damage deserves special attention because this will cause malfunctioning of cells and important mutations. Urocanic acid is among the normal oils secreted by the skin and acts as a natural sunscreen; however, when it absorbs UVB energy, it becomes *cis*-urocanic acid, which promotes suppression of the immune system and can promote the development of skin cancer. Vitamin E becomes inactivated by absorbing UVB rays. Proteins modified by advanced glycation end products can damage DNA. Advanced glycation end products accumulate on long-lived skin proteins such as elastin and collagen as a consequence of glycation. Advanced glycation end product proteins collect in the nucleus as well as the cytoplasm. DNA strand breaks occur from increased free radical activity as well as direct electron transfer between photoexcited advanced glycation end products and DNA. So as we age, we produce potent photosensitizers that make us age even more and cause more DNA damage! Not all chromophore interactions are damaging: an example is 7-dehydrocholesterol, which absorbs UVB energy and is converted to vitamin D in the keratinocytes.

On the other hand, UVA damages DNA through free radical action rather than absorption of energy by a chromophore. UVA rays are ubiquitous, plentiful, and can penetrate through clouds and window panes, so it is easy to understand that vitamin A in the skin is easily denatured by exposure to light. However, vitamin A is damaged because it is a chromophore and becomes inactive and cannot be reconstituted. In a paradoxical twist, UV light may also assist isomerization of all-*trans*-retinoic acid to *cis*-retinoic acid, which are both ligands for the genes expressing the effects of vitamin A. UVA, in addition, can activate genes at very low doses, and we experience this when we are trying to treat pigmentation problems. Very low–intensity light could activate the mechanisms responsible for inducing melanin production by melanocytes. Melanin absorbs UVA rays and all other light rays without damaging cells. NADH is important to the cells of our skin because it is a source of energy and gets altered into an inactive agent by absorbing UVA energy. Glutathione is an important antioxidant but depleted by UVA and that leads to a sensitization to UVA 334 nm (which inactivates vitamin A) and 365 nm and near-visible blue-violet light (405 nm, which inactivates vitamin C), as well as UVB 302 and 313 nm. Another paradox is that vitamin D is also sensitive to light and photodegrades easily once it has been formed in the skin. For this reason, people should not stay in the sun much longer than 20 minutes if they are intent on making vitamin D. Riboflavin and tryptophan both absorb UVA and, as a result, can increase the formation of free radicals.

Vitamin C (ascorbic acid) is a chromophore that is not affected so much by UV light (except in the battle against free radicals) but rather by blue light, which it absorbs and becomes deactivated.

The Role of Free Radicals in Photoaging

On the subatomic level, the absorption of energy can also result in electron changes with the generation of free radicals. If a photon should strike a vulnerable paired electron in the outer circuit of an oxygen atom, the electron is cast out of its circuit, and the molecule, in its quest for another electron, becomes a free radical. A free radical is in fact simply an atom with an unpaired electron that starts up a destructive concatenation of chemical reactions, involving tens of thousands of molecules in a fraction of a second, which may end up causing damage in the cell membranes or in the DNA of the cell. We must never forget the dangers of uncontrolled free-radical activity, so we should always ensure that our skin is rich in a wide variety of lipid- and water-soluble antioxidants. They have to be included in the skin care regimen and should be used both day and night.

FOCUSING ON CHROMOPHORES AND FREE RADICALS IN DEVELOPING COSMECEUTICALS

We know that only sun-damaged skin photoages. By understanding the chemical changes induced by exposure to sunlight, we can deduce that the most likely cause of photoaging is a chronic deficiency of essential chromophores in the exposed skin, combined with the effects of free radicals. Clearly, by understanding which molecules in skin are damaged by light, we should be able to design a cosmeceutical regime to combat photodamage and reverse its effects. The first molecules to come to mind are vitamins A and C, which could be described as the major vitamins of healthy skin.

For decades, we have realized that vitamin A is vital for healthy skin. Wise and Sulzberger (4) worked with vitamin A and realized that it was extremely unstable in light, and they suggested in 1938 that there is a local hypovitaminosis A in wrinkled skin. We now know that UVA rays, particularly at 334 nm, are responsible for photodecomposition of retinyl palmitate that is the main storage form of vitamin A in the skin (5). The plot thickens because we also know that vitamin A is the one key molecule essential for the normal growth and differentiation of all the important cells of the skin: keratinocytes, melanocytes, Langerhans cells, and fibroblasts. Cluver (6) was a pioneer in recognizing that vitamin A played an essential role in counteracting sun damage. He showed that every time we go out into sunlight, the photosensitive vitamin A molecule is denatured not merely in the skin but also in the blood. With time, investigations have demonstrated that vitamin A is not only good for aging skin but is actually essential. Women have an added disadvantage because blood levels of vitamin A drop when they menstruate (7). This means that skin levels are also lower, and so they are more vulnerable to photodamage during menstruation.

Retinyl palmitate, but not retinol, absorbs UV energy. Retinol is protected by its bond with a specific retinol-binding protein (8). A recently recognized effect of adequate doses of retinyl palmitate specifically within skin cells is to reduce the production of thymine dimers in the DNA. According to Antille et al. (9), "In human subjects, topical retinyl palmitate was as efficient as a sun protection factor 20 sunscreen in preventing sunburn erythema as well as the formation of thymine dimers. These results demonstrate that epidermal retinyl esters have a biologically relevant filter activity and suggest, besides their pleomorphic biologic actions, a new role for vitamin A that concentrates in the epidermis."

Vitamin A has a vast array of hormonal, physiological actions on the cells of the skin but is not (for practical purposes) an antioxidant, whereas vitamin C has some hormonal role on the DNA of the fibroblast by activating about four genes responsible for collagen production. It also has effects on the melanocyte by providing a reducing milieu to reduce the formation of melanin, but its main action is as an important antioxidant. Vitamin C is important for the reactivation of vitamin E that has been converted into a tocopheryl radical by quenching a free radical. Vitamin E plays an essential role as an antioxidant in safeguarding cellular membranes, and when it is applied topically, it augments photoprotection; however, this advantage only becomes clear a day or two after sun exposure. Patients using topical vitamin E get less sunburn and a lighter tan. Vitamin E is also light-sensitive and can be oxidized into an inactive form. Vitamin E, on the other hand, seems to have virtually no metabolic action at all and is only an antioxidant in the lipid phase of the cell.

This localized deficiency of vitamins A and C and skin antioxidants is insidious. Not all the vitamin A in the skin is destroyed, but it is instantaneous, and a single UV exposure could lower the levels of vitamin A in the skin where UVA can penetrate by 70–90% (10). The skin cell stores of retinyl palmitate are progressively diminished. Because retinoic acid is required for the formation of retinoid cellular and nuclear receptors, fewer retinoid receptors are produced on the cell membranes, and the retinoid metabolic pathways become less efficient. The keratinocytes produce less of the essential keratins and ceramides that ensure an effective chemical barrier for the skin. The horny layer becomes much thicker and rougher, with a basket-weave pattern instead of being compact, thinner, and denser. Irradiated keratinocytes release the precursors of matrix metalloproteinases (collagenases, elastases, and gelatinases). Normally, vitamin A controls the conversion of pre–matrix metalloproteinases secreted by keratinocytes and fibroblasts into active matrix metalloproteinases, but with a deficiency of vitamin A, UV irradiation stimulates the unimpaired release of metalloproteinases that then destroy collagen and the anchoring fibrils. Without vitamin A, the rete pegs become flattened. Langerhans cells need vitamin A to function, but if the vitamin A is inactivated by light, then they cannot function properly and recognize cells whose DNA has been damaged. These cells would normally be removed but clones of abnormal cells slowly start to develop and, years later, manifest as keratoses or skin cancer.

The melanocyte is stimulated to produce more melanin, but if there is adequate vitamin A, this is controlled for unexplained reasons, and the distribution of melanin in the skin is kept even. If the DNA of the melanocyte is damaged by irradiation, excessive amounts of melanin may be produced under lower light fluxes. These clones of cells are also not recognized by the Langerhans cells and grow into obvious splodges of darker pigment that are very resistant to treatment.

The fibroblast produces less glycosaminoglycans, so the skin feels drier, and wrinkles show up very easily. There is little value in looking at diet to replenish the depleted vitamin stores because that will take too long. Once the skin retinoids are depleted after a heavy exposure to sunlight, it takes several days before diet alone can restore the normal cutaneous retinoid levels (5). On the other hand, application of an active vitamin A cream can restore the normal levels within hours.

Ascorbic acid is water-soluble and is not stored in cells, so loss has to be replaced by the blood supply. Deficiencies of vitamin C permit more free radical damage but this does not show up clinically until significant damage has been done. There are no cellular receptors for ascorbic acid probably because its main action is as an antioxidant in extracellular fluid where it is closely associated with lipid membranes and can easily interact with vitamin E. Melanin is produced under oxidative conditions, so low levels of vitamin C would favor the development of pigment blemishes.

Vitamin E (D-tocopherol and derivatives) is probably the major antioxidant in the skin and is readily depleted after sun exposure (11). The normal network antioxidants of the skin are vitamin E, vitamin C, glutathione, coenzyme Q10, and α-lipoic acid. These are potentiated by flavonoids and carotenoids. Betacarotene, the plant form of vitamin A, is a powerful free radical quencher. Estimates suggest that one molecule of betacarotene can cope with 1000 free radicals. Lutein is another carotenoid that has particular value because it is a powerful absorber of blue light, which can severely damage cells. There are many other carotenoids that can also protect the skin. Sun exposure seriously depletes the levels of these essential antioxidants (12), so we are impelled to boost our antioxidant protection both topically and systemically. Panthenol is a coenzyme in fat and carbohydrate metabolism. It has other soothing effects on skin and is also a free radical quencher.

SELECTING COSMECEUTICAL INGREDIENTS

Cosmeceutical ingredients should be classified as follows:

- Those that are naturally found in the skin (e.g., chirally correct vitamins)
- Phytonutrients not normally found in skin but have physiological benefits (e.g., green tea polyphenols)
- Designed molecules (e.g., peptides not normally found in nature but that have physiological actions due to their cytokine activity)

SCIENTIFICALLY PROVEN COSMECEUTICAL INGREDIENTS

Although it is not feasible to make an encyclopedic list of all known cosmeceuticals, we can concentrate on the most widely used cosmeceuticals, which are briefly given here.

Vitamins and Antioxidants

Vitamin A, as retinoic acid, retinol, retinyl aldehyde, and retinyl esters, was the first cosmeceutical ingredient that was brought to our attention. Kligman had been researching the treatment of acne with retinoic acid (vitamin A acid, or tretinoin) in the 1960s, and over time, he noticed that his patients developed healthy skin. By 1986, he was able to report for the first time in history that a topically applied product had reduced wrinkles (13). This report was followed by another landmark paper produced under the guidance of Voorhees (14).

It has been established that a chronic deficiency of vitamin A lies at the heart of photoaging. We also know that vitamin C (ascorbic acid and its water and lipid-soluble variants) deficiency aggravates the effects of vitamin A deficiency as far as collagen and melanin are concerned. Because vitamins A, C, and E (tocopherol) and other network antioxidants [carotenoids, flavonoids, coenzyme Q10 or idebenone, dehydrolipoic acid (α-lipoic acid), green tea, peptides, AHAs, and β-hydroxy acids (BHAs)] are the fundamental molecules that determine the development or repair of actinic damage to create a function cosmeceutical for photoaged skin, one has to include topical replenishment of these vitamins. Of course, prevention is better than cure, so we should start using these vitamins on our skin from a very early age. I believe that we need to dose skin with vitamin A and the associated antioxidants very soon after we are first exposed to sunlight and to keep doing so for the rest of our lives. This means that the skin will never suffer from transient deficiencies of vitamins A and C and become more resistant to the development of skin cancers.

Which vitamin A? Medical literature reports for retinoid replenishment of the skin are virtually confined to retinoic acid despite the fact that there are a number of other chemical forms of vitamin A. In 2000, Varani et al. reported that a cosmetic ingredient (retinol) was able to minimize photoaging (15). Saurat's team concentrated on retinyl aldehyde (16) because retinyl aldehyde is one metabolic step away from retinoic acid, and although it is a cosmetically approved ingredient, its structural proximity to retinoic acid would give it an added advantage over retinol. Retinoic acid is generally classed as the medicinal form of vitamin A because of its rather harsh topical effects. All-*trans*-retinoic acid and some of its isomers are the ligands that interact with the DNA, but the fact remains that retinoic acid is not usually found extracellularly. Topical applications of retinoic acid do raise the levels of retinoic acid in the skin, but at the same time, the retinyl palmitate levels are also increased probably because of the reduction of the conversion of retinyl palmitate to retinol and retinaldehyde. Retinoic acid is irritant to skin and causes a marked retinoid reaction if there are inadequate retinoid receptors on the cell walls. Normal cellular physiology favors only minute quantities of retinoic acid within cells. Retinyl esters can be converted to retinol, then to retinyl aldehyde, and finally to retinoic acid. The step from retinyl aldehyde to retinoic acid is not reversible, so whatever retinoic acid is presented to the cell, it has to remain as retinoic acid and be metabolized and interact in the nucleus as the ligand for retinoid acid receptors (RAR and RXR and their subtypes). Should there be more than the cell can use, it cannot be stored as a retinyl ester. On the other hand, retinol and retinyl aldehyde are easily converted to retinyl esters. It also seems that the larger the retinyl ester storage, the higher the levels of retinoic acid. Retinyl esters may in fact be the driving force in the metabolism of vitamin A. That means that one does not have to use retinoic acid to get the effects of retinoic acid (17). Applying retinyl aldehyde or retinol, or retinyl esters such as retinyl palmitate or retinyl acetate to the skin will give similar results to retinoic acid but at physiological doses of retinoic acid. However, investigation has shown that when retinol or retinyl aldehyde is applied to the skin, then virtually all is converted to retinyl esters, and very little is converted to retinoic acid. If you scan the cosmetic advertisements, then you will get the impression that the only version of vitamin A that works is retinol. However, retinol is irritant to cell membranes and is normally found free only in tiny doses in the skin. It is the form used for transport of vitamin A from the liver, through the blood to the body. However, virtually all the retinol applied to skin will be converted to retinyl palmitate and build up the stores of vitamin A in the skin cells (18).

Retinaldehyde advertisements focus on the fact that it is only one step away from retinoic acid and imply that it is a simple step to the active version of vitamin A.

However, once again, enzymes convert virtually all the topically applied retinaldehyde into retinyl palmitate, and only a tiny fraction actually gets converted into retinoic acid.

The esters of vitamin A (e.g., retinyl palmitate or acetate) are milder, active, and more easily tolerated by the skin. Jarret (19) showed that retinyl acetate was similar but more active than retinoic acid (20), with fewer side effects.

We have to use the form of vitamin A that is easiest for our patients to use, and I believe that for initial stages, we should use retinyl palmitate because it is effective and will give all the effects of retinoic acid provided it is used in adequate concentration (21). For more intense treatments in patients who have adapted their skin to vitamin A, we can use retinyl acetate, retinaldehyde, or retinol. My experience indicates that although patients are reluctant to continue using retinoic acid daily, there is no problem with the continual use of retinyl acetate or retinyl palmitate. I have used retinol at higher doses, but not everyone can use it. Clinical experience has shown that retinol cannot easily be used at levels higher than 10,000 IU g%, whereas retinyl acetate and retinyl palmitate can be used as high as 50,000 IU g% both morning and evening for many years without any deleterious effects.

Which vitamin C? The ideal cosmeceutical care regime includes vitamin C (L-ascorbic acid), but it is unstable and rapidly decomposes. Ascorbic acid is commercially available as a dry powder (dehydroascorbic acid), which is relatively stable and white. When ascorbic acid powder is exposed to light and air, it slowly decomposes to oxidized ascorbic acid, which is brown. When ascorbic acid crystals are mixed in water, the solution fairly rapidly (over a period of weeks) decomposes to dehydroascorbic acid. Therefore, a solution of ascorbic acid, even in a gel, has a limited shelf life and should be used within 3 to 6 weeks. Ascorbic acid acts like an AHA, which interacts on the adhesion of the corneocytes and increases the penetration into the deeper layers of the skin. Ascorbic acid does not easily permeate the stratum corneum and passes with difficulty into the cell wall because it is a water-soluble molecule, and there are no receptors on the cell wall for ascorbic acid. However, magnesium (or sodium) L-ascorbyl phosphate is also water-soluble but is taken up into cells much more effectively. Inside the cells, the compound is readily converted to L-ascorbic acid, phosphate, and magnesium (sodium) (22). These solutions are also more stable than conventional ascorbic acid and can last up to 200 days before there is any appreciable loss of activity (23). Lower concentrations (compared with ascorbic acid) are required to get the same amount of ascorbic acid into the cell.

Ascorbic acid is too aggressive for people with sensitive skin, although they can use ascorbyl esters and, if the right dose is being used, will get more vitamin C into their cells. Patients with pigmentation problems should avoid any product that peels the skin because they need a thick horny layer to protect melanocytes. Ascorbic acid is an exfoliant, so I recommend that patients with melasma or other pigmentation problems should use ascorbyl esters. Better results may be achieved using an oil-soluble complex of ascorbic acid, ascorbyl tetraisopalmitate, which is extremely stable. This fat-soluble molecule passes more readily through the stratum corneum than L-ascorbic acid and achieves up to 10-fold more vitamin C in the cell. This leads to more effective control of melanin formation, greater collagen deposition, and more efficient antioxidant protection. Ascorbyl tetraisopalmitate combined with vitamin A gives rapid smoothening and lightening of the skin without any irritation. Of course, if it should also be combined with a wide antioxidant brigade and effective UVA protection.

Because vitamins A and E absorb UV light in the region that is responsible for most of its deleterious effects, both should be included when formulating a cosmeceutical. Topical vitamin A (in mouse skin) has been shown to prevent the UV-induced epidermal hypovitaminosis A, whereas topical vitamin E prevents oxidative stress and cutaneous and systemic immunosuppression elicited by UV. These natural epidermal vitamins A and E of the skin can be reinforced by topical application of natural retinoids and α-tocopherol (24). Botanical compounds, such as green tea (25), offer an expanding range of antioxidants that qualify as cosmeceuticals, and these are discussed elsewhere in this volume.

Surgeons are bombarded with claims about the magical effects of various products to rejuvenate skin. Because of the fundamental importance of vitamins A, C, and E and other antioxidants, if a skin care range does not include them, then it cannot claim to be true skin care. The burgeoning problem of stratospheric ozone depletion means that virtually everyone who ventures into sunlight will get more destruction of their cutaneous antioxidant system and, therefore, be at greater risk of photodamage. This may be the underlying reason for the dramatic increase in melanoma and other skin cancers. In ideal circumstances, everyone should apply vitamin A and other antioxidants daily and should wear sun protective clothing to maintain skin health.

There are cosmeceutical ingredients that are not involved in photodamage but can be used to rejuvenate cells or stimulate more collagen formation. Molecules that act on the mitochondria can correct senescent cells [e.g., idebenone, coenzyme Q10, dehydrolipoic acid (25)]. Coenzyme Q10 (ubiquinone) has the ability to prevent many of the detrimental effects of photoaging. The processes of aging and photoaging are associated with lower levels of antioxidants in mitochondria and an increase in cellular oxidation (26). Topical coenzyme Q10 was found to be effective against UVA and significantly suppressed collagenase in human dermal fibroblasts and reduced wrinkle depth (27). Coenzyme Q10, idebenone, and kinetin are not as effective in photoprotection compared with vitamins C and E (28).

Active Peptides

Recent research has shown that active peptides such as palmitoyl pentapeptide (Matrixyl)® and palmitoyl hexapeptide (Dermaxyl)® have a special value in stimulating the production of collagen and elastin. They are both made of a sequence of amino acids normally found in collagen and elastin. Palmitoyl pentapeptide stimulates about 16 genes in skin cells, which is only a fraction of the number of genes that vitamin A favorably stimulates in the skin. The peptides are not an alternative to vitamin A and should be used in conjunction with the vitamin. Copper peptides facilitate healing of tissues and may assist in remodelling of collagen. Probably the most appropriate indication for copper peptides is on skin injured by peeling, laser, or dermabrasion.

AHAs and BHAs

AHAs have been the most misused and misunderstood molecules in skin rejuvenation. They do have a role in smoothening skin, mainly as a peeling agent, but they should not be considered as true cosmeceuticals. AHAs are water-soluble and can only penetrate the outer stratum corneum unless higher concentrations are used to induce an acid peeling effect. They are effective in desquamating skin, increasing cell turnover, and stimulating keratinocyte growth.

AHAs modify the barrier function of the skin as their main function rather than influence the metabolism of the keratinocyte, and these changes are not the same for all AHAs but are more marked in those with antioxidant activity (29). An important concern about AHAs is that they may sensitize skin to UV damage. This, however, is transient and disappears on cessation of treatment (30).

Glycolic acid has been shown in vitro to stimulate the production of collagen (31). Epidermal and dermal remodeling of the extracellular matrix can result from high concentrations. Longer treatment intervals may result in collagen deposition as suggested by the measured increase in mRNA (32). These effects seem related to the concentration and low pH.

Lactic acid has great value in enhancing the natural moisturizing factors and is much kinder to skin than glycolic acid (33). Lactic acid does have effects on the metabolism of the cell, and even when supplied as lactates at a higher pH, they can still induce changes to skin by improving hydration. Lactic acid may also have an important role in stimulating the release of cytokines by keratinocytes (34). Lactic acid also inhibits tyrosinase and therefore reduces pigmentation. However, both glycolic and lactic acid are only modestly successful in reducing photoaging (35). They do impair the natural protection from the sun, and they should always be used in conjunction with vitamin A. Their role is more as an adjuvant than an actual therapeutic agent, except in the case of acne where they help to control infection and reduce obstruction of follicles.

Both AHA and BHA have effects on desmosomes and promote desquamation. BHAs may be more effective because they are lipid-soluble, penetrate the stratum corneum, and may penetrate into comedones. They also have the benefit of being more effective at lower doses.

Hormones

The advantages of using estrogen to thicken skin and recondition it in the menopausal phase are well-known. Vitamins cannot play the role of hormones and growth factors, so we have to use hormones when they are required, and hopefully future cosmetics will also include essential growth factors. At this stage, cosmeceuticals can only use phytoestrogens, but because these molecules do stimulate estrogen receptors, there is confusion about their use in patients with breast cancer.

CLINICAL USE OF COSMECEUTICALS

Many surgeons make the mistake of believing that youthful skin can be achieved using drastic measures such as laser resurfacing, heavy peels, or other techniques that destroy the epidermis. Medical practitioners, in particular dermatologists, cosmetic, and plastic surgeons, should have an understanding of cosmeceuticals so that they can guide their patients in the use of effective cosmeceuticals to treat photoaging. Cosmetic surgery alone cannot create a convincingly youthful impression. The skin does not simply have to be smooth; it should look fresh, glowing, and show few or no signs of accumulated photodamage. Using scientifically targeted cosmeceuticals, one can normalize skin, and cosmetic surgery can achieve a more harmonious appearance as well as much more effective rejuvenation. An effective cosmeceutical will first restore normal function to keratinocytes. This usually results in healthier-looking skin, and results can match those achieved by more complicated treatments (36). Unfortunately, even the most powerful cosmeceutical will not smooth skin as much as we wish it would, neither will melasma reliably disappear. For these reasons, we often have to resort to more major procedures to get the best results.

The first step is to use treatments augmented by enhanced penetration through the epidermis. We can enhance penetration by carefully formulating products so that more of the active ingredient gets down to the target areas, but this is not enough to obtain greater tightening of the skin and other positive changes. For greater penetration, one can use iontophoresis, low-frequency sonophoresis (LFS), or physical interference with the barrier properties of the stratum corneum (e.g., microneedling, microdermabrasion).

Iontophoresis

Galvanic current is useful if a selected molecule such as vitamin A or ascorbic acid can be ionized into positively and negatively charged ions. A charged electrical current repels similarly charged ions into the skin, the cells, and even right into their mitochondria. This can cause about 400% better penetration than simple topical applications. Treatments should be done for a minimum of 20 minutes once or twice a week for 24–30 treatments. This is a very successful method for treating photoaging but has to be done by an experienced therapist/nurse.

LFS

LFS uses sounds at about 20 kHz at an effective intensity to create cavitation of the lipid bilayers of the skin. Cavitation develops rapidly and is maintained for several hours after treatment. Adding treatments with LFS as described by Mitragotri (37) but adapted (Environ® Ionzyme® DF machine; Environ Skin Care, Cape Town, South Africa) for use in the skin care salon, up to 4000% better penetration may occur after only 3 minutes of treatment and quite dramatically rejuvenate skin (38). Of course, this will only happen if rational cosmeceuticals are used. LFS should not be confused with ultrasound (about 1.1 MHz), which does not have the same powerful properties. The advantage of LFS is that it can be used on nonpolar molecules. Treatments are best done once or twice a week for about 24–30 times, and the best results seem to occur in combination with iontophoresis.

Microneedling

Microneedling of skin offers a means to enhance penetration. Holes are made only through the stratum corneum, so this is not painful, and patients are requested to use it daily before applying their skin care. Significant improvement may be achieved in those patients who are diligent about using the tool everyday for about 3–5 minutes. The results are because of enhanced penetration of vitamins A and C and other active agents, not microtrauma.

There are a number of other ancillary procedures to rapidly smoothen and lighten skin. The following treatments aim to induce tightening of the skin and/or lightening of the skin. They all work by controlled damage to either individual cells or all the cells of the epidermis or the dermis. Their benefits arise from the induction of the natural healing process with the release of various growth factors. The safest use of these various treatments is when the trauma or energy is the lowest, and cosmeceuticals can augment the results. By combining these traumatic treatments with the chemical effects of vitamin A (normal maturation of cells), vitamin C, and antioxidants, one can expect

· healthier keratinocytes with faster healing of the epidermis;
· a thicker epidermis;
· better control of pigmentation and the prevention of postinflammatory hyper-pigmentation;
· more intense collagen deposition from direct stimulation of the responsible genes;
· healthier collagen with topical vitamin C;
· thicker dermis with better support for blood vessels;
· healthier blood supply to facilitate healing and growth;
· greater elastin and collagen formation with added peptides, such as palmitoyl pentapeptide and palmitoyl hexapeptide.

SUMMARY

Cosmeceuticals have changed the world of skin care. It no longer makes sense to use simple plant extracts in skin care creams. The use of molecules derived from plants requires that they be highly refined and available in standard concentrations with scientifically proven effects. Cosmeceutical skin care is essential to minimize the ravages of the environment and may be used to complement facial cosmetic surgery and other operations that intend to rejuvenate skin anywhere on the body. By understanding the basics of the science of skin care cosmeceuticals, one can design cosmeceutical products that the end user can rely on to make smooth, fresh glowing skin that shows few signs of accumulated photodamage. Many doctors make the mistake of believing that they can achieve youthful skin by using AHAs, heavy peels, or other drastic techniques that destroy the epidermis measures such as laser resurfacing. The epidermis is far too important and complex to be destroyed or tortured into becoming smooth. For the first time in history, the general public has the chance to rehabilitate damaged skin at the same time as preventing photoaging. Healthy keratinocytes are ultimately responsible for a beautiful, resilient skin. The first aim of cosmeceuticals must be to rehabilitate photoaged, inefficient keratinocytes and create a normal healthy epidermis that then sets up the possibility of improving the dermis.

Vitamin A, especially in its ester form, gives all the benefits of retinoic acid without the irritation. Its role is both preventative against photoaging as well as regenerative. Antioxidants work hand in hand with vitamin A and also complement sun protection but act only in preventing photoaging to a degree. Vitamin A may be considered as the agent that sets up a healthy skin and also organizes the "collagen factories," but without vitamin C, healthy woven collagen will not be laid down. Because collagen deposition lies at the very heart of rejuvenating skin, vitamins A and C should always be used together. Iontophoresis and LFS enhance penetration of vitamins and active peptides and can help surgeons achieve realistic rejuvenation.

Numerous machines have been developed to try and build up the dermal collagen and elastin, but it has been repeatedly observed that rationally designed cosmeceuticals can achieve results similar to those seen from treatments using these machines. Cosmeceutical skin care is relatively inexpensive and will become more effective in controlling the environmentally induced skin damage.

REFERENCES

1. Toyoda M, Bhawan J. Ultrastructural evidence for the participation of Langerhans cells in cutaneous photoaging processes: a quantitative comparative study. J Dermatol Sci 1997; 14:87–100.
2. Craven N, Watson R, Jones C, et al. Clinical features of photodamaged human skin are associated with a reduction of collagen VII. Br J Dermatol 1997; 137:344–350.
3. Fisher GJ, Wang ZQ, Datta SC, et al. Pathophysiology of premature skin aging induced by ultraviolet light. N Engl J Med 1997; 337:1419–1428.
4. Wise F, Sulzberger MB. Yearbook of Dermatology 1938:282.
5. Berne B, Nilsson M, Vahlquist A. UV irradiation and cutaneous vitamin a: an experimental study in rabbit and human skin. J Invest Dermatol 1984; 83:401–404.
6. Cluver EH, Politzer WM. Sunburn and vitamin A deficiency. S A J Sci 1965; 61:306 309.
7. Lithgow DM, Politzer WM. Vitamin A in the treatment of menorrhagia. S Afr Med J 1977; 51(7):191–193.
8. Tang G, Webb A, Russel RM, et al. Epidermis and serum protect retinol but not retinyl esters from sunlight-induced photodegradation. Photodermatol Photoimmunol Photomed 1994; 10:1–7.
9. Antille C, Tran C, Sorg O, et al. Vitamin A exerts a photoprotective action in skin by absorbing ultraviolet B radiation. J Invest Dermatol 2003; 121(5):1163–1167.
10. Berne A, Vahlquist A, Fischer T, et al. UV treatment of uremic pruritis reduces the vitamin A content of the skin. Eur J Clin Invest 1984; 14:203–206.
11. Thiele JJ, Schroeter C, Hsieh SN, et al. The antioxidant network of the stratum corneum. Cur Probl Dermatol 2001; 29:26–42.
12. Verschooten L, Claerhout S, Laethem AV, et al. New strategies of photoprotection. Photochem Photobiol 2006 Jul-Aug; 82(4):1016–23.
13. Kligman LH. Photoaging. Manifestations, prevention, and treatment. Dermatol Clin. 1986; 4(3):517–528.
14. Weiss JS, Ellis CN, Headington JT, et al. Topical tretinoin improves photoaged skin. A double-blind vehicle-controlled study. JAMA. 1988; 259(4):527 532. Erratum in: JAMA 1988; 260(7):926. JAMA 1988; 259(22):3274.
15. Varani J, Warner RL, Gharaee-Kermani M, et al. Vitamin A antagonizes decreased cell growth and elevated collagen-degrading matrix metalloproteinases and stimulates collagen accumulation in naturally aged human skin. J Invest Dermatol 2000; 114(3): 480–486.
16. Tran C, Sorg O, Carraux P, et al. Topical delivery of retinoids counteracts the UVB-induced epidermal vitamin A depletion in hairless mouse. Photochem Photobiol 2001; 73:425–431.
17. Jarrett A, Spearman RI. Vitamin A and the skin. Br J Dermatol 1970; 82:197–199.
18. Antille C, Tran C, Sorg O, et al. Penetration and metabolism of topical retinoids in ex vivo organ-cultured full-thickness human skin explants. Skin Pharmacol Physiol 2004; 17:124–128.
19. Jarrett A, Spearman RIC. Histochemistry of the Skin-Psoriasis. London U.K.: English Universities Press, 1964.
20. Jarrett A, Wrench R, Mahmoud B. The effects of retinyl acetate on epidermal proliferation and differentiation. I. Induced enzyme reactions in the epidermis. Clin Exp Dermatol 1978; 3:173–188.
21. Spearman RI, Jarrett A. Biological comparison of isomers and chemical forms of vitamin A (retinol). Br J Dermatol 1974; 90:553–560.
22. Elmore AR. Final report of the safety assessment of L-ascorbic acid, calcium ascorbate, magnesium ascorbate, magnesium ascorbyl phosphate, sodium ascorbate, and sodium ascorbyl phosphate as used in cosmetics. Int J Toxicol 2005; 24(Suppl. 2):51–111.
23. Kobayashi S, Takehana M, Itoh S, et al. Protective effect of magnesium-L-ascorbyl-2 phosphate against skin damage induced by UVB irradiation. Photochem Photobiol 1996; 64:224–228.
24. Sorg O, Tran C, Saurat J-H. Cutaneous vitamins A and E in the context of ultraviolet- or chemically-induced oxidative stress. Skin Pharmacol Appl Skin Physiol 2001; 14: 363–372.

25. Beitner H. Randomized, placebo-controlled, double blind study on the clinical efficacy of a cream containing 5% alpha-lipoic acid related to photoageing of facial skin. Br J Dermatol 2003; 149:841–849.

26. Blatt T, Lenz H, Koop U, et al. Stimulation of skin's energy metabolism provides multiple benefits for mature human skin. Biofactors 2005; 25:179–185.

27. Hoppe U, Bergemann J, Diembeck W, et al. Coenzyme Q10, a cutaneous antioxidant and energizer. Biofactors 1999; 9:37–378.

28. Tournas JA, Lin FH, Burch JA, et al. Ubiquinone, idebenone, and kinetin provide ineffective photoprotection to skin when compared to a topical antioxidant combination of vitamins C and E with ferulic acid. J Invest Dermatol 2006; 126:1185–1187.

29. Berardesca E, Distante F, Vignoli GP, et al. Alpha hydroxyacids modulate stratum corneum barrier function. Br J Dermatol 1997; 137:934–938.

30. Kaidbey K, Sutherland B, Bennett P, et al. Topical glycolic acid enhances photodamage by ultraviolet light. Photodermatol Photoimmunol Photomed 2003; 19:21–27.

31. Moy LS, Howe K, Moy RL. Glycolic acid modulation of collagen production in human skin fibroblast cultures in vitro. Dermatol Surg 1996; 22:439–441.

32. Bernstein EF, Lee J, Brown DB, et al. Glycolic acid treatment increases type I collagen mRNA and hyaluronic acid content of human skin. Dermatol Surg 2001; 27:429–433.

33. Smith WP. Epidermal and dermal effects of topical lactic acid. J Am Acad Dermatol 1996; 35(3 Pt. 1):388–391.

34. Rendl M, Mayer C, Weninger W, et al. Topically applied lactic acid increases spontaneous secretion of vascular endothelial growth factor by human reconstructed epidermis. Br J Dermatol 2001; 145:3–9.

35. Stiller MJ, Bartolone J, Stern R, et al. Topical 8% glycolic acid and 8% L-lactic acid creams for the treatment of photodamaged skin. A double-blind vehicle-controlled clinical trial. Arch Dermatol 1996; 132:631–636.

36. Fernandes D. Pre- and post-operative skin care. In: Panfilov G, ed. Aesthetic Surgery of the Facial Mosaic. Heidelberg: Springer, 2006; 492–502.

37. Mitragotri S, Edwards DA, Blankschtein D, et al. A mechanistic study of ultrasonically-enhanced transdermal drug delivery. J Pharm Sci 1995; 84:697–706.

38. Fernandes D. Understanding and treating photoaging. In: Peled I, Manders E, eds. Esthetic Surgery of the Face. London: Taylor & Francis, 2004; 227–240.

5 Biology of Skin Pigmentation and Cosmetic Skin Color Control

Chong Jin Loy and Raman Govindarajan

Johnson & Johnson Asia Pacific, Singapore Research Center, Singapore

INTRODUCTION

The color of skin is an important attribute that has often changed the course of history and, unfortunately, still "colors" the way we interact in human society. This review covers various aspects of cutaneous melanin pigmentation in man. It also highlights lacunae in current knowledge and brings into focus questions that are not answered by current opinion and known facts. Current controversies are also commented upon. This is a concise review of a vast body of literature, and readers are referred to more exhaustive treatises given at the end of the chapter.

HUMAN SKIN COLOR

Pigmentation is a widely occurring phenomenon in nature and plays important roles in the appearance and biology of all living organisms. For example, being endowed with certain color pigments affords environmental advantages to the organism, such as camouflage, visual communication, prey avoidance, reproductive success, or thermal regulation. In humans, skin pigmentation is the most dramatic visual difference in skin characteristics among different populations and has also evolved as a metaphor for race (1). Human skin color can range from almost black among some Africans to pinkish white among some Northern Europeans. This continuum in skin color is a blend resulting from the various skin chromophores: oxyhemoglobin in the superficial dermal capillaries (red), deoxygenated hemoglobin in the dermal venules (blue), dietary carotenoids (yellow-orange), bilirubin by-product of old red blood cells (yellow), and most importantly, melanin (black/brown). In addition, the surface microtexture and sebum in the skin affect the reflective properties of skin and thus impact the total overall perceived skin color.

The various shades of brown in dark and tanned skin are attributable to the amount of melanin in the epidermis. The synthesis of melanin and its fate in the epidermis is a complex biological process involving keratinocytes and melanocytes, immune system cells and soluble substances derived from cells in the epidermis and dermis (e.g., dermal fibroblasts) and from cells elsewhere in the body (e.g., pituitary and adrenal glands), and the amount of solar radiation exposure. In the absence of environmental influences, genetics determine the heritable skin color trait and is termed constitutive pigmentation. In contrast, facultative pigmentation refers to the additional skin color that is achieved as a result of increasing melanin production beyond constitutive pigmentation levels in response to exposure to solar radiation. Additional stimuli that lead to increases in melanin formation include hormones and growth factors as well as inflammation due to physical and chemical irritants, immune responses (contact dermatitis), and light interacting with chemicals in the skin (photodermatitis). Although, in many instances, the increase in response to external influences recedes upon removal of the stimulus, it is well known that certain examples of facultative pigmentation are either irreversible or are only partially reversible even upon removal of the external stimulus. Conversely, external influences may damage the melanin system to lead to hypopigmentation that is circumscribed or patchy and irregular.

HISTOLOGY AND GENERAL PHYSIOLOGY OF THE EPIDERMIS AND MELANIN PIGMENTARY SYSTEM

The epidermis (Fig. 1) comprises several layers of somatic ectoderm-derived keratinocytes at different stages of differentiation. Keratinocytes in the basal layer are composed of three populations of cells: the stem cells, transit amplifying cells, and cells committed to terminal differentiation. The latter move upward from the basal layer to form layers of progressively more differentiated cells, culminating in terminally differentiated keratinocytes located in the stratum corneum. Together, the keratinocytes constitute at least 80% of the epidermis. Intercalated among the keratinocytes are the mechanoreceptor Merkel cells, antigen-presenting Langerhans cells, and the melanin-producing melanocytes located on the basal lamina of the basal epithelial layer. Interestingly, melanocytes are derived from neural crest cells rather than the basal cells of epidermis (2). Melanoblasts from the neural crest migrate into the epidermis, uveal tract of the eye, leptomeninges, mucous membranes, hair bulb, mesentery, and inner ear and mature into melanocytes. In the extra-epidermal locations, except in the hair bulb, melanosomes are not transferred out, and for this reason, extra-epidermal melanocytes have been termed continent. The retinal pigment epithelial melanocytes are not derived from the neural crest but from the optic cup. In the epidermis, melanocytes residing in the dermoepidermal junction put out dendrites to transfer melanosomes to neighboring basal and suprabasal keratinocytes. Dendrites are never put out into the dermis. There are no other connections such as desmosomes or hemidesmosomes between keratinocytes and melanocytes. Each melanocyte services 16–32 keratinocytes (the epidermal melanin unit, EMU) but has contacts with only a few at any point. Interestingly, the number of melanocytes is similar for the same body region from light- and dark-skinned

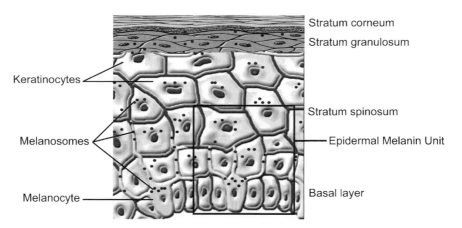

FIGURE 1   Structure of epidermis.

individuals (3). However, differences in melanocyte numbers are seen between body locations, with the genital area having the highest number and the abdomen having the lowest number per unit area of skin. UV-exposed skin has more melanocytes than unexposed skin, and it has been suggested that this difference may be contributed by dormant melanocytes that are subsequently recruited by UV or hormonal influences, leading to an apparent increase in the number of melanocytes. Some workers have also shown melanocyte proliferation in response to UV. Such increases could be because of direct effects of UV or secreted factors from UV-irradiated keratinocytes. Although pigment synthesis occurs within the melanocyte, most pigment within the skin is found in melanosomes within keratinocytes. As the keratinocytes mature and differentiate, they form an outermost dead layer of cells called the stratum corneum, where individual cells (squame) slough off, thus requiring continuous synthesis and intercellular transfer of melanosomes for maintaining pigmentation. The melanocyte remains at the basal layer normally and is a nonmotile cell. Under abnormal circumstances, localized proliferation (as in moles) or downward migration (with basal membrane incontinence) may occur, resulting in localized hyperpigmentation. Migration of melanocytes to areas where resident melanocytes have died has been documented. Age-dependent decrease in melanocyte number is known, and imbalances in number, dendricity, and EMU relationships are most likely the cause of age-related changes in pigmentation.

Definition of Melanin

A lack of precise chemical characterization of animal melanin has led to the description of almost any dark natural pigment, including those derived from plants and microbes (also known as allomelanins), as melanin. A principal point of difference between the two is that allomelanins are derived from the action of cell wall–bound phenolase, as opposed to a secreted or intracellular enzyme in animal melanins, on a locally available phenol. Allomelanins are poorly characterized and, indeed, could be a very heterogeneous group of molecules. Further, allomelanins are derived from single-electron oxidations, whereas melanins are derived from two-electron oxidations. Another important chemical distinction between plant and animal melanins is that animal melanins are derivatives of 5,6-dihydroxyindolequinones, whereas plant (allo) melanins are derivatives of catechol. Although it is possible to distinguish allomelanins from animal melanins, the definition of the latter remains vague: solvent-resistant brown/black (eumelanin) and red/yellow (pheomelanin) pigments that are derived from tyrosine that can be bleached by oxidants, can reduce ammoniacal solutions of silver, of indeterminate molecular weight, and generally bound to proteins. It was earlier believed that melanin was a linear polymer of indolequinone units. It is now generally accepted that there is branching, but no clear rules have been defined as to where the branching occurs.

Evolution of Epidermal Melanin in Animals

Most animals do not have a pigmented epidermis. They have colored hair fur that protects them from UV. In the early man, dehairing left him vulnerable to UV. We may inquire if the early man needed protection if he lived under a canopy and assuming that the life span was 35 years at best and if such conditions were enough for carcinomas to form and thus for natural selection to prefer more pigmented individuals. It raises the question whether pigmentation of the epidermis evolved to protect from UV or was primarily a sexual aid (as in fur color in animals), which later did serve to protect from UV. Four stages of melanin evolution have been described.

Stage I

Tyrosinase-derived orthoquinone (dopaquinone) and subsequent intermediates cyclodopa, dihydroxyindole (DHI), indolequinone are all reactive and probably cytotoxic. These were generated extracellularly as the enzyme was secreted out of the cell. Several functions have been ascribed to these intermediates, namely, participation in stress responses, as a primitive immune system, as defensive sprays, camouflaging ink in cephalopods, and cuticular hardening in insects.

Stage II

Once nature found these intermediates useful, she probably sought to make use of them within the cell. Modifications of tyrosinase transport, containment of intermediates within an organelle, and possibly new enzymes for the generation of DHI carboxylic acid (DHICA) evolved.

Stage III

This probably involved using the intermediates for a period and then nullifying their reactivity by polymerizing them and/or bringing in detoxifying steps such as conjugation with cysteine/glutathione and a concurrent curtailing of these processes to a limited number of cells that were inherently incapable of rapid division.

Stage IV

The development of transfer mechanisms that allowed removal from the body of the complex protein-bound polymer that the cells had no machinery to catabolize. This last stage has evolved only in the skin and hair because these are the only situations where perhaps major increases in the quantity of melanin produced has occurred over evolutionary time scales—possibly in response to exposure to cosmic UV rays. Keratinocytes are perhaps still learning to deal with these "foreign" organelles. It is important to note that this sequence of events is speculative, and the principal supporting facts are the presence of extracellular intermediates before genesis of melanosomes and transfer of melanosomes being seen selectively and much later (4).

Functions of Melanin

Table 1 shows the many functions that have been ascribed to melanin. Although these properties can be proven in the laboratory, some properties are probably not relevant, or it is not obvious how these properties can lead to functional effects in vivo. For example, because melanin is enclosed in melanosomes and not freely soluble in the cell, free-radical scavenging can occur only within the melanosome (i.e., free radicals generated upon exposure of the melanosome membrane to UV). It has, however, been observed that melanosomes move to the periphery of a cell when the cell is exposed to UV (5). This could be a mechanism to protect the cell against free radicals generated upon UV exposure of the cell membrane. If so, can melanin within melanosomes scavenge free radicals generated outside melanosomes? Many of the effects of melanin that are purported to be due to free radical scavenging effects have still to be proven, although there are circumstantial and epidemiological data supporting a good UV-protective role for melanin in skin. In addition, melanin composition (ratios or monomers units) and structure and therefore function may

TABLE 1 Properties of Melanin

Absorption of UV (phototoxic and photosensitizer)	Protects against oxidative stress
Photoprotection	Structural polymer
Scattering and density filter	Shields DNA against UV damage
Thermoregulation	Protects against photoaging
Free-radical quenching	Cation trap (binds to toxic drugs)
Protects against lipid peroxidation	Regulates vitamin D synthesis
prostaglandins D2 and E2	Camouflage and sexual appeal
Protects against photocarcinogenesis	

vary in different organs (e.g., retinal pigmented epithelium vs. skin), depending on the free radical quenching requirement in a given tissue (6,7).

Melanin Pigmentary System

For the purpose of understanding skin pigmentation, four stages of the melanin pigmentary system can be clearly defined. These stages possibly happen as one smooth process in vivo. Although it is convenient to study them separately, they are clearly linked, and research will reveal feedback control loops that operate across these stages (Fig. 2):

1. Biogenesis of melanosomes in melanocytes
2. Biosynthesis of melanin precursors and polymerization of melanin in melanocytes
3. Transfer of melanosomes to keratinocytes
4. Movement and degradation in keratinocytes

Melanosome Biogenesis

Melanin synthesis occurs within highly specialized membrane-bound organelles called melanosomes that are produced exclusively by melanocytes located at the base of the epidermis. Two major types of melanosomes are made and named

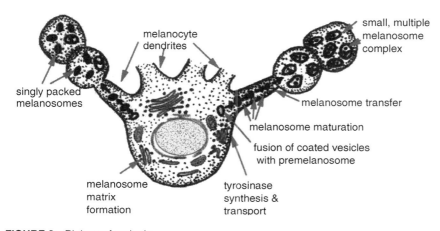

FIGURE 2 Biology of melanin.

according to the type of melanin they contain. The eumelanosome is large (200–900 nm in diameter) and ellipsoidal, with a highly ordered glycoprotein matrix that is integral to the production of the black or brown eumelanin pigments. The red or yellow pheomelanins are produced within smaller and spherical (700 nm in diameter) pheomelanosomes that are composed of a loosely aggregated and disordered glycoprotein matrix. The regulation of melanin synthesis and subsequent incorporation into and biogenesis of melanosomes have been studied extensively by microscopy, biochemistry, and immunohistochemical methods. Melanosome biogenesis has been classified into four stages (I–IV) based on morphology and degree of melanization. Melanosomes, which are thought to be of lysosomal lineage (8), are assembled in the smooth endoplasmic reticulum (ER) as colorless organelles, called premelanosomes. The tyrosinase complex, which comprises tyrosinase, tyrosinase-related proteins 1 and 2 (TRP-1 and TRP-2), OA1, pMel17, and Mart 1, and possibly other regulatory components, is synthesized in the rough ER, glycosylated in the Golgi apparatus, and targeted to the melanosome by a specific hexapeptide sequence Asn-Gln-Pro-Leu-Leu-Thr (9). This tyrosinase complex is then enveloped in coated vesicles (CVs) and transported toward premelanosomes/stage I/II melanosomes for fusion. CVs have an active tyrosinase, bear an acidic pH, and contain melanin monomers but no melanin polymer. It is not clear how the hexapeptide sequence of proteins in the CV is deciphered by the outer surface of the CV for actual fusion with the pre/early melanosome. It is possible that the hexapeptide sequence may be a signal for incorporation into CVs and all CVs are destined to fuse with premelanosomes.

Upon fusion of CVs with stage I/II melanosomes, melanin polymerization begins and progresses. The amount of melanin determines the stages of melanosome maturation. Stage I melanosomes in eumelanogenesis are spherical and contain amorphous proteinaceous material and a few vesicoglobular bodies/CVs. In stage II, they become ellipsoidal with organized lamellae and CVs. Although tyrosinase activity has been demonstrated in CVs, stage I/II melanosomes do not exhibit activity of the enzyme. This paradox is possibly because of the lack of adequate sensitivity of the methods used or inhibition/modulation of tyrosinase activity in the melanosomal milieu. It is not clear what causes the change in shape between stages I and II. It may be because of the organization of the lamellae, with some melanization occurring to cement the lamellar structure. Obvious melanization begins at stage III, and at stage IV, melanosomes are highly melanized and electron dense. Tyrosinase activity has not been detected in stage IV. No melanization occurs in the CVs, and these remain electron lucent. Pheomelanosomes are always spherical and do not exhibit lamellae. Numerous CVs are seen making it microgranular, and melanization occurs both inside and outside these CVs. Availability of thiol moieties may determine the nature of the melanosomes made (i.e., higher thiols may lead to more pheomelanosome formation (10). In response to UV radiation, the melanosomes move from their perinuclear position toward the periphery of the melanocytes and the dendrite tips and are then translocated into adjoining keratinocytes, where they will reside until they are shed with the stratum corneum as the keratinocytes mature. Despite the identification and characterization of several key enzymatic and structural melanosomal proteins, attempts to purify and identify other proteins in melanin-laden melanosomes have been extremely difficult and challenging, mainly because melanin impairs the solubilization of proteins associated with melanin polymers. To overcome this problem, various studies used early-stage melanosomes to maximize the opportunity to detect novel proteins. Several recent studies (11–13) investigated the distribution of melanosomal proteins in melanosomes from different stages (I–IV). However, more than 80% of the other proteins identified are components of lysosomes and other subcellular organelles, raising the possibility that many of these candidates may not be representative of bona fide melanosomal proteins. Alternatively, perhaps melanosomes and lysosomes indeed share many common features, as is widely accepted, such that differences in protein makeup is determined by only a small subset of organelle-specific components. Because melanosomes are derived from the ER, it may not be surprising that ER proteins continue to be found in melanosomes, and a so-called pure melanosomal preparation may never be found. OA1 is a Gprotein-coupled receptor (GPCR)-linked protein and is perhaps the only known intracellular membrane GPCR-linked protein, perhaps modulating organelle to cytosol communication (14). Thus, one could postulate that perhaps the melanosome is a primordial bacterium that was evolutionarily incorporated into melanocytes, similar to what has been proposed for the presence of mitochondria in cells. It would also be interesting to know if melanosomes have functional DNA. Further, one can ask if this bacterium indeed infects keratinocytes to protect the melanocyte from UV—an example of cellular symbiosis.

Biosynthesis of Melanin Precursors

Melanocytes produce two chemically distinct types of melanin pigments: dark-colored brown-black, insoluble eumelanin derived from the oxidative polymerization of dihydroxyindolequinones that can be found in almost every type of human skin and the light-colored red-yellow, alkali-soluble, sulfur-containing pheomelanin derived from cysteinyldopa which is abundant mostly in fair-skinned persons with red hair (15). The chemistry and enzymology of the biosynthetic pathway involved in the synthesis of the monomers that make up eumelanin and pheomelanin are now well understood and thought to be synthesized in vitro from tyrosine through the Raper-Mason enzymatic pathway (16–18) (Fig. 3). The conversion of tyrosine to melanin is a complex series of reactions. Tyrosinase, a key enzyme has at least two functions. It converts tyrosine (that has been selectively transported into the

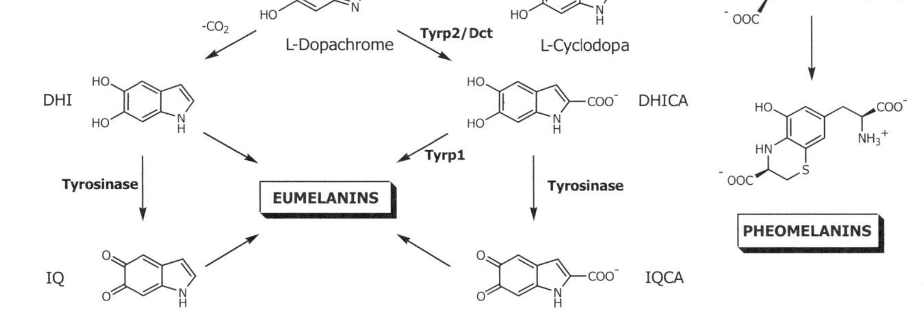

FIGURE 3 Raper-Mason enzymatic synthesis of melanin.

melanosome by a specific melanosome membrane protein (19) to dopa and then to dopaquinone. Two soluble forms, an insoluble form (bound to ER and Golgi apparatus), and a melanosome-bound form of tyrosinase are described as T1, T2, T3, and T4, respectively. Of these, 90% is the T3 form. These forms differ slightly in molecular weight possibly because of differences in glycosylation. Presumably, these are successive forms of each molecule of tyrosinase. Interestingly, tyrosinase has been used as a model to study protein processing and fate (20).

Tyrosinase, with two copper atoms and oxygen at its active site, binds a monohydric phenol (e.g., tyrosine) at its active site, which, by successive rearrangements, is converted to an orthoquinone (dopaquinone) and a deoxy enzyme. Orthoquinones are known for their ability to react with nucleophiles such as thiol or amino groups. The presence of an amino group in dopaquinone permits cyclization to yield cyclodopa, a transient product, due to rapid redox exchange yielding dopachrome (DC). DC can undergo spontaneous decarboxylation to yield DHI, which could then lead to generation of indolequinones. DHICA that is generated from DC by a tautomerase (TRP-2) or by metal ions is less easily oxidizable than DHI and probably requires the enzyme TRP-1 to be converted to an indolequinone. Uncolored indolequinones from DHI and DHICA then react with each other to generate the colored polymer. Eumelanins are derived from DHI and DHICA, whereas pheomelanins and trichromes are derived from cysteinyldopa/glutathionyldopa–derived benzothiazine units (Fig. 3). Melanogenic inhibitors have been reported but not well characterized. It is likely that these molecules have "fine-tuning" effects on the constitutive and facultative pathways. Some investigators speculate that all intermediates being reactive could participate in the formation of the melanin polymer. It is for this very reason that we still do not have a structure for melanin—each time a polymer is made, it is different from the one made before!

Regulation of tyrosine substrate availability in the melanosomes has also been postulated as a possible mechanism to influence the rate of melanin synthesis. Indeed, the cloning of a specific tyrosine transporter and its localization to the melanosome membrane is supportive of this notion (19,21). A cysteine transporter has also been identified in melanocytes and is thought to influence the switch to pheomelanin synthesis (22). Peroxidase and γ-glutamyl transpeptidase have all been implicated in the control of the type of melanin synthesized and in polymerization of oligomers (23). Some investigators believe that the activity of tyrosinase determines whether eumelanin will be formed or pheomelanin will be formed. A high tyrosinase activity results in eumelanin and a low tyrosinase activity results in pheomelanin.

Control of Melanin Polymerization

Although the preliminary steps in melanin synthesis are well characterized, the structure, composition, and polymerization/aggregation of the melanin monomers that lead to color remain poorly understood. This is partly because of its amorphous physical nature—mature melanin is composed of a combination of DHI, DHICA, and, possibly, other monomers as well, with great variability in the amount of these two precursors resulting in a featureless absorption spectrum (24). At the melanosomal pH of 5 or less, the synthesis of a colored monomer does not take place in vitro under controlled conditions (see below). A black pigment is easily formed even without tyrosinase at pH 7 and above. It was clear that a mechanism had to be defined for the conversation of uncolored monomers to a colored polymer at pH 5. There is one report in literature that ascribes a DHICA polymerase function to the product of the gene *pmel17* (25). We also knew from literature that CVs (see "Melanosome Biogenesis") were acidic and had an active tyrosinase and melanin monomers but no polymer. We hypothesized that melanosomal proteins played a key role in polymerization by providing local alkaline microenvironments in an overall acidic milieu. We showed that melanosomal proteins nonspecifically promoted polymerization in an acidic milieu possibly by proton abstraction by side groups of amino acids (dimerization of monomers: the initiation of polymerization requiring abstraction of protons) (26). The pH of the melanosome is known to fall further with progressive polymerization, and this, we believe, is an additional feedback loop that controls both tyrosinase activity and polymerization. The role of free radicals in polymerization cannot be excluded acting independently/concurrently or as part of the above-proposed mechanism.

We have further shown that proteins, depending on the nature of melanin formed and its interaction with protein, keep melanin in a soluble or insoluble form. We have thus hypothesized that initiation of polymerization and binding to proteins are independent but spatially and temporally related steps in polymerization. Also, the charges on proteins could aid in increasing the concentration of monomers locally, thus aiding polymerization. Additionally, we have shown that the two forms of melanin, soluble and insoluble, can be interconverted and do exist in cultured cells and that soluble melanin is more reactive than the insoluble form (12). Finally, we have speculated on why the pH of the melanosome is acidic. Based on molecular weight determinations of melanoproteins by gel permeation chromatography, we have shown that at an acidic pH, more melanins are protein bound and that protein-bound melanin is also less reactive (27). We speculate that nature maintains the pH of the melanosome below 5, at considerable energy cost, because at this pH, tyrosinase is less active, and melanin polymerization occurs intimately bound to proteins and not in the cytoplasm. Thus, reactivity of melanin is contained by this interaction. Containment of reactive species is easier when they are bound to protein because of diffusional constraints imposed by the high molecular weight of the melanoprotein complex. Further, because we have found protein-bound soluble melanin to be more reactive, we speculate that from uncolored monomers, soluble melanin is first formed, which, after subserving its function, is converted to an insoluble form and deposited on the melanosomal matrix. It is still unclear what functions reactive intermediates subserve. Clearly, if proteins play a role in polymerization, they probably determine the length, nature of branching, and size of the polymer, which, in turn, is expected to influence the UV-absorptive, free radical-quenching, and light-scattering properties of melanin and consequently constitutive and facultative pigmentation. We must question the general view that melanin, once made, is an unchangeable polymer. Perhaps during polymerization, there is a window when monomers are exchangeable (just as the two forms of melanin we have described are interconvertible). We also assume that no proteins other than those that came with the melanosome when it was transferred to keratinocytes play a role. Perhaps as evolution progressed, keratinocytes developed a mechanism to incorporate proteins into melanosomes that could affect the nature of melanin. Such intrakeratinocyte incorporation of proteins into melanosomes has not been described.

As alluded to earlier, most investigations study tyrosinase-mediated reactions at pH 6.8 (at which the enzyme is most active) instead of the melanosomal pH of 5 or below. At pH 6.8, there is a considerable lag phase before reaction products can be detected. This lag phase is seen only if tyrosine is used as substrate and not if dopa is used. In fact, the lag phase can be abolished by the addition of dopa, which thus raises the question of "where does the first molecule of dopa come from?" Devi et al. (28) have argued that a lag phase can actually be indefinite, and thus tyrosinase would have no activity. They have argued that this lag phase is an artifact of pH 6.8, but at melanosomal pH 5, the lag phase would not be evident. Recent data suggest that tyrosinase converts tyrosine directly to DQ, and dopa is generated from this DQ directly (by action of tyrosinase) or from the redox reaction of cyclodopa to DC. Although generation of dopa by this mechanism may help to overcome the lag phase, we propose that all investigations should be carried at the relevant pH (i.e., 5 or below).

The Molecular Weight of Melanin and the Nature of the Melanin Protein Interaction

Various methods have been used to determine the molecular weight of melanin. DHICA melanins synthesized in vitro have a molecular weight of 20,000 to 200,000 by gel permeation chromatography. These columns are calibrated using globular proteins, and the possibility of interaction of melanin with the column material leading to erroneous data is high. In vivo melanin is almost always protein bound, and the extent of binding to protein will affect molecular weight determination. Methods to remove protein have been harsh, which can affect the melanin itself, and data derived after such harsh treatments should be viewed with caution. Theoretically (in vivo and in vitro), poorly reactive, generally homogeneous monomer units can be made to form large polymers. The monomer units in melanin are highly reactive, and it is argued that such monomers units will not form large polymers (a fact borne out by advanced mass spectrometry data). However, melanins synthesized in vitro may be very different from melanin in vivo because the systems used for in vitro synthesis are quite simplistic. Various types of bonds have been claimed to exist between melanin and proteins. Charge interactions certainly occur because melanin is very negatively charged and, at melanosomal pH, many proteins will be positively charged. Weak molecular interactions will occur. Covalent bonds have been claimed to exist, which can arise out of interaction with thiol groups in proteins, free radical interactions, and, possibly, effects of UV. Metal ions also play an important role in the structural organization of the melanoprotein complex (29). The role of proteins in initiating, extending, binding, and giving stability to melanin cannot, in our view, be overemphasized—an area that has not been studied till now.

Types of Melanins

Two types of melanins are generally recognized: eumelanin and pheomelanin. Differences in the chemistry and the organelles that contain them, including the controversies and unanswered questions, have been detailed earlier. Pheomelanin is more soluble than eumelanin. The solubility of eumelanin depends on the ratio of DHICA oligomers to DHI oligomers, with the former being more soluble. Undoubtedly, the proteins intimately involved and the nature of interaction are determinants of solubility as well. Electron spin resonance and derivative high-performance liquid chromatography are the two methods commonly used to determine type of melanin. Some workers have used sulfur content as a measure of pheomelanin, but this is fraught with problems because the amount of cysteine in the proteins associated with melanin will affect the sulfur content of both melanins.

It has been shown that eumelanin and pheomelanin can be made by the same melanocyte (in the skin and hair). If this is the case, the question is, can they be incorporated into the same melanin polymer? Current opinion is that mixed melanins are both eumelanin and pheomelanin in the same cell. It is not clear if they are in the same melanosome. This, therefore, brings up another possibility—does the shape of melanosomes (elliptical or spheroidal) determine/contribute to the nature of polymer made because elliptical melanosomes are thought to contain eumelanin and spheroidal melanosomes are thought to contain pheomelanin? In chemical terms, it is not clear if pheomelanin is a polymer of purely cysteinyldopa/glutathionyldopa units or whether it only has a higher proportion of these units compared with very low or even absent cysteinyldopa/glutathionyldopa units in a putative pure eumelanin. Conversely, it is not clear if DHI/DHICA exist in a pure pheomelanin.

Although it has been accepted that melanin is synthesized only within melanocytes, recent data (30) suggest that colorless melanin monomers also accumulate outside the melanosomes in the basal layer of the epidermis, and UVA exposure converts the monomers into dark polymeric melanin. This could reflect the mechanism of immediate pigment darkening (IPD) response in skin to UV exposure, in which pigmentation is achieved quickly albeit only transiently (see below). In vitro, DHICA and 6-hydroxy-5-methoxyindole-2-carboxylic acid accumulated in keratinocytes and supernatants cocultured with melanocytes and produced brown melanin upon UVA exposure. This raises the question of the origin of these melanin precursor molecules. It is possible that these monomers are actually derived from melanocytes, which then "leach" into the intercellular space. Alternatively, keratinocytes, in proximity to neighboring melanocytes, and UV exposure may trigger intrinsic melanin synthetic machinery within keratinocytes that is yet to be discovered. Our initial findings suggest that key enzymes involved in the melanin synthesis pathway are not expressed in cultured keratinocytes or keratinocytes sampled from human skin by tape stripping.

Melanosome Trafficking

Melanosomes move in an orderly way into dendrites of melanocytes before their transfer to basal or suprabasal keratinocytes. Although this happens at a basal rate, UV exposure increases the movement and transfer rate of melanosomes. The size of melanosomes determines the number that will fit the tip of a dendrite. UV may also influence the width of a dendrite. Thus, a single melanosome or a group of smaller melanosomes may occupy the dendrite tip. The aggregated nature of melanosomes in white skin is thought to be because of a number of melanosomes occupying the dendrite tips when pinched off by keratinocytes. Much of our earlier understanding of melanosome trafficking came from studies looking at the mechanism that redistributes pigment granules in specialized amphibian melanophore cells to control color changes in response to the environment. In these cells, melanosomes undergo microtubule-dependent pigment aggregation to the cell center or dispersion throughout the cytoplasm along actin filaments, mediated by three types of molecular motors: kinesin 2, dynein, and myosin V (31,32). In mouse, the observation that three mutant loci (dilute, leaden, and ashen) encode genes that are required for the polarized transport of melanosomes to the neighboring keratinocytes (and eventually into coat hairs) revealed that they encode for actin-based melanosome transport motor (*MyoVa*), melanophilin (*Mlph*, also known as *Slac2-a*), and *rab27a*, respectively, to form part of the transport machinery that is responsible for the retrograde and anterograde movement of melanosomes in melanocytes (33–37). Defects in the human homologues of these three genes are associated with Griscelli syndrome, which is characterized by hypopigmentation of the skin and hair (38,39), providing strong evidence that spatial distribution of melanosomes in melanocytes, and perhaps also within keratinocytes post transfer, plays an important role in skin color. Whether a similar tripartite molecular motor is involved in the posttransfer shuttling of melanosomes in keratinocytes remains unanswered. Intriguingly, results from retinal pigmented epithelium suggest that expression of all three genes are detectable in retinal pigmented epithelia, but only Rab27a homozygous knock-out mice show evidence of abnormal melanosome distribution (40,41).

Melanosome Transfer and Degradation

There are several theories on the mechanism of melanosome transfer leading to changes in melanin content in the epidermis and hence skin pigmentation (42–44). One hypothesis postulates that melanocytes discharge melanosomes into the extracellular fluid and keratinocytes phagocytose them (45). Keratinocytes have been shown to phagocytose melanosomes and latex beads in vitro and in vivo (46–48). A second hypothesis is that melanosomes put out dendrites that inject melanosomes into keratinocytes (45). A third theory holds that melanocytes put out dendrites toward keratinocytes and the keratinocytes pinches off the dendrite tip. Depending on the actual mechanism of transfer, the transferred melanosomes can have only a melanosome membrane, a melanosome and melanocyte membrane, or a melanosome, melanocyte, and keratinocyte membrane (Fig. 4). Keratinocytes presumably lose melanosome acceptance competence upon differentiation.

These membrane-covered melanosomes are singly and large in Blacks and are small and aggregated in Whites. In Indian skin, we have observed both single and aggregated types, depending on the color of skin. It is noteworthy that the size of the single melanosome and the aggregated melanosomes are the same (roughly 1 μm), thus signifying a major role for melanin in absorbing visible light. Up to two membranes have been seen surrounding melanosomes in keratinocytes. The above findings and theories presuppose chemical signaling between the two cell types to cause directional dendrite growth from melanocytes toward keratinocytes, directed by specific signaling and surface molecules on each of the cell types. In culture, melanocytes are known to ignore keratinocytes near them and insert dendrites into keratinocytes that are relatively far away. They even appear to choose a particular region of the membrane to make actual contact. This indicates a high degree of specificity both in choice of keratinocytes and site on the keratinocyte membrane caused, no doubt, at a molecular level, by specific signaling and surface molecules on each of the cell types. That signaling mechanisms exist was shown in melanocyte-keratinocyte coculture experiments where activation of the proteinase-activated receptor 2 (PAR-2) by UV irradiation led to an increase in melanosome transfer through increase in melanosome phagocytosis by keratinocytes (47,49,50). In HaCaT keratinocytes, the extracellular amino-terminal domain of PAR-2 (member of PAR family of G-coupled transmembrane receptors) is cleaved by serine proteinases (e.g., trypsin) to expose a tethered ligand that subsequently activates the receptor. Significantly, activation of PAR-2 in vivo resulted in changes in pigmentation by modulating melanosome transfer, and the presence of serine proteinase inhibitors such as soy trypsin inhibitor is able to reduce melanosome transfer, albeit incompletely, suggesting that additional mechanisms may also be involved in phagocytosis/transfer of melanosomes by keratinocytes (49,50).

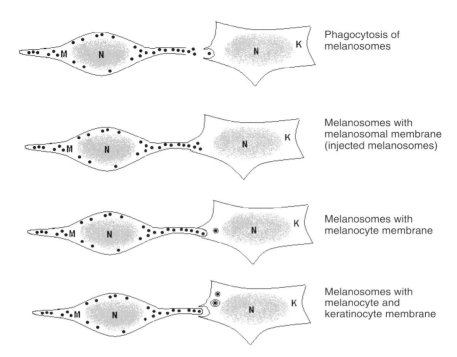

Phagocytosis of
melanosomes

Melanosomes with
melanosomal membrane
(injected melanosomes)

Melanosomes with
melanocyte membrane

Melanosomes with
melanocyte and
keratinocyte membrane

FIGURE 4 Melanosome transfer mechanisms.

Although there is no evidence to date to suggest that keratinocytes transfer melanosomes between themselves, it remains an interesting hypothesis that keratinocytes derived from individuals with different skin color may have different competencies in their ability to accept melanosomes from melanocytes. Such innate differences, if they exist, would play an important physiological role in determining individual skin color. Transfer occurs only at basal or suprabasal levels and at specific sites on the keratinocyte cell membrane and to only one or two keratinocytes of the EMU at a time, indicating a "state of acceptance" in receptive keratinocytes. Such "acceptance competence" could be a result of the exhibition of particular molecules at particular regions of the cell surface that are involved in transfer and such molecules being lost on differentiation. Such differences in the phagocompetency of keratinocytes at various states of maturation may perhaps account for the nonuniformity in in vitro uptake of latex beads by keratinocytes in culture (48–50). The transfer of melanosomes into keratinocytes is also the only physiological instance known of an organelle being transferred into a new host cell that harbors it and makes use of it. The fact that such an organelle transfer system exists and is conserved through mammalian evolution suggests that it serves important roles in pigmentation biology and confers advantage to keratinocytes. A question that arises from this is whether harboring a foreign organelle stimulates phagocytic and degradative mechanisms in the keratinocyte host cell? This together with differences in the nature of covering(s) of the transferred melanosome may, in fact, determine the physiological lifespan of melanosomes in the keratinocytes. Such a scenario could explain the presence of ill-defined melanin dust in fair Whites that are subsequently lost during epidermal desquamation, whereas intact melanosomes are found in the skin of blacks (42,51), suggesting that susceptibility of melanosomes to degradative enzymes or efficacy of such degradative processes may also contribute to the racial differences in skin color. Indeed, there is some evidence to suggest that human skin contains melanin-degrading enzymes that can affect skin color (52). Degradation of melanosomes is also observed in the turnover of melanosomes in retinal pigment epithelium (53). However, it was also noted that although the melanosomes have disintegrated, the melanin moiety remains intact and may require further oxidative decomposition via enzymes such as phagosomal NADPH oxidase (54). If by breaking the melanosome will stop absorption of visible light and skin color will reduce, melanosome degradation may be a route to skin lightening. Alternatively, one could view the melanosome as a foreign body in the keratinocyte. Upon uptake, the keratinocyte host cell, having phagocytic properties, could initiate degradative processes to digest the foreign body. The nature of membrane coverings of the melanosome could affect the longevity of the melanosome in the keratinocyte and recognition as a foreign body and therefore the triggering of degradative processes. This theory suggests that in Whites, the recognition (and therefore the covering membranes) is different than in dark skin.

One question that is raised is whether the transfer of melanosomes to keratinocytes is to actually confer a better protection to melanocytes, with keratinocytes also being secondarily protected? This possibility is supported by the fact that melanomas are almost unknown in non-Whites, whereas basal and squamous cell carcinomas are known in nonwhite populations, albeit at a lower incidence than in whites. The transfer process could thus be an example of cellular symbiosis.

Melanosomes Spatial Distribution and Skin Color

There are quantifiable differences in the degree of melanization and distribution of melanosomes in individuals of diverse ethnic background (55). In particular, the number, size, and packaging of the melanosomes within the keratinocytes of individuals from different ethnic background vary (56–60). In general, more deeply pigmented skin contains numerous large melanosomes in the cytosol of keratinocytes, predominantly over the nucleus, whereas lighter pigmentation is associated with small and less dense melanosomes that are clustered in membrane-bound groups of two to eight melanosomes. Depending on proposed mechanisms of transfer, a melanosome may have only a melanosomal membrane, a melanosome and melanocyte membrane, or a melanosome, melanocyte, and keratinocyte membrane (Fig. 4). Further, if taken up by lysosomes, it can also have a lysosomal membrane. Recent data indicate that melanosomes within Asian skin are distributed as a combination of individual and clustered melanosomes, and melanosome size correlates with ethnicity, where melanosomes are largest in dark African American skin, followed by Asian and white skin (61). An interesting observation is that regardless of donor origin, melanosomes are predominantly distributed individually by recipient keratinocytes from dark skin and in membrane-bound clusters by those from light skin, suggesting that factors within keratinocytes determine the distribution pattern of melanosomes (59). More importantly, the sizes of clustered and individually distributed melanosomes from either dark or light skin–derived melanocytes were not significantly different from each other within each type of recipient keratinocyte, in the range of visible light wavelength (~900nm), thus signifying a major role for melanin in absorbing visible light. Positioning of melanosomes within keratinocytes also appears to be involved in UVA-induced pigmentation where it was shown in vivo that melanosomes within keratinocytes disperse and migrate from their normal aggregated location around the nucleus toward the cell periphery upon UVA irradiation (5). Significantly, these changes were not observed in specimens exposed to melanogenic doses of UVB. The authors proposed that UVA wavelengths can selectively cause redistribution of melanosomes within keratinocytes, which accounts for the visually observed increase in IPD (see below) that develops soon after single exposures of UVA. Consistent with this hypothesis, it was also shown that there is no increase in melanosome transfer after IPD induction in full-thickness skin and epidermal sheets (62). Undoubtedly, this peripheral movement of melanosomes contributes to skin color change. Whether this movement is reversible has not been answered nor are the mechanisms that control movement in keratinocytes clear. Central clumping is a feature reported in black keratinocytes. This is possibly a default state. Numbers of melanosomes also may contribute to such a positioning. Melanosomes are thought to have a supranuclear position to protect the nucleus. If this were true, it seems strange that upon UV exposure, they would move away from the nucleus to near the cell membrane, unless, in a three-dimensional way, there would be a better cover for the cell if all the melanosomes in all the keratinocytes were lining the inner aspect of the cell membrane.

In summary, current available evidence indicate that differences in the degree of melanization, chemical differences in the melanin pigments themselves, and the spatial distribution of melanin laden melanosomes within the epidermal layers are critical factors in the visual gradation of skin color. Most of the work in the area of pigmentation of the skin has been confined to the processes within the melanocyte and, more recently, on melanosome transfer. There has been very little work on the fate of melanosomes after they are transferred to the keratinocytes. As mentioned above, other factors, such as integrity of transferred melanosomes and the presence of melanin degrading enzymes in the skin, may also be important to overall skin color.

REGULATION OF SKIN PIGMENTATION
Constitutive Pigmentation

Genes play important roles in constitutive skin color. Comparative studies in mouse with different coat color mutations have revealed that more than 150 genes have effects on pigmentation. Not all of these identified genes may have equivalents in humans. The prominent and well-characterized mouse genes include agouti, albino, brown, dilute, leaden, mottled, pink-eye dilute, silver, and slaty (Table 2) (63–65). In humans, pigmentation genes that are best studied are mutations that lead to the various forms of oculocutaneous albinism (66). However, these genes do not account for the normal variation in skin color among different populations. The major breakthrough can be attributed to the discovery that polymorphism in the gene encoding for the melanocortin 1 receptor (*MC1R*) was associated with red hair and fair skin phenotype among Europeans (67,68). Further evidence to suggest a role of *MC1R* in normal skin color variation is provided by findings that certain *MC1R* nucleotide sequence variants are more frequently found in Asian and African populations, in particular, the Arg163Gln variant, which occurs with an average frequency of 70% in East and Southeast Asian populations but in only about 5% in some European populations (69,70). In addition, polymorphism in the upstream promoter regions of the *MC1R* gene has also been linked to variations in population pigmentation (71,72). What remains to be determined, however, is the functional significance of

TABLE 2   Examples of Pigmentation Gene Mutants and Their Human Homologues

Gene mutation	Protein	Human locus	Phenotype	Function
Agouti (mouse)	Agouti signal protein	*ASIP*	Unknown	Morphology of melanosome, ratio of eumelanin/ pheomelanin
Albino (mouse)	Tyrosinase	*TYR*	OCA1	Tyrosinase and melanosome number
Brown (mouse)	Tyrosinase-related protein 1	*TRP1*	OCA3	Melanosome structure
Dilute (mouse)	Myosin Va	*MYO5A*	Griscelli syndrome	Melanosome transfer, dendrite structure/function
Leaden (mouse)	Melanophilin	*MLPH*	Griscelli syndrome	Melanosomes transport
Microphthalmia (mouse)	Transcription factor	*MITF*	Waardenburg syndrome type 2	Melanocyte differentiation
Mottled (mouse)	Cu^{2+}-transporting ATPase, α-polypeptide	*ATP7A*	Menkes disease	Availability of copper
Pink-eyed dilute (mouse)	P-protein	*OCA2*	OCA2	Melanin synthesis
Silver/Pmel17 (mouse)	Pmel17	*SILV*	Unknown	DHICA polymerization
Slaty (mouse)	Tyrosinase-related protein 2	*DCT*	Unknown	Dopachrome tautomerase
Underwhite (mouse)	Membrane-associated transporter protein	*MATP*	OCA4	Ion transporter, role in regulation of melanosome pH
Golden (zebra fish)	Slc24a5	*SLC24A5*	Unknown	Cation exchanger, regulates elanosome calcium uptake(?)

Abbreviations: DHICA, dihydroxyindole carboxylic acid; OCA1, oculocutaneous albinism type 1; OCA3, oculocutaneous albinism type 3; OCA4, oc.
Source: From Ref. 75.

these coding and promoter variants of *MC1R*. In conjunction with sequence variations in *MC1R* gene, population studies have also revealed that polymorphisms in the P (OCA2) and MATP (OCA4) genes are associated with determining the range of colors observed for skin (73,74).

The activities of melanogenic enzymes tyrosinase, *TRP1* and *TRP2*, are also subject to transcriptional control. Microphthalmia-associated transcription factor (*Mitf*), consisting of at least seven isoforms, belongs to the basic helix-loop-helix and leucine zipper class of transcription factor (76). They bind to the canonical CAT-GTG *Mitf* consensus motif located in the 5" flanking region of *TYR*, *TRP1*, and *TRP2* genes to regulate their expression levels (77–79). Mice with mutations in the *Mitf* locus are characterized by hearing loss, coat color dilution, white spotting, or complete loss of pigmentation due to defects in melanocyte development. In humans,

MITF gene mutations are most notably associated with the auditory-pigmentary syndromes known as Waardenburg syndrome type 2 (80,81).

Another compelling candidate for determining skin pigmentation comes from a study using zebra fish as a model to search for cancer genes (82). The authors noted a mutation called golden, which lightened the fish's normally dark melanin-rich stripes. The mutated gene shared 69% sequence homology and was functional conserved with the human *SLC24A5* gene, which encodes a putative cation exchanger that appears to localize to melanosomes. Further probing showed that *SLC24A5* has primarily two alleles that varied by one amino acid. Nearly all African and East Asians have an allele with alanine in a key locus, while 98% of Europeans carry the threonine allele. Most significantly, the authors found that within a population admixture that is representative of African and European ancestry, individuals homozygous for the threonine allele tended to have light skin, whereas those with the alanine were darkest, with heterozygotes in between, a pattern consistent with association of a genotype with a specific phenotype. However, this allelic variation in *SLC24A5* cannot be the only determinant of skin color because there are also considerable differences in skin pigmentation between Africans and East Asians who share the common alanine allele, suggesting that variations in other genes also affects skin color. Because *MC1R* is associated with red hair and fair skin among Europeans, it would be interesting to ask if permutations of different *MC1R* and *SLC24A5* variants have any influence on skin color variations among Europeans. At a functional level, cations, including protons, definitely play a role in melanin polymerization and structure, and these alleles may be playing an initial role in the amount and properties of melanin synthesis (29). Despite these intriguing findings, how different genes influence the spectrum of human skin color remains elusive.

UV-Induced Pigmentation

UV radiation is the most important external stimulus for modulating pigmentation. UV-induced skin darkening is divided into two categories: IPD and delayed tanning (DT). IPD occurs within minutes of UV exposure in whites and in a few hours in darker skin types and has an action spectrum in the UVA range (83). It begins as a pale blue-black discoloration in the exposed area that gradually fades to a brown color during a period of days depending on the UV dose and skin type. These changes are not because of new melanin synthesis or increased melanosome transfer but are rather thought to be the result of photooxidation of preexisting melanin precursors and redistribution of melanosomes from perinuclear to a peripheral location (5,62,84,85). IPD, therefore, does not confer photoprotection. IPD could also be because of changes in melanin solubility. Ou-Yang et al. (85) observed a significant UVA-induced in vitro and in vivo decrease in eumelanin absorbance spectra in the UV range accompanied by a concomitant increase in absorbance in the visible range from 450 to 800 nm. It would be tempting to speculate that this change in the visible range plays an important role in the free radical scavenging response of cells exposed to solar radiation, in particular UVA. DT, on the other hand, has a broader action spectrum including UVB and UVA, indicating that it is mechanistically distinct from IPD (86). DT could be a result of changes in all steps of the melanin pathway—numbers of melanocytes, amount of melanin, transfer rate, dendricity of melanocytes, increased melanin in keratinocytes with peripheral distribution. DT is characterized by a reddish brown discoloration that becomes deep brown/black, which may indicate an initial co-stimulation of erythema immediately after UV exposure that resolves over time. DT begins in 48 hours and can last several months. There is a wide range in DT response and persistence of the tan even within individuals with similar skin phenotypes (87,88). Effects of solar radiation in the visible and infrared regions on skin, and their influence on pigmentation, remain poorly studied. It should be noted that UVA-induced melanogenesis is two to three orders of magnitude less efficient per unit dose than UVB (89). The persistence of DT could be, in part, because of "memory of the insult" (i.e., postinflammatory hyperpigmentation that can lead to blotchy or uniform hyperpigmentation).

DT and Melanin Content

Although evidence indicates that DT involves new synthesis of melanin and stimulation of almost all steps in the melanin pathway, there is a clear lack of correlation between melanin content in the skin and the visible progression of the tan (60,88,90–92). For example, Tadokoro et al. (88) observed a significant change in skin color (assessed by eye and reflectance spectroscopy) within 7 days after UV exposure in subjects from different ethnic background but no significant increase in melanin content, determined by Fontana-Masson staining. Fontana-Masson staining depends upon the ability of melanin granules to reduce ammoniacal silver nitrate (93). It is possible that because of the nonlinear chemistry of Fontana-Masson staining and/or the variation in the redox state of melanin in each person/area is not uniform, its use to precisely quantify the amount of melanin in skin is limited, thus yielding melanin content measurements that are neither representative of color photography (i.e., visual register) of the skin complexion of subjects nor with measurements made by diffuse reflectance spectrometry that measures light reflectance at the skin surface (88). Alternatively, the data suggest that factors other than the total amount of melanin in the skin are also important for skin pigmentation.

Skin Phototypes

The ability to tan varies among individuals with different pigmentary phenotypes (Table 3) (94). Those with very light skin (phototypes I and II) burn easily and do not tan; those with dark skin (phototypes III–V) tan well upon sun exposure and do not burn. They have a higher ratio of eumelanin to pheomelanin than in lightly pigmented skin. However, questions have been raised about the clinical usefulness and accuracy of such a classification based on tanning response. For example, it has been repeatedly observed that color of skin does not correlate with ability to tan

TABLE 3 The Fitzpatrick Classification of Skin Phototypes

Skin phototype	Description	Skin color	Susceptibility to skin cancer
I	Never tan, always burn	Pale white	High
II	Tan minimally, always burn	Pale white	High
III	Tan gradually, burn moderately	White	Moderate
IV	Tan well, rarely burn	Light brown	Low
V	Tan well, burn minimally	Brown	Very low
VI	Tan deeply, never burn	Dark brown	Very low

in some phototype III, IV, and V skin (e.g., Indian skin). Even within a phototype (e.g., III, IV), we have observed a lack of tanning response. This inability to tan is not explained on the basis of simple photoprotection. The reason for such varied responses is not known and indicates that we still do not entirely understand the functional significance of skin pigmentation. Moreover, the Fitzpatrick classification is based predominantly on large numbers of white subjects and fewer dark-skinned subjects, and thus the findings, although applicable, could be skewed toward fair-skinned populations. Indeed, the authors believe that there are many subtypes within III, IV, and V, and type VI is very poorly studied. This created a paradox for the photoprotective role of melanin that has been proposed in that dark-skinned populations with higher melanin index are not necessarily completely protected from all the deleterious effects of UV radiation.

Endocrine, Paracrine, and Autocrine Factors

Skin pigmentation is also influenced by the action of hormones (95). An important influence on skin color is the activation of the *MC1R* on the cell surface of melanocytes by its ligands α-melanocyte–stimulating hormone (α-MSH) and adrenocorticotropic hormone (ACTH), derived from the proteolytic cleavage of proopiomelanocortin (POMC) produced in the intermediate lobe of the pituitary (96,97). Activation of *MC1R* leads to elevation of intracellular cAMP via activation of adenylate cyclase and results in increase in tyrosinase levels and eumelanin production. Abnormalities in ACTH and adrenal physiology result in changes in skin pigmentation. For example, in Addison's disease or ACTH-secreting tumors, skin hyperpigmentation and sometimes premature graying of the hair is presented; on the other hand, hypopituitarism leads to lowering of ACTH levels and hypopigmentation. Reduced testosterone levels have also been associated with skin lightening in that castrated men are characteristically pale and tan poorly (98). Hormonal changes during pregnancy and during some phases of the menstrual cycle lead to changes in cutaneous pigmentation (e.g., melasma) especially in the genital and malar areas, thus implicating the influence of estrogen and progesterone levels (99). Studies have shown that melanocytes express both receptors for estrogen and progesterone, but it is not clear if their effects are mediated through receptor or nonreceptor mechanisms or whether the hormones affect melanocytes proliferation or activates the melanogenic pathway. Other hormones/growth factors that have been clinically associated with changes in pigmentation include insulin, prostaglandins, leukotrienes, cytokines, growth factors, and thyroid hormones. UV augments the effects of most if not all agents that increase pigmentation. Melatonin from the pineal gland is probably the only important hormone that decreases pigmentation (100,101) via a mechanism that may involve reversing the actions of α-MSH.

Inflammation-Induced Pigmentation

The occurrence of postinflammatory hyperpigmentation indicates that inflammatory mediators also contribute to skin color. For example, cytokines interleukins (IL; IL-1α, IL-1β, IL-6) and tumor necrosis factor α (TNF-α) reduced tyrosinase and TRP-1 and TRP-2 protein levels in human melanocytes (102). Another group of inflammatory factors are the metabolites of arachidonic acid, the eicosanoids, which include prostaglandins. Prostaglandin F2α stimulates melanocyte dendricity as well as the activity and expression of tyrosinase, the rate-limiting step in melanin synthesis (103). In addition, it was also shown that melanocytes produce prostaglandin

TABLE 4   Keratinocyte-Derived Factors Involved in Melanogenesis

Keratinocyte-derived factors	Reference
IL	108
α-MSH	109
bFGF	110
NGF	111
ET-1	112
GM-CSF	108
ACTH	113
SCF	114
PGE-2/PGF-2a	115
POMC	116
NO	117, 118

Abbreviations: ACTH, adrenocorticotropic hormone; bFGF, basic fibroblast growth factor; ET-1, endothelin 1; GM-CSF, granulocyte-macrophage colony-stimulating factor; IL, interleukin; α-MSH, α-melanocyte stimulating hormone; NGF, nerve growth factor; NO, nitric oxide; SCF, stem cell factor; PGE-2/PGF-2a, prostaglandin E2/2a; POMC, proopiomelanocortin.

F2α in response to UV irradiation, suggesting that it is an autocrine factor for melanocyte function.

Signaling Between Melanocytes and Keratinocytes

Because melanocytes in vivo are surrounded by keratinocytes, it is reasonable to postulate that melanocyte function can be modulated by signals originating from keratinocytes (Table 4) (104). Keratinocytes exposed to UV up-regulate their IL-1α, IL-4, IL-8, IL-10, and IL-12, TNF-α, transforming growth factor α, endothelin 1 (ET-1), nerve growth factor (NGF), basic fibroblast growth factor (bFGF), granulocyte-macrophage colony-stimulating factor, MSH, POMC, nitric oxide, and prostaglandin E2. When exposed specifically with UVB, IL-1, IL-6, IL-8, IL-10, granulocyte-macrophage colony-stimulating factor, and TNF-α are secreted, and cells can progress to apoptosis or cell cycle phase arrest. Melanocytes exposed to UV up-regulate IL-10, arachidonic acid, diacyl glycerol, and α-MSH receptors. Internalization of α-MSH receptors by melanosomes also suggests specific and precise UV-induced communications between host cell and melanosomes (105). Other cells in the skin, endothelial cells, Langerhans cells, macrophages, and mast cells also respond to UV and make several active growth factors and lipid mediators. Undoubtedly, these too affect both keratinocytes and melanocytes. bFGF, NGF, ET-1, POMC, cyclic adenosine monophosphate, and theophylline-like drugs increase dendricity of melanocytes. bFGF, NGF, ET-1, POMC, epidermal growth factor, and phorbol esters increase proliferation of melanocytes. TNF-α, TGF-α, and interferon γ all reduce proliferation of melanocytes. Appropriate receptors on complementary cell type have also been identified for some growth factors. Although cytokine literature has been growing at a furious pace, one must not forget the importance of membrane-derived messenger molecules especially upon exposure to UV, some of which are enumerated above. Indeed, the primary stimulus to melanocytes may be signals from keratinocytes. The possibility of this cannot be overemphasized, because there are far more keratinocytes than melanocytes. Melanin in keratinocytes could also behave as a photoreceptor. Indeed, there is much in vitro evidence that demonstrates that melanocytes stimulate melanin synthesis upon exposure to the conditioned media from UV-irradiated keratinocytes. Interestingly, DNA photoproducts generated by UV-induced DNA repair have also been shown to increase melanogenesis (106,107).

Effects of Age on Skin Color

Although not as dramatic as change in skin color resulting from tanning, skin color does show considerable subtle variations throughout the life. Skin reflectometric studies show that skin becomes darker as people transit through puberty, concomitant with changes in hormonal levels, and lighten with onset of age (119,120). These changes appear to correlate with the capacity of melanocytes to produce melanin or, in some instances, the complete attrition of melanocytes as in the case of melanocytes in the hair follicles associated with graying or white hair (121). In addition to age-associated changes in melanocyte function and abundance, there are also qualitative and quantitative changes in elastic fibers, particularly in the sun-exposed facial region, resulting in increase in skin thickness and changes in skin tone (122). An interesting observation is that *Mitf* protein is dramatically down-regulated in senescent melanocytes in vitro, but expression of melanogenic genes such as tyrosinase, *TRP2*, and *PMEL17* is not affected (123). It is not clear if other transcription factors beside *Mitf* are responsible for the continued expression of these melanogenic genes. With age, the normal homeostasis of the EMU seems to be disturbed, with blotch/uneven pigmentation occurring.

Carotenoids

Some evidence suggests that carotenoids, in particular, the yellow-red colored betacarotene, lycopene, and lutein commonly found in a wide variety of fruits and vegetables contribute to normal skin color. These pigments enter the bloodstream through dietary consumption and get distributed to various parts of our body, including the dermis, epidermis, and even stratum corneum. Studies in Whites have shown that carotenoids in normal diet contribute to a significant skin "yellowness" and also provide photoprotective benefits that are linked to the concentration of carotenoids in the tissue (124). When associated with thinning of the skin, in general, with age, this would lead to a greater "visibility" of the pigments deposited deep in the dermis, leading to the "sallowness" of aging.

Drug-Induced Pigmentation

Pharmacological agents have also been shown to induce hyperpigmentation (125). Pigmentation-causing agents include nonsteroidal anti-inflammatory drugs, antimalarials, amiodarone, cytotoxic drugs, tetracyclines, heavy metals, and psychotropic drugs. The clinical features presented with these agents involve a large range of patterns and shades depending on the triggering molecule. Current therapy for drug-induced pigmentation is limited to cessation of offending drug use and sun avoidance.

HYPERPIGMENTATION DISORDERS

Age spots, postinflammatory spots, and melasma are dyschromias that are important in the point of view of cosmetic treatment. Although they present no disease or discomfort, they could be a cause of emotional and psychological stress among those that are afflicted. What follows is a brief description of each of these.

Age Spots
Synonyms of age spots include sun spots, solar lentigines, senile lentigines, and liver spots. Age spots are prevalent in low-grade phototype, thought to affect more than 90% of whites older than 60 years, and is linked strongly to sun exposure and age. They are presented as yellow–light brown to black macules on surfaces of the skin exposed to the sun (face, upper back, forearms, dorsum of the hands). Histologically, age spots are characterized by the presence of elongated epidermal rete ridges with heavy pigmentation in the basal layer. Electron microscopy revealed an increase in the number of active melanocytes and number and size of the melanosomal complexes in keratinocytes. Some have reported the presence of giant melanosomal complexes in melanocytes. Keratinocyte defects can be expected because an "age spot" persists even with differentiation, thus indicating that the progeny of keratinocytes persists in perpetuation of the "age spot." A keratinocyte memory can be postulated. Basement membrane defects are possible with diffusion of melanin into the dermis or transgression of melanin-bearing keratinocytes into the dermis (126). Treatment options include hydroquinone (2–4%), tretinoin (0.05–0.1%), tazarotene (0.1%), adapalene (0.1–0.3%), azelaic acid, and kojic acid. Laser treatment and intense pulsed light treatment have also shown to be effective.

Postinflammatory Hyperpigmentation
These are hyperpigmented lesions that appear after the resolution of inflammation in the skin, which may be due to infections, injury, allergy, cosmetic surgery, laser procedures. This is more common in Fitzpatrick skin types IV–VI. Found as discrete macules with hazy, feathered margins that vary in size and shape, they are histologically characterized as either epidermal melanosis (inflammation confined to the epidermis, where various lipid mediators of inflammation have been shown to increase the dendricity and amount of immunoreactive tyrosinase in the melanocytes) or as dermal melanosis (where the basal cell layer is destroyed, resulting in macrophages phagocytosing the degenerating basal keratinocyte and melanocytes with melanosomes, with these being abnormally retained in the dermis). Treatment options for epidermal melanosis include hydroquinone (2–4%), tretinoin (0.1%), corticosteroids, and keratolytics. Dermal melanosis is difficult to treat, but surgical removal or laser ablation has been used.

Melasma
Melasma manifests as increased pigmentation in the face, typically symmetric patches or macules are found on either side, with a tendency to occur on the sun-exposed areas of the face (cheeks, upper lips). This disorder is much more common in women than men (a ratio of 9:1) and in persons with high-grade phototype. Major etiologic factors include genetic influences, female sex hormones, and exposure to UV radiation. Histopathology findings indicate hyperpigmentation in all epidermal layers caused by an increase in melanin and also the number of active melanocytes. A flattening of the epidermal rete ridges has been reported, suggesting that keratinocytic proliferation may not be involved in melasma. Pathogenesis

is poorly understood. A recent study indicated that the high expression of α-MSH in keratinocytes of the melasmic lesions was a major factor. Treatment options are prevention using good broad-spectrum sunscreen, retinoids, α-hydroxy acids, and hydroquinone.

MELANIN PIGMENTATION AND PHOTOPROTECTION

Although it is clear that melanin synthesis in the epidermis is a physiological response upon exposure to UV, the primary function of melanin in the skin has yet to be firmly established. Melanin is thought to have a number of properties that are beneficial, including UV radiation absorption, light scattering, free radical scavenging, and immune modulation. Human epidermal melanin absorbs both UV and visible light. Melanin absorption increases linearly in the visible range (720–620 nm) and then exponentially toward the shorter wavelengths (600–300 nm) (127). Photoprotective effects of melanin are evidenced by epidemiological studies, which indicate that skin with higher melanin content (phototypes IV, good tanners; V, brown; and VI, black) have much lower incidence rates of skin cancer than people with comparatively lower levels of melanin in the epidermis (128). DNA represents the direct target for UV radiation damage. UV-induced damage leads to the formation of mutagenic dipyrimidine lesions such as cyclobutane pyrimidine dimers and pyrimidine(6–4)pyrimidone photoproducts (129,130). Failure to repair dipyrimidine lesions, as is the case in patients with the rare genetic disorder xeroderma pigmentosum, results in multiple skin cancers at an early age. Consistent with this notion that melanin mitigates the UV-induced photodamage to cells, it was postulated that melanin synthesis may be a damage response system, similar to the observed induction of SOS response in UV-irradiated *Escherichia coli* that resulted in increased efficiency of global nucleotide excision repair mechanism (131,132). Interestingly, Im et al. (133) reported that melanosomes isolated from human hair offered a sun protection factor of 3 against UVB when applied topically as a 25% preparation. Although this demonstrated that topical melanin is a poor sunscreen compared with currently available organic and inorganic sunscreens, it is nonetheless present 24 hours a day at different levels of the epidermis and can offer significant protection from solar radiation that impinges on our skin. One can hypothesize that melanin in keratinocytes really is present to protect the melanocytes from UV irradiation or that melanocytes and keratinocytes are in a sense symbiotic in protecting each other. More recently, it was proposed that eumelanin was the major factor in the photoprotective properties of melanin, which when induced in white skin types, results in a protection factor of about 2–3 against DNA photodamage and erythema (134). Using mouse models, Takeuchi et al. (135) showed that UV-irradiated melanin photosensitizes neighboring cells to UV-induced cell death as indicated by the presence of DNA double-strand breaks. Significantly, there was a three-fold higher frequency of DNA double-strand breaks in yellow mice than in black mice, suggesting that pheomelanin is a more potent photosensitizer than eumelanin, which may explain why blondes and red hair individuals are more susceptible to skin cancer.

Role of UV-induced pyrimidine dimers in skin pigmentation was demonstrated by several studies that evaluated the effects of thymidine dinucleotides (pTpT) on melanogenesis. Increased pigmentation and melanin content was observed when mice were treated with pTpT compared with control animals (106,136). Human melanoma cells also responded to pTpT by increasing pigmentation (137). Additional data indicate that pTpT directly activates the tumor suppressor gene p53, which, in turn, induces tyrosinase gene expression (138,139). Although the significance of these in vitro findings are yet to be understood in vivo, it has opened up the possibility of using small DNA fragments, in particular pTpT oligos, for use as photoprotective tanning agents that can mitigate the harmful effects of UV radiation (140). One should ask though if the levels of pTpT used in these studies are actually produced in vivo with conventional sun exposure. If the levels used in these studies are not physiological, the finding is of anecdotal significance, and mechanisms other than pTpT operate to induce pigmentation under physiological conditions.

IN PURSUIT OF THE IDEAL SKIN COLOR

Being the largest and most visible feature of the body, skin serves as an indicator of age, health, wealth, ancestry, and as a canvas for beauty decoration. For centuries, humans have tried to alter what heredity determines—either to darken or lighten skin color through various decorative cosmetic regimes, whether to hide unappealing features, enhance attractiveness, mask unsightly scars, or just to give the skin a healthy radiant blush. Deliberate sun exposure to get the perfect tan has become fashionable in the West, presumably to denote leisure time and hence economic independence and wealth. In the East, however, not having to work in the sun and thus being protected from the darkening effects of sun is the social equivalent. The biological end points are diametrically opposite, but the financial opportunities presented by our desire to look appealing to one another is the same—a global market for attractive skin color and healthy skin tone that is in the range of U.S. $2.5 to $3.5 billion. The cosmetics industry today is inundated with products that claim to alter skin color in various ways. Many of these products are available on supermarket shelves and through the booming health spa industry, network distribution channels, and the internet and attract billions in advertising dollars.

Skin Darkening

A tanned complexion has become a fashion statement in some societies to denote availability and affordability of leisure time. Tanning is naturally achieved through deliberate exposure to the sun or tanning beds in beauty salons. However, the down side of tanning is that excessive UV exposure results in accelerated skin aging and significant increase in squamous and basal cell carcinomas, especially in fair-skinned white populations. This quest for an aesthetic tan without photodamage to the skin has led to the evolution of artificial or "sunless" tanning products. Many of these products dye the skin using chemicals such as dihydroxyacetone (DHA). In use since the 1960s, DHA is a sugar that reacts with amino acids in the outer stratum corneum to form a brown complex that stains the skin, giving it a tanned appearance (141). This process, known as Maillard reaction, occurs frequently in food preparation and is responsible for the caramelization of sugar and the golden brown color of beer. Similarly, erythrulose darkens skin by deposition of brownish polymers termed melanoids (142), albeit requiring a longer time to see visible effects compared with DHA. Despite their widespread use as cosmetic skin darkening agents, sunless tanning products have their drawbacks. For example, the color obtained via these agents can be inconsistent if applied unevenly, leading to unappealing patchy appearance. In addition, because these products have no effect at all on melanogenesis, they do not provide any sun protection as compared with naturally tanned skin. Studies have shown that DHA only provides a sun protection factor of 3 at the most upon application and decreases to less than 2 for the five to seven days following application, despite the continued appearance of tanned skin (143). A recent study in young adults suggested that the use of sunless tanning products did not decrease rates of sunburning among the at-risk groups who were more inclined to use such products (144). Questions have been raised about the safety of long-term topical DHA application. Petersen et al. (145) demonstrated that DHA has genotoxic effects in in vitro tests with HaCaT keratinocytes, including DNA damage, exit from cell cycle, and increased apoptosis. Although these effects were observed at concentrations lower than were expected to be attainable in vivo, long-term clinical consequences of DHA use to darken skin has not been evaluated. Other topically applied coloring agents that have been explored include natural dyes such as lawsone (derived from the henna plant), mahakanni (from *Eclipta alba*), and rhubarb extract.

Because of the potential risks associated with DHA use, alternative approaches that attempt to increase pigmentation via increasing melanin density with simultaneous sun protection are currently under evaluation. Melasyn® (Vion Pharmaceuticals, Inc., New Haven, Connecticut, U.S.) is a group of plant-derived synthetic melanin (146). Because they mimic natural melanin, they are thought to offer photoprotection in addition to increasing topical melanin density. More notably, Melanotans are potent synthetic analogues of α-MSH that were initially created, synthesized, and developed at The University of Arizona and the Arizona Cancer Center (147). Melanotan I is a linear, full-length peptide (containing all 13 amino acids). Melanotan II is a shortened, circular version of the same peptide. Both show potent induction of tyrosinase in S91 melanoma cells, and recent clinical evaluation demonstrated that Melanotan I delivered by subcutaneous injection into the abdomen for three 10-day cycles for three months resulted in significant increase in melanin density in all subjects and reduced UV-induced sunburn in those with low baseline minimal erythemal dose (148). But because Melanotans require delivery via subcutaneous injection and are associated with side effects such as nausea, their wide use as tanning agents may not be acceptable. However, they do offer potentially exciting avenues for targeted cosmetic treatment of dermatological hypopigmentation or uneven pigmentation problems, especially if combined with less invasive delivery technologies such as dermabrasion.

Orally delivered tanning agents in the form of tanning pills are available. Approved as dietary supplements, they contain the orange pigment carotenoid (including betacarotene, cantaxanthin, or lycopene), which, when ingested, is deposited in the fat layers just below the skin, giving it the skin color. Unfortunately, there is no control of where the body deposits the ingested pigment, making these products unattractive. Similarly, topically applied melanosomes offer limited protection from UV effects (133), raising the question of whether melanin has to be inside keratinocytes and enclosed within melanosomes to provide protection against the harmful effects of UV. The fact that melanosomes are transferred intact into keratinocytes and are never observed deposited in the intracellular space supports the idea that once transferred into keratinocytes, melanosomes confer new functions/attributes to their host cell.

Skin Lightening

Although a tanned skin is desirable in some populations, fair skin in the eastern populations is indicative of economic wealth and freedom from laboring under the sun. Reduction of epidermal melanin is also desirable in many pathological conditions associated with skin, such as melasma, postinflammatory hyperpigmentation, and solar lentigines. These conditions are mainly characterized by excessive deposition

TABLE 5   Depigmentation Agents and Their Modes of Action

Depigmenting agent	Mode of action	Reference
2,5-Dihydroxybenzoic acid component of *Gentiana* root	Inhibits melanin synthesis in mouse melanocytes	152
All-*trans*-retinoic acid/tretinoin	Desquamation	153–155
Aloesin and aloe vera component	Inhibits mushroom tyrosinase	156, 157
α-Hydroxy acids (e.g., lactic acid, glycolic acid)	Desquamation	158
α-Tocopherol and derivatives	Tyrosinase inhibition, increases intracellular glutathione	159
Arbutin (extract of bearberry plant) and adeoxyarbutin	Inhibits DHICA polymerase activity, inhibits melanosome maturation	160, 161
Azelaic acid	Copper chelation	162
C2-ceramide	Decrease *MITF* expression	163
Chamomile extract	Prevention of black spots	164
Ellagic acid and pomegranate extract	Inhibits mushroom tyrosinase	165
Hydroquinone	Compete for tyrosine oxidation in activated melanocytes	166
Jojoba extract	Inhibits mouse tyrosinase	167
Kojic acid	Inactivate tyrosinase by copper chelation and suppressing tautomerization from DC to DHICA	168
L-Ascorbic acid (vitamin C) and derivatives	Interacts with copper ions at tyrosinase active site, reduce dopaquinone, blocks DHICA oxidation	169, 170
Licorice extract	Inhibits mouse tyrosinase	171
Lignin peroxidase	Melanin decomposition agent	172
Linoleic acid/α-linolenic acid	Suppression of melanin production in guinea pigs	173
Lipoic acid	Reduce MITF and tyrosinase promoter activities	174
Milk proteins (κ-casein)	Tyrosinase inhibition in B16 cells	175
Niacinamide	Inhibition of melanosome transfer, exfoliant	176
Optical brighteners	Optical brightener	151
PaSSO3Ca	Glycosylation/melanosomal protein processing	177
Peroxidase inhibitors—methimazole	Inhibits mushroom tyrosinase and peroxidase	178
Piperlonguminine from *Piper longum*	Down-regulation of tyrosinase expression via microphthalmia-associated transcription factor	179
Proanthocyanidin polyphenolic antioxidant from grape seed extract	Inhibition of tyrosinase	180
Resorcinol	Desquamation, keratolytic	181
Resveratrol (component of red wine)	Reduce *MITF* and tyrosinase promoter activities	173
RW-50353	Inhibition of PAR-2 cleavage	49
Salicylic acid	Desquamation	182, 183
Soybean extract (STI/BBI)	Inhibition of PAR-2 cleavage	184
Tranexamic acid, 4-amino-methylcyclohexanecarboxylic acid	Inhibition of melanin synthesis	185

Abbreviations: DC, dopachrome; DHICA, dihydroxyindole carboxylic acid; PAR-2, proteinase-activated receptor 2; PaSSO3Ca, calcium pantetheine sulfonate; STI/BBI, soy tripsin inhibitor/Bowman-Birk trypsin inhibitor.

of melanin in the epidermis, resulting in darkening of the affected area. A plethora of both synthetic and natural actives have been used as skin lightening agents via topical application (Table 5). These agents function by targeting components of the melanin biosynthetic pathway to interfere with melanin production at various levels, including presynthesis by inhibition of transcription, trafficking of melanogenic proteins, inhibition of melanin synthesis and polymerization, melanosomes transfer, blocking of the protease-activated PAR-2 pathway, and altering the position of melanosomes by agents such as nicotinamide. Others achieve depigmentation by enhancing desquamation to accelerate epidermal renewal, for example, topical retinoic acid and α-hydroxy acids. The different approaches for depigmentation have been dealt with in recent reviews (149–151). Inhibition of melanin synthesis remains the most common approach to skin lightening. However, many of these inhibitors are ineffective in vivo, although they show potency in in vitro tests. The challenge of many of these agents targeting melanin synthesis has been their availability in the basal epidermis where the melanocytes reside and where they are most effective. However, increasing their levels in formulations is often associated with allergy or contact sensitivity. Another approach has been to use melanosome transfer inhibitors (e.g., protease inhibitors that block the protease activated PAR pathway). A third approach has been to alter the position of melanosomes in keratinocytes by use of cyclic adenosine monophosphate–modulating agents such as niacinamide. The use of enhanced delivery technologies such as liposomes or dendrimer molecules and a better understanding of the skin barrier functions will allow more efficacious strategies for cosmetic intervention of hyperpigmentation and superior skin lightening products.

Other novel skin lightening strategies involve the use of optical brighteners that work by diffusing light to reduce the visual perception of skin imperfections such as cellulite, shadows, skin discolorations, and wrinkles (186). Unfortunately, they often do not offer long-lasting effects and require repeat application. Congenital forms of hyperpigmentation, such as café-au-lait spots, where melanin is deposited in the dermis) do not respond well to topical treatments and requires laser therapy. However, melanin intermediates in the dermal layer may be effectively targeted via judicious selection of suitable depigmentation agents (30). Other approaches that have received little attention include the use of intrinsic/extrinsic melanin degrading agents that target the preformed protein-bound melanin that resides within the different layers of epidermal keratinocytes. Finally, because UV does cause inflammation and this biological response leads indirectly to pigmentation, anti inflammatory agents are being used to mitigate the effects of UV.

CONCLUSION

Despite the availability of many cosmetic products that claim to address skin pigmentation, many are either ineffective or are slow to achieve their desired outcome and fall short of consumer expectations. Part of the reason for such unmet consumer needs arises from a lack of a comprehensive understanding of the physiological parameters, besides melanin deposition, that contribute to the overall appearance of skin color. For example, we know little about how underlying skin structures in the epidermis and dermis affect skin surface topology and light reflectance or the role of hormones in skin physiology associated with age-related changes in pigmentation. There is also a paucity of biological insight into the etiology of pigmentation defects that are of most concern (e.g., age spots, melasma, uneven pigmentation). In addition, environmental factors such as exposure to sun and environmental pollutants also impinge on skin pigmentation. Differences in the way attractive skin color is perceived in different populations also adds to the challenge of how aesthetically appealing skin color can be cosmetically achieved.

REFERENCES

1. Diamond J. Evolutionary biology: geography and skin color. Nature 2000; 435:283–284.
2. Parichy DM. Evolution of danio pigment pattern development. Heredity 2006; 97: 200–210.
3. Szabo G. The number of melanocytes in human epidermis. Br Med J 1954; 1:1016–1017.
4. Riley PA. The evolution of melanogenesis. In: Zeise L, Chedekel MR and Fitzpatrick TB, eds. Melanin: Its Role in Human Photoprotection. Overland Park, Kan: Valdenmar Publishing, 1995:1–10.
5. Lavker RM, Kaidbey KH. Redistribution of melanosomal complexes within keratinocytes following UV-A irradiation: a possible mechanism for cutaneous darkening in man. Arch Dermatol Res 1982; 272:215–228.
6. Hong L, Simon JD, Sarna T. Melanin structure and the potential functions of uveal melanosomes. Pigment Cell Res 2006; 19:465–466.
7. Meredith P, Sarna T. The physical and chemical properties of eumelanin. Pigment Cell Res 2006; 19:572–594.
8. Orlow SJ. Melanosomes are specialized members of the lysosomal lineage of organelles. J Invest Dermatol 1995; 105:3–7.
9. Vijayasaradhi S, Xu Y, Bouchard B, et al. Intracellular sorting and targeting of melanosomal membrane proteins: identification of signals for sorting of the human brown locus protein, gp75. J Cell Biol 1995; 130:807–820.
10. Prota G. Melanins and Melanogenesis. New York: Academic Press, 1992.
11. Kushimoto T, Basrur V, Valencia J, et al. A model for melanosome biogenesis based on the purification and analysis of early melanosomes. Proc Natl Acad Sci USA 2001; 98:10698–10703.
12. Sharma S, Wagh S, Govindarajan R. Melanosomal proteins - role in melanin polymerization. Pigment Cell Res 2002; 15:127–133.
13. Basrur V, Yang F, Kushimoto T, et al. Proteomic analysis of early melanosomes: identification of novel melanosomal proteins. J Proteome Res 2003; 2:69–79.
14. Schiaffino MV, Tacchetti C. The ocular albinism type 1 (OA1) protein and the evidence for an intracellular signal transduction system involved in melanosome biogenesis. Pigment Cell Res 2005; 18:227–233.
15. Hunt G, Kyne S, Ito S, et al. Eumelanin and pheomelanin contents of human epidermis and cultured melanocytes. Pigment Cell Res 1995; 8:202–208.
16. Raper HS. The tyrosinase-tyrosine reaction: production from tyrosine of 5: 6-dihydroxyindole and 5: 6-dihydroxyindole-2-carboxylic acid — the precursors of melanin. Biochem J 1927; 21:89–96.
17. Mason HS. The chemistry of melanin. III. Mechanism of the oxidation of dihydroxyphenylalanine by tyrosinase. J Biol Chem 1948; 172:83–99.
18. Prota G. Progress in the chemistry of melanins and related metabolites. Med Res Rev 1988; 4:525–556.
19. Potterf SB, Muller J, Bernardini I, et al. Characterization of a melanosomal transport system in murine melanocytes mediating entry of the melanogenic substrate tyrosine. J Biol Chem 1996; 271:4002–4008.
20. Wang N, Herbert DN. Tyrosinase maturation through the mammalian secretory pathway: bringing color to life. Pigment Cell Res 2006; 19:3–18.
21. Gahl WA, Potterf B, Durham-Pierre D, et al. Melanosomal tyrosine transport in normal and pink-eyed dilution murine melanocytes. Pigment Cell Res 1995; 8:229–233.
22. Potterf SB, Virador V, Wakamatsu K, et al. Cysteine transport in melanosomes from murine melanocytes. Pigment Cell Res 1999; 12:4–12.

23. Chaubal VA, Nair SS, Mogador MV. Type I gamma-GT mRNA is expressed in B16 melanoma and levels correlate with pigmentation. Pigment Cell Res 2002; 15:367–372.
24. Chedekel, MR. Photophysics and photochemistry of melanin. In: Zeise L, Chedekel MR and Fitzpatrick TB, eds. Melanin: Its Role in Human Photoprotection. Overland Park, Kan: Valdenmar Publishing, 1995:11–23.
25. Pawelek JM, Platt J, Pugliese PT, et al. Enzymatic and non enzymatic synthesis of melanins. In: Zeise L, Chedekel MR and Fitzpatrick TB, eds. Melanin: Its Role in Human Photoprotection: Overland Park, Kan: Valdenmar Publishing, 1995:109–115.
26. Wagh S, Ramaiah A, Subramanian R, et al. Melanosomal proteins promote melanin polymerization. Pigment Cell Res 2000; 13:442–448.
27. Mani I, Sharma V, Tamboli I, et al. Interaction of melanin with proteins—the importance of an acidic intramelanosomal pH. Pigment Cell Res 2001; 14:170–179.
28. Devi CC, Tripathi RK, Ramaiah A. pH-dependent interconvertible allosteric forms of murine melanoma tyrosinase. Physiological implications. Eur J Biochem 1987; 166:705–711.
29. Liu Y, Simon JD. Metal-ion interactions and the structural organization of *Sepia* eumelanin. Pigment Cell Res 2005; 18:42–48.
30. Maeda K, Hatao M. Involvement of photooxidation of melanogenic precursors in prolonged pigmentation induced by ultraviolet A. J Invest Dermatol 2004; 122:503 –509.
31. Rogers SL, Tint IS, Fanapour PC, et al. Regulated bidirectional motility of melano-phore pigment granules along microtubules in vitro. Proc Natl Acad Sci USA 1997; 94:3720–3725.
32. Kashina A, Rodionov V. Intracellular organelle transport: few motors, many signals. Trends Cell Biol 2005; 15:396–398.
33. Mercer JA, Seperack PK, Strobel MC, et al. Novel myosin heavy chain encoded by murine dilute coat color locus. Nature 1991; 349:709–713.
34. Wilson SM, Yip R, Swing DA, et al. A mutation in Rab27a causes the vesicle transport defects observed in ashen mice. Proc Natl Acad Sci USA 2000; 97:7933–7938.
35. Matesic LE, Yip R, Reuss AE, et al. Mutations in Mlph, encoding a member of the Rab effector family, cause the melanosome transport defects observed in leaden mice. Proc Natl Acad Sci USA 2001; 98:10238–43.
36. Strom M, Hume AN, Tarafder AK, et al. A family of Rab27-binding proteins. J Biol Chem 2002; 277:25423–25430.
37. Fukuda M. Versatile role of Rab27 in membrane trafficking: focus on the Rab27 effector families. J Biochem (Tokyo) 2005; 137:9–16.
38. Pastural E, Ersoy F, Yalman N, et al. Two genes are responsible for Griscelli syndrome at the same 15q21 locus. Genomics 2000; 63:299–306.
39. Ménasché G, Ho CH, Sanal O, et al. Griscelli syndrome restricted to hypopigmentation results from a melanophilin defect (GS3) or a *MYO5A* F-exon deletion (GS1). J Clin Invest 2003; 112:450–456.
40. Gibbs D, Azarian SM, Lillo C, et al. Role of myosin VIIa and Rab27a in the motility and localization of RPE melanosomes. J Cell Sci 2004; 117:6473–6483.
41. Futter CE. The molecular regulation of organelle transport in mammalian retinal pigment epithelial cells. Pigment Cell Res 2006; 19:104–111.
42. Wolff K. Melanocyte-keratinocyte interactions in vivo: the fate of melanosomes. Yale J Biol Med 1973; 46:384–396.
43. Seiberg M. Keratinocyte-melanocyte interactions during melanosome transfer. Pigment Cell Res 2001; 14:236–242.
44. Van Den Bossche K, Naeyaert JM, Lambert J. The quest for the mechanism of melanin transfer. Traffic 2006; 7:769–778.
45. Yamamoto O, Bhawan J. Three modes of melanosome transfer in Caucasian facial skin: hypothesis based on an ultrastructural study. Pigment Cell Res 1994; 7:158–169.
46. Wolff K, Konrad K. Phagocytosis of latex beads by epidermal keratinocytes in vivo. J Ultrastruct Res 1972; 39:262–280.
47. Sharlow ER, Paine CS, Babiarz L, et al. The protease-activated receptor–2 upregulates keratinocyte phagocytosis. J Cell Sci 2000; 113:3093–3101.
48. Virador VM, Muller J, Wu X, et al. Influence of alpha-melanocyte–stimulating hormone and ultraviolet radiation on the transfer of melanosomes to keratinocytes. FASEB J 2002; 16:105–107.

49. Seiberg M, Paine C, Sharlow E, et al. The protease-activated receptor 2 regulates pigmentation via keratinocyte-melanocyte interactions. Exp Cell Res 2000; 254:25–32.
50. Seiberg M, Paine C, Sharlow E, et al. Inhibition of melanosome transfer results in skin lightening. J Invest Dermatol 2000; 115:162–167.
51. Wolff K, Honigsmann H. Are melanosome complexes lysosomes? J Invest Dermatol 1972; 59:170–176.
52. Mammone T, Marenus K, Muizzuddin N, et al. Evidence and utility of melanin degrading enzymes. J Cosmet Sci 2004; 55:116–117.
53. Schraermeyer U. Does melanin turnover occur in the eyes of adult vertebrates? Pigment Cell Res 1993; 6:193–204.
54. Borovansky J, Elleder M. Melanosome degradation: fact or fiction. Pigment Cell Res 2003; 16:280–286.
55. Barsh GS. What controls variation in human skin color? PLoS Biol 2003; 1:19–22.
56. Szabo G, Gerald AB, Pathak MA, et al. Racial differences in the fate of melanosomes in human epidermis. Nature 1969; 222:1081–1082.
57. Konrad K, Wolff K. Hyperpigmentation, melanosome size, and distribution patterns of melanosomes. Arch Dermatol 1973; 107:853–860.
58. Jimbow K, Fitzpatrick TB, Wick MM. Biochemistry and physiology of melanin pigmentation. In: Goldsmith SA, ed. Physiology, Biochemistry, and Molecular Biology of the Skin. 3rd ed. Vol. 2. New York: Oxford University Press, 1991:873–909.
59. Minwalla L, Zhao Y, Le Poole IC, et al. Keratinocytes play a role in regulating distribution patterns of recipient melanosomes in vitro. J Invest Dermatol 2001; 117:341–347.
60. Alaluf S, Atkins D, Barrett K, et al. Ethnic variation in melanin content and composition in photoexposed and photoprotected human skin. Pigment Cell Res 2002; 15:112–118.
61. Thong HY, Jee SH, Sun CC, et al. The patterns of melanosome distribution in keratinocytes of human skin as one determining factor of skin color. Br J Dermatol 2003; 149:498–505.
62. Honigsmann H, Schuler G, Aberer W, et al. Immediate pigment darkening phenomenon. A reevaluation of its mechanisms. J Invest Dermatol 1986; 87:648–652.
63. Sturm RA, Teasdale RD, Box NF. Human pigmentation genes: identification, structure and consequences of polymorphic variation. Gene 2001; 277:49–62.
64. Bennett DC, Lamoreux ML. The Color Loci of Mice—A Genetic Century. Pigment Cell Res 2003; 16:333–344.
65. Oetting WS, Bennett DC. Mouse Coat Color Genes. International Federation of Pigment Cell Societies, April 6, 2006. (Accessed October 5, 2007, at www.ifpcs.umn.edu/micemut .htm.)
66. Oetting WS. Albinism Database. International Albinism Center, University of Minnesota, April 6, 2004. (Accessed October 5, 2007, at www.albinismdb.med.umn.edu/.)
67. Valverde P, Healy E, Jackson I, et al. Variants of the melanocyte-stimulating hormone receptor gene are associated with red hair and fair skin in humans. Nature Genet 1995; 11:328–330.
68. Makova K, Norton H. Worldwide polymorphism at the MC1R locus and normal pigmentation variation in humans. Peptides 2005; 26:1901–1908.
69. Rana BK, Hewett-Emmett D, Jin L, et al. High polymorphism at the human melanocortin 1 receptor locus. Genetics 1999; 151:1547–1557.
70. Harding RM, Healy E, Ray AJ, et al. Evidence for variable selective pressures at MC1R. Am J Hum Genet 2000; 66:1351–1361.
71. Makova KD, Ramsay M, Jenkins T, et al. Human DNA sequence variation in a 6.6-kb region containing the melanocortin 1 receptor promoter. Genetics 2001; 158:1253–1268.
72. Smith AG, Box NF, Marks LH, et al. The human melanocortin-1 receptor locus: analysis of transcription unit, locus polymorphism and haplotype evolution. Gene 2001; 281:81–94.
73. Shriver MD, Parra EJ, Dios S, et al. Skin pigmentation, biogeographical ancestry and admixture mapping. Hum Genet 2003; 112:387–399.
74. Yuasa I, Umetsu K, Watanabe G, et al. MATP polymorphisms in Germans and Japanese: the L374F mutation as a population marker for Caucasoids. Int J Legal Med 2004; 118:364–366.
75. http://ifpcs.med.umn.edu/micemut.htm.
76. Levy C, Khaled, Fisher DE. MITF: master regulator of melanocyte development and melanoma oncogene. Trends Mol Med 2006; 12:406–414.

77. Hodgkinson CA, Moore KJ, Nakayama A, et al. Mutations at the mouse microphthalmia locus are associated with defects in a gene encoding a novel basic-helix-loop-helix-zipper protein. Cell 1993; 74:395–404.
78. Amae S, Fuse N, Yasumoto K, et al. Identification of a novel isoform of microphthalmia-associated transcription factor that is enriched in retinal pigment epithelium. Biochem Biophys Res Commun 1998; 247:710–715.
79. Takeda K, Shibahara S. Transcriptional regulation of melanocyte function. In: Nordlund JJ, Boissy RE, Hearing VJ, King RA, Oetting WS, Ortonne JP, eds. The Pigmentary System. 2nd ed. Malton, MA: Blackwell Publishing, 2006:242–260.
80. Hughes AE, Newton VE, Liu XZ, et al. A gene for Waardenburg syndrome type 2 maps close to the human homologue of the microphthalmia gene at chromosome 3p12-p14.1. Nat Genet 1994; 4:509–512.
81. Tassabehji M, Newton VE, Read AP. Waardenburg syndrome type 2 caused by mutations in the human microphthalmia (MITF) gene. Nat Genet 1994; 8:251–255.
82. Lamason RL, Mohideen MA, Mest JR, et al. SLC24A5, a putative cation exchanger, affects pigmentation in zebrafish and humans. Science 2005; 310:1782–1786.
83. Irwin C, Barnes A, Veres D, et al. An ultraviolet radiation action spectrum for immediate pigment darkening. Photochem Photobiol 1993; 57:504–507.
84. Routaboul C, Denis A, Vinche A. Immediate pigment darkening: description, kinetic and biological function. Eur J Dermatol 1999; 9:95–99.
85. Ou-Yang H, Stamatas G, Kollias N. Spectral responses of melanin to ultraviolet A irradiation. J Invest Dermatol 2004; 122:492–496.
86. Parrish JA, Jaenicke KF, Anderson RR. Erythema and melanogenesis action spectra of normal human skin. Photochem Photobiol 1982; 36:187–191.
87. Tadokoro T, Kobayashi N, Zmudzka BZ, et al. UV-induced DNA damage and melanin content in human skin differing in racial/ethnic origin and photosensitivity. FASEB J 2003; 17:1177–1179.
88. Tadokoro T, Yamaguchi Y, Batzer J, et al. Mechanisms of skin tanning in different racial/ethnic groups in response to ultraviolet radiation. J Invest Dermatol 2005; 124:1326–1332.
89. Auletta M, Gange RW, Tan OT, et al. Effect of cutaneous hypoxia upon erythema and pigment responses to UVA, UVB, and PUVA (8-MOP+UVA) in human skin. J Invest Dermatol 1986; 86:649–652.
90. Wakamatsu K, Ito S. Evaluation of melanin-related metabolites as markers of solar ultraviolet-B radiation. Pigment Cell Res 2006; 19:460–464.
91. Coelho SG, Miller SA, Zmudzka BZ, et al. Quantification of UV-induced erythema and pigmentation using computer-assisted digital image evaluation. Photochem Photobiol 2006; 82:651–655.
92. Miller SA, Coelho SG, Zmudzka BZ, et al. Reduction of the UV burden to indoor tanners through new exposure schedules: a pilot study. Photodermatol Photoimmunol Photomed 2006; 22:59–66.
93. Bancroft JD, Stevens A. Theory and Practice of Histological Techniques. Edinburgh, UK: Churchill Livingstone, 1982.
94. Fitzpatrick TB. The validity and practicality of sun-reactive skin types I through VI. Arch Dermatol 1988; 124:869–871.
95. Slominski A, Tobin DJ, Shibahara S, et al. Melanin pigmentation in mammalian skin and its hormonal regulation. Physiol Rev 2004; 84:1155–228.
96. Suzuki I, Im S, Tada A, et al. Participation of the melanocortin-1 receptor in the UV control of pigmentation. J Invest Dermatol Symp Proc 1999; 4:29–34.
97. Rouzaud F, Kadekaro AL, Abdel-Malek ZA, et al. MC1R and the response of melanocytes to ultraviolet radiation. Mutat Res 2005; 571:133–152.
98. Edwards EA, Hamilton JB, Duntley SQ, et al. Cutaneous vascular and pigmentary changes in castrate and eunuchoid men. Endocrinology 1941; 28:119–128.
99. Shah MG, Maibach HI. Estrogen and skin. An overview. Am J Clin Dermatol 2001; 2:143–150.
100. McElhinney DB, Hoffman SJ, Robinson WA, et al. Effect of melatonin on human skin color. J Invest Dermatol 1994; 102:258–259.
101. Nordlund JJ, Lerner AB. The effects of oral melatonin on skin color and on the release of pituitary hormones. J Clin Endocrinol Metab 1977; 45:768–774.

102. Abdel-Malek Z, Swope V, Collins C, et al. Contribution of melanogenic proteins to the heterogeneous pigmentation of human melanocytes. J Cell Sci 1993; 106:1323–1331.

103. Scott G, Jacobs S, Leopardi S, et al. Effects of PGF2alpha on human melanocytes and regulation of the FP receptor by ultraviolet radiation. Exp Cell Res 2005; 304:407–416.

104. Hirobe T. Role of keratinocyte-derived factors involved in regulating the proliferation and differentiation of mammalian epidermal melanocytes. Pigment Cell Res 2005; 18:2–12.

105. Lerner AB, Moellmann G, Varga VL, et al. Action of melanocyte-stimulating hormone on pigment cells. Cold Spring Harbor Conf Cell Prolif 1979; 6:187–197.

106. Eller MS, Ostrom K, Gilchrest BA. DNA damage enhances melanogenesis. Proc Natl Acad Sci USA 1996; 93:1087–1092.

107. Gilchrest BA, Park HY, Eller MS, et al. Mechanisms of ultraviolet light-induced pigmentation. Photochem Photobiol 1996; 63:1–10.

108. Swope VB, Abdel-Malek Z, Kassem LM, et al. Interleukins 1 alpha and 6 and tumor necrosis factor-alpha are paracrine inhibitors of human melanocyte proliferation and melanogenesis. J Invest Dermatol 1991; 96:180–185.

109. Chakraborty AK, Funasaka Y, Slominski A, et al. Production and release of proopiomelanocortin (POMC) derived peptides by human melanocytes and keratinocytes in culture: regulation by ultraviolet B. Biochim Biophys Acta 1996; 1313:130–138.

110. Halaban R, Langdon R, Birchall N, et al. Basic fibroblast growth factor from human keratinocytes is a natural mitogen for melanocytes. J Cell Biol 1988; 107:1611–1619.

111. Yaar M, Grossman K, Eller M, et al. Evidence for nerve growth factor-mediated paracrine effects in human epidermis. J Cell Biol 1991; 115:821–828.

112. Imokawa G, Yada Y, Miyagishi M. Endothelins secreted from human keratinocytes are intrinsic mitogens for human melanocytes. J Biol Chem 1992; 267:24675–24680.

113. Imokawa G, Yada Y, Kimura M, et al. Granulocyte/macrophage colony-stimulating factor is an intrinsic keratinocyte-derived growth factor for human melanocytes in UVAinduced melanosis. Biochem J 1996; 313:625–631.

114. Hachiya A, Kobayashi A, Ohuchi A, et al. The paracrine role of stem cell factor/c-kit signaling in the activation of human melanocytes in ultraviolet-B–induced pigmentation. J Invest Dermatol 2001; 116:578–586.

115. Scott G, Leopardi S, Printup S, et al. Proteinase-activated receptor–2 stimulates prostaglandin production in keratinocytes: analysis of prostaglandin receptors on human melanocytes and effects of PGE2 and PGF2a on melanocyte dendricity. J Invest Dermatol 2004; 122:1214–1224.

116. Tsatmali M, Ancans J, Yukitake J, et al. Skin POMC peptides: their actions at the human MC-1 receptor and roles in the tanning response. Pigment Cell Res 2000; 13(Suppl. 8): 125–129.

117. Weller R. Nitric oxide: a key mediator in cutaneous physiology. Clin Exp Dermatol 2003; 28:511–514.

118. Lasalle MW, Igarashi S, Sasaki M, et al. Effects of melanogenesis-inducing nitric oxide and histamine on the production of eumelanin and pheomelanin in cultured human melanocytes. Pigment Cell Res 2003; 16:81–84.

119. Nordlund JJ. The lives of pigment cells. Dermatol Clin 1986; 4:407–418.

120. Montagna W, Carlisle K. Structural changes in ageing skin. Br J Dermatol 1990;122(Suppl.35): 61–70.

121. Nishimura EK, Granter SR, Fisher DE. Mechanisms of hair graying: incomplete melanocyte stem cell maintenance in the niche. Science 2005; 307:720–724.

122. Takema Y, Yorimoto Y, Kawai M, et al. Age-related changes in the elastic properties and thickness of human facial skin. Br J Dermatol 1994; 131:641–648.

123. Schwahn DJ, Xu W, Herrin AB, et al. Tyrosine levels regulate the melanogenic response to alpha-melanocyte–stimulating hormone in human melanocytes: implications for pigmentation and proliferation. Pigment Cell Res 2001; 14:32–39.

124. Alaluf S, Heinrich U, Stahl W, et al. Dietary carotenoids contribute to normal human skin color and UV photosensitivity. J Nutr 2002; 132:399–403.

125. Dereure O. Drug-induced skin pigmentation. Epidemiology, diagnosis and treatment. Am J Clin Dermatol 2001; 2:253–262.

126. Noblesse E, Nizard C, Cario-Andre M, et al. Skin ultrastructure in senile lentigo. Skin Pharmacol Physiol 2006; 19:95–100.
127. Kollias N, Sayre RM, Zeise L, et al. Photoprotection by melanin. J Photochem Photobiol B 1991; 9:135–160.
128. Scotto J, Fraumeni JF Jr. Skin (other than melanoma). In: Schottenfeld D, Fraumeni JF Jr, eds. Cancer Epidemiology and Prevention. Philadelphia: W.B. Saunders, 1982.
129. Chadwick CA, Potten CS, Nikaido O, et al. The detection of cyclobutane thymine immers, (6-4) photolesions and the Dewar photoisomers in sections of UV-irradiated human skin using specific antibodies, and the demonstration of depth penetration effects. J Photochem Photobiol B 1995; 28:163–170.
130. Young AR, Chadwick CA, Harrison GI, et al. The similarity of action spectra for thymine immers in human epidermis and erythema suggests that DNA is the chromophore for erythema. J Invest Dermatol 1998; 111:982–988.
131. Crowley DJ, Hanawalt PC. Induction of the SOS response increases the efficiency of global nucleotide excision repair of cyclobutane pyrimidine immers, but not 6-4 photoproducts, in UV-irradiated *Escherichia coli*. J Bacteriol 1998; 180:3345–3352.
132. Eller MS, Gilchrest BA. Tanning as part of eukaryotic SOS response. Pigment Cell Res 2000; 13(Suppl. 8):94–97.
133. Im S, Lee S, Hann SK, et al. The ultraviolet B protection effects of topically applied melanosomes onto human skin. Yonsei Med J 1991; 32:330–334.
134. Agar N, Young AR. Melanogenesis: a photoprotective response to DNA damage? Mutat Res 2005; 571:121–132.
135. Takeuchi S, Zhang W, Wakamatsu K, et al. Melanin acts as a potent UVB photosensitizer to cause an atypical mode of cell death in murine skin. Proc Natl Acad Sci USA 2004; 101:15076–15081.
136. Eller MS, Yaar M, Gilchrest BA. DNA damage and melanogenesis. Nature 1994; 372:413–414.
137. Pedeux R, Al-Irani N, Marteau C, et al. Thymidine dinucleotides induce S phase cell cycle arrest in addition to increased melanogenesis in human melanocytes. J Invest Dermatol 1998; 111:472–477.
138. Eller MS, Maeda T, Magnoni C, et al. Enhancement of DNA repair in human skin cells by thymidine dinucleotides: evidence for a p53-mediated mammalian SOS response. Proc Natl Acad Sci USA 1997; 94:12627–12632.
139. Khlgatian MK, Hadshiew IM, Asawanonda P, et al. Tyrosinase gene expression is regulated by p53. J Invest Dermatol 2002; 118:126–132.
140. Gilchrest BA, Eller MS. DNA photodamage stimulates melanogenesis and other photoprotective responses. J Investig Dermatol Symp Proc 1999; 4:35–40.
141. Maibach HI, Kligman AM. Dihydroxyacetone: a suntan simulating agent. Arch Dermatol 1960; 82:505–507.
142. Simpson GL, Ortwerth BJ. The non-oxidative degradation of ascorbic acid at physiological conditions. Biochim Biophys Acta 2000; 1501:12–24.
143. Faurschou A, Wulf HC. Durability of the sun protection factor provided by dihydroxy-acetone. Photodermatol Photoimmunol Photomed 2004; 20:239–242.
144. Brooks K, Brooks D, Dajani Z, et al. Use of artificial tanning products among young adults. J Am Acad Dermatol 2006; 54:1060–1066.
145. Petersen AB, Wulf HC, Gniadecki R, et al. Dihydroxyacetone, the active browning ingredient in sunless tanning lotions, induces DNA damage, cell-cycle block and apoptosis in cultured HaCaT keratinocytes. Mutat Res 2004; 560:173–86.
146. Pawelek JM. Approaches to increasing skin melanin with MSH analogs and synthetic melanins. Pigment Cell Res 2001; 14:155–160.
147. Levine N, Sheftel SN, Eytan T, et al. Induction of skin tanning by subcutaneous administration of a potent synthetic melanotropin. JAMA 1991; 266:2730–2736.
148. Barnetson RS, Ooi TK, Zhuang L, et al. [Nle4-D-Phe7]-alpha-melanocyte–stimulating hormone significantly increased pigmentation and decreased UV damage in fair-skinned Caucasian volunteers. J Invest Dermatol 2006; 126:1869–1878.
149. Briganti S, Camera E, Picardo M. Chemical and instrumental approaches to treat hyper-pigmentation. Pigment Cell Res 2003; 16:101–110.

150. Parvez S, Kang M, Chung HS, et al. Survey and mechanism of skin depigmenting and lightening agents. Phytother Res 2006; 20:921–934.
151. Solano F, Briganti S, Picardo M, et al. Hypopigmenting agents: an updated review on biological, chemical and clinical aspects. Pigment Cell Res 2006; 19:550–571.
152. Dooley TP, Gadwood RC, Kilgore K, et al. Development of an in vitro primary screen for skin depigmentation and antimelanoma agents. Skin Pharmacol 1994; 7:188–200.
153. Nair X, Parah P, Suhr L, et al. Combination of 4-hydroxyanisole and all trans retinoic acid produces synergistic skin depigmentation in swine. J Invest Dermatol 1993; 101:145–149.
154. Kimbrough-Green CK, Griffiths CE, Finkel LJ, et al. Topical retinoic acid (tretinoin) for melasma in black patients. A vehicle-controlled clinical trial. Arch Dermatol 1994; 30:727–733.
155. Griffiths CE, Finkel LJ, Ditre CM, et al. Topical tretinoin (retinoic acid) improves melasma. A vehicle-controlled, clinical trial. Br J Dermatol 1993; 129:415–421.
156. Piao LZ, Park HR, Park YK, et al. Mushroom tyrosinase inhibition activity of some chromones. Chem Pharm Bull Tokyo 2002; 50:309–311.
157. Jones K, Hughes J, Hong M, et al. Modulation of melanogenesis by aloesin: a competitive inhibitor of tyrosinase. Pigment Cell Res 2002; 15:335–340.
158. Smith W. The effects of topical L (+) lactic acid and ascorbic acid on skin whitening. Int J Cosmetic Sci 1999; 21:33–40.
159. Marmol VD, Solano F, Sels A, et al. Glutathione depletion increases tyrosinase activity in human melanoma cells. J Invest Dermatol 1993; 101:871–874.
160. Chakraborty AK, Funasaka Y, Komoto M, et al. Effect of arbutin on melanogenic proteins in human melanocytes. Pigment Cell Res 1998; 11:206–212.
161. Boissy RE, Visscher M, DeLong MA. DeoxyArbutin: a novel reversible tyrosinase inhibitor with effective in vivo skin lightening potency. Exp Dermatol 2005; 8:601–608.
162. Sarkar R, Bhalla M, Kanwar AJ. A comparative study of 20% azelaic acid cream monotherapy versus a sequential therapy in the treatment of melasma in dark-skinned patients. Dermatology 2002; 205:249–254.
163. Kim DS, Kim SY, Chung JH, et al. Delayed ERK activation by ceramide reduces melanin synthesis in human melanocytes. Cell Signal 2002; 14:779–785.
164. Skin color improver. Kao Corporation, Japan. European Patent 0904772, 1999.
165. Shimogaki H, Tanaka Y, Tamai H, et al. In vitro and in vivo evaluation of ellagic acid on melanogenesis inhibition. Int J Cosmetic Sci 2000; 22:291–303.
166. Palumbo A, d'Ischia M, Misuraca G, et al. Mechanism of inhibition of melanogenesis by hydroquinone. Biochim Biophys Acta 1991; 23:85–90.
167. Composition and method to whiten skin. Kao Corporation, Japan. U.S. Patent 7025957, 2004.
168. Kahn V. Effect of kojic acid on the oxidation of DL-DOPA, norepinephrine, and dopamine by mushroom tyrosinase. Pigment Cell Res 1995; 8:234–240.
169. Gukasyan GS. Study of the kinetics of oxidation of monophenols by tyrosinase. The effect of reducers. Biochemistry (Mosc) 2002; 67:277–280.
170. Ros JR, Rodriguez-Lopes JN, Garcia-Canovas F. Effect of L-ascorbic acid on the monophelase activity of tyrosinase. Biochem J 1993; 295:309–312.
171. Yokota T, Nishio H, Kubota Y, et al. The inhibitory effect of glabridin from liquorice extracts on melanogenesis and inflammation. Pigment Cell Res 1998; 11:355–361.
172. Methods of producing lignin peroxidase and its use in skin and hair lightening. Kao Corporation, Japan. U.S. Patent 20060051305, 2006.
173. Ando H, Ryu A, Hashimoto A, et al. Linoleic and a-linolenic acids lighten UV-induced hyperpigmentation of the skin. Arch Dermatol Res 1998; 290:375–381.
174. Lin CB, Babiarz L, Liebel F, et al. Modulation of microphthalmia-associated transcription factor gene expression alters skin pigmentation. J Invest Dermatol 2002; 119:1330–1340.
175. Nakajima M, Shinoda I, Samejima Y, et al. κ- suppresses melanogenesis in cultured pigment cells. Pigment Cell Res 1996; 9:235–239.
176. Hakozaki T, Minwalla L, Zhuang J, et al. The effect of niacinamide on reducing cutaneous pigmentation and suppression of melanosome transfer. Br J Dermatol 2002; 147:20–31.
177. Franchi J. Depigmenting effects of calcium D-pantetheine-S-sulfonate on human melanocytes. Pigment Cell Res 2000; 13:165–171.

178. Kasraee K. Depigmentation of brown guinea pig skin by topical application of methimazole. J Invest Dermatol 2002; 118:205–207.
179. Kim KS, Kim JA, Eom SY, et al. Inhibitory effect of piperlonguminine on melanin production in melanoma B16 cell line by downregulation of tyrosinase expression. Pigment Cell Res 2006; 19:90–98.
180. Yamakoshi J, Otsuka F, Sano A, et al. Lightening effect on ultraviolet-induced pigmentation of guinea pig skin by oral administration of a proanthocyanidin-rich extract from grape seeds. Pigment Cell Res 2003; 16:629–638.
181. Shimizu K, Kondo R, Sakai K, et al. Novel vitamin E derivative with 4-substituted resorcinol moiety has both antioxidant and tyrosinase inhibitory properties. Lipids 2001; 36:1321–1326.
182. Swinehart JM. Salicylic acid ointment peeling of the hands and forearms. Effective nonsurgical removal of pigmented lesions and actinic damage. J Dermatol Surg Oncol 1992; 18:495–498.
183. Grimes PE. The safety and efficacy of salicylic acid chemical peels in darker racial-ethnic groups. Dermatol Surg 1999; 25:18–22.
184. Paine C, Sharlow E, Liebel F, et al. An alternative approach to depigmentation by soybean extracts via inhibition of the PAR-2 pathway. J Invest Dermatol 2001; 116:587–595.
185. Maeda K, Naganuma M. Topical *trans*-4-aminomethylcyclohexanecarboxylic acid present ultraviolet radiation-induced pigmentation. J Photochem Photobiol 1998; 47:136–141.
186. Optical brightener as a bleaching agent. Japanese Patent 2006206602, 2006.

Evidence-Based Cosmeceutical Therapy

Maria Miteva
Skin Physiology Laboratory, Department of Dermatology, Friedrich Schiller University of Jena, Jena, Germany

Joachim W. Fluhr
Skin Physiology Laboratory, Department of Dermatology, Friedrich Schiller University of Jena, Jena and Bioskin, Berlin, Germany

UNDERSTANDING THE SKIN BARRIER FUNCTION

The stratum corneum (SC), the outer permeability barrier of the skin, is continuously exposed to physical and chemical agents from the environment. As a highly specialized structure, it is essentially impermeable to water, except for a small but vital flux serving to maintain its hydration and flexibility (1). As discussed in Chapters 7 and 24 of this volume, the SC is a very resilient tissue. The physical barrier to permeation through the skin, located in the SC, is primarily a function of the long-chain lamellar lipids that fill the intercellular space between the corneocytes. To account for such barrier properties and for the hydrophilic and hydrophobic pathways through the skin barrier, an alternative model to the "brick-and-mortar" model, the domain mosaic model, has been proposed (2). This model envisages the barrier lipids as existing predominantly in crystalline domains, surrounded by grain borders of lipids in a liquid crystalline state. The latter provide an effective barrier that allows a small, but controlled, water loss through the liquid interdomains, which is sufficient to keep the SC keratin hydrated. Perturbation in the barrier due to the use of organic solvents, detergents, or mechanical abrogation leads to an altered water flux and initiates a cascade of events within the underlying epidermis to promote barrier recovery. The principal response to minor repeated or severe barrier disruption comprises a temporary increase in the biosynthesis of all major lipid species in the epidermis, enhanced cytokine production, inflammatory events involving the deeper layers of the skin and the endothelium, epidermal hyperplasia, and abnormal keratinization.

RISK FACTORS FOR CUTANEOUS DAMAGE: WHAT SHOULD THE SKIN BE "AWARE OF"?

Sunlight, coupled with living in an oxygen-rich atmosphere, causes unwanted and deleterious stresses on skin (3). Photoaging (extrinsic skin aging) is a term coined to describe the changes in the skin as a result of the superposition of chronic sun damage upon intrinsic (chronologic) aging. The most severe consequence of photodamage is skin cancer, whereas less severe impacts result in wrinkling, scaling, roughness and dryness of the skin, and mottled hypopigmentation/hyperpigmentation.

Recently, experimental studies brought about advances in understanding the immediate cellular responses and functional abnormalities of photoaged skin (4–7). In general, chronically irradiated skin is metabolically hyperactive, thus giving rise to epidermal hyperplasia and neoplasia, increased production of elastic fibers (solar elastosis), accelerated breakdown and synthesis of collagen, and enhanced inflammatory processes (8). Initially, UV radiation (UVR) is absorbed by skin-specific chromophores (nucleic acids, and proteins), whereupon photoproducts between adjacent pyrimidine bases on one strand of DNA are created. The latter account for the blockage of the RNA transcription mechanisms and the activation of the p53 protein, which in cases of overwhelming DNA damage induces direct apoptosis of the irradiated keratinocytes (6, 9). In the surviving cells, the primary response to the DNA photodamage is the repair of the photolesions by means of nucleotide excision repair. If a mutation occurs in the p53 gene, the keratinocytes may lose their ability to undergo cell death upon high-dose UVR exposure and lead to further clonal expansion, resulting in actinic keratoses, squamous cell, or basal cell carcinoma. In addition to the direct effects of UVR on DNA, the generation of reactive oxygen species through endogenous photosensitization of intracellular chromophores represents another crucial mechanism of immediate and chronic photodamage. Neutrophils are generally increased in photodamaged skin and produce superoxide anion and hydrogen peroxide, thus contributing further to the load of reactive oxygen species in photoaging (10,11). Hence, damage to DNA with supervening mutagenesis seems to be the major consequence of UV-induced oxidative reaction. The oxidative stress further activates metalloproteinases and mitogen-activated protein kinases and stimulates the expression and secretion of cytokines. Degradation of the collagen framework and inhibition of the procollagen synthesis as well as modification of the cellular proteins and lipids occur. The chronic accumulation of such deviated cell components may result in tissue aging.

Because of its location at the interface between body and environment, SC is frequently and directly exposed not only to UVR but also to other outside forces such as air pollutants, chemical oxidants, smoking, and microorganisms (12,13). Because the integrity of the SC lipids and proteins play a key role in maintaining an adequate barrier function, the protection of the latter from harmful oxidation is the primary objective of a network of cellular enzymatic and nonenzymatic antioxidants, which keep oxidative damage to cells at a minimum (3). In times of increased oxidative stress, however, the protective control may be insufficient, and oxidative damage may occur. Free radicals (superoxide anion, peroxyl, and hydroxyl radicals) are considered the most relevant oxidative "aggressors" because they are extremely chemically reactive and short-lived and react instantaneously. Other reactive molecules (molecular oxygen, singlet oxygen, and hydrogen peroxide), although not free radicals per se, can also initiate oxidative reactions and generate free radical species (3). It has been suggested that vitamin E (α-tocopherol) is the most important lipid-soluble antioxidant in human tissues, because apart from its defence against lipid peroxidation, it is considered necessary to stabilize lipid bilayers, SC lipid bilayers particularly (13). The highest levels of α-tocopherol have been detected in the lower SC with sharply decreasing concentrations toward the skin surface. In analogy, the concentrations of ascorbate within SC show a 10-fold increase while tracing down to its lower parts. Similar gradients have been established for other antioxidants (glutathione and uric acid) in experimental mouse models (14). Because the outer layers of the SC are more susceptible to lipid/protein oxidation, direct topical delivery of antioxidants aimed to enrich the physiological reservoir is desirable.

Apart from natural (photo)aging, daily manipulations such as regular skin cleansing with soaps and detergents create another exogenous mechanism for barrier damage. The aim of a washing process is to remove or reduce dust particles, microorganisms, and odorous substances (15,16). The resident skin flora can be significantly reduced by a washing process. The antiseptic effect of washing is gained independently from the function of soaps and detergents through the removal of dust and dandruff material from the skin and as well as reduction of bacteria. The surfactants in modern cleansing products are anionics, nonionics, and amphoterics, each with a specific active profile (17). The dermatological effects of surfactants on skin can be attributed to four fundamental mechanisms affecting barrier homeostasis of the skin and other physiological factors: (1) adsorption to skin surface, (2) removal of skin components, (3) penetration into deeper skin layers, and (4) cytotoxic effects on living cells in the epidermis. Hence, there is a broad variety of parameters that may be affected by surfactant or surfactant-containing formulations (17). Shortly after the application of a dilute surfactant solution, a SC swelling occurs. The water uptake can be detected from zero to 15 minutes after washing by measuring SC hydration (18). However, after long-term application of surfactants, a reversed effect occurs, namely dehydration of the SC. Ultrastructural studies after long-duration exposure and repetitive exposure for three days to surfactant-containing formulations (sodium lauryl sulfate, SLS) have revealed damage to the nucleated epidermis and alterations in the lower parts of the SC. At this level, the extrusion and transformation of lamellar body–derived lipids into lamellar bilayers are disrupted. However, the upper portions of the SC display intact intercellular lipid layers contradicting the long-standing belief that surfactants damage the skin by delipidization (19). Particularly, the effect of surfactants on the surface lipids of the skin damages the epidermal barrier function, especially on predamaged skin. Hence, the washing procedure is of particular importance to patients who, per se, have reduced barrier lipids, impaired barrier function, and lower SC water content (e.g., persons with atopic dermatitis or dry/sensitive skin) (20–22). Sensitive skin is considered a special condition in which there is reduced tolerance and high incidences of adverse reactions to frequent or prolonged use of cosmetic products. Therefore, individuals with sensitive skin should change their washing behavior and use mild acidic cleansing products (23). Recently, it was shown that an acidic SC pH is crucial for maintaining barrier homeostasis and SC integrity (24,25).

COSMECEUTICALS—DEFINITIONS AND REGULATIONS

Cosmeceuticals are considered to be the fastest growing segment of natural personal care industry (26,27). Variability of interpretations and definitions of cosmeceuticals and related products exist, most of them, although overlapping, implicate new hues in the correct understanding of this concept (see Chapter 1). According to the U.S. Federal Food, Drug, and Cosmetic Act, a cosmetic is defined as "an article intended to be rubbed, poured, sprinkled, sprayed on, introduced into or otherwise applied to the human body or any part thereof for cleansing, beautifying, promoting attractiveness or altering the appearance." A drug, on the other hand, is defined as an article "intended for use in the diagnosis, cure, mitigation, treatment, or prevention of disease in man." In 1938, the U.S. Congress enacted a statute that officially defined cosmetics and drugs in specific terms: formal criteria were set for classifying a product as either a drug or a cosmetic. No intermediate category was countenanced, and this remains the law (28). According to Kligman, who first coined the term cosmeceutical some 20 years ago, the term "recognizes the new realities of skin care products, emphasizing their functional aspects" (28). Lavrijsen and Vermeer (29) also noted that a separate group of products were neither pure drugs nor cosmetics and should be called cosmeceutics. They suggested that products intended for use in traditional cosmetic indications, with little pharmaceutical activity and potential side effects, should be termed cosmeceuticals. Further, the efficacy of such products should be verified in well-defined studies, the requirements of which should be as strict as those for the assessment of drugs.

Presently, no Food and Drug Administration (FDA) definition of cosmeceutical exists since it is not a category recognized by this organization. In general, cosmeceuticals are cosmetic products claimed or proven to have biologic activity (30). Variations on the theme cosmeceuticals sometimes render abstract definitions such as "a marriage between cosmetics and pharmaceuticals," "cosmetic-pharmaceutical hybrids intended to enhance beauty through ingredients providing additional health-related function or benefit," "a catchword for in-between, drug-like miracle products," "quasi-drugs," and so forth. In reality, cosmeceuticals are mainly designed to address the major causes of skin aging—photodamage and oxidative stress.

Cosmetics are not regulated by the FDA; they do not require testing or approval because they are not considered to have biologic activities. Discovering biologic activity in an ingredient automatically reclassifies the product as a drug, which, in turn, demands many expensive and time-consuming premarket studies (30). Therefore, a great number of cosmetic companies do not test the ingredients in their products for pharmacological activity to avoid the oversight of federal and European law. Hence, such products fall outside the regulations of existing classifications, especially if the manufacturer or distributor is guarded on label claims (31). Unfortunately, the efficacy of new emerging cosmeceutical ingredients has not been sufficiently proven in appropriate clinical study settings.

To cope with the steadily increasing number of cosmeceutical ingredients, Kligman has offered the following guidance to the dermatologist (32): (1) Can the active ingredient penetrate the SC and be delivered in sufficient concentrations to its intended target in the skin over a time course consistent with its mechanism of action? (2) Does the active ingredient have a specific biochemical mechanism of action in the target cell or tissue in human skin? (3) Are there published, peer-reviewed, double-blinded, placebo-controlled, statistically significant clinical trials to substantiate the efficacy claims? Otherwise summarized, the desirable features any cosmeceutical agent is supposed to fulfill are efficacy, safety, formulation stability, novelty, patent protection, metabolism within skin, and inexpensive manufacture (27). Evidence-based product claims are always recommendable.

SUITABLE COSMETIC VEHICLES

Skin delivery of dermatological drugs depends considerably on the vehicles with which they are applied, which may either enhance or retard penetration. Updated knowledge of the clinical effects of cosmetic vehicles on skin may provide further understanding of how cosmeceuticals function. Cosmeceutical moisturizers, which go beyond moisturizing because of their additional benefits, are the most common over-the-counter product.

Different therapeutic and physiological functions of cosmetic vehicles are well recognized and have been recently reviewed (33). Research has shown that the composition of cosmetic vehicles is of great importance for the specific treatment of some skin diseases because the vehicle is no longer considered simply as a drug carrier or delivery system but rather as an essential component of successful topical treatment. Thus, adapting the type and composition of cosmetic vehicles, either as adjuvant treatment [e.g., ceramide-dominant barrier-repair mixture in atopic dermatitis (34)] or as a delivery system according to the disease status, is a modern pharmacological approach. Vehicles for dermatological and cosmetic uses can be divided into different classes according to their composition (Fig. 1), although the classification of commercially available products is often difficult or impossible based solely upon product labeling.

Dermatological and cosmetic vehicles exert number of effects, in and on the skin, including skin hydration, skin cooling, and barrier effect (33). The relative cooling effect can be attributed to the amount of water and/or alcohol in the emulsion system(s) and to water "activity," more precisely, the amount of freely evaporating water that is liberated in the early phase after topical application. Moreover, the emulsion structure (e.g., liquid crystals) and the presence of hydrotropes determine the water-liberation properties. This effect is more pronounced when the vehicle is formed by an aqueous or hydroalcoholic phase or when these are present within the external phase of the formulation (e.g., lotions, hydrogels, or oil-in-water emulsions).

Cosmetic vehicles are also known to influence the hydration of the SC, for which at least three different mechanisms have been proposed: First, the cosmetic vehicle can exert a direct hydrating effect by liberating water from the formulation itself (35). In this way, moisturizers actively increase the water content of the skin. Second, the occlusive effect of the formulation can influence SC hydration, especially in long-term applications. Emollients are designed to smooth the skin and increase the water content indirectly by creating an occlusive film on the skin surface, which traps the water in the upper layers of the SC. Third, by absorbing water from the vehicle itself, surface water, or water evaporation, highly hygroscopic compounds such as glycerol or hydrotropes such as hyaluronic acid or trimethylglycine, can increase SC hydration (36).

In addition, vehicles can exert an emollient (relipidizing or regreasing) effect, which is of great importance in the postexposure treatment of skin conditions, where cracked, rigid, or rough skin surface is the main problem. Furthermore, lipid-rich formulations improve skin distensibility, whereas creams and gels with lower lipid content have a more pronounced effect on short-term skin hydration (37). Of note is that formulations intended for facial use should avoid urea because of its irritative potential (38). For patients showing allergic reactions to constituents of dermatological or cosmetic vehicles, most fragrances, lanolin (wool wax), and paraben preservatives should be avoided when possible. Propylene glycol has also been reported to be a potential irritant (39).

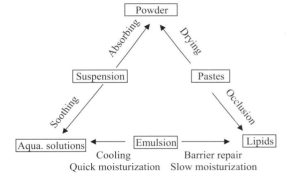

FIGURE 1 Revised "phase triangle" for dermatological vehicles. Such a classification has been useful in facilitating the choice of a vehicle for specific skin diseases according to the function of their different components.

In conclusion, classical vehicles in dermatology are amphiphilic systems containing high quantity of emulsifiers that, in turn, may have a negative effect in long-term application or counteract the positive features of vehicles. A new approach is the use of hydrogenated polydecenes, which are oligomers of decene with branched isoparaffinic structures completely saturated after full hydrogenation. Polydecenes are soluble in most nonpolar solvents and can be blended with common lipids, spread easily, do not interfere negatively with the skin barrier, and are not occlusive (40).

EVIDENCE-BASED COSMECEUTICAL THERAPY—
FEASIBLE OR FABULOUS?

Bringing research findings into clinical practice requires constant and rigorous updating of physicians who tend to remain adherent to traditional interventions even when better opportunities are available. On the other hand, physicians may be forced by commercial pressure to apply new treatment regimens that still lack substantial evidence of their validity (41). In the past decade, evidence-based medicine became a generally accepted method for bringing the results of research and medical practice together. It uses the following steps: (1) formation of a clear clinical question, (2) searching the literature for relevant articles, (3) assessing (clinical appraisal) validity and usefulness, (4) implementation of useful findings in clinical practice, and (5) evaluation of performance (42). Dermatology is considered a highly empirical field of medicine, and therapeutic interventions are based simply "on experience" in many instances (43). A recently published trial (41) reported that most of the patients in the study sample received evidence-based care, yet 36% underwent interventions lacking substantial experimental evidence. However, the dermatologist may find it difficult to discern the validity of the overwhelming amount of reports constantly published because many trials are performed with flawed designs and advance unreliable results or unwarranted conclusions. Case series fall into that category particularly because they are exposed to the risk of drawing conflicting conclusions and showing "effectiveness" of treatments that are purely due to phenomena such as the placebo effect, selection bias, and regression toward the mean (41).

Regarding evidence-based cosmeceutical application, it is important to consider the following facts. First, the steadily increasing interest in "natural," "hypoallergenic," and homeopathic compounds has created awareness of a multitude of new cosmeceutical ingredients. Second, the efficacy and safety of many of these ingredients has not been adequately tested because of the desire of cosmetic companies to keep them classified as cosmetics. Furthermore, to avoid expensive and time-consuming in vivo studies on human subjects, companies prefer to invest in in vitro studies. In vitro models are designed to mimic the reaction of in vivo skin, while being simple, rapid, and safe, and are recommended as a screening procedure for new product candidates. However, there are few in vitro models established that examine the effects of cosmeceutical ingredients on photoaging because the skin changes due to UVR are multiple and cannot be closely duplicated in vitro (44). It should also be noted that there are no animal models that can simulate perfectly the penetration of a topical product in humans (45). Even extensive laboratory testing cannot reproduce the complex pattern of skin aging and exposure to various toxins in the everyday life. Animal testing is or will be banned for testing cosmetics and cosmeceuticals.

BIOENGINEERING METHODS IN THE OBJECTIVE ASSESSMENT OF COSMETIC (COSMECEUTICAL) EFFECTS

Conventional bioengineering methods ensure accurate, highly reproducible results and have, therefore, gained popularity in experimental dermatology and cosmetic science. This is because of several facts: (1) being noninvasive, such measurements are considered ethical and, therefore, applicable in human settings; (2) they provide objective and quantifiable biophysical information on skin reactions such as irritation and cosmetic efficacy and, thus, reduce the subjective nature of the clinical observation arising from interobserver differences; (3) even subclinical effects, capable of predicting the onset of skin irritation, although invisible to naked eye, could be detected with bioengineering assessment; (4) by correlating the results obtained with the clinical readings, more profound and precise measurement can be achieved, (5) multidevice testing is recommendable because a single instrument provides only information on a certain skin parameter (46). One disadvantage of bioengineering methods, as suggested in the assessment of protective moisturizers, is that the results might sometimes be influenced by methodological difficulties (47). Bioengineering methods applied in cosmetic sciences aim at investigating different parameters. Most commonly assessed are transepidermal water loss (TEWL), skin hydration (corneometry), pH, skin elasticity (cutometry, reviscometry, optical profilometry), skin thickness (ultrasound), ultrastructural assessment of the skin surface (confocal multiphoton microscopy), and others.

Nowadays, the measurement of TEWL is the most reliable method used by many laboratories to characterize the water barrier function of the skin, both in physiological and pathological conditions, to perform predictive irritancy tests and evaluate the therapeutic efficacy of skin care systems (48–50). Although different methods for TEWL assessment exist, the open unventilated chamber technique based on the instrumental calculation of the water evaporation gradient within the SC is used in most commercially available devices (51). Individual related variables that may influence TEWL values are age, anatomical sites, physical, thermal or emotional sweating, and body temperature (49).

The assessment of skin hydration is one of the most important measurements for testing the efficacy of cosmetic products on the skin surface. A corneometer is a capacitance-based measuring device operating at low frequency (40–75 Hz) that is sensitive to relative dielectric changes of a material placed in contact with the electrode surface. The SC itself is a dielectric medium dependent on its water content. Individual variables interfering with the values obtained are regional differences in SC water content, body hair, and age (52) as well as room humidity and temperature. Skin surface irregularities and agents other than water (e.g., urea, salts) can also influence the results (47).

An acidic pH is critical for barrier homeostasis, in part because two key lipid-processing enzymes (β-glucocerebrosidase and acidic sphingomyelinase), which generate a family of ceramides from glucosylceramide and sphingomyelin precursors, respectively, exhibit low pH optima (25). Furthermore, an acidic pH clearly promotes SC integrity and cohesion (53). Endogenous or physiological factors, unrelated to pathological features, which influence skin pH are race, anatomical site, sex, age, and circadian rhythm, as well as sweating, skin temperature, and sebum. Furthermore, washing procedures have an alkalizing effect on the skin surface pH. Therefore, the application of neutral or acidic skin care systems (cleanser and emollient with pH 5.5) is considered less harmful to the surface pH and should be applied particularly to subjects with sensitive skin.

The epidermis, the fibrous collagen and elastin network of the dermis, and the hypodermis determine the biomechanical properties of the skin. Measurements of these properties have been used extensively to evaluate treatments designed to fight the effects of skin aging (54). The Reviscometer® RVM 600 (Courage & Khazaka, Cologne, Germany) is a device for the determination of the skin elasticity. The measuring principle is based on a resonance running time evaluation of the mechanical wave propagation in the skin. The wave propagates differently according to the state of skin hydration and elasticity. Variables such as dermal thickness and subepidermal tissue composition as well as age and/or solar exposure may influence the results.

The Cutometer® SEM 575 skin elasticity meter (Courage & Khazaka) is a suction device designed to measure the vertical deformation of the skin using an optical system (55). A vacuum pump is used to exert linearly increasing negative pressure at about 200 to 500 mbar upon the skin surface followed by abrupt negative pressure termination initiating the relaxation period. The depth of skin penetration into the measuring probe is detected through an optical sensor system and the relaxation recovery time, which depends on the elasting properties of the skin, is calculated.

Ultrasound techniques use a variety of instruments that can easily and objectively measure epidermal and dermal thickness. An automatic mode is used to define the outer epidermal boundary and the inner dermal/subcutaneous fat boundary. After manual selection of the boundaries, mean thickness is calculated automatically by the software. Nevertheless, the use of ultrasound measurements in photoaging is of questionable value because no significant correlation has been determined between skin thickness and parameters such as roughness, wrinkles, and pigmentary lesions, which are known to improve after effective antiaging therapy.

Skin microrelief changes with aging. Image analysis techniques (such as skin replica optical profilometry) are designed to quantify cutaneous relief. A soft dental impression material (silicone polymer) is placed onto the skin to obtain a "skin replica," which is analogous to a topographic map in reverse (56). The replica is side illuminated, in a standardized way, and the shadows generated correspond to peaks and valleys that can be assessed quantitatively by means of computer image analysis software for the evaluation of skin roughness and wrinkling.

The confocal laser scan microscopy (e.g., DermaInspect®; JenLab, Jena, Germany) represents a new noninvasive method aimed at studying the morphological and functional details of the skin (57). A thorough screening within the epidermis and the dermis to the extent of investigating cellular details is feasible. The method was recently suggested to be a reliable technique in the overall assessment of cutaneous photoaging (58).

COMMONLY USED COSMECEUTICAL INGREDIENTS

The number of cosmeceutical ingredients has drastically risen during the past few years (Table 1). Although the FDA does not have authority to approve cosmetic product ingredients, there are certain compounds that are prohibited or whose usage is restricted by federal regulations (Title XXI of the Code of Federal Regulations, Parts 250.250 and 700.11–700.23) (Table 2). Evidence-based validation of the purported benefits of cosmeceuticals is difficult. Because there are many cosmeceutical ingredients, we shall concentrate on a few recent scientific reports regarding the most commonly used ingredients.

TABLE 1 The Most Commonly Used Cosmeceutical Ingredients and Their Purported Effects

Cosmeceutical	Function
Retinoids	Antioxidants and activate specific genes and proteins
α-Hydroxy acids	Increase epidermal exfoliation and increase dermal collagen deposition
Antioxidants	Neutralize free radicals and protect cell membranes
Vitamin C	Antiaging potential — inhibit melanogenesis and promote collagen synthesis
Vitamin E	Moisturizing effect and weak photoprotective potential
Panthenol	Humectant properties
Lipoic acid	Able to recycle other antioxidants
Ubiquinone (coenzyme Q10)	Exhibits antiapoptotic activity and inhibits the expression of collagenase
Niacinamide	Antitumor activity; promotes increased epidermal turnover and exfoliation
Dimethylaminoethanol	Improves skin firmness and lift sagging skin; diminishes cross-linking of proteins
Spin traps	Interact with reactive free radicals and augment the effect of antioxidant enzymes
Melatonin	Yields antimutagenic, UV-protective, and oncostatic effects
Catalase	Imparts antioxidative activity in the skin
Glutathione	Fundamental as an antioxidant
Superoxide dismutase	Decreases UV erythema and damage
Peroxidase	Additional antibacterial activity
Glycopyranosides	Potent free-radical scavengers with further cardioprotection and neuroprotection
Polyphenols	Inhibit UV-induced tumorigenesis; reduce UV erythema and sunburn cells
Cysteine	Protects against UV-induced immunosuppression and tumorigenesis
Allantoin	Promotes cell proliferation and healing process
Furfuryladenine	Acts as a growth factor — increases epidermal thickness and collagen synthesis
Uric acid	Has a sparing action in plasma ascorbate
Carnosine	Has also metal ion-scavenging activities
Depigmenting agents	Inhibit melanogenesis at different stages
Phenolic compounds	
Nonphenolic compounds	
Combination formulas	
Others	
Botanicals	Exert effects through the mechanisms of antioxidants, α-hydroxy acids, etc.
Glycosaminoglycans	Stimulate epidermal regeneration and wound healing
Anticellulites	Yield lipolysis
Enzymes	Exfoliate keratotic skin; reduce UV-induced carcinogenesis
Growth factors	Increases epidermal thickness and collagen synthesis; accelerate wound healing
Hormones	Retard skin aging through reversing skin tone and elasticity
Botulinum A exotoxin	Eliminate wrinkles through blocking the sympathetic muscle innervations
Peptides	Stimulate collagen and extracellular matrix production; yield copper in the tissues
Antimicrobical agents	Inhibit microorganisms and microbial decomposition in perspiration
Topical anesthetics/antipruritics	Relieve local discomfort and reduce pruritus
Hair removal/hair loss therapy	Hydrolyze and disrupt hair keratins' bonds/act like hormones
Scar management	Modulate collagenase kinetics

Vitamin A, retinol, and retinoids are probably the most prevalent cosmeceuticals on the market and are mainly applied in extrinsic aging (photoaging). The retinoids have two important functions: (1) they act as antioxidants and (2) they activate specific genes and proteins, thus exerting several biologic effects, including regulation of growth and differentiation of epidermal cells, inhibition of tumor promotion in experimental models, decreasing inflammation, and stimulating the immune system (59). Retinoic acid (tretinoin), used as an antiacne therapy in the past two decades, is effective as an antiphotoaging treatment (60,61). It is now known that tretinoin reverses photoaging by exerting epidermal and dermal effects such as decreasing wrinkling, improving skin texture, decreasing actinic keratoses and lentigines (62) as well as improving the appearance of striae (63). Furthermore, in vitro cell culture studies have shown that retinoic acid stimulates the growth of keratinocytes and fibroblasts and the extension of the extracellular matrix, respectively (64). Retinol is a prodrug derived from vitamin A that can be converted into retinoic acid within the skin. Because of its exemption from FDA regulations, it has become a very fashionable ingredient in cosmeceutical moisturizers, so that counterclaims of "retinol-free" products are now appearing (65). In vitro and in vivo studies have shown that the pharmacological effects of retinol are similar to these of tretinoin, although better cutaneous penetration and less irritation have been demonstrated (66,67). Retinaldehyde, the immediate precursor of retinoic acid, has demonstrated reduction of wrinkling and skin roughness in double blind clinical studies (68). Furthermore, clinical open and controlled studies proved that regular use of retinaldehyde diminished the cutaneous consequences of photoaging and was superior to the vehicle, as evidenced by the profilometric study of skin replicas (69). Tazarotene is a third-generation retinoid with rapid and comprehensive efficacy in the treatment of photodamaged skin. A large double-blind, vehicle-controlled study showed that fine and course wrinkles, mottled hyperpigmentation, lentigines, elastosis, pore size, irregular hypopigmentation, and tactile roughness significantly improve after 24 weeks of treatment (70,71).

The most popular antioxidants in the cosmetic industry are the so-called network antioxidants that work synergistically to protect the body against the ravages of free radicals. Vitamins C and E, glutathione, lipoic acid (α-lipoic acid, ALA), and coenzyme Q10 (CoQ10) are the five network antioxidants specified at this time. Topical antioxidants have to fulfill specific requirements such as having increased stability,

TABLE 2 Cosmeceutical Ingredients Currently Prohibited or Restricted by Regulation

Ingredient	Potential toxicity
Hexachlorophene	Neurotoxic effects
	Ability to penetrate human skin
Mercury compounds	Accumulation in the body
	Skin irritation
	Allergic reactions
	Neurotoxicity
Bithionol	Photocontact sensitization
Halogenated salicylanilides	Photocontact sensitization
Chlorofluorocarbon propellants	Hazardous to human health
Chloroform	Plausible carcinogenicity
Vinyl chloride	Plausible carcinogenicity
Zirconium-containing complexes	Lung toxicity
Methylene chloride	Plausible carcinogenicity

appropriate vehicle formulation for skin delivery, photoprotection, and the ability to reduce pigment abnormalities, photoaging changes, and skin cancer. There are many in vivo studies on the antioxidant and photoprotective properties of vitamin C. Comprehensive summaries have recently been published (72,73). Because of its ability to neutralize free radicals and protect cell membranes, vitamin C is now considered a popular antiaging compound, gaining further continuous support in the scientific literature. Several recent double-blind clinical studies have revealed significant clinically apparent and instrumentally assessed improvement of wrinkles with vitamin C therapy (74–76). In addition, topical vitamin C has been shown to inhibit melanogenesis and be helpful as a mono/combined treatment in the therapeutic approach to melasma (77,78). Furthermore, in the skin, vitamin C plays a vital role in the metabolism of collagen. It is necessary for the hydroxylation of lysine and proline in procollagen, thus promoting collagen synthesis and aging repair. In vitro studies have shown that increased fibroblast synthesis is obtained when vitamin C is added to the culture medium (79). Recent in vivo studies on humans have generated clinical and ultrastructural data that elastic tissue repair, enhanced density of dermal papillae, and significant increase in the density of the skin microrelief in photoaged skin could be achieved with topical application of vitamin C (75,80,81). The stimulatory effects on collagen production are also believed to be useful in the prevention and treatment of striae alba, particularly if combined with other commercial topical agents (82). Despite the interesting laboratory research, there are still some drawbacks—designing proper formulations of vitamin C is a very challenging process, and many companies have elected to use cheaper, ineffective formulations. Most preparations are very unstable on exposure to UVR and air, and oxidation occurs rapidly. Even if products are formulated properly and stable, many of them do not penetrate the SC.

Apart from protecting cell membranes and scavenging free radicals, vitamin E (tocopherols and tocotrienols) has been touted as an excellent moisturizer, giving increased softness and smoothness to the skin (30,83). It has also been promoted for its photoprotective and anticarcinogenic effects and particularly for reducing erythema, edema, sunburn, sunlight-induced immunosuppression, and DNA adduct formation when applied before UVR exposure. A summary of the photoprotective effects of vitamin E on the skin has been recently published (72). However, controversy exists as to whether vitamin E is capable of providing significant protection against UV-induced damage to skin because most of these studies have been performed on animals and have produced equivocal results (3,72). It appears that despite the controversy and conflicting results, the evidence-based literature as a whole defines vitamin E as an antioxidant with weak photoprotective activity. Combinations with other antioxidants such as vitamin C are therefore recommended (84–87). Furthermore, vitamin C protects vitamin E from oxidation in the tissues. In brief, reversion of skin UV-induced erythema and edema by topical vitamin E, particularly if applied after acute UVR exposure, has not been proven feasible in humans (3,30). It may be assumed that UVR-induced free radicals react with the skin biomolecules and lead to rapid photodamage that cannot be inhibited by topically applied antioxidants because they cannot reach the site of action in therapeutic amounts quickly enough.

ALA is a new antioxidant recognized as suitable for the treatment and prevention of skin aging (88). The effectiveness of ALA is based on its metabolite, dihydrolipoic acid (DHLA), which is formed by the reduction of ALA. DHLA is considered the most powerful anti-inflammatory cell-protective antioxidant discovered in vitro to date. It is also able to recycle other antioxidants, such as vitamins C and E and glutathione (89,90). Furthermore, ALA is absorbed well through human skin. Studies on mice have shown that ALA in a lecithin base is capable of reducing UVB-induced erythema twice as quickly as skin treated with a lecithin base alone (91). However, a recent in vivo study on animal skin was unable to demonstrate detectible photoprotection against solar simulated radiation when using either ALA alone or in combination with vitamins C and E (92). Furthermore, a commercial formulation of ALA provided no protection. The investigators speculated that ALA absorbs UVR in the UVA spectrum, whereupon ALA is oxidized to its free radical and subsequently destroyed. Conversion to DHLA is, therefore, inefficient and there is little interaction with vitamins C and E to significantly augment their photoprotective properties.

CoQ10 (ubiquinone) is a naturally occurring antioxidant present in all human cells as a part of the electron transportation chain responsible for energy production. Apart from inhibition of lipid peroxidation in both cell membranes and serum low-density lipoproteins, CoQ10 has recently been found to exhibit antiapoptotic activity (93). An age-related decline of CoQ10 levels has been detected in both animals and humans (94). There is a lack of evidence regarding the protective role of CoQ10 in photoaged skin, with a single study being repeatedly cited in the literature (95). In this study, CoQ10 yielded antioxidant protection against UVA-mediated oxidative stress in human keratinocytes and was also able to suppress the expression of collagenase in human dermal fibroblasts after UVR, thus preventing the detrimental consequences in photoaging. More research is needed to substantiate the antiphotoaging potential of CoQ10 as well as to legitimize its effectiveness as a moisturizer additive.

α-Hydroxy acid (AHA) formulations comprise the second most available cosmeceutical on the market. Although their mechanisms of action are not thoroughly elucidated, AHAs are considered useful in treating skin aging because of their ability to enhance epidermal exfoliation, thus thinning SC and improving surface flexibility (30). Additional claimed effects of AHAs, based on the results of human clinical applications, include increased epidermal ceramide synthesis, increased transglutaminase expression in dermal dendrocytes, increased epidermal and dermal hyaluronic acid, and increased collagen deposition in the papillary dermis. The latter is questionable because in vivo studies on photoaged mice have failed to demonstrate enhanced collagen synthesis upon AHA application (96). However, scientific evidence to support the above stated claims is rather incomplete and controversial.

More than 60 botanicals are marked in cosmeceutical formulations, the most important of them pertaining to dermatological use being teas, soy, pomegranate, date, grape seed, pycnogenol, horse chestnut, German chamomile, circumin, comfrey, allantoin, fern extracts, and aloe (see Chapter 24 for a discussion of the chemistry of natural ingredients). However, only green and black tea, soy, pomegranate, and date have featured in published clinical trails for the treatment of extrinsic aging (97). Soy isoflavones (genistein and daidzein) function as phytoestrogens when consumed orally and have been credited with estrogenic properties such as increasing epidermal thickness and promoting collagen synthesis, thus rejuvenating photoaged skin. Increased dermal collagen and hyaluronan levels have been detected in cultured human fibroblasts (98). However, such claims are controversial. Soy preparations lack estrogen activity when applied topically because they are present as isoflavone glycosides. These glycosides are converted into free isoflavones in the gut after oral consumption. This will have implications for the topical use of soy (3). Several in vivo studies on mice have suggested that genistein significantly inhibits oxidative DNA damage and proto-oncogene expression as well as UV-induced changes in photoaged skin (99,100). In human epidermis, genistein was shown to inhibit UVR-induced apoptotic changes (101). In conclusion, although evidence concerning the cosmeceuticals effects of soy extracts exists, it is limited to animal studies or in vitro studies on human cultures.

Green tea is a popular ingredient in many beauty products mainly because it is a potent source of polyphenols. These have been widely investigated for anticarcinogenic potential and have yielded promising results in animal models. However, epidemiological studies on humans have failed to show any protection against tumorigenesis, with the exception of squamous cell carcinoma of the skin (102,103). Although evidence is mounting for the effectiveness of green tea polyphenols as antioxidants, more powerful than vitamins C and E, most products containing these ingredients have not been tested in controlled clinical studies (30). It has been demonstrated in vitro that polyphenols can limit UV-induced lipid peroxidation in skin and reduce oxidation of proteins as well as inhibit carcinogenesis and selectively increase apoptosis in UVB-induced skin tumors in mice (104). In vivo studies on mouse and human skin have also shown that tea polyphenols reduce UV-induced erythema and sunburn cell formation in a concentration-dependent pattern (105,106). Furthermore, a recent double-blind, placebo-controlled trial showed significant histological improvement in the elastic tissue content of photoaged skin under a combination regimen of topical and oral green tea (107). An advantage of green tea as a cosmeceutical ingredient is that it appears safe, and no side effects have been reported (30).

New ingredients of specific interests to cosmeceutical manufacturers are growth factors (GFs) and cosmeceutical peptides. GFs are regulatory proteins that mediate signaling pathways between and within cells. While assuming that GF have shown positive effects on wound healing (108) and that photodamaged skin is similar to a chronic wound that may not progress to complete tissue remodeling, a recent pilot study evaluated the effects of GF on photodamaged skin (109), and 78.6% of the patients treated with a mixture of multiple GF showed clinical improvement of wrinkle score at 60 days, substantiated objectively using optical profilometry. Furthermore, new collagen formation, improved epidermal thickness and skin hydration, and decreased roughness, dyspigmentation, and blotchiness were documented in a larger study on GF effects in photodamaged skin (110). Although the topical use of GF is still an emerging therapeutic approach, these initial data suggest that dermal collagen production and clinical improvement in photodamage appear relevant. Three types of peptides (signal, carrier, and neurotransmitter-inhibiting peptides) are now recognized as active cosmeceutical ingredients. The concept has evolved from research into wound healing and studies on growth stimulation of human skin fibroblasts. The primary objective of all biochemical and cellular research on peptides is to prove that if peptides are stabilized in cosmeceuticals and adequately delivered to the viable epidermis, they may stimulate collagen and extracellular matrix production via activation of protein kinases, yield copper necessary for the proper completion of wound healing and enzyme functioning, and decrease ion-mediated facial muscle contractions (111). However, evidence is still lacking on whether cosmeceutical peptides have the potential to improve the appearance of aging skin.

CONCLUSION

In conclusion, for the benefit of cosmeceuticals to be realized, the final product must be stable, sufficiently absorbed into the skin, and biologically active at the selected target. Even with clearly effective cosmeceuticals, in most cases, manufacturers take the decision not to claim them as therapeutically beneficial because that would result in scrutiny by FDA and consideration of the product as a drug. Furthermore, if a product is widely and judiciously advertised and if improvement of the appearance of the skin is noticed, the product will become a commercial success and escape the cost of FDA approval. However, if true physiological changes are occurring with cosmeceuticals, as has been evidenced for some, it is only a matter of time before the FDA requires verification of the effectiveness, safety, and potential toxicity of the active ingredients (111). It is, therefore, important that companies are encouraged to perform double-blind, placebo-controlled studies. This will endow patients with safer therapeutic approaches as well as provide stronger evidence for companies' claims and increase sales by physician recommendations.

REFERENCES

1.   Harding C. The stratum corneum: structure and function in health and disease. Dermatol Therapy 2004; 17:6–15.
2.   Forslind B. A domain mosaic model of the skin barrier. Acta Derm. Venereol. 1994; 74(1):1–6.
3.   Pinnell SR. Cutaneous photodamage, oxidative stress, and topical antioxidant protection. J Am Acad Dermatol 2003; 48:1–19.
4.   Bernerburg M, Plettenberg H, Krutmann J. Photoaging of human skin. Photodermatol Photoimmunol Photomed 2000; 16:239–244.
5.   Hadshiew IM, Eller MS, Gilchrest BA. Skin aging and photoaging: the role of DNA damage and repair. Am J Contact Dermat 2000; 11:19–25.
6.   Trautinger F. Mechanisms of photodamage of the skin and its functional consequences for skin aging. Clin Exp Dermatol 2001; 26:573–577.
7.   McGregor WG. DNA replication, and UV mutagenesis. J Invest Dermatol Symp Proc 1999; 4:1–5.
8.   Kligman LH. Photoaging. Manifestations, prevention, and treatment. Clin Geriatr Med 1989; 5(1):235–251.
9.   Ljungman M, Zhang F. Blockage of RNA polymerase as a possible trigger for UV-light induced apoptosis. Oncogene 1996; 13:823–831.
10. Kochevar IE, Moran M, Granstein RD. Experimental photoaging in C3H/HeN, C3H/HeJ, and Balb/c mice: comparison in extracellular matrix components and mast cell numbers. J Invest Dermatol 1994; 103:797–800.
11. Kawanishi S, Hiraku Y. Sequence specific DNA damage induced by UVA radiation in the presence of endogenous and exogenous sensitizers. Curr Probl Dermatol 2001; 29:74–82.
12. Thiele JJ, Podda M, Packer L. Tropospheric ozone: an emerging environmental stress to skin. Biol Chem 1997; 378:1299–1305.
13. Thiele JJ. Oxidative targets in the stratum corneum. Skin Pharmacol Appl Skin Physiol 2001; 14(Suppl. 1):87–91.
14. Weber SU, Thiele JJ, Cross CE, et al. Vitamin C, uric acid and glutathione gradients in murine stratum corneum and their susceptibility to ozone exposure. J Invest Dermatol 1999; 113:1128–1132.
15. Subramanyan K. Role of mild cleansing in the management of patient skin. Dermatol Ther 2004; 17:26–34.
16. Fluhr JW, Gloor M, Gehring W. Physiology of skin cleaning and functional mechanism bath oils in irritant contact dermatitis. In: Berardesca PE, Pigatto M, eds. Proceedings of the 3rd International Symposium (ISICD). Milan, Italy: Medical Publishing & New Media, 2000:291–307.
17. Fluhr JW, Ennen J. Standardized washing models: facts and requirements. Skin Res Technol 2004; 10:141–143.
18. Wilhelm KP, Cua AB, Wolff HH, et al. Surfactant-induced stratum corneum hydration in vivo: prediction of the irritation potential of anionic surfactants. J Invest Dermatol 1993; 101:310–315.

19. Fartasch M, Schnetz E, Diepgen TL. Characterization of detergent-induced barrier alterations—effect of barrier cream on irritation. J Invest Dermatol Symp Proc 1998; 3:121–127.
20. Muizzuddin N, Marenus KD, Maes DH. Factors defining sensitive skin and its treatment. Am J Contact Dermat 1998; 9:170–175.
21. Seidenari S, Francomano M, Mantovani L. Baseline biophysical parameters in subjects with sensitive skin. Contact Dermatitis 1998; 38:311–315.
22. Bornkessel A, Flach M, Arens-Corell M, et al. Functional assessment of a washing emulsion for sensitive skin: mild impairement of stratum corneum hydration, pH, barrier function, lipid content, integrity and cohesion in a controlled washing test. Skin Res Technol 2005; 11:53–60.
23. Loden M, Buraczewska I, Edlund F. Irritation potential of bath and shower oils before and after use: a double-blind randomized study. Br J Dermatol 2004; 150:1042–1047.
24. Fluhr JW, Kuss O, Diepgen T, et al. Testing for irritation with a multifactorial approach: comparison of eight non-invasive measuring techniques on five different irritation types. Br J Dermatol 2001; 145:696–703.
25. Hachem JP, Crumrine D, Fluhr J, et al. pH directly regulates epidermal permeability barrier homeostasis, and stratum corneum integrity/cohesion. J Invest Dermatol 2003; 121:345–353.
26. Millikan LE. Cosmetology, cosmetics, cosmeceuticals: Definitions and regulations. Clin Dermatol 2001; 19(4):371–374.
27. Harish D, Kaushik D, Gupta M, et al. Cosmeceuticals: an emerging concept. Indian J Pharmacol 2005; 37(3):155–159.
28. Kligman AM. Cosmeceuticals: a broad-spectrum category between cosmetics and drugs. In: Elsner P, Maibach H, eds. Cosmeceuticals and Active Cosmetics. Drugs Versus Cosmetics. Boca Raton, Fla: Taylor & Francis, 2005:1–9.
29. Lavrijsen APM, Vermeer BJ. Cosmetics and drugs. Is there a need for a third group: cosmeceuticals? Br J Dermatol 1991; 124:503–504.
30. Lazarus MC, Baumann LS. The use of cosmeceutical moisturizers. Dermatol Therapy 2001; 14:200–207.
31. Brody H. Relevance of cosmeceuticals to the dermatologic surgeon. Dermatol Therapy 2005; 31:796–798.
32. Kligman D. Cosmeceuticals. Dermatol Clin 2000; 18:609–615.
33. Fluhr JW, Rigano L. Clinical effects of cosmetic vehicles on skin. J Cosmet Sci 2004; 55(2):189–205.
34. Chamlin SL, Kao J, Frieden IJ, et al. Ceramide-dominant barrier repair lipids alleviate childhood atopic dermatitis: changes in barrier function provide a sensitive indicator of disease activity. J Am Acad Dermatol 2002; 47(2):198–208.
35. Blichmann CW, Serup J, Winther A. Effects of single application of a moisturizer: evaporation of emulsion water, skin surface temperature, electrical conductance, and skin surface (emulsion) lipids. Acta Derm. Venereol 1989; 69(4):327–330.
36. Fluhr JW, Gloor M, Lehmann L, et al. Glycerol accelerates recovery of barrier function in vivo. Acta Derm Venereol 1999; 79(6):418–421.
37. Jemec GB, Wulf HC. Correlation between the greasiness and the plasticizing effect of moisturizers. Acta Derm Venereol 1999; 79(2):115–117.
38. Agner T. An experimental study of irritant effects of urea in different vehicles. Acta Derm Venereol Suppl 1992; 177:44–46.
39. Funk SO, Maibach H. Propylene glycol dermatitis: re-evaluation of an old problem. Contact Dermatitis 1994; 31(4):236–241.
40. Rigano L, Muukkonen P. Problem solving emollients: high-tech hydrogenated poly-decenes in diseased skin treatment. 20th World Congress of Dermatology, Paris, 2002.
41. Abeni D, Girardelli CR, Masini C, et al. What proportion of dermatological patients receive evidence-based treatment? Arch Dermatol 2001; 137:771–776.
42. Rosenberg A, Donald A. Evidence-based medicine, an approach to clinical problem-solving. Br Med J 1995; 310:1122–1126.
43. Bigby M. Snake oil for the 21st century. Arch Dermatol 1998; 134:1512–1514.
44. Kligman LH, Kligman AM. Photoaging-retinoids, alpha hydroxy acids and antioxidants. In: Gabard B, Elsner P, Surber C, Treffel P. eds. Dermatopharmacology of Topical

Preparations. A Product-Development Orientated Approach. Berlin Heidelberg: Springer Verlag, 1999; 383–400.

45. Zhai H, Maibach H. Testing and efficacy of barrier creams. In: Fluhr JW, Elsner P, Berardesca E, Maibach HI, eds. Bioengineering of the Skin. Boca Raton, Fla: CRC Press, 2005.

46. Berardesca E. Bioengineering methods in the objective evaluation of cosmetic effects. XIII International Symposium on Contact Dermatitis, Uruguay, 2001.

47. Jemec GB, Na R, Wulf HC. The inherent capacitance of moisturizing creams: a source of false positive results? Skin Pharmacol Appl Skin Physiol 2000; 13:182–187.

48. Primavera G, Fluhr JW, Berardesca E. Standardization of measurements and guidelines. In: Fluhr JW, Elsner P, Berardesca E, Maibach HI, eds. Bioengineering of the Skin. Water and the Stratum Corneum. Boca Raton, Fla: CRC Press, 2005:83–95.

49. Rogiers V. EEMCO Group. EEMCO guidance for the assessment of transepidermal water loss in cosmetic sciences. Skin Pharmacol Appl Skin Physiol 2001; 14:117–128.

50. Pinnagoda J, Tupker RA, Agner T, et al. Guideliness for transepidermal water loss (TEWL) measurment. Contact Dermatitis 1990; 22:164–178.

51. Fluhr JW, Feingold KR, Elias PM. Transepidermal water loss reflects permeability barrier status: validation in human and rodent in vivo and ex vivo models. Exp Dermatol 2006; 15(7):483–492.

52. Berardesca E, EEMCO Group, EEMCO guidance for the assessment of stratum corneum hydration: electrical methods. Skin Res Technol 1997; 3:126–132.

53. Fluhr JW, Kao J, Jain M, et al. Generation of free fatty acids from phospholipids regulates stratum corneum acidification and integrity. J Invest Dermatol 2001; 117:44–51.

54. Smalls LK, Wickett RR, Visscher M. Effect of dermal thickness, tissue composition, and body site on skin biomechanical properties. Skin Res Technol 2006; 12:43–49.

55. Cua AB, Wilhelm KP, Maibach HI. Elastic properties of human skin: relation to age, sex and anatomical region. Arch Dermatol Res 1990; 282:283–288.

56. Lévêque JL. EEMCO guidance for the assessment of skin topography. J Eur Acad Dermatol Venereol 1999; 12:103–114.

57. Koenig K, Reimann I. High-resolution multiphoton tomography of human skin with subcellular spatial resolution and picosecond time resolution. J Biomed Opt 2003; 8(3):432–439.

58. Lin SJ, Wu R Jr, Tan HY, et al. Evaluating cutaneous photoaging by use of multiphoton fluorescence and second harmonic generation microscopy. Opt Lett 2005; 30(17): 2275–2277.

59. Keller KL. Uses of vitamins A, C, and E and related compounds in dermatology. J Am Acad Dermatol 2000; 39(4 Pt 1):611–625.

60. Kligman LH. Effects of all-trans-retinoic acid on the dermis of hairless mice. J Am Acad Dermatol 1986; 15:779–785.

61. Weiss JS, Ellis CN, Headington JT, et al. Topical tretinoin in the treatment of aging skin. J Am Acad Dermatol 1988; 19(1 Pt 2):169–175.

62. Kligman AM. Cosmetics: a dermatologist looks to the future: promises and problems. Dermatol Clin 2000; 18:699–709.

63. Kang S. Topical tretinoin therapy for management of early striae. J Am Acad Dermatol 1998; 39(2 Pt 3):S90–S92.

64. Varani J, Fisher GJ, Kang S, et al. Molecular mechanisms of intrinsic skin aging and retinoid induced repair and reversal. J Invest Dermatol 1998; 3(1):57–60.

65. Cunnigham JW. Cosmeceuticals in photoaging. In: Elsner P, Maibach HI eds. Cosmeceuticals and Active Cosmetics. Drugs Versus Cosmetics. Boca Raton, Fla: Taylor & Francis, 2005:262–277.

66. Kang S, Duell EA, Fisher GJ, et al. Application of retinol to human skin in vivo induces epidermal hyperplasia and cellular retinoid binding proteins characteristic of retinoic acid, but without measurable retinoic levels of irritation. J Invest Dermatol 1995; 105(4): 549–556.

67. Duell EA, Kang S, Voorhees JJ. Unoccluded retinol penetrates human skin in vivo more effectively than unoccluded retinyl palmitate or retinoic acid. J Invest Dermatol 1997; 109:301–305.

68. Saurat JH, Didierjean L, Masgrau E, et al. Topical retinaldehyde on human skin: biologic effects and tolerance. J Invest Dermatol 1994; 103(6):770–774.

69. Creidi P, Humbert Ph. Clinical use of topical retinaldehyde on photoaged skin. Dermatology 1999; 199(Suppl. 1):49–52.

70. Kang S, Leyden JJ, Lowe NJ, et al. Tazarotene cream for the treatment of facial photodamage: a multicenter, investigator-masked, randomized, vehicle-controlled, parallel comparison of 0.01%, 0.025%, 0.05% and 0.1% tazarotene creams with 0.05% tretinoin emollient cream applied once daily for 24 weeks. Acta Dermatol 2001; 137(12):1597–1604.

71. Sefton J, Kligman AM, Kopper C, et al. Photodamage pilot study: a double-blind, vehicle-controlled study to assess the efficacy and safety of tazarotene 0.1% gel. J Am Acad Dermatol 2000; 43(4):656–663.

72. Thiele JJ, Dreher F. Antioxidant defense systems in skin. In: Elsner P, Maibach HI, eds. Cosmeceuticals and Active Cosmetics. Drugs Versus Cosmetics. Boca Raton, Fla: Taylor & Francis, 2005:37–88.

73. Farris PK. Topical vitamin C: a useful agent for treating photoaging and other dermatological conditions. Dermatol Surg 2005; 31(7 Pt 2):814–817.

74. Traickovich SS. Use of topical ascorbic acid and its effects on photodamaged skin topography. Arch Otolaryn Head Neck Surg 1999; 125:1091–1098.

75. Humbert PC, Haftek M, Creidi P, et al. Topical ascorbic acid on photoaged skin. Clinical, topographical and ultrastructural evaluation: double-blind study vs. placebo. Exp Dermatol 2003; 12(3):237–244.

76. Fitzpatrick RE, Rostan EF. Double-blind, half-face study comparing topical vitamin C and vehicle for rejuvenation of photodamage. Dermatol Surg 2002; 28(3):231–236.

77. Kameyama K, Sakai C, Kondoh S, et al. Inhibitory effect of magnesium L-ascorbyl-2-phosphate (VC-PMG) on melanogenesis in vitro and in vivo. J Am Acad Dermatol 1996; 34(1):29–33.

78. Seite S, Bredoux C, Compan D, et al. Histological evaluation of a topically applied retinol-vitamin C combination. Skin Pharmacol Appl Skin Physiol 2005; 18(2):81–87.

79. Geesin JC, Darr D, Kaufman R, et al. Ascorbic acid specifically increases type I and type III procollagen messenger RNA levels in human skin fibroblasts. J Invest Dermatol 1998; 90:420–424.

80. Sauermann K, Jaspers S, Koop U, et al. Topically applied vitamin C increases the density of derma papillae in aged human skin. BMC Dermatol 2004; 4(1):13.

81. Nusgens BV, Humbert P, Rougier A, et al. Topically applied vitamin C enhances the mRNA level of collagens I and III, their processing enzymes and tissue inhibitor of matrix metalloproteinase 1 in the human dermis. J Invest Dermatol 2001; 116:853–859.

82. Ash K, Lord J, Zukowski M, et al. Comparison of topical therapy for straie alba (20% glycolic acid/0.05% tretinoin versus 20% glycolic acid/10% L-ascorbic acid). Dermatol Surg 1998; 24(8):849–856.

83. Draelos ZD. Therapeutic moisturizers. Dermatol Clin 2000; 18:597–607.

84. Zhai H, Behnam S, Villarama CD, et al. Evaluation of the antioxidant capacity and preventive effects of a topical emulsion and its vehicle control on the skin response to UV exposure. Skin Pharmacol Physiol 2005; 18(6):288–293.

85. Lin JY, Selim MA, Grichnick JM, et al. UV photoprotection by combination topical antioxidants vitamin C and vitamin E. J Am Acad Dermatol 2003; 48(6):866–874.

86. Jurkiewicz BA, Bissett DL, Buettner GR. Effect of topically applied tocopherol on ultraviolet radiation-mediated free radical damage in skin. J Invest Dermatol 1995; 104(4):484–488.

87. Damiani E, Rosati L, Castagna R, et al. Changes in ultraviolet absorbance and hence in protective efficacy against lipid peroxidation of organic sunscreens after UVA irradiation. J Photochem Photobiol 2006; 82(3):204–213.

88. Podda M, Zollner TM, Grundmann-Kollmann M, et al. Activity of alpha-lipoic acid in the protection against oxidative stress in skin. Curr Probl Dermatol 2001; 29:43–51.

89. Ortial S, Durand G, Poeggeler B, et al. Fluorinated amphiphilic amino acid derivatives antioxidant carriers: a new class of protective agents. J Med Chem 2006; 49(9):2812–2820.

90. Perricone NV. Pharmacologic cognitive enhancers. Skin Aging 1998; 6:68–74.
91. Podda M, Rallis M, Traber MG, et al. Kinetic study of cutaneous and subcutaneous distribution following topical application of (7,8-14C)rac-alpha-lipoic acid onto hairless mice. Biochem Pharmacol 1996; 52:627–633.
92. Lin JY, Lin FH, Burch JA, et al. Alpha-lipoic acid is ineffective as a topical antioxidant for photoprotection of skin. J Invest Dermatol 2004; 123(5):996–998.
93. Papucci L, Schiavone N, Witort E, et al. Coenzyme Q10 prevents apoptosis by inhibiting mitohondrial depolarization independantly of its free radical scavenging property. J Biol Chem 2003; 278(30):28220–28228.
94. Beyer RE, Ernster L. The antioxidant role of coenzyme Q. In: Lenaz G, Barnabei O, Battinc M, eds. Highlights in Ubiquinone Research. London, U.K.: Taylor & Francis, 1990:191–213.
95. Hoppe U, Bergemann J, Diembeck W, et al. Coenzyme Q10, a cutaneous antioxidant and energizer. BioFactors 1999; 9(2–4):371–378.
96. Kligman LH, Sapadin AN, Schwartz E. Peeling agents and irritants, unlike tretinoin, do not stimulate collagen synthesis in the photoaged hairless mice. Arch Dermatol Res 1996; 288:615–620.
97. Thornfeldt C. Cosmeceuticals containing herbs: fact, fiction, and future. Dermatol Surg 2005; 31(7 Pt. 2):873–880.
98. Sudel KM, Venzke K, Mielke H, et al. Novel aspects of intrinsic and extrinsic aging of human skin: beneficial effects of soy extracts. Photochem Photobiol 2005; 81(3):581–587.
99. Wei H. Photoprotective action of isoflavone genistein: models, mechanisms, and relevance to clinical dermatology. J Am Acad Dermatol 1998; 39(2 Pt. 1):271–272.
100. Kim SY, Kim SJ, Lee JY, et al. Protective effects of dietary soy isoflavones against UV-induced skin aging in hairless mouse model. J Am Coll Nutr 2004; 23(2):157–162.
101. Wang Y, Zhang XS, Lebwohl M, et al. Inhibition of ultraviolet B (UVB)-induced c-Fos and c-Jun expression in vivo by a tyrosine kinase inhibitor genistein. Carcinogenesis 1998; 19:649–654.
102. Katiyar SK, Mukhtar H. Tea consumption and cancer. World Rev Nutr Diet 1996;79: 154–184.
103. Hakim IA, Harris RB, Weisgerber UM. Tea intake and squamous cell carcinoma of the skin: influence of type of tea beverages. Cancer Epidemiol Biomarkers Prev 2000; 9: 727–731.
104. Kim SY, Hwang JS, Cho YK, et al. Protective effects of (–)-epigallocatechin-3-gallate on UVA-and UVB-induced skin damage. Skin Pharmacol Appl Skin Physiol 2001; 14: 11–19.
105. Saliou C, Rimbach G, Moini H, et al. Solar ultraviolet-induced erythema in human skin and nuclear factor-kappa-B-dependent gene expression in keratinocytes are modulated by a French maritime pine bark extract. Free Radic Biol Med 2001; 30:154–160.
106. Vayalil PK, Mittal A, Hara Y, et al. Green tea polyphenols prevent ultraviolet light-induced oxidative damage and matrix metalloproteinases expression in mouse skin. J Invest Dermatol 2004; 122:1480–1487.
107. Chiu AE, Chan JL, Kern DG, et al. Double-blind, placebo-controlled trial of green tea extracts in the clinical and histologic appearance of photoaging skin. Dermatol Surg 2005; 31(7 Pt. 2):855–860.
108. Goldman R. Growth factors and chronic wound healing: past, present, and future. Adv Skin Wound Care 2004; 17:24–35.
109. Fitzpatrick RE, Rostan EF. Reversal of photodamage with topical growth factors: a pilot study. J Cosment Laser Ther 2003; 5:25–34.
110. Fitzpatrick RE. Endogenous growth factors as cosmeceuticals. Dermatol Surg 2005; 31:827–831.
111. Lupo MP. Cosmeceutical peptides. Dermatol Surg 2005; 31:832–836.

7 Skin Hydration—A Key Determinant in Topical Absorption

Michael S. Roberts
School of Medicine, University of Queensland, Princess Alexandra Hospital, Woolloongabba, Queensland, Australia

Joke Bouwstra
Leiden/Amsterdam Center for Drug Research, Leiden, the Netherlands

Fabrice Pirot and Françoise Falson
Faculté de Pharmacie, Université de Lyon, Lyon, France

INTRODUCTION

Skin hydration, a major determinant of percutaneous absorption, refers to the extent of hydration in the outermost layer of the skin, the stratum corneum (SC). SC moisture levels, transepidermal water loss (TEWL), skin elasticity, and SC cell turnover are perhaps four of the key measures for skin conditioning. The extent of skin hydration is largely dependent on the water gradient across the SC from the largely aqueous viable epidermal tissues and the external environment, as well as on the amount of water held in the SC. The normal functioning of the SC is also dependent on an appropriate SC hydration. The level of SC hydration influences each step in the SC formation, maturation, and exfoliation, including the formation of resilient corneocytes and highly organized intercellular lipids and the generation of water binding components. These processes, as well as the final step of corneodesmolysis that mediates exfoliation, are often disturbed by disease and adverse environmental conditions, resulting in dry, flaky skin conditions. Although this chapter focuses on the role of skin hydration in the ingress and egress of solutes through the skin, it should be noted that skin hydration also affects the appearance, flexibility, and feel (texture) of the skin. Aspects on the biophysical interaction of water and the SC have been previously addressed elsewhere (1) and, in this update of that chapter, are only addressed to a limited extent.

BIOCHEMICAL ASPECTS ASSOCIATED WITH SKIN HYDRATION

SC water content is dependent on four key processes: SC water binding, SC barrier properties, water gradient across the SC, and viable epidermal SC transporter function (Fig. 1). Products seeking to hydrate the SC on application to the skin generally seek to modify one of the first three processes.

SC water binding is facilitated by the presence of natural intracellular hygroscopic and water-soluble agents within the corneocytes, a complex mixture commonly referred to as the natural moisturizing factor (NMF). NMF makes up ~10% of the corneocyte mass and generates the osmotic force that attracts water in the corneocyte. The main components of NMF are amino acids (~40%), mineral ions (e.g., sodium, potassium, calcium, magnesium; ~18%), pyrrolidone-5-carboxylic

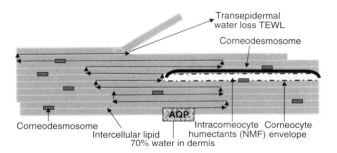

FIGURE 1 Schematic diagram of factors affecting SC hydration including SC water binding to intracorneocyte humectants, SC intercellular lipid barrier pathway, water gradient across the SC (leading to transepidermal water loss), and viable epidermal SC transporters (AQP) function. *Abbreviations*: AQP, aquaglyceroporin; NMF, natural moisturizing factor; SC, stratum corneum; TEWL, transepidermal water loss.

acid (~12%), lactate (~12%), sugars (e.g., glucose; ~8%), urea (~7%), and other water-soluble ions (~8.5%) formed within the corneocytes by degradation of the histidine-rich protein known as filaggrin and the SC maturation process (2). SC water binding may be facilitated by the penetration and retention of topically applied product ingredients in the SC that can enhance water uptake into SC and their retention therein. Such ingredients are referred to as moisturizers or humectants. The second group restores normal water loss from the SC by acting as a barrier against possible environmental insults that may damage the SC and cause water loss. These agents are usually partially or fully occlusive. Partially occlusive products include the emollients, which are oils and lipids that spread easily and may change the lipid organization in SC (3). Newer products also modify enzymatic processes associated with SC maturation and exfoliation. A more detailed examination of skin moisturizers for dry skin is presented in Chapter 22.

Skin hydration is also facilitated by the nature of the SC barrier in which water transport through the SC is retarded as a consequence of the highly organized SC intercellular lipid lamellae and the long path length through these lamellae around the long, flat, and interdigitating corneocytes (Fig. 1). The lipid organization within the lipid lamellae is predominantly as an orthorhombic crystalline phase. An additional major determinant of skin hydration is the water gradient across the SC, determined largely by relative humidity (RH) or effective RH at the outermost SC surface created by the topical products used. At a normal RH, the approximate SC water level is 15% to 20% of its dry weight. Soaking, occlusion, and high humidity may increase water content further—up to 300% to 400% of the dry weight after extensive soaking or hydrating at 100% RH. As a consequence, the appearance of the SC surface, or its topology, varies with SC hydration. Figure 2 shows the desorption profiles for water from SC after various degrees of hydration (4). The initial rapid loss is because of surface water and water that is present in the intercellular regions at this very high water levels. The rapid desorption for delipidized membranes suggests that the corneocyte envelope may have been disrupted so that the osmotic gradient between the cells and the outside is destroyed or that penetration across the intercellular lipid lamellae forms the rate-limiting step for water desorption. After the first phase of surface water loss, water trapped by NMF in the corneocytes is lost by desorption gradually during several hours. The final 5% to 10% is very slowly desorbed, suggesting that they are bound to the polar side chain groups of keratin.

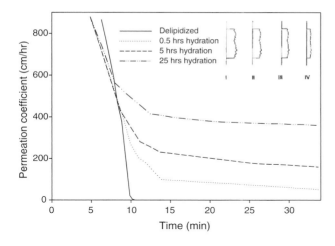

FIGURE 2 Water desorption curves for human stratum corneum after different treatments. *Source*: Adapted from Ref. 3.

The SC has been described as an ideal osmometer in that SC water capacity can be shown to be directly related to the external osmotic pressure (Fig. 3) (5). The SC is also able to absorb and retain humectant materials such as glycerol and urea. Osmolyte pretreatment of SC can therefore be shown to increase SC osmolarity and SC hydration for a given osmotic pressure (Fig. 3). SC hydration and can be shown to be correlated with osmotic pressure of the applied solutions (Fig. 3A). In addition, the retained humectant materials also reduce the magnitude of outward water transfer and net evaporation (5).

Water transport across the tight junctions between the stratum granulosum and SC is facilitated by the water-glycerol transporting protein aquaglyceroporin (AQP). The strictly water channels, AQP1 and AQP5, appear not to be highly expressed in human skin, whereas AQP3, which appears to selectively facilitate glycerol and urea transport, and AQP10 are highly expressed in mammalian epidermal keratinocytes epidermis. Interestingly, epidermal edema was correlated to the absence of AQP3 in experimental eczema and hyperplasia (6). The relationship between the reduced glycerol content of SC and epidermis of AQP3-deficient mice and the dry, inelastic skin in AQP3-null mice has been attributed to the humectant properties of glycerol. This finding supports the inclusion of glycerol in cosmetic products for dry skin (7).

SC HYDRATION AND TOPOLOGY

Figure 4 shows a scanning electron microscopy view of the topology of the skin before and after hydration for 16 hours by an occlusive saran wrap dressing. Hydration leads to a swelling and developing of folds in the SC, reflecting up to a 50% increase in surface area (8). Other methods can also be used to characterize hydration effects on skin topology and include analysis of SC by tape stripping to provide an analysis of consecutive SC layers and biopsy or shave biopsy of skin layers down to the hypodermis or, in the latter case, the papillary dermis. A range of microscopy techniques can be used to define three-dimensional surface topography. Procedures used include naked eye observations, photography, and video microscopes as well as the usually more invasive confocal microscopy, three-dimensional stylus, and white-light interferometry (9). The skin topography is characterized by wrinkles and microrelief, the latter comprising a number of rectilinear grooves varying in depth and orientation (Fig. 5). Changes

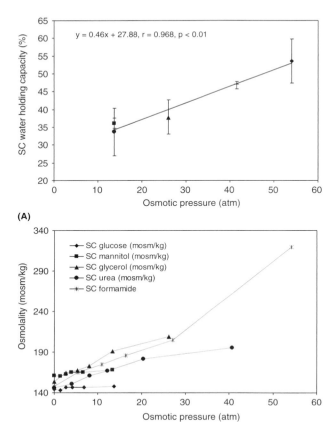

(A)

(B)

FIGURE 3   SC hydration (**A**) and osmolality (**B**) is directly related to osmotic pressure of applied solutions. *Source*: Adapted from Ref. 5.

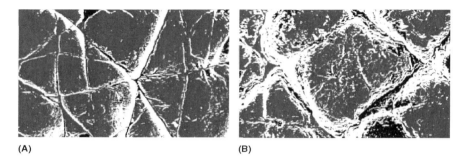

(A)   **(B)**

FIGURE 4   Scanning electron microscopy (×100) demonstrating the microtopography of normal human skin before and after a 16-hour application of Saran™ Wrap. *Source*: From Ref. 1.

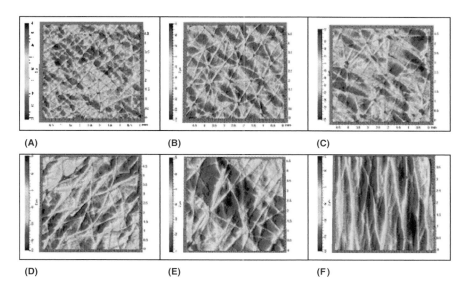

(A)   (B)   (C)

(D)   (E)   (F)

FIGURE 5   Skin line morphology of volar forearm during aging. (**A**) 30–40 years old; (**B**) 41–50 years old; (**C**) 51–60 years old; (**D**) 61–70 years old; (**E–F**) >71 years old. *Source*: Adapted from Ref. 10.

in the SC microrelief arise, in part, from collagen fibers in the dermis moving from a tangled stretched (anisotropic) state in the young to an isotropic one (at about 50 years old) in which the collagen is reorganized to be in a mainly parallel orientation. As a consequence, older skin is often associated with deep skin furrows and sagging skin. SC surface parameters are characterized by parameters such as length and total area covered by creases, wrinkle heights and depths, and number of pores (9,10). In young and in hydrated skin, cutaneous furrows or lines are homogenously distributed (anisotropy), whereas in older or delipidized skin, cutaneous furrows are mainly in one direction (isotropy). Widened furrows appear as visible wrinkles. Figure 6 shows examples of skin microrelief obtained for hydrated and delipidized skin.

More direct measurement of hydration is based on either skin capacitance or conductance using various frequencies and electrodes. Skin capacitance mapping is a relatively new technique that enables the distribution of water across the surface of the skin to be visualized (11,12). However, because an integral value is provided for skin depth, no information can be provided on localization in skin depth. Figure 7 shows an example of normal, hydrated, and psoriatic skin with varying hydration. Areas of increased hydration appear darker as characterized by a higher skin capacitance (12). The psoriatic lesion is characterized by a mixture of dry (light area = low capacitance), hydrated (medium level capacitance), and a highly hydrated (darker area = high capacitance); the sharply circumscribed, highly hydrated area corresponds to an inflammatory area (13). Skin capacitance mapping has recently been used to show that surfactant treatments can lead to rapid water swelling of corneocytes/SC (12).

SC HYDRATION AND WATER DISTRIBUTION IN SC

The distribution of water in the SC has been examined by a number of workers. Figure 8 shows that the water content is lowest at the external SC surface and increases

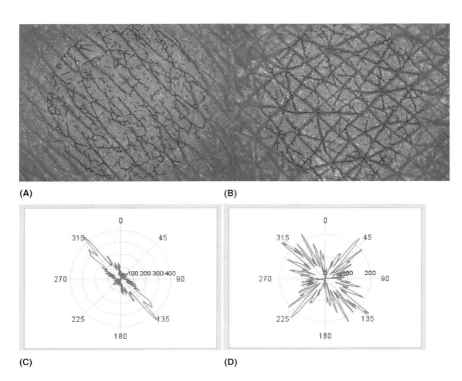

FIGURE 6   Skin microrelief for (**A**) acetone-delipidized skin and (**B**) hydrated skin (5-minute application of a nanoemulsion) and the corresponding roses for distribution (www.labo-lalicorne.com/en/07_about_skin/micro_relief.htm), defining the distribution and lengths of the lines for (**C**) delipidized skin and (**D**) hydrated skin.

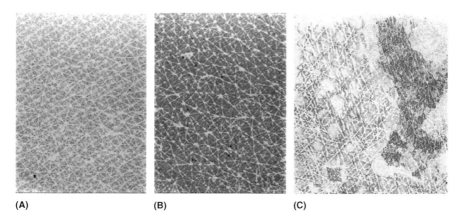

FIGURE 7   Capacitance imaging of the ventral side of the forearm (**A**) before and (**B**) 60 minutes after application of a moisturizing cosmetic and (**C**) in a psoriatic lesion. *Source*: From Refs. 12, 13.

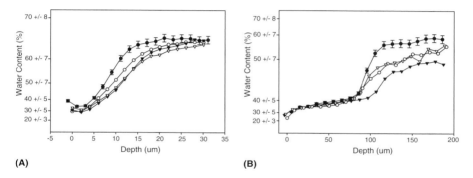

(A)   **(B)**

FIGURE 8 Four examples of in vivo water concentration profiles of the stratum corneum on (**A**) the volar aspect of forearm and (**B**) the thenar region. *Source*: Adapted from Ref. 14.

progressively as the viable epidermis is approached (14). The X-ray diffraction pattern of the SC, shown in Figure 9, shows a strong peak and a shoulder on the right hand side, which are both due to the lipid lamellae in the SC. Minimal change in the position of the strong peak is evident when the diffraction pattern of dry SC sheets is compared with that of 300% hydrated SC. Hence, almost no swelling of the lamellae is observed, which indicates that at high water levels, water is located either in the intercellular regions in separate domains or trapped in corneocytes.

    Figure 10 shows high-magnification cryo-scanning electron microscopy (cryo-SEM) images of SC hydrated to various levels and follows on former work we have previously reported (15). These images are obtained by slicing the skin perpendicular to the skin surface. In Figure 10A, SC hydrated to 17% w/w water by embedding

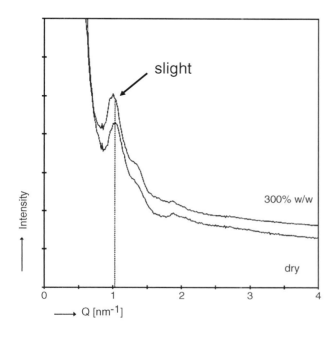

FIGURE 9 X-ray diffraction curve: intensity of the scattered X rays as function of the hydration. In this graph, dry SC is compared with SC sheet hydrated over water during 24 hours, after which the sheet has been measured immediately. *Abbreviation*: SC, stratum corneum.

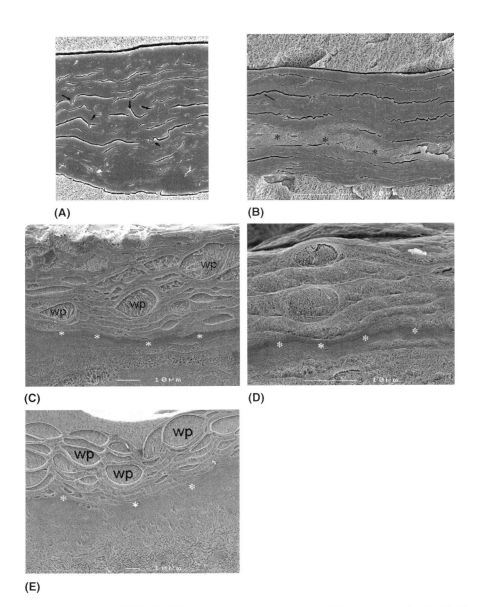

FIGURE 10   Cryo-SEM: (**A**) SC hydrated to 17% w/w water. SC sheet is embedded in tissue freezing medium. Arrows indicate undulations of cells. (**B**) SC hydrated to 70% w/w. White arrows indicate undulations. (**C**) Human skin after 48 hours of equilibration at 100% RH. White asterisks refer to non-swelling region. (**D**) Human skin after 15 hours of passive diffusion in an iontophoresis cell in an isotonic phosphate buffer solution. White asterisks refer to nonswelling region. (**E**) Human skin after six hours of passive diffusion followed by nine hours of iontophoresis. *Abbreviations*: RH, relative humidity; SC, stratum corneum; wp, water pools in the intercellular regions.

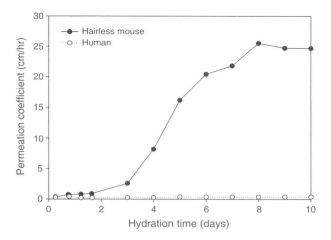

FIGURE 11   Hairless and human stratum corneum hydration during a 10-day period of hydration. *Source*: Adapted from Ref. 17.

the SC sheet in tissue-freezing medium. The image shows the tissue freezing medium in the top and bottom parts of the image with individual cells being visible. The low contrast indicates the absence of water pools and that no free water is present in the SC sheet. Arrows indicate undulations of cells. In contrast, freeze drying of water leads to an increase in sample surface relief, with dark regions corresponding to holes (lower regions) in the surface. In Figure 10B, when SC is hydrated to 70% w/w of its dry weight, it is apparent that slightly swollen cells exist in the center of the SC and that water is present, as indicated by the higher contrast (see black asterisks). The keratin network in this region is visible by white lines. It is notable that the appearance of the SC in the upper and lower SC that is similar to that seen in dry skin, indicating a lower water content in these regions. For the first time, three regions of skin hydration were identified in the SC. The white arrows indicate undulations, which are still present. A further increase in hydration levels in SC

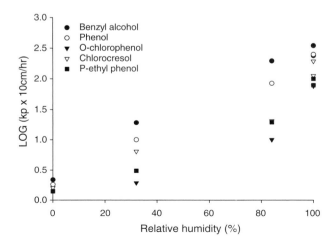

FIGURE 12   Phenolic compound permeability coefficients in human epidermis as a function of RH. *Abbreviation*: RH, relative humidity. *Source*: Adapted from Ref. 18.

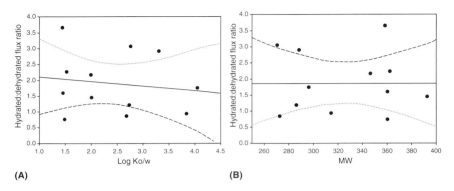

(A)   **(B)**

FIGURE 13 Comparison of hydration and dehydration on human skin flux of a series of steroids with (**A**) varying lipophilicity (log $K_{o/w}$ for octanol-water) and (**B**) size (MW). *Abbreviation*: MW, molecular weight. *Source*: Adapted from Ref. 21.

results not only in an increase hydration of the corneocytes but also in the formation of water pools in the intercellular regions (16). However, even at these very high water levels, a non-swelling region is present in the deepest SC regions as indicated by the white asterisks in Figure 10C. Cryo-SEM after 15 hours of passive diffusion in an iontophoresis cell in an isotonic phosphate buffer solution shows a swollen keratin network in corneocytes but again no swelling in the deepest corneocytes regions (Fig. 10D) or formation of water pools. This might be because of the isotonic solution instead of 100% RH in the environment. In contrast, iontophoresis leads to the formation of water pools in the intercellular regions (Fig. 10E), suggesting an SC hydration during iontophoresis (17). More recent work, also using cryo-SEM, again concluded that the SC exists as three functional zones, each with different water penetration and binding potentials (18). They proposed that the second zone was the functional SC barrier.

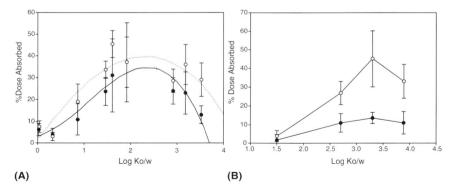

(A)   **(B)**

FIGURE 14 Occlusivity does not uniformly enhance penetration of solutes with varying octanol water partition coefficient (log $K_{o/w}$) across human skin in vivo: (**A**) phenols and (**B**) steroids. Open symbols, occluded; closed symbols, unoccluded. *Source*: Adapted from Ref. 22.

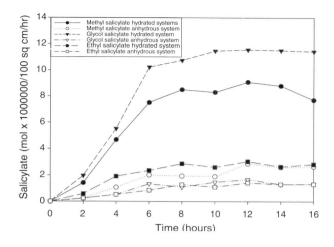

FIGURE 15 Effect of hydration on absorption of salicylate esters. *Source*: Adapted from Ref. 23.

SKIN TRANSPORT AND SC HYDRATION

SC hydration arises from water diffusing through the skin from a much-hydrated dermis to an ambient environment with variable RH. Also associated with an increase in water content is an increase in elasticity and SC permeability.

The choice of SC in skin penetration studies is very dependent on the conditions of use (19). Figure 11 shows that the SC permeability coefficient for human skin is relatively constant for 3 days, which for hairless mouse skin increases greatly after 24 hours. We have suggested that skin hydration may affect skin permeation by several orders of magnitude (20) as shown in Figure 12. In that work, the same solution was used for the donor- and receptor-side compositions and water activity expressed in terms of the effective RH generated by them. As we reviewed previously, increasing the percent RH has been shown to markedly increase the absorption for

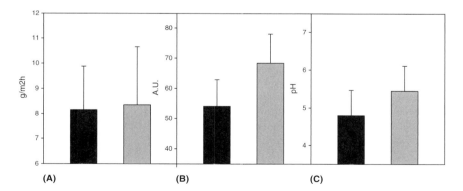

FIGURE 16 (**A**) TEWL, (**B**) capacitance, and (**C**) pH values (mean ± SD) in infants and adults at the volar forearm. *Significant with respect to adult skin. *Abbreviations*: A.U., arbitrary units by the instrument; TEWL, transepidermal water loss. *Source*: Adapted from Ref. 28.

a range of other solutes including aspirin, fusidic acid, methylethylketone, various corticosteroids, polar solutes, and more lipophilic solutes (1).

Most recently, Hikima and Maibach (21) examined the ratio of fluxes and lag times for a range of solutes and concluded that hydration enhancements were independent of lipophilicity and molecular weight. Figure 11 shows the results obtained for flux. These findings are consistent with the summary we had reported previously (1). Bucks and Maibach (22) had also reported a similar percent change in the dose absorbed for phenolic compounds with a log octanol-water partition coefficient range of 0 to ~4 (Fig. 14A). However, they concluded that a solute structure was evident for the steroids, with the more lipophilic steroids showing a greater enhancement by occlusion than the more polar ones (Fig. 14B). In contrast, as shown in Figure 13 for the salicylates, hydration aided the penetration of the more polar glycol salicylate than the more lipophilic methyl or ethyl salicylates (23).

The weight of current evidence suggests that enhancement of skin permeability is relatively independent of solute structure. Indeed, Tang et al. concluded that skin hydration increased skin permeability by inducing new pores and reducing the tortuosity of existing pores during a 4-hour hydration period. Importantly, they suggested that average pig SC pore radii remained relatively constant at ~26 Å for 48 hours (24). Hydration, both the reservoir effects in the skin, and later, occlusion, can also affect the retention and release of solutes from the SC (25,26). Given the likely larger reservoir effect in the SC for lipophilic solutes (25), such solutes would be expected to show a greater release on rehydration of the skin.

SC HYDRATION AND OTHER ASPECTS OF SKIN TRANSPORT

The vapor pressure of water above the skin that arises from this water leaving the SC is used to estimate the TEWL. A normal TEWL is about 0.5 $\mu L/cm^2/hr$. In principle, TEWL is a complementary measure of skin permeability. The permeability constant of water through SC is ~0.5×10^{-3} cm/hr, which corresponds to a flux from pure water of 0.2 $mg/m^2/hr$ (1). The self-diffusion of water is about 5 orders of magnitude less than that in the SC (1). The relationship between TEWL and percutaneous absorption has recently been reviewed (27). They concluded that, "the weight of evidence confirms a relationship between TEWL (water transport) to percutaneous absorption," but much remains to be learned. For example, the penetration route for water and other substances through SC is not necessarily the same.

The importance of the TEWL-percutaneous relationship is that TEWL may be a predictor for percutaneous absorption of solutes being applied to different skins in vivo and for which percutaneous absorption data are not available. There are numerous examples, such as the one presented here, on skin function with age (Fig. 16) (28) that show the value of recognizing TEWL as a measure of percutaneous absorption. A number of reviews and recent publications detail the associations between various skin diseases and altered skin barrier function as expressed by an increase in TEWL, a decrease in water-binding properties, and a reduction in skin surface lipids, specifically levels of ceramides (29–31).

CONCLUSION

Water is the most natural penetration enhancer and the agent most able to rectify abnormalities in skin function. Products that can assist in its function are discussed in Chapter 22.

ACKNOWLEDGMENT

One of the authors (M.R.) thanks the Australian National Health and Medical Research Council (NHMRC) for support.

REFERENCES

1. Roberts MS, Walker M. Water—the most natural penetration enhancer. In: Walters KA, Hadgraft J, eds. Skin Penetration Enhancement. New York: Marcel Dekker, 1993:1–30.
2. Rawlings AV, Matts PJ. Stratum corneum moisturization at the molecular level: an update in relation to the dry skin cycle. J Invest Dermatol 2005 Jun; 124(6): 1099–110.
3. J. Caussin, J. Wiechers, J.A. Bouwstra, Interactions of lipophilic moisturisers and stratum corneum lipids, Annual Controlled Release Society Meeting, Long Beach, 2007.
4. Scheuplein RJ, Morgan LJ. "Bound water" in keratin membranes measured by a microbalance technique. Nature 1967; 29:456–458.
5. Pirot F, Falson F, Maibach HI. Stratum corneum: an ideal osmometer? Exo Derm 2006; 3:339–349.
6. Boury-Jamot M, Sougrat R, Tailhardat M, et al. Expression and function of aquaporins in human skin: Is aquaporin-3 just a glycerol transporter? Biochim Biophys Acta 2006;1758:1034–1042.
7. Hara-Chikuma M, Verkman AS. Aquaporin-3 functions as a glycerol transporter in mammalian skin. Biol Cell 2005 Jul; 97(7):479–86.
8. Harris DR, Papa CM, Stanton R. Percutaneous absorption and the surface area of occluded skin. A scanning electron microscopic study. Br J Dermatol 1974; 91:27–32.
9. Rosén B-G, Blunt L, Thomas TR. On in-vivo skin topography metrology and replication techniques. J Phys. Conf Ser 2005; 13:325–329.
10. Zahouani H, Vargiolu K. Skin line morphology: tree and branches. In: Agache P, Humbert Ph, eds. Measuring the skin. Berlin-Heidelberg: Springer-Verlag, 2004.
11. Batisse D, Giron F, Lévêque JL. Capacitance imaging of the skin surface. Skin Res Technol 2006; 12:99–104.
12. E Xhauflaire-Uhoda, C Piérard-Franchimont, GE Piérard Skin capacitance mapping of psoriasis. J Eur Acad Dermatol Venereol 2006; 20:1261–1265.
13. Xhauflaire-Uhoda E, Haubrechts C, Loussouarn G, Lévêque JL, SaintLéger D, Piérard GE. Skin capacitance imaging and corneosurfametry. A comparative assessment of the impact of surfactants on stratum corneum. Contact Dermatitis 2006; 54: 249–253.
14. Caspers PJ, Lucassen GW, Carter EA, Bruining HA, Gerwin J, Puppels GJ. In vivo confocal Raman microspectroscopy of the skin: noninvasive determination of molecular concentration profiles. J Invest Dermatol 2001; 116:434–442.
15. Bouwstra JA, de Graaff A, Gooris GS, Nijsse J, Wiechers JW, van Aelst AC. Water distribution and related morphology in human stratum corneum at different hydration levels. J Invest Dermatol 2003; 120:750–758.
16. Bouwstra, JA, Groenink HW, Kempenaar JA, Romeijn S, Ponec, M. Water distribution and natural moisturising factor content in human skin equivalents is regulated by environmental relative humidity. J Invest Dermatol (in press).
17. Fatouros DG, Groenink HW, de Graaff, AM, van Alelst, AC, Koerten HK, Bouwstra JA. Visualization studies of human skin in vitro/in vivo under the influenze of an electric field. Eur J Pharm Sci. 2006; 29:160–170.
18. Richter T, Peuckert C, Sattler M, et al. Dead but highly dynamic—the stratum corneum is divided into three hydration zones. Skin Pharmacol Physiol 2004; 17:246–257.
19. Bond JR, Barry BW. Hairless mouse skin is limited as a model for assessing the effects of penetration enhancers in human skin. J Invest Dermatol 1988; 90:810–813.
20. Roberts MS. Structure-permeability considerations in percutaneous absorption. In: Scott RCt, Guy RH, Hadgraft J, Bodde HE, eds. Prediction of Percutaneous Penetration—Methods, Measurement and Modelling. Vol 2. London: IBC Technical Services, 1991:210–228.
21. Hikima T, Maibach H. Skin penetration flux and lag-time of steroids across hydrated and dehydrated human skin in vitro. Biol Pharm Bull 2006; 29:2270–2273.

22. Bucks D, Maibach H. Occlusion does not uniformly enhance penetration in vivo. In: Bronaugh RL, Maibach HI, eds. Percutaneous Absorption. 4th Edition. Boca Raton: Taylor & Francis, 2005:81–105.

23. Wurster DE, Kramer SF. Investigation of some factors influencing percutaneous absorption. J Pharm Sci 1961 Apr; 50:288–293.

24. Tang H, Blankschtein D, Langer R. Prediction of steady-state skin permeabilities of polar and nonpolar permeants across excised pig skin based on measurements of transient diffusion: characterization of hydration effects on the skin porous pathway. J Pharm Sci 2002; 91:1891–907.

25. Roberts MS, Anissimov YG, Cross SE. Factors affecting the formation of a skin reservoir for topically applied solutes. Skin Pharmacol Physiol 2004; 17(1): 3–16.

26. Pellanda C, Strub C, Figueiredo V, Rufli T, Imanidis G, Surber C. Topical bioavailability of triamcinolone acetonide: effect of occlusion. Skin Pharmacol Physiol 2007; 20:50–56.

27. Levin J, Maibach H. The correlation between transepidermal water loss and percutaneous absorption: an overview. J Control Release 2005; 103:291–99.

28. Giusti F, Martella A, Bertoni L, Seidenari S. Skin barrier, hydration, and pH of the skin of infants under 2 years of age. Pediatr Dermatol 2001; 18: 93–96.

29. Lebwohl M, Herrmann LG. Impaired skin barrier function in dermatologic disease and repair with moisturization. Cutis 2005; 76(6 Suppl.):7–12.

30. Rim JH, Jo SJ, Park JY, Park BD, Youn JI. Electrical measurement of moisturizing effect on skin hydration and barrier function in psoriasis patients. Clin Exp Dermatol 2005; 30:409–413.

31. Tomita Y, Akiyama M, Shimizu H. Stratum corneum hydration and flexibility are useful parameters to indicate clinical severity of congenital ichthyosis. Exp Dermatol 2005; 14:619–624.

8 Epidemiology of Skin Barrier Function: Host and Environmental Factors

Greg G. Hillebrand
Procter & Gamble, Cincinnati, Ohio, U.S.A.

R. Randall Wickett
James L. Winkle College of Pharmacy, University of Cincinnati, Cincinnati, Ohio, U.S.A.

INTRODUCTION

The skin's vital role as a protective barrier is often considered the most important of its many functions. Skin protects against mechanical injury, UV radiation damage, microbial infection, and permeation of harmful chemicals. In addition to protecting the body from these environmental insults, the skin also prevents rapid dehydration by slowing down the evaporative loss of internal water (see Chapter 7). Although the skin has many different protective barrier functions, it is the skin's ability to limit the movement of molecules, including water, from both inside-to-outside and from outside-to-inside, that is perhaps most commonly associated with the word "barrier." Amazingly, this permeability barrier function is localized almost entirely in the skin's outmost layer, the paper-thin stratum corneum (SC), a highly organized assembly of lipid-depleted corneocytes embedded in a lipid-enriched extracellular matrix (1–4).

The influence of various intrinsic (host) factors, such as age, sex, and race, or extrinsic (environmental) factors, such as lifetime sun exposure, diet, and lifestyle, on skin health and skin barrier properties is of particular interest. The study of such relationships falls under the general heading of epidemiology, and in this chapter, we will discuss the epidemiology of the skin barrier function. Most of the previous work in this area has concentrated on host factors, especially race, age, and body site. It is well-accepted that the efficiency of the SC's permeability barrier varies tremendously over different body sites. What is less well understood, and remains the focus of continued effort, is the variability in the skin's barrier properties across different ethnic populations and age groups. Starting as far back as 1919 with the studies by Marshall et al. (5) who investigated the relative susceptibility of black versus white skin to irritation by mustard gas, the scope of our understanding of the factors associated with skin barrier function has been steadily expanding to include nonwhite populations over a much wider age range, from the prenatal to the elderly (6–8).

Most of the work in this area involves the use of objective methods to compare the skin barrier properties of a sample group from one population to that of another at a single point in time. The early pioneering cross-sectional surveys used very small sample sizes that often yielded conflicting results that were difficult to interpret. In hindsight, it is not surprising that the base sizes of the earlier studies were so small. At the time these studies were conducted, the list of known host and environmental factors that could potentially affect skin barrier function was relatively short. Further, the large variance between individuals within a population relative to the small difference between populations was yet to be appreciated. Still, the ramifications of this previous and more recent research remains important and far reaching, for the results observed and conclusions made are usually extrapolated to the entire parent population of the sample group under study, which may have important practical implications in, for example, the way drugs are dosed or skin care products are formulated for one ethnic group or another (9,10). This is not to say that these earlier small base size studies were without value. On the contrary, our knowledge and understanding about the variability of the skin barrier has benefited greatly from this previous research because it helps guide the design of future more definitive studies.

In the last several years, the list of host and environmental factors that can potentially influence the skin's permeability barrier has greatly increased and will certainly continue to grow (e.g., nutrition and diet, history of cosmetic product use, history of sun exposure, season, hour of day, place of residence, and psychological stress). In this chapter, we try to recap the voluminous amount of previous literature on the epidemiology of the skin barrier function and offer suggestions for future work.

METHODS

As the body's interface with the external world, the skin's protective barrier prevents the movement of molecules, including water, in both directions, that is from inside-to-outside and from outside-to-inside. Each direction of this two-way street can be independently and objectively measured. The most commonly used end point for measuring the inside-to-outside direction in vivo is water evaporation at the skin surface, or transepidermal water loss (TEWL) (11,12). In fact, TEWL is so commonly used that standards are in place to define exactly how the measurement should be done (13–17). In this way, TEWL measurements can be more easily compared from one laboratory to another. The in vivo measurement of barrier function in the other direction (i.e., outside to inside) is more difficult and involves measuring the penetration of specific compounds across the permeability barrier into the body either directly or indirectly through a biological response.

Transepidermal Water Loss

From the classic experiment by Pinson in 1942 (18), comparing insensible perspiration from the skin on contralateral body sites with and without sweat glands inactivated by formaldehyde to our modern-day evaluations of skin-surface water evaporation, TEWL is taken as a true reflection of SC barrier function only when there is no sweat gland activity and the skin surface is dry (7). This is achieved by conducting measurements in controlled temperature and humidity environments, typically 21°C, 50% relative humidity (RH) with subjects at rest. Basal or baseline TEWL is the resting rate of evaporative loss of water through normal nonperturbed skin. Although variation is observed from one body site to another, basal TEWL is low in normal healthy intact human skin. Basal TEWL is a primary end point used to dimension the variability in skin barrier function across age, body site, ethnicity, and other factors. Although in vitro evidence has challenged the validity of the assumption that TEWL is predictive of the skin's permeability to topical penetrants (19), more recent validation studies support the generally agreed conclusion that TEWL is the current best objective measure of the skin's barrier to evaporative water loss (20,21).

The three instruments most commonly used to noninvasively measure TEWL are the Tewameter® evaporimeter (Courage & Khazaka, Cologne, Germany), the Dermalab TEWL module (Cortex Technologies, Hadsund, Denmark), and the ServoMed® evaporimeter (Servomed, Varberg, Sweden). All of these instruments are open-chamber devices of the type first reported by Hammarlund et al. (22). Correlation between data obtained using these instruments is excellent (21), but the absolute numbers do not agree because of slight differences in probe geometry (16,23). Values obtained with the ServoMed Evaporimeter are consistently lower than those obtained with the other instruments (16).

Just as a person with heart disease may be symptom-free and exhibit a normal EKG at rest but may show the heart abnormality under exercise-induced stress, basal TEWL may not reveal underlying deficiencies in an individual's barrier function. In the cutaneous stress test, barrier disruption (the stress) is typically accomplished by acute tape stripping or topical detergent/solvent treatment. Various parameters can be measured during and after barrier disruption including the number of tape strips needed to remove the SC, TEWL after each tape strip (or series of tape strips), the amount of SC removed, or the time it takes for the SC barrier function to return to baseline conditions (11,24–26). Both basal and stress TEWLs have been used to understand the variability in the skin barrier across many of the factors we will discuss.

Percutaneous Absorption

Compared with measuring TEWL, the in vivo measurement of percutaneous penetration is more difficult. One approach is to measure the biological response of the skin after topical application of a known irritant. Because both percutaneous penetration of the irritant and a biological response are required to reach the experimental end point (e.g., erythema or vasodilatation), the specific assessment of percutaneous penetration becomes more complicated. For reviews on the racial differences in susceptibility to skin irritation, see those by Robinson (27), Modjtahedi and Maibach (28), and Robinson (29). Given the large interindividual variance in barrier function combined with large interindividual variance in irritant susceptibility, it is not surprising that it is difficult to repeat studies on the response of various populations to irritants (30). A more direct approach to measuring percutaneous penetration is to follow the excretion of topically applied radiolabeled drugs over time. We review several in vivo studies that used radiolabeled agents to compare percutaneous penetration across ethnicity and body site.

In addition to the physiological parameters of TEWL and percutaneous absorption, various structural parameters related to the SC barrier have also been quantified as a function of age, body site, and ethnicity. These include the overall SC thickness, number of cell layers, corneocyte surface area, lipid content and composition, number of sweat glands and sweat pores, number of vellus hair follicles, and others.

Cross-Sectional Surveys: Size Does Matter

Medical science falls under two broad classes of research, experimental medicine and epidemiology. Experimental medicine involves the assessment of a defined treatment intervention on the progression of disease in a prospective format; the double-blind, randomized, vehicle-controlled clinical trial is the definitive experimental clinical method to prove cause of disease or treatment efficacy. Epidemiology, on the other hand, does not involve treatment intervention and relies solely on the observation of populations either retrospectively (looking back), prospectively (from this point forward), or at a single point in time, otherwise known as a cross-sectional design. To determine the similarities and differences of skin barrier properties across various host and environmental factors, many of the studies we will discuss used a cross-sectional design.

For example, in a simple theoretical study, the objective might be to compare the barrier function of Asian with white skin. The investigator might design a survey to measure TEWL on the forearm skin of a sample group of Chinese American women to that of an age-matched group of white American women during the second week of August. In this design, the researcher has matched the two groups for age, sex, ethnicity, nationality, and season of year. Forearm TEWL would be objectively measured according to a standardized protocol on every individual in the Chinese group and every individual in the white group. The mean TEWL values for each group would be compared using a two-tailed independent samples t test to determine the ratio of the difference between the two group means and the SD of the difference. If the ratio is large and we have 95% confidence to reject the null hypothesis ($P < 0.05$), we call the difference statistically significant. If the difference were found to be statistically significant, the investigator might conclude that Asian skin and white skin have different barrier properties.

This conclusion might be valid if the researcher were careful to consider the many pitfalls that accompany observational studies of this type (31). Unintentional subject selection bias can easily invalidate a study. Cross-sectional studies must be done on representative samples of the population if generalizations from the findings are to have any validity. Observational studies are particularly prone to selection bias when subject selection is nonrandom and/or the parent populations for the two groups are inherently different in some way. For example, in the example case above, if the Chinese Americans had lived most of their lives in San Francisco and the white Americans had lived most of their lives in Los Angeles, then any differences found in TEWL might be explained by differences in lifetime place of residence and have no relation to ethnicity.

Another very important aspect concerning the design of cross-sectional surveys of skin condition is sample size, and we would like to take time to discuss this in more detail using an example case study because many of the studies we will review have vastly different sample sizes. A type I error (α) occurs when the observed difference between the sample means is found to be statistically significant when, in fact, there is no real difference between the parent population means. The confidence level ($1 - \alpha$) increases as the power of the study decreases, and the power of a study decreases as (1) the interindividual variance increases, (2) the sample size decreases, (3) the actual difference in the means decreases, and/or (4) the acceptable level of risk, α, decreases.

We recently measured basal TEWL on the forearms of 452 normal healthy Chinese women, ages 10 to 70 years (n = 75, or 76/decade), who had lived most of their lives in northern (Beijing) China. All measurements were conducted in a room controlled for temperature ($21 \pm 1°C$) and RH ($50 \pm 5\%$) during the first two weeks of November, 2006. The same trained operator conducted all the measurements using the Tewameter evaporimeter according to a standardized protocol. After the subjects had acclimated to the room conditions for 45 minutes, three separate TEWL measurements were taken from each subject's middle volar forearm. All measurements were performed with the arm resting in a large open-top Plexiglas™ box to prevent air currents from interfering with the measurement. The mean of the three measurements was used as the final forearm TEWL value for that particular subject.

TABLE 1 Forearm TEWL for Chinese Women by Age Group: Mean, SD, and COV

	Age group						
	10–19	20–29	30–39	40–49	50–59	60–70	Average
Subjects	n = 76	n = 75	n = 75	n = 75	n = 76	n = 75	
TEWL	6.82	7.20	7.86	7.98	7.68	6.90	7.41
SD	2.30	2.53	2.75	2.62	2.38	2.07	2.44
COV (%)	33.7	35.2	35.0	32.8	31.0	29.9	33.0

Abbreviations: COV, coefficient of variance; SD, standard deviation; TEWL, transepidermal water loss. (GGH, unpublished data)

The mean *intra*individual coefficient of variance (COV) calculated from the three TEWL measurements across all 452 subjects was 7.8%, slightly lower than that observed by Shah et al. (12) for the open-chamber Tewameter evaporimeter.

Table 1 shows the mean TEWL ± SD for each 10-year age group. The mean *inter*individual COV for each age group was essentially unchanged across the age ranges surveyed showing an overall mean of 33%. This interindividual COV was in general agreement with that found previously by other groups. Fluhr et al. (32), observed a mean baseline TEWL of 8.5 with a SD of 2.9 (COV = 34.1%) on the ventral forearm of 12 white volunteers. Oestmann et al. (33) and Barel and Clarys (15) reported slightly lower (19% and 23.5%, respectively) interindividual variation (COV), whereas Marrakchi and Maibach (34) reported slightly higher (46%) interindividual variation for forearm TEWL in the groups of subjects enrolled in those studies.

These data allow us to calculate the sample size needed to provide 80% power to observe statistical significance ($P < 0.05$) for any predicted difference in mean forearm TEWL between similarly behaving sample groups (Table 2). As a low-end estimate of the potential difference we might expect to observe between population means, we can look to the in vitro studies of Wilson et al. (35). The researchers hoped to avoid problems associated with in vivo measurements, such as eccrine sweating and differences in body temperature by measuring TEWL on skin specimens taken from the inner thigh skin of 12 whites to that of 10 African Americans. The subjects ranged in age from 5 to 72 years and had a mean age of 40 years. Both male and female subjects provided skin for the study. The two groups were age- and sex-matched. African American skin showed 1.1 times (10%) higher ($P < 0.01$) in vitro TEWL compared with excised white skin.

Table 2 shows that to have 80% power to observe a 10% difference between the mean basal TEWL for a group of African Americans and the mean basal TEWL for a group of whites in vivo with statistical significance ($P < 0.05$, two-sided, independent *t* test), the sample size required would be at least 172 people for each leg of the study,

TABLE 2 Sample Size Requirements as a Function of the Mean Difference in Basal Forearm TEWL[a]

Predicted difference in TEWL	Required sample size per leg (independent *t* test)	Required sample size (paired *t* test)
10%	172	88
20%	44	24
30%	20	12
40%	12	8
50%	8	6

[a]assumes 80% power, $P < 0.05$, COV=33%.
Abbreviations: COV, coefficient of variance; TEWL, transepidermal water loss.

a total of 344 people! As the expected difference between mean TEWL for each group increases, the sample size needed to show statistical significance decreases. For paired comparisons, substantially smaller base sizes are required. In cross-sectional surveys of skin condition, size does matter!

HOST FACTORS
Ethnicity
Many cross-sectional surveys have been conducted aimed at comparing basal TEWL, stress TEWL, and/or percutaneous absorption across different ethnic populations (36). Here, we will discuss, in chronological order, the results of 11 such surveys organized by the end point measured: first, the basal TELW results, then the stress test results, and, finally, the percutaneous absorption results.

In 1988, Berardesca and Maibach (37) compared in vivo TEWL on the back skin of 10 African American versus 10 White American male subjects with a mean age of 30 years. No significant difference in basal TEWL was observed. In parallel work, Berardesca and Maibach (38) compared basal TEWL on the forearm of Hispanics (n = 7, age 27.8 ± 4.5 years) and White (n = 9, age 30.6 ± 8.8 years). No significant difference in basal TEWL was observed. Takahashi et al. (39) followed with a large base-size study comparing basal TEWL on 258 whites from the United Kingdom, 277 Whites from France, 180 Whites from the United States, and 77 Japanese from Japan. The study was conducted in February in the United Kingdom, France, and United States and in December in Japan. The subjects were all female and ranged in age from 10 to 69 years. No significant difference in basal TEWL was observed between the Japanese and Whites.

In 1991, Berardesca et al. (40) reported a study comparing basal TEWL on a group of 15 Blacks, 12 Whites, and 12 Hispanics on the volar and dorsal forearm. TEWL on the volar forearm was found to be 2.55 ± 0.19 for blacks, 2.75 ± 0.33 for Whites, and 2.93 ± 0.33 for Hispanics, but none of the differences were statistically significant because of the large interindividual variability. In a 1993 abstract, Sugino et al. (41) reported that the basal TEWL was in decreasing order: African American > White ≥ Hispanic ≥ Asian. That same year, Kompaore et al. (42) reported on another small base size study comparing forearm TEWL on a three groups of subjects, seven black men, eight whites (six men and two women), and six Asian men. The age of the subjects ranged from 23 to 32 years, and the study was conducted in France. Although there was no significant difference in basal TEWL between Asian and black skin, both Asian and black skin showed 1.3 times higher basal TEWL than that of white skin ($P < 0.01$).

In 1996, Warrier et al. (43) compared the skin biophysical properties of female African Americans versus White Americans between the ages of 18 and 45 years. Forty-five subjects of each race were recruited and screened for skin color with the Minolta Chromameter® (Konica Minolta, Osaka, Japan). The 30 white subjects with the highest L^* values and the 30 African American subjects with the lowest L^* values were selected for the measurement phase of the study. The two groups were approximately matched for age. TEWL measurements were made on the right medial cheek, mid volar forearms, and lateral mid lower legs during the winter months from December to February in Cincinnati, Ohio, U.S.A. using the ServoMed evaporimeter (Fig. 1). Basal TEWL was found to be significantly lower in the African American skin versus that of White skin on the legs and cheeks but not significantly different on the forearm. Capacitance, a measure of skin hydration, was found to be significantly higher on the cheeks of African Americans as well. Figure 1 also shows the typical difference between TEWL on the face compared with the forearms and legs.

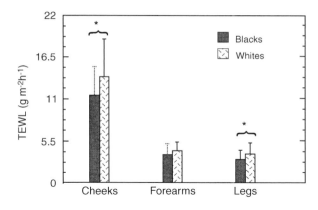

FIGURE 1 Baseline transepidermal water loss (TEWL) on the cheeks, forearms, and legs of black and white subjects (mean ± SD). *Source*: From Ref. 43.

Subsequently, Berardesca et al. (25) also reported no significant difference in basal forearm TEWL from a study comparing 10 female white Americans with 8 female African Americans with a mean age of 42 years. In another small base-size study, Singh et al. (44) did not observe a significant difference in forearm basal TEWL among Whites, Hispanics, Asians, and African Americans (five male and five female subjects in each group). The subjects ranged in age from 10 to 80 years. Whites showed higher basal TEWL than that of the other three ethnic groups, but the difference was not statistically significant.

In 2002, Aramaki et al. (45) also found that white skin showed significantly higher TEWL than that of Asian skin. In that work, basal TEWL was measured on the forearms of 22 Japanese women and 22 white German women. Groups were balanced for age (mean age, 26 years), and the study was conducted in Marburg, Germany. But that same year, Yosipovitch and Theng (46) and Yosipovitch et al. (47) reported no significant difference in forearm basal TEWL when comparing four different subpopulations of Asian ethnic groups with Whites (13 Chinese, 7 Malay, 10 Indian, and 9 white; mean age, 34 years).

Most recently, a large base size study was carried out to compare TEWL and barrier strength among Whites (n = 114), African Americans (n = 63), and Asians (n = 155) (48). The results suggested that the African Americans have lower basal TEWL compared with Whites and Asians, in agreement with Warrier et al. (43). However, the differences observed were not reported to be statistically significant. The researchers also found that the number of tape strips needed to increase TEWL > 18 $g/m^2/hr$ was in rank order: African Americans > Whites > Asians with the difference between African Americans and Asians being statistically significant.

In summary, the mixed findings of the 11 in vivo studies we reviewed that addressed the question of ethnic variability in basal TEWL prevent a firm conclusion regarding the relationship between ethnicity and skin barrier function (as measured by basal TEWL). Seven of the studies reported no significant difference in basal TEWL among the ethnic groups under study. Of the three studies reporting a significant difference between Blacks and Whites, two reported finding significantly higher basal TEWL in Blacks compared with Whites, and one reported finding significantly higher TEWL in Whites compared with Blacks. For the comparison between Asian skin and white skin, the results were also mixed. One study reported significantly higher basal TEWL in white skin, and one study reported significantly higher TEWL in Asian skin. We interpret these data to suggest that the actual difference in basal TEWL between ethnic populations is small and difficult to reproducibly demonstrate in a survey. Any difference that may exist between ethnic groups is overwhelmed by the large interindividual differences within those ethnic groups.

The cutaneous stress test has also been used to compare differences in barrier function between ethnicities. Twenty years ago, Berardesca and Maibach (37) performed a cutaneous stress test on African American and white male subjects. They observed that the African American male subjects (n = 10) have a higher TEWL increase on back skin in response to sodium lauryl sulfate (SLS) treatment compared with white male subjects (n = 9). However, the difference in the means was only statistically significant when the skin had been preoccluded with plastic film. Similar findings were observed by the two investigators comparing the TEWL response to SLS treatment in Hispanics versus Whites; Hispanics were more responsive to SLS when the skin was preoccluded (38). Five years later, Kompaore et al. (42) measured TEWL after either 8 or 12 tape strips on the forearm and found that Asians had up to 1.7 times higher TEWL after tape stripping compared with Whites. There was no significant difference between black skin and Asian skin.

In 1995, Reed et al. (49) reported on the number of tape strips needed to perturb the barrier and the rate of barrier repair in white (n = 8), Asian (n = 6), and African American (n = 4) skin. The subjects were of both sexes. There was no significant difference between ethnic groups for the number of tape strips needed to perturb the barrier, nor were there any significant differences between groups in the rate of barrier repair. However, when the researchers grouped the subjects according to skin types, they found that it took more tape strips to perturb the barrier of skin types V and VI compared with skin types II and III. Skin types V and VI also recovered more quickly compared with skin types II and III. Subjects with skin type I were excluded.

Berardesca et al. (25) measured TEWL after tape stripping the forearm skin of African American women (n = 8) and white American women (n = 10). The mean age of the two groups was 42 years. TEWL was significantly higher in the African American group after three and six tape strips (the upper SC layers), but there was no significant difference in TEWL between groups after 9, 12, and 15 strips (the deeper SC layers).

In a study comparing Japanese (n = 22) with white (n = 22) women with a mean age of 26 years, Aramaki et al. (45) found that the Japanese showed lower TEWL after SLS-induced barrier disruption on the forearm compared with Whites ($P < 0.05$). This result mirrored the findings for basal TEWL for the two groups; the Japanese women showed significantly lower basal TEWL compared with the white women. On the other hand, Yosipovitch and Theng (46) and Yosipovitch et al. (47) did not observe a significant difference between a group of Asians and a group of Whites for TEWL after tape stripping.

In summary, as was the case with baseline TEWL, the results for ethnic difference in SC barrier function as determined by the cutaneous stress test TEWL are also mixed. This is not surprising given the variety of protocols used to stress the skin barrier and the variety of end points used to measure the response of the individual to the stress. Although the stress test TEWL method is a useful tool to assess the efficacy of topical treatments for accelerating barrier repair in controlled clinical trials (50,51), its use for differentiating population differences in barrier properties is a challenge.

Several researchers have measured percutaneous absorption of topically applied molecules across ethnic groups. For many of these studies, the end point measured was the skin's biological response to a topically applied drug. For example, vasodilatation in response to topical methyl nicotinate has been used to compare the barrier properties of Asian (n = 13), black (n = 7), and white (n = 8) skin (52). Both male and female subjects were enrolled. All the subjects were living in France at the time. Vasodilatation in response to the test treatment was objectively measured by laser Doppler velocimetry which avoids the difficulty of trying to measure irritant-induced erythema on dark-colored skin. The lag time between application of the test agent and vasodilatation was used as a measure of the permeability barrier. Using this method, the authors found that black skin showed the longest lag time, then white skin, then Asian skin. After tape stripping (12 strips for each group), the rank order for lag times remained the same (although the percent decrease in lag time was greater for Asians than for Whites or Blacks). The authors concluded that black skin was less permeable than white and Asian skin. These results are consistent with those observed a few years earlier by Berardesca and Maibach (53).

The observed differences in lag time to vasodilatation after treatment with methyl nicotinate might have been partly or solely because of differences in SC barrier function. However, because the end point measured is a biological response, other explanations could also account for the observed differences including population differences in blood vessel reactivity to the test agent. Guy et al. (54) points out that there may be racial differences in the vasodilatation response to methyl nicotinate. Because of this, Leopold and Maibach (55) took a different approach to try and measure the actual drug flux through the SC under steady-state conditions. In this method, glass chambers containing the drug are mounted onto the skin site (upper arm), and the amount of drug depleted during a 6-hour period is measured. Leopold and Maibach compared the flux of methyl nicotinate in healthy female Whites, Hispanics, Blacks, and Asians (n = 12 for each group). The authors observed that drug flux increased in the following order: Blacks < Asians < Whites < Hispanics with the difference between Blacks and Hispanics reaching statistical significance.

A more direct approach to measure the SC barrier to topical penetrants is to use radiolabeled topically applied drugs. In this approach, the radiolabeled drug is applied to the skin, and the amount of drug penetrated is measured in the urine, feces, and/or blood. Wickrema-Sinha et al. (56) used this method to measure percutaneous absorption of tritiated diflorasone diacetate. The authors compared a group of white men (n = 3) with a group of African American men (n = 3) between the ages of 26 and 46 years. Considering the extremely small sample size, it is not surprising that no significant difference between ethnic groups was observed.

Wedig and Maibach (57) used ^{14}C-labeled dipyrithione to measure skin penetration in four white and four black male subjects. Absorption was measured by urinary excretion during the course of 1 week after a single topical dose. Mean absorption in the black subjects was 34% less compared with the white subjects.

Lotte et al. (58) also used a radiolabeled approach to follow the penetration of ^{14}C-benzoic acid, ^{14}C-caffeine, and ^{14}C-acetylsalicylic acid through the upper outer arm skin of African Americans (n = 6–8, number depended on the compound tested), white Americans (n = 9), and Chinese American (n = 6–7). Urinary excretion of radiolabel was monitored during the 24-hour period after dosing. No statistically significant differences were found between ethnic groups for percutaneous penetration of any of the tested compounds.

The most direct way to measure the skin barrier to percutaneous absorption without the confounding variables of metabolism, blood flow, or biological response is to use excised skin from cadavers. Bronaugh et al. (59) developed a relatively simple method to determine the skin barrier integrity by measuring the water permeability constant using tritiated water. As part of the overall effort to establish this method, the researchers compared the barrier integrity of abdominal skin samples taken from male and female Whites (n = 23) with that of African Americans (n = 10), ages 40–70 years. There was no significant difference in water permeation between the two ethnic groups.

Various constituents of the SC have been quantified in the skin of people representing different population groups. SC lipids, especially the ceramide component, have been extensively studied because their essential role in maintaining a healthy skin barrier (60,61). Meguro et al. (62) showed there is an inverse relationship between epidermal SC ceramides and TEWL.

La Ruche and Cesarini (63) and Rienertson and Wheatley (64) found that the lipid content of the SC was higher in Blacks versus Whites. Sugino et al. (41) found significant differences in ceramide levels with the lowest levels in Blacks (10.7 ± 4.7 µg/mg), then whites (20.4 ± 8.1 µg /mg), then Hispanics (20.0 ± 4.3 µg/mg). Sugino et al. (41) also found that the SC ceramide level was inversely proportional to TEWL and directly proportional to water content further supporting the physiological relevance of this SC lipid with barrier function. Hellemans et al. (48) reported lower ceramide levels in the skin of African American subjects.

Structural features of the SC from different ethnic populations have also been compared, including corneocyte cell size. In Whites, it has been suggested that corneocyte size is an important factor related to TEWL and percutaneous absorption of topically applied compounds (65). Greater permeability was associated with smaller corneocyte size. However, Fluhr et al. (66) observed no such correlation between corneocyte size and TEWL or hydration. Corcuff et al. (67) measured corneocyte surface area in the SC of Whites, Blacks, and Chinese (n = 18–25/group), with a mean age of 31, 33.5, and 26.5 years, respectively. There was no significant difference among black, white, and Asian skin for corneocyte surface area. One difference that was found was significantly higher (2.5-fold) spontaneous desquamation in Blacks versus both Whites and Chinese.

Several researchers have compared the skin thickness of the SC of Blacks to that of Whites. La Ruche and Cesarini (63), Thomson (68), Freeman (69), and Lock-Anderson et al. (70) all found no significant difference in the SC thickness between African American and white skin. Although skin thickness at a particular body site is not significantly different among ethnic groups, the number of cell layers at that body site may be related to ethnicity. Weigand et al. (71) took 4-mm punch biopsies from the lumbar skin from 17 African Americans and 15 Whites (biopsies were from both live subjects and cadavers with a mix of sex) and compared for the number cell layers. Cryostat-frozen sections of the biopsy samples were prepared for microscopy by expanding the SC with NaOH followed by staining with methylene blue. They found significantly more cell layers in the SC of African Americans (21.8 ± 2.7) compared to that of Whites (16.7 ± 2.0). The number of layers was not related to the degree of pigmentation. Also, more tape strips were required to remove the SC of black skin compared with white skin. The authors suggested that compared to white skin, the black skin SC layers had greater cellular cohesion compared with Whites.

The transcutaneous pathways of percutaneous absorption of topically applied substances include not only direct diffusion through the lipid domains of the SC but also through pathways provided by hair follicles and sweat glands. Ethnic differences in hair follicle density and/or size could therefore contribute to differences in skin penetration (72). There are clearly tremendous ethnic differences in the terminal hair characteristics and hair follicle structure on the scalp. Sperling (73) measured the scalp hair density of a group of African Americans (n = 22; mean age, 31.7 years) to a group of whites (n = 12; mean age, 34.6 years). The scalp hair density in African Americans was found to be significantly lower than that in Whites.

Mangelsdorf et al. (74) studied vellus hair follicular size and density at different body sites in African Americans (n = 10), Asians (n = 6), and whites (n = 10). On the forehead, which showed the highest density of vellus hair follicles of any body site, whites showed significantly higher density compared with African Americans followed by Asians. La Ruche and Cesarini (63) as well as Jorgenson et al. (75) have reported that the number of sweat glands and sweat pores in black and white skin is identical.

Age

Earlier, in Table 1, we showed the mean forearm TEWL for Chinese female subjects in each 10-year age group from 10 to 70 years. Analysis of variance reveals there is a statistically significant difference between groups ($P = 0.008$). The post hoc analysis (least significant difference) showed the 10–19-year age group mean is significantly less ($P < 0.05$) than the 30–39-, 40–49-, and 50–59-year age group means. The 60–70-year age group mean was also significantly less than the 30 to 39, 40 to 49, and 50 to 59 age group means. With these data, expressed in this way, we might conclude that skin barrier function on the forearm of Chinese women living in Beijing decreases from the teens to the 40s (as gleaned from the 17% increase in TEWL) and thereafter increases.

Figure 2 shows the scatter plot for these same data; each point is one of the 452 subjects in the study. The line is a quadratic regression fit to the data. With the added perspective of the relatively wide range of TEWL values observed across the sample population, the relative difference between the teens and the middle-aged years does not now seem so impressive. Indeed, without the quadratic regression fit to help aid the interpretation (right graph), one might conclude there is no clinically important change in forearm TEWL across age in Chinese women,

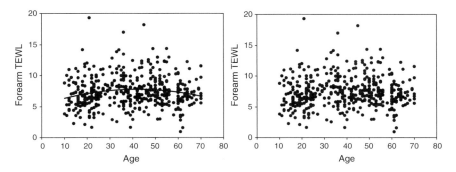

FIGURE 2 Basal forearm TEWL across age with (left) and without (right) the quadratic regression fit (GGH, unpublished data). *Abbreviation*: TEWL, transepidermal water loss.

a conclusion markedly different from what we made in the previous paragraph using the same data.

There is another important aspect concerning cross-sectional surveys across age that we feel is frequently missed and needs to be pointed out. Let us assume the observed differences in mean basal TEWL values for the different age groups shown in Table 1 are real and clinically important. Our initial conclusion would be that forearm TEWL on Chinese women changes with increasing age, first increasing and then decreasing as Chinese women grow older. But is age the only variable here? We must remember that the women in our sample lived during vastly different cultural periods of modern China. Those in the oldest age group were born between 1936 and 1946, whereas those in the youngest age group were born between 1988 and 1997. An alternative and perhaps equally valid explanation for the observed results is that the women in the different age groups experienced different environmental factors during their lifetime (e.g., sun, diet, stress), depending on when they were born, and that the differences in exposure to these factors accounts for the observed differences in mean TEWL and has nothing to do with human aging. The adage, "correlation does not necessarily mean causation" must be reminded over and over when interpreting data such as those in Table 1.

Although the data in Table 1 and Figure 2 suggest a significant association between age and basal TEWL, at least for normal healthy Chinese women, most researchers have not observed an association of this host factor with barrier function as measured by basal TEWL albeit with much smaller base sizes (76–78). Roskos and Guy (79) observed no difference in basal TEWL between a group of young (n = 13, 19–42 years) and old (n = 9, 69–85 years) white men and women. However, the time for the skin to return to basal TEWL levels after 24 hours of occlusion with a polypropylene chamber (to achieve complete SC hydration) was much longer for the old group compared with the young group.

In an interesting intrafamilial study by Fluhr et al. (80), basal TEWL and several other biophysical measurements were taken on the volar forearm of 44 children (mean age, 3.5 years; range, 1–6 years) and one of their parents (mean age, 34.6 years). Although the subjects all had atopic dermatitis, the researchers were prudent to ensure there was no difference with respect to the clinical atopy score between the adult and child groups. Further, the test areas (volar forearms) were free of eczematous lesions. The mean basal TEWL for the children (5.4 ± 2.5 g/m^2/hr) was not significantly different from that of their parents (6.2 ± 3.5 g/m^2/hr). In fact, there was no difference in several of the measured skin biophysical properties including capacitance, conductance, water-holding capacity, and yellowness (b^*). The authors summarize that "based on the almost identical values for the parameters of TEWL, SC hydration and pH value, the skin physiology of the child differs very little in SC hydration and barrier function from that of adults."

Takahashi et al. (39) measured basal TEWL on 258 Whites from the United Kingdom, 277 Whites from France, 180 Whites from the United States, and 77 Japanese from Japan. Basal TEWL was observed to decline with increasing age. Skin surface conductance, a measure of SC hydration, tended to increase with age. The scaling score on the cheek significantly decreased with increasing age. The surface area of corneocytes on the cheek increased with age.

Marrakchi and Maibach (34) compared basal TEWL on the face, neck, and forearm between a group of young adults (n = 10; mean age, 25.2 years; range, 19–30 years) and older adults (n = 10; mean age, 73.7 years; range, 70–81 years). In addition, the same skin sites were challenged with 2% SLS under occlusion for one hour.

TEWL was measured at baseline and at 23 hours after patch removal. The mean change from baseline in TEWL was determined at the different body sites in both the young and old groups. For all the skin sites tested, the young group showed a larger SLS-induced TEWL change from baseline than the older group, with the chin and nasolabial area being significantly different. The authors did not report the basal TEWL values at each site for each age group.

Ten years earlier, Shriner and Maibach (81) conducted a very similar study and measured basal TEWL at several locations on the face as well as on the neck and forearm for a small group of middle-aged adults (n = 10; mean age, 37.8 years; range, 23–47 years) and older adults (n = 5; mean age, 76 years; range, 72–90 years). Basal TEWL was consistently lower in the older age group, but the difference was not statistically significant. This was consistent with a comparison between a small group of young adult women (n = 7, age = 25.9 ± 1.4 years) and elderly women (n = 8, age = 74.6 ± 1.9 years); there was no significant difference between young and elderly groups (82).

Wilhelm et al. (8) measured basal TEWL at several body sites in 14 young adults (26.7 ± 2.8 years) and 15 adults (70.5 ± 13.8 years). Basal TEWL was significantly lower in the older age group at most skin sites tested.

Rogers et al. (84) studied the change in SC lipids with age in 49 white women between the ages of 21 and 60. Eight sequential tape strips from the hands, face, and leg were collected, and the SC lipids (fatty acids, cholesterol, and ceramides) were separated and quantified using high-performance thin-layer chromatography and scanning densitometry. There was a significant decrease in all major lipid classes with increasing age; however, the ratio of the different lipids remained constant. All the ceramide species declined with increasing age on the face and hand.

SC thickness has not been found to change significantly with age. In a study of 301 Japanese men and women ranging in age from 1 to 97 years, Ya-Xian et al. (85) counted cell layers in frozen 6-μm-thick sections stained and expanded in alkaline solution and found no relationship between SC thickness and age in female subjects and a slight trend toward thicker SC with age in men ($P = 0.67$). A similar conclusion was reached (i.e., no change in SC thickness with age) by Batisse et al. (86) who used confocal imaging to quantify and compare the SC thickness of 16 young adult women (mean age, 21 ± 2 years) with 18 older adult women (mean age, 65 ± 2 years); the mean SC thickness was 15 ± 3 and 17 ± 3 μm, respectively.

Body Site

The study of barrier function variability across the skin regions of the human body has a tremendous advantage compared with the study across age and ethnicity in that each subject serves as their own control, thereby allowing for paired comparisons. This translates into much greater statistical power at less cost (sample size) compared with unpaired comparisons (Table 2). Perhaps that is partly why barrier function has been so well-studied and better understood at different body sites across a wide age range, from neonates (87) to adults (85).

It is well-known that the relative efficiency of the skin barrier is not uniform across the body. Forty years ago, Feldman and Maibach (88) reported on the regional variation in skin permeability using ^{14}C-labeled hydrocortisone (HC) in vivo. Subjects (all male) had a known amount of HC, spiked with ^{14}C-labeled HC, applied to various parts of their body using acetone as a solvent. Urine was collected for five days and analyzed for [14]C. Large regional variations in absorption were observed. Using the ventral forearm as the control site, the highest absorption was observed on scrotal areas (42 times that of the ventral forearm), whereas the lowest absorption was observed on the heel of the foot, similar to the earlier findings of Smith et al. (89). The authors noted that in hairy areas, follicular absorption may be greater than transepidermal absorption.

Dupuis et al. (90) measured TEWL and percutaneous absorption of ^{14}C-labeled benzoic acid on the upper back, upper outer arm, chest, anterior thigh, abdomen, and forehead of men (six men per site). After dosing at each site, urine was collected during the next 4 days and counted. TEWL was measured after the benzoic acid treatment on a contralateral site. There was a strong relationship between basal TEWL and total benzoic acid penetration in 4 days ($r = 0.97$), indicating that TEWL was predictive of penetration. The permeability of benzoic acid varied according to body site in the following order: back < arm < chest < thigh < abdomen < forehead. The authors point out that although the forehead was two to three times more permeable to water and benzoic acid than the other sites tested, the difference in SC thickness between sites is very small (91).

In a large base size study of Japanese men (n = 158) and women (n = 143), ranging in age from 1 to 97 (mean age, 42 years), Ya-Xian et al. (85) quantified the relationship between the number of SC cell layers and TEWL at various body sites. TEWL was highest on the eyelid, then the cheek, then the upper arm, abdomen, back, and extensor thigh. There were great individual differences in the number of cell layers in the SC even from the same site. The number of cell layers was smallest on genital skin (6 ± 2), whereas in skin from most locations of the trunk and extremities, it was between 10 and 20 layers. The skin of the palmoplantar areas is extremely thick, from 50 layers on the palm to as high as 86 layers on the heel. The SC of the extremities showed a higher number of cell layers than that of the trunk. The SC of the face, neck, and scalp tended to be thinner than that of the trunk. There was no difference between sexes. There was no correlation between the number of cell layers and age for the back, abdomen, and anterior surface of the thigh. There was a significant increase in the number of cell layers on the cheek with increasing age for men. The variation in SC thickness may help explain the higher sensitivity of the face and neck to topical formulations (81) as well as the finding that the barrier function of scrotal skin is much less than that of abdominal skin (89).

Not only is there tremendous variability in barrier function between body regions, there can also be tremendous variability within a given region such as the face or arm. Marrakchi and Maibach (34) recently mapped skin barrier function (basal TEWL) on the face (cheek, chin, forehead, nasolabial, nose, and perioral area) of 20 volunteers (12 white and 8 Hispanic). At baseline, the nasolabial fold area (a facial site commonly used for stinging tests) showed the highest TEWL value at 28.74 ± 8.56 $g/m^2/hr$, while the forehead showed half that value (14.10 ± 5.71 $g/m^2/hr$). The rank order was, from highest to lowest, nasolabial > perioral > chin > nose > cheek > forehead > neck > forearm. Ten years earlier, Shriner and Maibach (81) measured baseline TEWL at the same facial locations in a group of young adults (n = 10; mean age, 37.8 years; range, 23–47 years). In that study, the perioral area showed the highest baseline TEWL value followed by the nose and nasolabial areas. Shah et al. (12), in a small study of four women and five men (ages 27–70 years), found that TEWL was much lower on the forearm than on the forehead. The center of the forehead had higher TEWL values than the sides of the forehead, and the forearm near the wrist had higher values than near the elbow.

Interestingly, forearms may not be symmetrical when it comes to barrier function. Although there is no significant difference between the right and left forearms for basal TEWL (15,33), there is a significant difference between dominant and non-dominant forearms (i.e., right- or left-handed) (92).

The correlation between baseline TEWL and the subsequent change in TEWL after exposure to one-hour occlusive challenge with 2% SLS in water has been examined (34). Some regions of the face (cheek and chin) are more sensitive to SLS (assessed by change in TEWL) than others. Interestingly, the authors found a significant correlation between basal TEWL and the susceptibility of the skin site to SLS irritation at some skin sites, suggesting that basal TEWL may be predictive of the percutaneous absorption of the topical irritant.

Menstrual Status

Kikuchi et al. (93) did not observe a difference in pre- versus post-menopause women for basal TEWL on either the cheek or the flexor forearm. TEWL was measured on 26 premenopausal (mean age, 36 ± 9 years) and 13 postmenopausal (mean age, 59 ± 11 years) Japanese women.

Fluhr et al. (64) measured corneocyte surface area, TEWL, SC hydration, water-holding capacity, and moisture accumulation velocity in 33 premenopausal women (mean age, 41 ± 4.4 years), 21 postmenopausal women (mean age, 50.6 ± 4.9 years), and 25 men (mean age, 44.0 ± 5.5 years). There was no significant difference in basal TEWL or the hydration parameters among groups. There was a significant difference among groups for corneocyte surface area, but the authors did not observe a correlation between surface area and TEWL or hydration. The body site where these measurements were conducted was missing from the report.

Harvell et al. (94) measured the change in basal TEWL on the volar forearm and the upper back of nine healthy women ages 19 to 46 years (mean age, 32 years) with normal menstruations and cycle lengths in the normal range. The women were not taking contraceptives. Basal TEWL on both the forearm and the back was significantly higher on the day of the month of minimal estrogen/progesterone secretion (just before the onset of menses) as compared with the day of maximal estrogen secretion (just before ovulation). These data, although only on a small base size sample, suggest that skin barrier function is slightly compromised before the onset of the menses as compared with the days just before ovulation.

Agner et al. (95) also found significant differences for the skin response to SLS challenge as assessed by TEWL at different days in the menstrual cycle. The response was significantly stronger for women (n = 29) on their first day of their menstrual cycle compared with days 9 to 11. More recently, in a larger base study, Muizzuddin et al. (129) measured the skin barrier strength during the cycle and found that barrier strength was the weakest on days 22 to 26, the days before menses, corroborating the findings of Harvell et al. (94).

Sex

Most of the evidence suggests there is little, if any, difference in barrier function (basal TEWL) between the sexes at most body sites (82,84,96).

Body Mass Index

Forearm TEWL was measured on 63 subjects (39 women and 23 men) equally divided into three groups of low (<25), middle (25–30), and high (>30) body mass index (BMI) ranges (97). Each group was matched for sex, age, and Fitzpatrick skin

TABLE 3   Basal Forearm TEWL as a Function of BMI

BMI	Baseline	24-hour water	24-hour 0.25% SLS	24-hour 0.5% SLS
<25	6.9	8.4	22	33.4
25–30	8.8	9.0	24.3	29.3
>30	11.5[a]	11.0	30.1	36.1

[a]Significantly different from < 25 BMI group ($P < 0.05$).
Abbreviations: BMI, body mass index; SLS, sodium lauryl sulfate. *Source*: From Ref. 97.

type. Subjects were in good health and free of skin abnormalities in the test area. Measurements were at baseline before applying 60 μL of water, 0.25% SLS, or 0.5% SLS under occlusion for 48 hours using Large Finn Chambers® (Epitest Ltd., Hyrlä, Finnland). Twenty-four hours after removing the patch, a second TEWL measurement was taken (Table 3). The most obese individuals (BMI > 30) showed significantly higher basal forearm TEWL compared with the underweight/normal BMI group (BMI < 25, Table 3). There was no significant difference between groups for TEWL after either water or the two concentrations of SLS treatment. The authors note that the subjects with high BMI also had significantly higher skin blood flow. Because changes in skin blood flow do not affect baseline TEWL (17), the observed difference in mean TEWL between obese and underweight/normal individuals are likely associated with differences in barrier function. With the increased prevalence of human obesity in many developed countries around the word, much more work is needed in this area to confirm these results.

ENVIRONMENTAL FACTORS
Season of Year
Kikuchi et al. (93) showed that baseline TEWL was significantly higher on the cheek and the forearm in the winter than in the summer months (Fig. 3). In that work, TEWL was measured on exactly the same 39 Japanese women (mean age, 44 years; range, 24–78 years) in the summer (August 14 to October 9) versus winter (December 16 to April 15) months. The subjects were subdivided into premenopausal and post-menopausal groups. There were 26 women in the younger premenopausal group (mean age, 36 years) and 13 women in the older postmenopausal group (mean age, 59 years). Compared with the summer months, there was a significant ($P < 0.0001$) increase in TEWL across all the subjects in the study during the winter on both the cheek and the forearm, with the cheek showing the larger change. Indeed, on the cheek, the change was remarkable in the older postmenopausal age group woman: 5.3 ± 1.9 g/m²/hr in the summer versus 10.5 ± 5.0 g/m²/hr in the winter. Interestingly, despite this marked seasonal change in cheek TEWL, there was no significant difference in cheek SC hydration as determined by electrical conductance. Finally, there was no significant seasonal variation in corneocyte size or skin surface lipids observed in this study.

Akasaka et al. (98) measured the change in TEWL on the forearm in 11 male and 11 female Japanese subjects and showed that TEWL was lowest in the spring (April) and fall (October).

Seasonal variation in skin permeability is suggested by the results of Frosch et al. (99), where they showed that skin weal formation as a result of DMSO treatment was much more pronounced in the winter months than in the summer months.

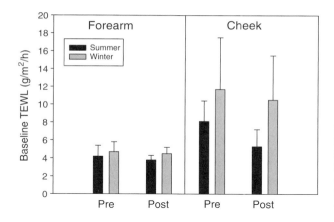

FIGURE 3 Seasonal change in baseline TEWL (mean ± SD) on the cheek and forearm as a function of menopausal status. *Abbreviations*: Pre, premenopausal; Post, postmenopausal. *Source*: From Ref. 93.

There are also dramatic seasonal variations in SC lipids (84). SC lipids were measured in August, April, and January in 26 white women. The sample sizes were not consistent at each time point—the summer time point had 26 subjects, the spring time point had 5 subjects, and the winter time point had 17 subjects. The authors observed that all the lipid species assayed were decreased in the winter season compared with the summer season; the relative amount of each of the lipid classes did not change from winter to summer season. There was a 20% decrease in ceramide 1 linoleate levels in winter versus summer. The amount of ceramide 1 linoleate relative to ceramide 1 oleate was 1.74 in the winter but fell to 0.51 in the summer. These marked seasonal changes in SC lipids observed by Rogers et al. (84) are in stark contrast to the findings of Yoshikawa et al. (100) where no seasonal changes in lipid levels were observed.

Abe et al. (101) studied the change in epidermal water loss (EWL) and skin lipids with changing seasons. Twenty-four (12 men and 12 women; ages 19–55 years) participated in their study and were observed during the course of several months. Baseline EWL on the forearm as well as total surface lipid was measured in October, January, April, and July. Measurements were made in the morning hours. Maximum EWL values occurred in July, and the minimum occurred in January. The value in July was 1.8 times that observed in January ($P < 0.001$). The authors admit that sweating could have contributed to the high EWL and were thus careful to classify the measurement as evaporative water loss and not TEWL. Total lipid, squalene, free cholesterol, and total cholesterol in the surface lipid film also peaked in July and showed a trough in January. Because sweating could have confounded the results of the TEWL measurement, we will not include these results in our overall assessment.

Although it is generally considered that exposure to low humidity during winter leads to decreased barrier function and increased TEWL, Chou et al. (102) reported that factory workers exposed to ultralow humidity at work (RH < 1.5%) actually had reduced TEWL compared with cohorts working a normal RH environment.

Time of Day (Circadian)

More than 35 years ago, Spruit (103) found that TEWL was higher in the afternoon than in the morning. Yosipovitch et al. (104) also measured TEWL during the course of a day and found a peak in the late afternoon. In a study of eight male subjects,

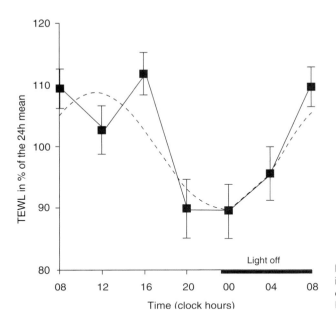

FIGURE 4   Circadian variations in baseline TEWL on the cheeks of white women. *Source*: From Ref. 106.

ages 19 to 23 years, Denda and Tsuchiya (105) found that basal TEWL showed its highest value during the early morning hours (03:00 hours). However, the authors do note that the difference in TEWL from the other time points was not statistically significant. Barrier recovery was significantly lower during the period between 20:00 and 23:00 hours compared with that at other time points.

In 2001, Le Fur et al. (106) reported results of round-the-clock skin surface measurements on a group of eight white women (mean age, 24 ± 3 years). The researchers were thorough and included subjects who were on the same phase of their menstrual cycle (luteal phase) and were nonsmokers. Exclusion criteria were comprehensive and considered ongoing and previous skin disease, pregnancy/breastfeeding, oral contraceptive use, alcohol use, and eating spicy food during the study. Subjects were put on a strict skin care program for both the body and face one week before collecting measurements, and all subjects wore the same cotton clothes during the measurement phase. Subjects were put on the same diurnal lighting schedule with lights on at 08:00 hour and lights off at midnight during the 48-hour study. The fluorescent lighting was carefully controlled, so that all subjects were exposed to exactly the same lux on their face and forearms. The subjects ate the same "standardized meals," which were served at fixed hours. Rooms were controlled for temperature and humidity. The subjects were allowed to read, write, and watch TV.

The researchers reported significant circadian rhythms for TEWL on both the face ($P = 0.0005$) and forearm ($P = 0.03$). Baseline TEWL ranged from 9.9 to 19.2 g/m^2/hr on the face and from 5.9 to 10.4 g/m^2/hr on the forearm (Fig. 4). Cosinor analysis of the data (collected every 4 hours during the 24-hour period) showed that TEWL on the cheek peaks at 11:20 ± 2.5 hours and shows a minimum at midnight. The forearm data, although slightly different from the cheek data, also showed a minimum at midnight.

More recently, in a study of 11 people of mixed ethnicity and sex, Yosipovitch et al. (107) found that TEWL, both baseline measurements and those taken three hours after tape stripping, was at a maximum at 11:00 hours and at a minimum between 05:00 and 08:00 hours. Skin blood flow on the forearm also exhibited a daily rhythm with a characteristic minimum found around 08:00 hours.

It is clear that TEWL undergoes significant daily rhythms. The changes range ±10% from the overall daily mean. The exact basis for these daily changes is not clear but does not seem to be explained simply by changes in skin temperature. Whatever the basis, the fact that TEWL (and several other biophysical parameters) shows daily rhythms implies that time of day is an important consideration in clinical design.

Nutrition and Diet

Clearly, good nutrition is important for healthy skin (108), and a diet deficient in vitamins, minerals, or essential fatty acids will manifest in a variety of skin diseases with concomitant change in barrier function (109,110). It is beyond the scope of this review to cover this topic in detail.

In the last few years, more attention is being focused on the concept of "beauty-from-within" skin care and the role of diet and nutrition in maintaining healthy skin. So-called beauty drinks are becoming more and more popular, but controlled clinical trials that prove the efficacy of these products are still lacking.

Mac-Mary et al. (111) assessed the value of additional water intact on skin hydration in healthy subjects. In that work, a total of 80 subjects (44 women and 36 men, mean age of 56) partook in the study. Each participant was asked to drink 1 L of water per day for 42 days, in addition to their normal water consumption. There was no control group for comparison. The study was conducted from April to June. The temperature of the room in which measurements were made varied from 20 to 24°C. Baseline TEWL was measured before and after the period of additional water consumption. TEWL significantly increased from a mean of 2.80 g/m²/hr at baseline to 3.16 g/m²/hr at 42 days. The authors acknowledge that the lack of a control group limits interpretation of the results.

Preclinical studies on the effect of certain diets on barrier function have addressed vitamin supplementation and alcohol consumption. Watson et al. (112) found that a diet supplemented with pantothenate, choline, nicotinamide, histidine, and inositol was able to significantly reduce TEWL in dogs after nine weeks. Brand et al. (113) found that chronic alcohol consumption in rats increased the transdermal absorption of several herbicides. Squier et al. (114) found that the diffusion coefficients (K_p) for both tritiated water and the tobacco carcinogen, nitrosonornicotine, increased significantly for rats on the ethanol supplemented diet.

During two months of dietary borage oil supplementation, forearm TEWL values decreased from 7.65 ± 2.96 to 7.2 ± 2.58 and finally to 6.82 ± 2.29 g/m²/hr (115). Water content of the SC increased slightly from 67.6 ± 9.9 to 69.1 ± 13.6 corneometer units, but the difference was not statistically significant. There was no control group in the study.

History of Cosmetic Product Use

Misra et al. (116), later reviewed by Ananthapadmanabhan et al. (117), used infrared spectroscopy and electron microscopy to show how multiple washes with a traditional high-alkalinity soap causes damage to the lamellar structure of the SC compared with washing with either water or a neutral/slightly acidic synthetic detergent bar. The investigators go on to show how barrier function, as assessed by TEWL, can be compromised by the use of a regular body wash compared with a moisturizing body wash.

Loden (118) showed that treatment for 10 or 20 days with a moisturizer containing 10% urea significantly reduced basal TEWL relative to the control nontreated skin site. Pretreatment with 10% urea also decreased the susceptibility to irritation from SLS. The observed decrease in TEWL and lower irritation response to SLS after long-term treatment with urea were unexpected in view of the keratolytic, hydrating, and permeability-increasing properties of urea. Indeed, shorter term treatment with 10% urea formulation increased TEWL although statistical significance was not achieved.

In a study on the effect of switching to an acid syndet bar for cleansing and regularly using a moisturizing lotion to treat the dry skin of a group of elderly nonatopic patients, Thune et al. (119) found that after one week of treatment, TEWL decreased and skin hydration increased.

Climate and History of Chronic Sun Exposure

Despite general agreement that chronic sun exposure has little effect on the integrity of the skin barrier, there is a surprising dearth of information that actually proves this conclusion. Comparing baseline TEWL or percutaneous absorption on sun-exposed versus sun-protected body sites is typically complicated by the inherent body site variation in the skin barrier as discussed earlier, thereby confounding interpretation of results (120). The ideal experiment would be to compare anatomically identical regions that have been either exposed or protected from chronic UV radiation on the same individuals.

An interesting study from the group at Tohoku University attempted to do just that (121). They compared basal TEWL on the right and left hands of 12 Japanese male golfers who regularly wore golfing gloves over the years (from 4 to 25 years of playing 18 holes of golf at least twice a month during the morning to early afternoon). All of the golfers were right-handed and played golf with a glove on their left hand. There was no significant difference in basal TEWL values between the exposed right and protected left hand.

Declercq et al. (122) compared the barrier strength and SC structure of people living in the hot and dry climate of Arizona in June (27% RH) versus peer groups living in New York or Oevel, Belgium (both 80% RH) in July. Skin exposed to the hot, dry environment showed better skin barrier functions and lower basal TEWL. They concluded that human skin can adapt to a low humidity environment by increasing epidermal barrier function and modulating desquamation.

Psychological Stress

Most of the evidence regarding the relationship between psychological stress and barrier function shows no relationship to basal TEWL but a strong relationship to barrier function repair. Garg et al. (123) found that medical students who were under extreme psychological stress during final examination week showed a significant increase in the time required for SC barrier recovery after barrier disruption by tape stripping. The preexamination low-stress period was in January, shortly after winter vacation. The examination period was in February during final examinations and the postexamination period was in mid-March. There was a good correlation between the rate of barrier repair and the perceived psychological stress as measured using validated stress assessment questionnaires. The perceived stress returned to normal after the examinations as did the rate of barrier repair.

Aioi et al. (124) showed that mice under the stress imposed by confinement in very crowded environmental conditions (high population density of 40 mice/cage) versus mice living under standard cage density conditions (5 mice/cage) had declined in several barrier function parameters, including increased TEWL, decreased skin surface conductance, increased skin permeability of indomethacin and nicotinic acid amide, and a decrease in SC ceramides and pyrrolidone carboxylic acid.

In an interesting study of the impact of chronic psychological stress, Muizzuddin et al. (125) compared the skin barrier function of a group (n = 28) of women who were going through marital separation/divorce with a control group (n = 27) of happily married or single women. There was no significant difference between groups for basal TEWL on the cheek. However, the researchers found that the women under the stress had a slower rate of barrier repair after tape stripping; there was an excellent relationship between the rate of repair and the level of stress at both 3 and 24 hours after tape stripping (Fig. 5).

Other forms of stress, such as sleep deprivation and psychological interviews, have been shown to delay barrier repair after tape stripping (126). In particular, the stress of a job interview was associated with a significant increase in basal TEWL on the cheek. There was no significant difference in basal TEWL on the forearm before and after stress by sleep deprivation, psychological interview, or exercise.

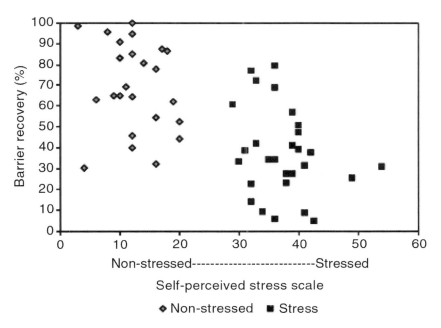

FIGURE 5 Self-perceived stress versus barrier recovery three hours after tape stripping on the cheek. *Source*: From Ref. 125.

SUMMARY AND RECOMMENDATIONS

There are many host and environmental factors significantly associated with skin barrier function. We have focused most of our review on those studies using methods that specifically measure the integrity of the SC barrier in normal healthy skin. The primary measure we considered to be most indicative of barrier function was basal TEWL. The measurement of basal TEWL is widely used and standardized so that studies can be more easily compared with one another. Barrier repair after barrier perturbation (the cutaneous stress test) was also viewed as a good measure of barrier function that might not be apparent with baseline measurements. However, the rate of barrier repair after an external insult such as tape stripping or detergent challenge might be considered more a measure of wound healing rather than a measure of barrier efficiency. Finally, we reviewed studies that used percutaneous absorption as a measure of barrier function, especially those that used radiolabeled drugs to directly follow transdermal penetration versus those that had the added complexity of a using biological response such as vasodilatation.

Several factors have been found to be significantly associated with skin barrier function. These include body site, season of year, diet, stress, time of day, history of cosmetic product use, menstrual status, BMI, and climate. For some factors, the difference between sample population means is quite small relative to the inter-individual variance within the sample population. These would include ethnicity, age, and gender. Regarding age, while the change in basal TEWL with age is small, the available data suggests that the rate of barrier repair following barrier perturbation declines with increasing age. Interestingly, many of the factors we have listed as being significantly associated with barrier function are environmental factors. We anticipate that the study of the influence of environmental factors on skin barrier health will continue to be an important research focus in the coming years.

We would like to echo many of the excellent suggestions made by Waller and Maibach (127,128) regarding the conduct of future studies in this area. As we discussed by example, studies should have adequate statistical power to discriminate differences. The potential for selection bias in the study design needs to be carefully thought through. Selection bias can be reduced or eliminated completely if the clinical is designed with consideration for the many host and environmental factors that can confound interpretation of the results. Methodologies, both clinical and instrumental, should be standardized to bring more consistency from study to study, and reports should describe the details as best as possible so that others can better interpret the results.

ACKNOWLEDGEMENTS

The authors would like to thank Dr. Zhiwu Liang for his helpful review and critique of the manuscript.

REFERENCES

1. Winsor T, Burch GE. Differential roles of layers of human epigastric skin on diffusion of water. Arch Intern Med 1944; 74:428–444.
2. Elias PM. Stratum corneum defensive functions: an integrated view. J Invest Dermatol 2005; 125:183–200.

3. Elias PM, Choi EH. Interactions among stratum corneum defensive functions. Exp Dermatol 2005; 14:719–726.
4. Wickett RR, Visscher, MO. Structure and function of the epidermal barrier. Am J Infect Control 2006; 34:S98–110.
5. Marshall EK, Lynch V, Smith HV. Variation in susceptibility of the skin to dichloroethylsulfide. J Pharmacol Exp Ther 1919; 12:291–301.
6. Taylor SC. Skin of color: biology, structure, function, and implications for dermatologic disease. J Am Acad Dermatol 2002; 46:S41–S62.
7. Wesley NO, Maibach HI. Racial (ethnic) differences in skin properties. Am J Clin Dermatol 2003; 4:843–860.
8. Rawlings AV. Ethnic skin types: are there differences in skin structure and function? Int J Cos Sci 2006; 28:79–93.
9. Berardesca E, Maibach HI. Sensitive and ethnic skin: a need for special skin-care agents? Dermatol Clin 1991; 9:89–92.
10. Wesley NO, Maibach HI. Racial (ethnic) differences in skin properties: can skin care be universal? Cosmet Toiletries 2003; 118:30–37.
11. Zhai H, Dika E, Goldovsky M, Maibach HI. Tape-stripping method in man: comparison of evaporimetric methods. Skin Res Technol 2007; 13:207–210.
12. Shah JH, Zhai H, Maibach HI. Comparative evaporimetry in man. Skin Res Technol 2005; 11:205–208.
13. Pinnagoda J, Tupker RA, Agner T, Seurp J. Guidelines for transepidermal water loss (TEWL) measurement. A report from the Standardization Group of the European Society of Contact Dermatitis. Contact Dermatitis 1990; 22:164–178.
14. Pinnagoda J, Tupker RA. Measurement of the transepidermal water loss. In: Serup J, Jemec GBE, eds. Handbook of Non-Invasive Methods and the Skin. Boca Raton, Fla: CRC Press, 1995:173–178.
15. Barel AO, Clarys P. Comparison of methods for measurement of transepidermal water loss. In: Serup J, Jemec GBE, eds. Handbook of Non-Invasive Methods and the Skin. Boca Raton, Fla: CRC Press, 1995:179–184.
16. Barel AO, Clarys P. Study of the stratum corneum barrier function by transepidermal water loss measurements: comparison between two commercial instruments: Evaporimeter and Tewameter®. Skin Pharmacol 1995; 8:186–195.
17. Rogiers V. EEMCO guidance for the assessment of transepidermal water loss in cosmetic sciences. Skin Pharmacol Appl Skin Physiol 2001; (14):117–128.
18. Pinson EA. Evaporation from human skin with sweat glands inactivated. Am J Physiol 1942; 187:492–503.
19. Chilcott RP, Dalton CH, Emmanuel AJ, Allen CE, Bradley ST. Transepidermal water loss does not correlate with skin barrier function in vitro. J Invest Dermatol 2002; 118:871–875.
20. Levin J, Maibach H. The correlation between transepidermal water loss and percutaneous absorption: an overview. J Controlled Release 2005; 103:291–299.
21. Fluhr JW, Feingold KR, Elias PM. Transepidermal water loss reflects permeability barrier status: validation in human and rodent *in vivo* and *ex vivo* models. Exp Dermatol 2006; 15:483–492.
22. Hammarlund K, Nilsson GE, Oberg PA, Sedin G. Transepidermal water loss in newborn infants. I. Relation to ambient humidity and site of measurement and estimation of total transepidermal water loss. Acta Paediatr Scand 1977; (66):553–562.
23. Grove G, Grove M, Zerweck C, Pierce E. Comparative metrology of the evaporimeter and the DermaLab TEWL probe. Skin Res Technol 1999; 5:1–8.
24. Bashir SJ, Chew AL, Anigbogu A, Dreher F, Maibach HI. Physical and physiological effects of stratum corneum tape stripping. Skin Res Technol 2001; 7:40–48.
25. Berardesca E, Pirot F, Singh M, Maibach H. Differences in stratum corneum pH gradient when comparing white Caucasian and black African-American skin. Br J Dermatol 1998; 139:855–857.
26. Loffler H, Dreher F, Maibach HI. Stratum corneum adhesive tape stripping: influence of anatomical site, application pressure, duration and removal. Br J Dermatol 2004; 151:746–752.
27. Robinson MK. Population differences in skin structure and physiology and the susceptibility to irritant and allergic contact dermatitis: implications for skin safety testing and risk assessment. Contact Dermatitis 1999; 41:65–79.

28. Modjtahedi SP, Maibach HI. Ethnicity as a possible endogenous factor in irritant contact dermatitis: comparing the irritant response among Caucasians, blacks, and Asians. Contact Dermatitis 2002; 47:272–278.
29. Robinson MK. Update on racial differences in susceptibility to skin irritation and allergy. In: Berardesca E, Leveque J, Maibach HI, eds. Ethnic Skin and Hair. New York: Informa Healthcare, 2007:123–134.
30. Robinson MK. Racial differences in acute and cumulative skin irritation responses between Caucasian and Asian populations. Contact Dermatitis 2000; 42:134–143.
31. Hillebrand GG, Levine MJ, Miyamoto KM. The age-dependent changes in skin condition in ethnic populations from around the world. In: Berardesca E, Leveque J, Maibach HI, eds. Ethnic Skin and Hair. New York: Informa Healthcare, 2007:105–122.
32. Fluhr JW, Dickel H, Kuss O, Weyher I, Diepgen TL, Berardesca E. Impact of anatomical location on barrier recovery, surface pH and stratum corneum hydration after acute barrier disruption. Br J Dermatol 2002; 146:770–776.
33. Oestmann E, Lavrijsen APM, Hermans J, Ponec M. Skin barrier function in healthy volunteers as assessed by transepidermal water loss and vascular response to hexyl nicotinate: intra- and inter-individual variability. Br J Dermatol 1993; 128:130–136.
34. Marrakchi S, Maibach HI. Sodium lauryl sulfate-induced irritation in the human face: regional and age-related differences. Skin Pharmacol Physio 2006; 19:177–180.
35. Wilson D, Berardesca E, Maibach HI. In vitro transepidermal water loss: differences between black and white human skin. Br J Dermatol 1988; 119:647–652.
36. Primavera G, Berardesca E. Biophysical properties of ethnic skin. In: Berardesca E, Leveque J, Maibach HI, eds. Ethnic Skin and Hair. New York: Informa Healthcare, 2007:13–18.
37. Berardesca E, Maibach HI. Racial differences in sodium lauryl sulfate induced cutaneous irritation: black and white. Contact Dermatitis 1988; 18:65–70.
38. Berardesca E, Maibach HI. Racial differences in sodium laural sulphate induced cutaneous irritation: comparison of white and Hispanic subjects. Contact Dermatitis 1988; 19:136–140.
39. Takahashi M, Watanabe H, Kumagai H, Nakayama Y. Physiological and morphological changes in facial skin with aging (II). J Soc Cosmet Chem Japan 1989; 23:22–30.
40. Berardesca E, de Rigal J, Levique JL, Maibach HI. In vivo biophysical characterization of skin physiological differences in races. Dermatologica 1991; 182:89–93.
41. Sugino K, Imokawa G, Maibach HI. Ethnic differences of stratum corneum lipid in relation to stratum corneum function. J Invest Dermatol 1993; 100:587 (abstract only).
42. Kompaore F, Marty JP, Dupont C. In vivo evaluation of the stratum corneum barrier function in blacks, Caucasians and Asians with two noninvasive methods. Skin Pharmacology 1993; 6:200–207.
43. Warrier AG, Kligman AM, Harper RA, Bowman J, Wicket RR. A comparison of black and white skin using noninvasive methods. J Soc Cosmet Chem 1996; 47:229–240.
44. Singh J, Gross M, Sage B, Davis HT, Maibach, HI. Effect of saline inotophoresis on skin barrier function and cutaneous irritation in four ethnic groups. Food Chem Toxicol2000; 38:717–726.
45. Aramaki J, Kawana S, Effendy I, Happle R, Loffler H. Differences in skin irritation between Japanese and European women. Br J Dermatol 2002; 146:1052–1056.
46. Yosipovitch G, Theng CTS. Asian skin: its architecture, function, and differences from Caucasian skin. Cosmet Toiletries 2002; 117:57–62.
47. Yosipovitch G, Goon ATJ, Chan YH, Goh CL. Are there any differences in skin barrier function, intregrity and skin blood flow between different subpopulations of Asians and Caucasians? Exog Dermatol 2002; 1:302–306.
48. Hellemans L, Muizzuddin N, Declercq L, Maes D. Characterization of stratum corneum properties in human subjects from a different genetic background. J Invest Dermatol 2005; 124:A62. (abstract only)
49. Reed JT, Ghadially R, Elias PM. Skin type, but neither race nor gender, influence epidermal permeability barrier function. Arch Dermatol 1995; 131:1134–1138.
50. Zettersten EM, Ghadially R, Feingold KR, Crumrine D, Elias PM. Optimal ratios of topical stratum corneum lipids improve barrier recovery in chronologically aged skin. J Am Acad Dermatol 1997; 37:403–408.
51. Visscher MO, Hoath SB, Conroy E, Wickett RR. Effect of semipermeable membranes on skin barrier repair following tape stripping. Arch Dermatol Res 2001; 293:491–499.

52. Kompaore R, Tsuruta H. In vivo differences between Asian, black and white in the stratum corneum barrier function. Int Arch Occup Environ Health 1993; 65(Suppl. 1):S223–S225.
53. Berardesca E, Maibach HI. Racial differences in pharmacodynamic response to nicotinates in vivo in human skin: black and white. Acta Derm Venereol (Stockh) 1990; 70:63–66.
54. Guy RH, Tur E, Bjerke S, Maibach HI. Are there age and racial differences to methyl nicotinate-induced vasodilatation in human skin? Dermatology 1985; 12:1001–1006.
55. Leopold CS, Maibach HI. Effect of lipophilic vehicles on in vivo skin penetration of methyl nicotinate in different races. Int J Pharm 1996; 139:161–167.
56. Wickrema-Sinha AJ, Shaw RS, Weber DJ. Percutaneous absorption and excretion of tritium-labeled diflorasone diacetate, a new topical corticosteroid in the rat, monkey and man. J Invest Dermatol 1978; 71:372–377.
57. Wedig JH, Maibach HI. Percutaneous penetration of dipyrithione in man: effect of skin color (race). J Am Acad Dermatol (1981); 5:433–438.
58. Lotte C, Wester RC, Rougier A, Maibach HI. Racial differences in the in vivo percutaneous absorption of some organic compounds: a comparison between black, Caucasian and Asian subjects. Arch Dermatol Res 1993; 284:456–459.
59. Bronaugh RL, Stewart RF, Simon M. Methods for in vitro percutaneous absorption studies VII: use of excised human skin. J Pharm Sci 1986; 75:1094–1097.
60. Elias PM, Menon GK. Structural and lipid biochemical correlates of the epidermal permeability barrier. Adv Lipd Res 1991; 24:1–26.
61. Uchida Y, Hamanaka S. Stratum corneum ceramides: function, origins, and therapeutic applications. In: Elias PM, Feingold KR, eds. Skin Barrier. New York: Taylor & Francis, 2006:43–64.
62. Meguro S, Arai Y, Masukawa Y, Uie K, Tokimitsu I. Relationship between covalently bound ceramides and transepidermal water loss (TEWL). Arch Dermatol Res 2000; 292:463–468.
63. La Ruche G, Cesarini JP. Histology and physiology of black skin. Ann Dermatol Venereal 1992; 119:567–574.
64. Rienertson RP, Wheatley VR. Studies on the chemical composition of human epidermal lipids. J Invest Dermatol 1959; 32:49–59.
65. Rougier A, Lotte C, Corcuff P, Maibach HI. Relationship between skin permeability and corneocyte size according to anatomic site, age and sex in man. J Soc Cosmet Chem 1988; 139:15–26.
66. Fluhr JW, Pelosi A, Lazzerina S, Dikstein S, Berardesca E. Differences in corneocyte surface area in pre- and post-menopausal women. Skin Parmacol Appl Skin Physio 2001; 14:10–16.
67. Corcuff P, Lotte C, Rougier A, Maibach HI. Racial differences in corneocytes. A comparison between black, white and oriental skin. Acta Derm Venereol (Stockh) 1991; 71:146–148.
68. Thomson ML. Relative efficiency of pigment and horny layer thickness in protecting the skin of Europeans and Africans against solar ultraviolet radiation. J Physiol (London) 1955; 127:236–246.
69. Freeman RG, Cockerell EF, Armstrong J, Knox JM. Sunlight as a factor influencing the thickness of the epidermis. J Invest Dermatol 1962; 39:295–297.
70. Lock-Anderson J, Therkildsen P, de Fine Olivarius F, et al. Epidermal thickness, skin pigmentation and constitutive photosensitivity. Photodermatol Photoimmunol Photomed 1997; 13:153–158.
71. Weigand DA, Haygood C, Gaylor GR. Cell layers and density of negro and Caucasian stratum corneum. J Invest Dermatol 1974; 62:563–568.
72. Otberg N, Richter H, Schaefer H, Blume-Peytave U, Sterry W, Lademann J. Variations of hair follicle size and distribution in different body sites. J Invest Dermatol 2004; 122:14–19.
73. Sperling MD. Hair density in African Americans. Arch Dermatol 1999; 135:656–658.
74. Mangelsdorf S, Otberg N, Maibach HI, Sinkgraven R, Sterry W, Lademann J. Ethnic variation in vellus hair follicle size and distribution. Skin Pharmacol Physiol 2006; 19:159–167.
75. Jorgenson RJ, Salinas CF, Dowben JS, St John DL. A population study on the density of palmar sweat pores. Birth Defects Orig Artic Ser 1988; 24:51–63.
76. Grice KA, Bettley FR. Skin water loss and accidental hypothermia in psoriasis, ichthyosis and erythroderma. Br Med J 1967; 4:195–198.

77. Kligman AM. Perspectives and Problems in Cutaneous Gerontology. J Invest Dermatol 1979; 73:39–46.
78. Leveque JL, Corcuff P, de Rigal J, Agache P. In vitro studies on the evolution of physical properties of the human skin with age. Int J Dermatol 1984; 23:322.
79. Roskos K, Guy RH. Assessment of skin barrier function using transepidermal water loss: effect of age. Pharm Res 1989; 6:949–953.
80. Fluhr JW, Pfisterer S, Gloor M. Direct comparison of skin physiology in children and adults with bioengineering methods. Pediatric Dermatol 2000; 17:436–439.
81. Shriner DL, Maibach HI. Regional variation of nonimmunologic contact urticaria. Functional map of the human face. Skin Pharmacol 1996; 9:312–321.
82. Cua AB, Wilhelm KP, Maibach HI. Cutaneous sodium lauryl sulphate irritation potential: age and regional variability. Br J Dermatol 1990; 123:607–613.
83. Wilhelm KP, Cua AB, Maibach HI. Skin aging. Effect on transepidermal water loss, stratum corneum hydration, skin surface pH, and casual sebum content. Arch Dermatol 1991; 127:1806–1809.
84. Rogers J, Harding C, Mayo A, Banks J, Rawlings A. Stratum corneum lipids: the effect of ageing and the seasons. Arch Dermatol Res 1996; 288:765–770.
85. Ya-Xian Z, Suetake T, Tagami H. Number of cell layers of the stratum corneum in normal skin—relationship to the anatomical location on the body, age, sex and physical parameters. Arch Dermatol Res 1999; 291:555–559.
86. Batisse D, Bazin R, Baldeweck T, Querleux B, Lévêque JL. Influence of age on the wrinkling capacities of skin. Skin Res Technol 2002; 8:148–154.
87. Yosipovitch G, Maayan-Metzger A, Merlob P, Sirota L. Skin Barrier Properties in Different Body Areas in Neonates. Pediatrics 2000; 106:105–108.
88. Feldman RJ, Maibach HI. Regional variations in percutaneous penetration of ^{14}C-cortisol in man. J Invest Dermatol 1967; 48:181.
89. Smith JG, Fisher RW, Blank H. The epidermal barrier. A comparison between scrotal and abdominal skin. J Invest Dermatol 1961; 36:337–343.
90. Dupuis D, Rougier A, Lotte C, Wilson D, Maibach HI. In vivo relationship between percutaneous absorption and transepidermal water loss according to anatomic site in man. J Soc Cosmet Chem 1986; 37:351–357.
91. Holbrook KA, Odland GF. Regional differences in the thickness (cell layers) of the human stratum corneum: an ultrastructural analysis. J Invest Dermatol 1974; 62:415–222.
92. Treffel P, Panisset F, Faivre B, Agache P. Hydration, transepidermal water loss, pH and skin surface parameters: correlations and variations between dominant and non-dominant forearms. Br J Dermatol 1994; 130:325–328.
93. Kikuchi K, Kobayashi H, Le Fur, I, Tschachler E, Tagami H. The winter season affects more severely the facial skin than the forearm skin: comparative biophysical studies conducted in the same Japanese females in later summer and winter. Exog Dermatol 2002; 1:32–38.
94. Harvell J, Hussona-Saeed I, Maibach HI. Changes in transepidermal water loss and cutaneous blood flow during the menstrual cycle. Contact Dermatitis 1992; 27:294–301.
95. Agner T, Damm P, Skouby SO. Menstrual cycle and skin reactivity. J Am Acad Dermatol 1991; 24:566–570.
96. Cua AB, Wilhelm KP, Maibach HI. Frictional properties of human skin: relation to age, sex and anatomical region, stratum corneum hydration and transepidermal water loss. Br J Dermatol 1990; 123:473–479.
97. Loffler H, Aramaki JUN, Isaak E. The influence of body mass index on skin susceptibility to sodium lauryl sulphate. Skin Res Technol 2002; 8:19–22.
98. Akasaka T, Yoshida A, Fukuda S, Takeuchi T, Katsuzaki N. Yearly changes in the physiological function of the skin. Environ Dermatol 2002; 9:1–10.
99. Frosch PJ, Duncan S, Kligman AM. Cutaneous biometrics I. The response of human skin to dimethyl sulphoxide. Br J Dermatol 1980; 102:263–274.
100. Yoshikawa N, Imokawa G, Akimoto K, Jin K, Higaki Y, Kawashima M. Regional analysis of ceramides within the stratum corneum in relation to seasonal changes. Dermatology 1994; 188:207–214.
101. Abe T, Mayuzumi J, Kikuchi N, Arai S. Seasonal variation in skin temperature, skin pH, evaporative water loss and skin surface lipid values on human skin. Chem Pharm Bull (Tokyo) 1980; 28:387–392.

102. Chou TC, Shih TS, Tsai JC, Wu JD, Sheu HM, Chang HY. Effect of occupational exposure to rayon manufacturing chemicals on skin barrier to evaporative water loss. J Occup Health 2004; 46:410–417.
103. Spruit D. The diurnal variation of water vapor loss frrm the skin in relation to temperature. Br J Dermatol 1971; 84:66–70.
104. Yosipovitch G, Xiong GI, Haus E, Sackett-Lunden L, Ashkenazi I, Maibach HI. Time-dependent variations of the skin barrier function in humans: transepidermal water loss, stratum corneum hydration, skin surface pH and skin temperature. J Invest Dermatol 1998; 110:20–23.
105. Denda M, Tsuchiya T. Barrier recovery rate varies time-dependently in human skin. Br J Dermatol 2000; 142:881–884.
106. Le Fur I, Reinberg A, Lopez S, Morizot F, Mechkouri M, Tschachler E. Analysis of circadian and ultradian rhythms of skin surface properties of face and forearm of healthy women. J Invest Dermatol 2001; 117:718–724.
107. Yosipovitch G, Sackett-Lundeen L, Goon A, Huak CY, Goh CL, Haus E. Circadian, ultradian (12 h) variations of skin blood flow and barrier function in non-irritated and irritated skin—effect of topical corticosteroids. J Invest Dermatol 2004; 122:824–829.
108. Boelsma E, Hendriks HFG, Roza L. Nutritional skin care: health effects of micronurients and fatty acids. Am J Clin Nutr 2001; 73:853–864.
109. Ruiz-Maldonado R, Orozco-Covarrubias L. Nutritional Diseases. In: Bolognia JL, Jorizzo JL, Rapini RP, eds. Dermatology. Edinburgh: Mosby, 2003:699–709.
110. Rawlings AV, Scott IR, Harding CR, Bowser PA. Stratum corneum moisturization at the molecular level. J Invest Dermatol 1994; 103:731–741.
111. Mac-Mary S, Creidi P, Marsaut D, et al. Assessment of effects of an additional dietary natural mineral water uptake on skin hydration in healthy subjects by dynamic barrier function measurements and clinic scoring. Skin Res Technol 2006; 12:199–205.
112. Watson A, Fray TR, Bailey J, Baker CB, Beyer SA, Markwell PJ. Dietary constituents are able to play a beneficial role in canine epidermal barrier function. Exp Dermatolol 2006; 15:74–81.
113. Brand RM, Charron AR, Dutton L, et al. Effects of chronic alcohol consumption on dermal penetration of pesticides in rats. J Toxicol Environ Health 2004; 67:153–161.
114. Squier CA, Kremer MJ, Wertz PW. Effect of ethanol on lipid metabolism and epithelial permeability barrier of skin and oral mucosa in the rat. J Oral Pathol Med 2003; 32:595–599.
115. Brosche R, Platt D. Effect of borage oil consumption on fatty acid metabolism, trans-epidermal water loss and skin parameters in elderly people. Arch Gerontol Geriatr 2000; 139–150.
116. Misra M, Ananthapadmanabhan KP, Hoyberg K, Gursky RP, Prowell S, Aronson MP. Correlation between surfactant-induced ultrastructural changes in epidermis and transepidermal water loss. J Soc Cosmet Chem 1997; 48:219–234.
117. Ananthapadmanabhan KP, Moore DJ, Subramanyan K, Misra M, Meyer F. Cleansing without compromise: the impact of cleansers on the skin barrier and the technology of mild cleansing. Dermatol Ther 2004; 17:16–25.
118. Loden M. Urea-containing moisturizers influence barrier properties of normal skin. Arch Dermatol Res 1996; 288:103–107.
119. Thune P, Nilsen T, Hanstad IK, Gustavsen T, Lovig Dahl H. The water barrier function of the skin in relation to the water content of stratum corneum, pH and skin lipids. The effect of alkaline soap and syndet on dry skin in elderly, non-atopic patients. Acta Derm Venereol 1988; 68:277–283.
120. Saijo S, Hashimoto-Kumasaka K, Takahashi M, et al. Functional changes of the stratum corneum associated with aging and photoaging. J Soc Cosmet Chem 1991; 42:379–383.
121. Kikuchi-Numagami K, Suetake T, Yanai M, Takahashi M, Tanaka M, Tagami H. Functional and morphological studies of photodamaged skin on the hands of middle-aged Japanese golfers. Eur J Dermatol 2000; 10:277–281.
122. Declercq L, Muizzuddin N, Hellemans L, et al. Adaptation response in human skin barrier to a hot and dry environment. J Invest Dermatol 2002; 119:716.
123. Garg A, Chren MM, Sands LP, et al. Psychological stress perturbs epidermal permeability barrier homeostasis. Implications for the pathogenesis of stress-associated skin disorders. Arch Dermatol 2001; 137:53–59.

124. Aioi A, Okuda M, Matsui M, Tonogaito H, Hamada K. Effect of high population environment on skin barrier function in mice. J Dermatol Sci 2001; 25:189–197.
125. Muizzuddin N, Matsui MS, Marenus KD, Maes DH. Impact of stress of marital dissolution on skin barrier recovery: tape stripping and measurement of *trans*-epidermal water loss (TEWL). Skin Res Technol 2003; 9:34–38.
126. Altmus M, Rao B, Dhabhar FS, Ding W, Granstein RD. Stress-induced changes in skin barrier function in healthy women. J Invest Dermatol 2001; 117:309–317.
127. Waller JM, Maibach HI. Age and skin structure and function, a quantitative approach (I): blood flow, pH, thickness, and ultrasound echogenicity. Skin Res Technol 2005; 11:221–235.
128. Waller JM, Maibach HI. Age and skin structure and function, a quantitative approach (II): protein, glycosaminoglycan, water, and lipid content and structure. Skin Res Technol 2006; 12:145–154.
129. Muizzuddin N, Marenus KD, Schnittger SF, Sullivan M, Maes DH. Effect of systemic hormonal cyclicity of skin. J Cos Sci 2005; 56:311–21.

9 Permeability Through Diseased and Damaged Skin

Daniel A. W. Bucks

Dow Pharmaceutical Sciences, Inc., Petaluma and Department of Dermatology, School of Medicine, University of California, San Francisco, San Francisco, California, U.S.A.

INTRODUCTION

Healthy mammalian skin provides a relatively efficient barrier to egress of endogenous compounds, particularly water, and the ingress of exogenous material. The outer layer of the skin (stratum corneum, the horny layer) is associated with the major barrier properties of the skin (1,2). One of the major physiological functions of the skin is the prevention of dehydration. The rate of water loss through skin to the surface, transepidermal water loss (TEWL), is a direct measure of the integrity of the stratum corneum barrier. Intact, normal skin of healthy subjects has a TEWL level of ~4 $g/m^2/hr$. Many examples demonstrating a good correlation of elevated TEWL with increased penetration of topically applied compounds follow.

Bos and Meinardi (3) have recently proposed that it seems logical to restrict the development of new innovative compounds to a molecular weight (MW) lower than 500 Da when topical dermatological therapy, percutaneous systemic therapy, or vaccination is the objective. Their arguments for this "500-Da rule" are the following: (1) virtually all common contact allergens are lower than 500 Da; (2) the most commonly used drugs in topical therapy are all lower than 500 Da; and (3) all known topical drugs used in transdermal drug delivery systems are lower than 500 Da. However, compromised skin barrier function is directly related with complications seen in several dermatological disorders and has been associated with compounds having MWs much greater than 500 Da penetrating the skin. Also, perturbation or disruption of normal skin barrier function has been employed as a means to increase bioavailability of topically applied compounds (4). Topical drug application has been used to target drug delivery to the epidermis, dermis, and deeper tissues as well as for systemic delivery (5). As discussed below, cutaneous diseases as well as physical disruption can significantly compromise stratum corneum barrier function, correspondingly affect skin permeability, and effectively shift the MW cutoff for sufficient skin penetration to molecules of larger size.

DISEASED SKIN BARRIER FUNCTION

Clinical manifestation of the condition of the skin should dictate the relevant type of topical formulation in which a given drug is administered. Although formulation composition has a significant impact on treatment outcome, it generally does not influence the penetration of drug across the stratum corneum more than 10- to 20-fold (6). This section will summarize the dermatological disease conditions of dermatitis, ichthyosis, psoriasis, and acne vulgaris and respective studies characterizing the barrier function of the skin associated with that cutaneous disease state.

Dermatitis (Eczema)

Dermatitis can be grouped into two broad categories based on immunology: atopic dermatitis (endogenous eczema) and contact/allergic contact dermatitis (exogenous eczema).

Atopic Dermatitis

Atopic dermatitis is often associated with asthmatics and sufferers of hay fever. The skin of the atopic is characterized by papules, bouts of itching, and lichenification (leathery induration and thickening of the skin with hyperkeratosis). Complications include dissemination over the entire body and generalized pustulation due to infection with herpes simplex virus (7). The involved eczematous skin of an atopic has an elevated TEWL relative to the uninvolved skin. Likewise, the TEWL of the uninvolved skin of an atopic is elevated relative to the skin of normal, healthy subjects (8,9). Impairment of barrier function as measured by TEWL is strongly correlated with the percutaneous absorption of hydrocortisone (10). Hydrocortisone skin penetration after topical application to patients with atopic dermatitis ranged from 4% to 19% of the applied dose (11). Comparatively, hydrocortisone percutaneous penetration after a single application in healthy adult males ranged from 0.3% to 3% of the applied dose (12) and after multiple daily applications in healthy adult males $3 \pm 1\%$ (mean + SD) of the applied dose (13).

The occurrence of skin barrier dysfunction in atopic dermatitis has also been demonstrated (14) by the increased stratum corneum permeability of theophylline and the increased wealing response to dimethyl sulfoxide of lesional skin compared with nonlesional atopic skin and skin from normal healthy subjects. Theophylline passed through the excised stratum corneum of lesional skin, nonlesional atopic skin, and normal skin at rates of 12.5 ± 2.5, 9.8 ± 2.7, and 4.9 ± 1.4 µg/mL/hr (mean $\pm$ SEM), respectively. The dimethyl sulfoxide–induced weal grades (mean $\pm$ SEM) in lesional skin, nonlesional atopic skin, and normal skin were 2.87 ± 0.21, 0.74 ± 0.18, and 0.62 ± 0.23, respectively, on a 0 (no weals) to 4 (solid, tense weals) grading scale.

Hata et al. (9) assessed the epidermal barrier function of clinically normal-appearing skin of patients with atopic dermatitis relative to that of healthy subjects. They applied a mixture of lipid- and water-soluble dyes to the skin and measured the disappearance rate through the stratum corneum, in vivo, using photoacoustic spectrometry. Dyes penetrated faster in the clinically normal skin of atopic dermatitis patients compared with healthy subjects. Furthermore, penetration rates of the hydrophilic dyes tended to increase in proportion to the severity of the disease and significantly correlated with the serum IgE levels in the severe atopic dermatitis patients. The authors conclude that the clinically normal-appearing skin of patients with atopic dermatitis has an abnormal barrier function that may predispose them to inflammatory processes evoked by irritants and allergens, especially their water-soluble elements.

Contact/Allergic Dermatitis (Contact Eczema)

Allergic dermatitis is induced by cutaneous contact with toxic substances and is clinically expressed as erythema, papules, and vesicles, oozing, scaling, crusts, and hyperkeratosis (thickened, scaly stratum corneum) (7). As with atopic dermatitis, TEWL is elevated at the site of inflammation. Sodium lauryl sulfate (SLS) is an anionic surfactant commonly used to induce contact dermatitis in animals as well as humans. The degree of barrier disruption associated with SLS exposure is generally dose dependent and can be assessed by the increase in TEWL. Benfeldt (15) reported a 46-fold increase in human percutaneous penetration of salicylic acid after exposure to 1% SLS and a 146-fold increase after exposure to 2% SLS.

The effect of SLS-induced contact dermatitis on the in vivo percutaneous penetration of ^{14}C-labeled hydrocortisone, indomethacin, ibuprofen, and acitretin was evaluated in hairless guinea pigs (16). Systemic absorption (skin penetration) was determined by urinary and fecal elimination. Stratum corneum levels were determined by tape stripping. Viable epidermal-dermal levels were determined from punch biopsies obtained after stratum corneum removal. Penetration through SLS-treated skin was significantly increased for hydrocortisone (2.6-fold), ibuprofen (1.9-fold), and indomethacin (1.6-fold) but not for acitretin. Interestingly, drug levels in the viable epidermis-dermis measured at 24 hours from dose application were 70% lower in SLS-treated skin than normal skin for hydrocortisone, not changed for acitretin, and higher for indomethacin (3.2-fold) and ibuprofen (1.4-fold). The general assumptions that skin penetration and tissue levels are higher in diseased skin were not consistently demonstrated with this animal model.

Tsai et al. (17) evaluated the dependence of polyethylene glycol (PEG) size on mouse skin permeation with sodium dodecyl sulfate (SDS) treatment. The percutaneous penetration of PEG 300, 600, and 1000 oligomers (range 230 to 1400 Da) increased as a function of TEWL (range, 3–37 $g/m^2/hr$), with the penetration enhancement more prominent with the larger molecules. Before barrier disruption, molecules larger than 414 Da did not appreciably penetrate the mouse skin.

The effect of irritant dermatitis on human percutaneous penetration of salicylic acid was evaluated in vivo using microdialysis (18). Mild and severe dermatitis was induced using 1% and 2% SLS exposure for 24 hours, respectively. A 46-fold increase in salicylic acid penetration with mild dermatitis and a 146-fold increase in penetration with severe dermatitis were observed relative to the penetration of salicylic acid through untreated, normal skin.

The effects of pretreating human cadaver skin with two known skin irritants, norephedrine and imipramine, on the in vitro percutaneous absorption of three model compounds (caffeine, indomethacin, and hydrocortisone) with diverse physicochemical properties was evaluated by Nangia et al. (19). Skin pretreatment with norephedrine increased the permeation of caffeine and hydrocortisone twofold and fourfold, respectively, whereas absorption of indomethacin declined by an order of magnitude. Pretreatment with imipramine increased the permeation of caffeine and hydrocortisone by an order of magnitude but did not affect indomethacin skin permeation. In vivo studies demonstrated that only norephedrine treatment increased TEWL, whereas imipramine treatment was the more severe irritant as judged by erythema. Not surprisingly, the authors conclude that the mechanisms associated with alterations in skin barrier function induced by irritants are rather complex.

Ichthyosis

The name ichthyosis was suggested by the scaly, fishlike (ichthys) appearance of the skin. The name referring to fish is a misnomer because this diseased skin state more closely resembles that of an alligator or snake (7). Ichthyosis is a group of inherited and acquired dermatoses characterized by hyperkeratosis and a reduction in barrier function as demonstrated by a significant increase in TEWL (15,20). One should expect increased percutaneous penetration of topically applied compounds to the involved skin of patients relative to that of normal, healthy individuals.

Psoriasis

Psoriasis is a defective skin reaction to intrinsic factors and is characterized by sharply defined red lesions with silvery scales and epidermal hyperproliferation (plaques) that primarily occur at the elbow, knee, side of the scalp, and the perianal region but can also arise in other regions. Skin irritation due to injury or trauma can give rise to new lesions (7). The barrier function of involved psoriatic skin is diminished as demonstrated by elevated TEWL that returns to normal with disease remission (21).

The reduced barrier function of involved psoriatic skin would suggest that percutaneous penetration of topically applied compounds would increase, but this is not always observed. The degree of potential penetration enhancement has been dependent upon experimental methods (such as pretreatment removal of the plaque before compound application), vehicle, and the use of occlusion (22). The presence of a thick, hyperkeratotic plaque may alter reservoir capacity of the skin and, thereby, alter percutaneous penetration (15).

The percutaneous absorption of radiolabeled triamcinolone acetonide in ointment or cream formulations was evaluated in skin of normal, healthy subjects and in psoriatic skin in vivo by Schaefer et al. (23). The stratum corneum of normal individuals stores up to 30% of the steroid after topical application. This is followed by a rapid penetration of triamcinolone acetonide into the viable epidermis and dermis. In normal skin, the viable epidermis reaches levels of 5 to 30 μM of tissue, and the dermis reaches levels of 0.8 to 1 μM. In psoriatic skin, the viable epidermis and dermis levels were 3 to 10 times higher than that of normal skin. The authors note that this magnitude of increase in viable tissue levels lies within the same range as that achieved after the removal of the stratum corneum by tape stripping before application.

White et al. (24) evaluated the penetration of large-MW, 15-mer, oligonucleotides in psoriatic patients relative to normal volunteers using live confocal microscopy and fluorescence microscopy of fixed sections of skin. They found oligonucleotide penetration through the stratum corneum of the psoriatic skin but not normal skin. The oligonucleotides were localized in psoriatic skin to the nucleus of the large parakeratotic cells as well as smaller basal and suprabasal keratinocytes. However, in normal skin, the oligonucleotides were observed in the stratum corneum and little or no oligonucleotide in the viable epidermis. The authors conclude that oligonucleotides penetrate psoriatic skin through areas of severe barrier function impairment followed by lateral oligonucleotide spread throughout the viable epidermis.

Gould et al. (25) evaluated the permeation of the recombinant protein plasminogen activator inhibitor type 2 (PAI-2) from hydroxyethylcellulose gels through the stratum corneum of involved and uninvolved skin of patients with plaque-type psoriasis. PAI-2 is the major plasminogen activator inhibitor of the epidermis and is correlated with keratinocyte differentiation and suppression of keratinocyte proliferation. PAI-2 (MW ~ 46,500 Da) was formulated into two gels, one containing propylene glycol as a penetration enhancer. The effect of occlusion was also evaluated. Permeation of ^{123}I-labeled PAI-2 into the viable tissues was determined after a 6-hour topical exposure and subsequent removal of the stratum corneum by repetitive tape stripping. Under occlusive and nonoccluded exposure conditions, penetration of PAI-2 into viable psoriatic skin was 10-fold higher than uninvolved skin ($P = 0.007$ and $P = 0.001$, respectively). Furthermore, penetration of PAI-2 into viable psoriatic skin under nonoccluded conditions was enhanced by propylene glycol.

Interestingly, occlusion of the formulation containing propylene glycol significantly (P = 0.001) reduced PAI-2 penetration into viable psoriatic skin (possibly because of substantial losses into the occlusive dressing).

The in vivo percutaneous absorption of ^{14}C-labeled hydrocortisone, formulated in 0.5% hydrocortisone cream (Cort-Dome®; Bayer Pharmaceutical Inc., West Haven, Connecticut, U.S.A.), was evaluated in four patients with psoriasis and six normal, healthy volunteers (26). Sixty microliters of cream were applied over 45.6 cm^2 of sharply defined erythematous plaques with silvery scales on the dorsal forearm. These were believed to be stable plaques. The same site of application and area were used in the normal volunteers. Participants were instructed not to wash the site of application for 24 hours. Percutaneous absorption was determined by the urinary excretion of ^{14}C monitored for 7 days from dose application. An average of 2.3 ± 1.4% (±SD) of the applied dose was absorbed by the psoriatic patients, whereas 2.5 ± 1.2% was absorbed by normal, healthy subjects. The authors concluded that, for presumably stable psoriatic plaques, the percutaneous absorption of hydrocortisone is the same as normal skin from healthy subjects.

Ghadially et al. (27) assessed skin barrier function, lamellar body structure, and extracellular lamellar body formation in untreated patients with different psoriatic phenotypes. Normal stratum corneum barrier formation requires the synthesis and secretion of lamellar body contents followed by the extracellular processing of these lamellar body contents into the lamellar bilayers that reside between the keratinocytes of the stratum corneum. Subjects with erythroderma and active plaque psoriatic phenotypes displayed elevated TEWL, increased numbers of epidermal lamellar bodies (of which many failed to be secreted), and extracellular domains largely devoid of lamellar body material. In contrast, patients with chronic plaque psoriasis and sebopsoriasis displayed a lower increase in TEWL, normal numbers of lamellar bodies (with only a few remaining unsecreted), and abundant amounts of extracellular lamellar body material (although a normal bilayer pattern was not observed). The authors conclude that these findings are consistent with the hypothesis that both the initial appearance of psoriasis and associated changes in the disease phenotype are driven by alterations in stratum corneum barrier function.

Jaeger (28) has proposed that because of the high rates of penetration and TEWL in psoriatic lesions, one could reduce the periods of application and occlusion, respectively, in corticosteroid treatment. He reported that in 11 patients, an application period of 3–5 minutes followed by occlusion for 20 minutes was as effective as classical long-term corticosteroid treatment. In addition, the reduction in duration of exposure and occlusion led to a reduction in the amount of steroid absorbed by the healthy skin. He concluded that "short contact therapy" would probably minimize steroid absorption by uninvolved skin surrounding the psoriatic lesions and, thereby, reduce the risk of side effects associated with topical treatment with potent corticoids.

Shani et al. (29) measured the in vivo skin penetration of electrolytes in healthy volunteers and in psoriatic patients after bathing in the Dead Sea or in simulated bath salt solutions. The serum levels of bromine, rubidium, calcium, and zinc were significantly increased from baseline only in the psoriatic patients after daily bathing for 4 weeks in the Dead Sea. Therefore, psoriatic patients have a compromised skin barrier to electrolyte penetration from hypertonic solutions relative to healthy volunteers.

Acne Vulgaris

Acne typically appears at puberty and involves nearly 80% of teenagers. Early acne may be the first sign of approaching puberty and is provoked by the androgenic hormones that stimulate the sebaceous glands (7). However, the actual cause of acne is multifactorial and can affect people well beyond their adolescent years. Clinically, acne affects cutaneous areas with large sebaceous glands (face, back, and upper anterior chest). Abnormal epidermal differentiation (keratinization) is involved with comedone formation. Yamamoto et al. (30) have proposed that the impaired water barrier function observed with acne skin is a result of the lower sphingolipid content (ceramides and free sphingosine) of the skin. This impaired water barrier function is then postulated as being responsible for comedone formation because barrier dysfunction is accompanied by hyperkeratosis of the follicular epithelium.

Acne lesions consist of closed (white) or open (black) comedones, papules, pustules, nodules, and abscesses. The abscesses may form channels under the skin, which then form fistulas to discharge pus on the skin surface (7). It should be noted that there are multiple forms of acne besides acne vulgaris (a form of endogenous acne) and that these individual manifestations of acne are typically grouped into the following classifications: endogenous acne, acne medicamentosa, and acne due to "other extraneous causes."

There are numerous topical acne products commonly available and used by patients. But, despite the high prevalence of this disease and the number of people afflicted at one point or another in their life, there is very little work published concerning compound percutaneous absorption in acne-involved skin, let alone relative to noninvolved or normal skin. Akhavan and Bershad (31) have recently reviewed the use of topical acne drugs and concluded that when used appropriately, prescription topical retinoids (such as tretinoin, adapalene, and tazarotene) and topical antimicrobials (such as clindamycin and erythromycin) result in miniscule amounts of drug in the systemic circulation. The extent of systemic availability after topical application of tretinoin and clindamycin is 5% to 7% and 8%, respectively (32). However, topical clindamycin has been rarely associated with diarrhea, and there have been two cases of pseudomembranous colitis reported. Birth defects have occurred in two patients treated with tretinoin and one patient treated with the more recently introduced adapalene; causation by the retinoid was not proven. Topical use of 20% azelaic acid is associated with relatively high systemic exposure. However, systemic exposure to azelaic acid resulting from topical exposure is presumed innocuous because it is a normal dietary constituent, and endogenous levels are not altered by topical use. Benzoyl peroxide, salicylic acid, sulfur, and sodium sulfacetamide are used in concentrations of 2% or more and exhibit some degree of percutaneous absorption. These agents are considered safe. Other than local skin irritation, local allergic contact dermatitis from benzoyl peroxide occurs in ~2.5% of patients, and rarely, local and systemic hypersensitivity reactions from sodium sulfacetamide can occur.

BARRIER FUNCTION OF PHYSICALLY COMPROMISED SKIN

Procedures that disrupt stratum corneum integrity should result in reduced skin barrier function. Scott et al. (33) measured the permeability of water (in vivo and in vitro) and the histology of rat skin after mild, superficial epidermal alterations: I, skin abrasion using the blunt edge of a scalpel blade; II, sandpaper abrasion; III, adhesive tape stripping; IV, suction blister top removal. Water permeation (loss of barrier function) increased after each procedure (IV > III > II > I), and the epidermis regenerated in biphasic manner. The rapid first phase of recovery corresponded with the development of a scab and a corresponding decrease in water permeation. The second phase was more gradual and consisted of the gradual thickening of the stratum corneum and a return to normal barrier function. The amount of time to return to normal was dependent upon the amount of initial stratum corneum removed. A similar process has been shown to occur in human skin with stratum corneum barrier disruption resulting from means other than physical removal. Changes in skin barrier function associated with physical disruption of the stratum corneum by delipidization and tape stripping are discussed below.

Delipidization

Organic solvent extraction can remove barrier-critical lipids from the stratum corneum. The delipidized skin has an increased TEWL (34) and typically enhanced permeability to exogenously applied hydrophobic and hydrophilic materials. The barrier properties of acetone-delipidized mouse skin to compounds with varying hydrophobic/hydrophilic properties (varying octanol–water partition coefficient, $K_{o/w}$) was evaluated by Tsai et al. (35). Delipidization enhanced the skin penetration of hydrophilic and amphipathic compounds (sucrose, caffeine, and hydrocortisone) but did not increase the penetration of highly lipophilic compounds (estradiol and progesterone). The optimal $K_{o/w}$ of compounds for skin penetration appeared to decrease with increased barrier disruption as measured by TEWL.

The effect of acetone delipidization treatment on changes to the MW cutoff of compound penetration of the skin was also evaluated (36) using mouse skin and PEG oligomers with varying MW. As with surfactant (SDS) or tape stripping treatment, the percutaneous penetration of PEG 300, 600, and 1000 oligomers increased as a function of increase in TEWL. The penetration enhancement afforded by barrier disruption was more prominent with the larger molecules. Enhancement in penetration of the largest molecules, the PEG 1000 oligomers, after acetone treatment was not as great as that observed after skin barrier disruption using SDS or tape stripping (17).

Interestingly, Bucks et al. (37) reported, in a clinical study designed to mimic occupational exposure, that delipidization of the palm with 1:1:1-trichloroethane did not effect the percutaneous penetration of hydrocortisone. These results may be due, in part, to the morphological differences in the stratum corneum of the palm relative to the rest of the body. Benfeldt (15) studied the effect of acetone delipidization and reported a 2.2-fold increase in salicylic acid penetration in humans and a decrease (although not significant) in hairless rats. Chloroform/methanol delipidization of hairless guinea pigs resulted in a 5.2- and 2.7-fold increase in hydrocortisone and benzoic acid penetration, respectively (38).

Changes to the in vivo skin penetration of topically applied salicylic acid after a 3-minute treatment of human skin by gently wiping with cotton buds soaked in 100% acetone were evaluated by Benfeldt et al. (18) using microdialysis. Acetone treatment resulted in a significant 2.2-fold increase in salicylic acid penetration.

Tape Stripping

Cells comprising the stratum corneum can be physically removed from the epidermis by the firm application and subsequent quick removal of adhesive tape. This procedure is referred to as tape stripping, and repetitive tape stripping can remove the stratum corneum of most individuals down to what has been described as the glistening layer of skin, which is wet or weepy in appearance. TEWL at the glistening layer in normal, healthy humans is significantly increased (15- to 30-fold) from a baseline of 4 to 8 $g/m^2/hr$ before tape stripping to 120 $g/m^2/hr$ at the glistening layer (39). Trypan blue staining demonstrates that the stratum corneum barrier is essentially removed by tape stripping to the glistening layer (40).

The tape stripping technique has been useful in dermatological research for selectively and exhaustively removing the stratum corneum (39). Tape-stripped skin has been used as a model standardized injury in wound healing research (41,42), and the technique has been used to study epidermal growth kinetics (43,44). Various aspects of intact, partially stripped, and fully stripped skin permeability, including estimates of diffusional resistance within the skin, have been reported (1,40,45–49).

Enhanced skin penetration after tape stripping has been demonstrated by many investigators. Moon et al. (38) observed a twofold increase in benzoic acid and a threefold increase in hydrocortisone penetration of hairless guinea pig skin after tape stripping. Salicylic acid penetration in hairless rats and humans was increased 180- and 157-fold, respectively, by tape stripping (15,18).

Changes in the dependence of PEG MW on mouse skin permeation after tape stripping was evaluated by Tsai et al. (17). As with SDS and acetone treatment, the percutaneous penetration of PEG 300, 600, and 1000 oligomers increased as a function of increase in TEWL, with penetration enhancement more prominent with the larger molecules. The MW dependence of PEG penetration was practically the same between tape-stripped and SDS-treated mouse skin.

Bucks et al. (40) evaluated the effect of repetitive cellophane tape stripping on the in vitro percutaneous absorption of [^{3}H]hydrocortisone and [^{14}C]inulin using human abdominal skin. Ten tape strippings neither appreciably increased skin staining after application of Trypan blue nor enhanced the penetration of either compound. Twenty-five sequential tape strips resulted in pronounced staining by Trypan blue and a 5.3- and 13-fold increase in [^{3}H]hydrocortisone and [^{14}C]inulin skin penetration, respectively. Feldmann and Maibach (50) have demonstrated a 32-fold increase in hydrocortisone penetration in man with tape stripping followed by occlusion.

CONCLUSIONS

The skin permeation results summarized above suggest that macromolecules (e.g., peptides, proteins, oligonucleotides, antibiotics) would have significantly greater bioavailability after topical application to diseased or wounded skin relative to the surrounding intact, healthy skin. This suggests the possibility of targeted delivery of drugs consisting of large molecules (>500 Da) to treat diseased skin. The diseased skin, with its compromised barrier properties, would allow the ingress of a large therapeutic agent, whereas penetration from the surrounding skin with a normal barrier would be significantly reduced. Under this hypothesis, as the diseased skin heals to form the normal barrier associated with an intact stratum corneum, significantly less high-MW drug would penetrate after repetitive topical treatment. Bioavailability and systemic body burden of large-MW therapeutic agents would decrease at a greater rate as the skin condition improves relative to drugs with MW less than 500 Da.

It is this intact, healthy stratum corneum that precludes skin penetration of most topically applied compounds, and as the MW of the compound increases, the ability of the stratum corneum to exclude penetration increases. Studies have shown that damaging the integrity of the stratum corneum leads to an increase in the bioavailability of topically applied agents. The more extensive the disruption of the stratum corneum, the greater the level of skin penetration achieved. Many of the techniques used to disrupt the stratum corneum are transient in nature, allowing a temporary portal of entry for topically applied agents before the natural regeneration of the intact stratum corneum. Stratum corneum disruption techniques are typically physical in nature and include tape stripping, cyanoacrylate stripping, sandpaper abrasion, and needle abrasion. These physical disruptive techniques realistically have very limited utility in the treatment of patients with normal stratum corneum barrier function, but these techniques can function as applicable models of probable barrier compromised skin after cutaneous injury. However, the more recent microneedle technique of physically compromising stratum corneum integrity by punching numerous, very small, and very short holes in the skin holds great promise as a means to increase the bioavailability of topically applied compounds. Microneedle technology represents a much more controlled and elegant form of abrasion-facilitated compound penetration of the skin that may well be applicable for the physician's office and/or patient's home use. This technology is discussed in Chapter 44 of this volume.

REFERENCES

1. Blank IH. Further observations on factors which influence the water content of the stratum corneum. J Invest Dermatol 1953; 21:259–269.
2. Scheuplein RJ, Blank IH. Permeability of the skin. Physiol Rev 1971; 51:702–747.
3. Bos JD, Meinardi MM. The 500 Dalton rule for the skin penetration of chemical compounds and drugs. Exp Dermatol 2000; 9:165–169.
4. Schaefer H, Stuttgen G, Zesch A, et al. Quantitative determination of percutaneous absorption of radiolabeled drugs in vitro and in vivo by human skin. Curr Probl Dermatol 1978; 7:80–94.
5. Roberts MS. Targeted drug delivery to the skin and deeper tissues: role of physiology, solute structure and disease. Clin Exp Pharmacol Physiol 1997; 24:874–879.
6. Schaefer H, Redelmeier TE. Skin Barrier: Principals of Percutaneous Absorption. Basel, Switzerland: Karger, 1996.
7. Steigleder GK, Maibach HI. Dermatology. Chicago, Il: Year Book Medical Publishers, 1980.
8. Werner Y, Lindberg M. Transepidermal water loss in dry and clinically normal skin in patients with atopic dermatitis. Acta Derm Venereol 1985; 65:102–105.
9. Hata M, Tokura Y, Takigawa M, et al. Assessment of epidermal barrier function by photoacoustic spectrometry in relation to its importance in the pathogenesis of atopic dermatitis. Lab Invest 2002; 82:1451–1461.
10. Aalto-Korte K, Turpeinen M. Transepidermal water loss and absorption of hydrocortisone in widespread dermatitis. Br J Dermatol 1993; 128:633–635.
11. Aalto-Korte K, Turpeinen M. Quantifying systemic absorption of topical hydrocortisone in erythroderma. Br J Dermatol 1995; 133:403–408.
12. Maibach HI. In vivo percutaneous penetration of corticoids and unresolved problems in their efficacy. Dermatologica 1976; 152(Suppl.):11–25.
13. Bucks D, Maibach H. Occlusion does not uniformly enhance penetration in vivo. In: Bronaugh RL and Maibach HI, eds. Percutaneous Absorption. 3rd ed. New York: Marcel Dekker, 1999:81–105.
14. Yoshiike T, Aikawa Y, Sindhvananda J, et al. Skin barrier defect in atopic dermatitis: increased permeability of the stratum corneum using dimethyl sulfoxide and theophylline. J Dermatol Sci 1993; 5:92–96.

15. Benfeldt E. In vivo microdialysis for the investigation of drug levels in the dermis and the effect of barrier perturbation on cutaneous drug penetration. Acta Derm Venereol (Stockh) 1999; 206(Suppl.):1–59.
16. Wilhelm KP, Surber C, Maibach HI. Effect of sodium lauryl sulfate–induced skin irritation on in vivo percutaneous penetration of four drugs. J Invest Dermatol 1991; 97(5):927–932.
17. Tsai JC, Shen LC, Sheu HM, et al. Tape stripping and sodium dodecyl sulfate treatment increase the molecular weight cutoff of polyethylene glycol penetration across murine skin. Arch Dermatol Res 2003; 295(4):169–174.
18. Benfeldt E, Serup J, Menne T. Effect of barrier perturbation on cutaneous salicylic acid penetration in human skin: *in vivo* pharmacokinetics using microdialysis and non-invasive quantification of barrier function. Br J Dermatol 1999; 140:739–748.
19. Nangia A, Camel E, Berner B, et al. Influence of skin irritants on percutaneous absorption. Pharm Res 1993; 10:1756–1759.
20. Lavrijsen APM, Oestmann E, Hermans J, et al. Barrier function parameters in various keratinization disorders: transepidermal water loss and vascular responses to hexyl nicotinate. Br J Dermatol 1993; 129:547–554.
21. Marks J, Rogers S, Chadkrirk B, et al. Clearance of chronic plaque psoriasis by anthralin — subjective and objective assessment and comparison with photochemotherapy. Br J Dermatol 1981; 105(Suppl. 20):96–99.
22. Wester RC, Maibach HI. Percutaneous absorption in diseased skin. In: Maibach HI, Surber C, eds. Topical Corticosteroids. Basel, Switzerland: Karger, 1992:128–141.
23. Schaefer H, Zesch A, Stuttgen G. Penetration, permeation, and absorption of triamcinolone acetonide in normal and psoriatic skin. Arch Derm Res 1977; 258:241–249.
24. White PJ, Gray AC Fogarty RD, et al. C-5 Propyne-modified oligonucleotides penetrate the epidermis in psoriatic and not normal human skin after topical application. J Invest Dermatol 2002; 118:1003–1007.
25. Gould AR, Sharp PJ, Smith DR, et al. Increased permeability of psoriatic skin to the protein, plasminogen activator inhibitor 2. Arch Dermatol Res 2003; 295:249–254.
26. Wester RC, Bucks DAW, Maibach HI. In vivo percutaneous absorption of hydrocortisone in psoriatic patients and normal volunteers. J Am Acad Dermatol 1983; 8:645–647.
27. Ghadially R, Reed JT, Elias PM. Stratum corneum structure and function correlates with phenotype in psoriasis. J Invest Dermatol, 1996; 107:558–564.
28. Jaeger L. Psoriasis treatment with betamethasone dipropionate using short-term application and short-term occlusion. Acta Derm Venereol 1986; 66:84–87.
29. Shani J, Barak S, Levi D, et al. Skin penetration of minerals in psoriatics and guinea-pigs bathing in hypertonic salt solutions. Pharmacol Res Commun 1985; 17:501–512.
30. Yamamoto A, Takenouchi K, Ito M. Impaired water barrier function in acne vulgaris. Arch Dermatol Res 1995; 287:214–218.
31. Akhavan A, Bershad S. Topical acne drugs: review of clinical properties, systemic exposure, and safety. Am J Clin Dermatol 2003; 4:473–492.
32. van Hoogdalem EJ. Transdermal absorption of topical anti-acne agents in man; review of clinical pharmacokinetic data. J Eur Acad Dermatol Venereol 1998; 11(Suppl. 1):S13–S19; discussion S28–S29.
33. Scott RC, Dugard PH, Doss AW. Permeability of abnormal rat skin. J Invest Dermatol 1986; 86:201–207.
34. Menczel E. Delipidization of the cutaneous permeability barrier and percutaneous penetration. In: Smith EW, Maibach HI, eds. Percutaneous Penetration Enhancers. Boca Raton, Fla: CRC Press, 1995:383–392.
35. Tsai JC, Sheu HM, Hung PL, et al. Effect of barrier disruption by acetone treatment on the permeability of compounds with various lipophilicities: implications for the permeability of compromised skin. J Pharm Sci 2001; 90(9):1242–1254.
36. Tsai JC, Hung PL, Sheu HM. Molecular weight dependence of polyethylene glycol penetration across acetone-disrupted permeability barrier. Arch Dermatol Res 2001; 293(6):302–307.
37. Bucks DA, Maibach HI, Menczel E, et al. Percutaneous penetration of hydrocortisone in humans following skin delipidization by 1:1:1 trichloroethane. Arch Dermatol Res 1983; 275:242–245.

38. Moon KC, Wester RC, Maibach HI. Diseased skin models in the hairless guinea pig: in vivo percutaneous absorption. Dermatologica 1990; 180:8–12.
39. Tsai JC, Weiner ND, Flynn GL, et al. Properties of adhesive tapes used for stratum corneum stripping. Int J Pharm 1991; 72:227–231.
40. Bucks D, Marshall B, Lund T, et al. Stratum corneum, epidermis and dermis barrier function: implications in the development of topical products containing large molecular weight drugs. 2005 AAPS National Biotechnology Conference. Arlington, Va: American Association of Pharmaceutical Scientists.
41. Pinkus H. Examination of the epidermis by the strip method of removing horny layers. I. Observations on thickness of the horny layer, and on mitotic activity after stripping. J Invest Dermatol 1951; 16:383–386.
42. Pinkus H. Examination of the epidermis by the strip method of removing horny layers. II. Biometric data on regeneration of the human epidermis. J Invest Dermatol 1952; 19:431–447.
43. Downes AM, Matoltsy AG, Sweeney TM. Rate of turnover of the stratum corneum in hairless mice. J Invest Dermatol 1967; 49:400–405.
44. Porter D, Shuster S. A new method for measuring replacement of epidermis and stratum corneum in human skin. J Invest Dermatol 1967; 49:251–255.
45. Monash S. Location of the superficial epithelial barrier to skin penetration. J Invest Dermatol 1957; 29:367–376.
46. Monash S, Blank IH. Location and reformation of the epithelial barrier to water vapor. Arch Dermatol 1958; 78:710–714.
47. Flynn GL, Durrheim H, Higuchi WI. Permeation of hairless mouse skin II: Membrane sectioning techniques and influence on alkanol permeabilities. J Pharm Sci 1981; 70:52–56.
48. Behl CR, Linn EE, Flynn GL, et al. Permeation of skin and eschar by antiseptics. I. Baseline studies with phenol. J Pharm Sci 1983; 72:391–397.
49. Bronaugh RL, Stewart RF. Methods for in vitro percutaneous absorption studies V: Permeation through damaged skin. J Pharm Sci 1985; 74:1062–1066.
50. Feldmann RJ, Maibach HI. Penetration of 14C hydrocortisone through normal skin: the effect of stripping and occlusion. Arch Dermatol 1965; 91:661–666.

10 Targeting the Pilosebaceous Gland

Guang Wei Lu, Susan Ciotti, and Satyanarayana Valiveti
Pfizer Global Research and Development, Ann Arbor, Michigan, U.S.A.

Jeffrey E. Grice and Sheree E. Cross
Therapeutics Research Unit, School of Medicine, University of Queensland, Princess Alexandra Hospital, Woolloongabba, Queensland, Australia

INTRODUCTION

When one speaks of targeting of skin appendages using topically applied agents/products, one is referring to one or another (or both) of two skin structures—hair follicles (pilosebaceous units) and/or eccrine sweat glands. Very little information has been published concerning drug delivery to/through eccrine sweat glands, whereas follicular drug delivery has received a considerable amount of research attention in recent years. This review is mainly concerned with the body of literature covering targeted follicular drug delivery. Successful targeting, as the phrase is used here, simply means getting more drug molecules into the specified appendage of action than can be delivered with conventional dosage forms (delivery systems). At the same time, it implies restricting the amount of drug that reaches therapeutically uninvolved sites, most particularly, the systemic circulation. Targeted follicular delivery would be useful to stem hair loss or promote new hair growth. In principle, topically applied agents can reach the hair bulb by either transfollicular or transepidermal route, with the former involving drug diffusion through the upper reaches of the pilosebaceous gland and the latter involving secondary local/systemic distribution into hair follicles. In fact, both pathways occur simultaneously in most cases, but the relative contribution of each pathway to the overall delivery seemingly should vary substantially depending upon the physicochemical properties of the therapeutic agent, the nature of its formulation, the specific site of topical application, and the elapsed time after topical dosing.

Targeted drug delivery to the hair follicle can be managed by two quite different ways—the first being a formulation approach and the second being a molecule modification approach (1). Several researchers using the formulation approach have established that improved localized delivery of drugs to the hair follicle can be achieved by varying the compositions of applied formulations (2–13). In one case, the gains in localized delivery were achieved through the application of a system containing a particulate carrier (13) and in another case by using sebum-miscible excipients in the topical preparation (14). In contrast, the molecule modification approach involves a tailoring of the physicochemical properties of a drug molecule, such as its size, polarity (lipophilicity), polar surface area, solubility parameter, and/or charge, any of which has a potential to modulate delivery into the hair follicle (1,15). To fully appreciate how these different approaches might be used, one has to come to working terms with the structure and physiology of the hair follicle. These critical aspects will not be reviewed in any detail here, as they are already discussed extensively in the literature (1,3,15–19).

PILOSEBACEOUS GLAND

The human body is virtually covered with hair and thus with hair follicles (pilosebaceous glands). Each pilosebaceous gland consists of an actual hair follicle, the outer projection of which, a hair, is visible to the eye, and one or more sebaceous glands that are buried approximately 50 to 100 μm below the surface of the skin (20,21). A very active gland, the hair follicle (Fig. 1) is a very complex appendage. At its base, one finds the hair bulb. It is in the hair bulb that the hair shaft (hair) is formed. Along with the stratum corneum, which covers 99% of the surface of the skin, and fingernails and toenails, hair is a keratinized structure. Cells in the bulb divide and migrate toward the center of the bulb. As they migrate, fibrous structures are woven within the cytoplasm. They rigidify as they lose vitality to become the building blocks of the hair shaft. Mitosis of cells at the hair bulb largely regulates hair growth. The fabric of hair is nothing other than that of a compact of devitalized, keratinized cells.

Irregularly shaped sebaceous glands are attached about two-thirds of the way up the follicle. These produce the oily secretion known as sebum. Like the hair shaft, sebum is also a product of cell division and specialization. Sebaceous stem cells at the periphery of the gland divide continuously. Daughter cells then migrate toward the center of the gland, in this course synthesizing vacuoles of lipid. Eventually they fill with lipid, whereupon they die and rupture. Sebum is all the substance that is left of them.

Over most of the body, a hair shaft is formed deep within each follicle; it extends all the way through the follicle and out of the body. Hair grows at different rates and for different durations, depending on the location of the body. The hair

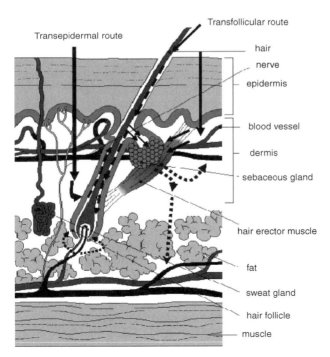

FIGURE 1 Structure of the human skin and route of drug transport to the hair follicle and sebaceous gland.

shaft is enveloped by several distinct layers of tissue, first, the inner root sheath; then, the outer root sheath; and finally, an outermost acellular "basement" membrane termed the glassy membrane. The pilosebaceous gland is an epidermal structure. This is shown by the fact that its outer root sheath is a keratinized layer that is continuous with the rest of the epidermis. The inner root sheath ends about halfway up the follicle. Because the hair shaft is scaly, hair growth helps to convey sebum to the skin surface and keep the sebaceous channel open.

The flasklike sebaceous glands are outgrowths of epithelial cells as well. Ducts join these multilobular holocrine glands to the upper part of the follicular canal. Sebum has to flow out from the central part of the gland and through the ducts to reach the skin surface.

Sebaceous Glands

Human sebaceous glands as described above are coupled to prominent hair follicles (Fig. 1). However, sebaceous glands are also found across the relatively hairless surfaces of the face, the forehead, and the nape of the back (20,21). Indeed, facial skin is estimated to have in excess of 450 sebaceous glands per square centimeter, the greatest density of these glands anywhere on the body. They are not present on the palms of the hands and soles of the feet. Those located on the mid back, forehead, and face are larger and more numerous than elsewhere. The hair shafts of the associated follicles in these locations tend to be tiny, almost microscopic, although the sebaceous glands themselves are especially large. Because these particular sebaceous glands dominate the follicles they are associated with, they are known as sebaceous follicles. As mentioned, in areas of prominent hair, the ducts of sebaceous glands open into the hair follicles beneath the surface of skin. Sebaceous follicles seemingly open directly on the surface of the skin. Synthesis and release of oily sebum are the only functions of these glands. This acts as a skin emollient and sealant. Thus, sebaceous glands are classified as holocrine glands.

It has been pointed out that sebum production by these glands involves cell proliferation, migration, and specialization. Beginning with mitosis along the outer margin of the gland, the process takes about three weeks. The lag time between cell death with sebum liberation and the appearance of sebum on the surface of the skin is only about 8 days (22). Human sebum is comprised of triglycerides (57.5%), wax esters (26%), squalene (12%), cholesterol esters (3%), and cholesterol (1.5%) (23). It is rich in neutral, nonpolar fats at the time of its inception within the follicle. However, the triglycerides produced within sebocytes and released on their demise are, to some extent, hydrolyzed by bacteria before sebum reaches the skin surface. By the time sebum exits the glands, it is replete with free fatty acids. Indeed, it is estimated that approximately a third of sebum is free fatty acids when it reaches the skin surface. Once sebum has entered the hair follicle, it takes approximately 14 hours to appear on the skin surface (24). It is expressed from follicles at a rate of about 0.1 mg/cm^2/hr. It has been estimated that the collective area of the openings of follicles on the skin ranges from 0.1% to 1% of the total skin surface. Using these figures, the actual flow of sebum out of the glands is projected to be about 10 to 100 mg/cm^2/hr. The buildup of sebum on the skin surface measures about 0.5 mg/cm^2 (22). In addition to the emollient/sealant functions of sebum that keep the stratum corneum pliable and prevent water loss from the body, sebum also helps protect the body from infection as a result of the free fatty acids it contains (25). These acidify the surface, providing the skin with what is often known as the acid mantle.

Potential Targets Within the Pilosebaceous Unit

The pilosebaceous unit has several physicochemical domains that can be targeted, including its sebaceous glands, its bulge region, and its follicular papilla. Follicular delivery, as the term is most often used, conjures up a picture of a drug diffusing out from an application to the skin surface, into the opening of the follicular channel, and down through the tissues of the follicle, all these steps necessary to reach a follicular target site. This view actually strictly defines the transfollicular route. In general, drug molecules reaching specified target sites in a follicle reach the sites by taking advantage of several transport pathways, including the transfollicular pathway. Local diffusion from the surrounding tissues invariably makes its contribution to follicular delivery as does a drug that works its way back into the sebaceous gland from the systemic circulation. Over and above the properties of drug molecules and formulations, the contribution of each pathway to the drug level at a target site depends upon the remoteness of the target by way of the pathway, the mass the tissue or substance offering the pathway, the physical nature of the local tissue or substance that is the pathway, and the vasculature subserving the target site. Because of the different natures of the subtissues, it would be possible for follicular drug delivery to play an appreciable role in targeting sebaceous glands, but at the same time for the same drug applied in the same vehicle to play only a minimal role with respect to the drug reaching the follicle papilla. Therefore, different delivery strategies have to be developed based on the actual target location within a follicle.

The effectiveness of follicular drug delivery can be controlled by partitioning of drug molecules into the opening of the pilosebaceous gland and diffusion of the molecules through the substance of the gland. It might also be effective to deliver the drug in question through the skin surface lying between and surrounding follicles. In other words, in addition to molecular diffusion vertically down the follicular duct, molecules might also spread out laterally through the various layers of the skin that surround the follicles to reach the deeper regions of the hair follicles. For the first 200–500 µm, the molecules taking the transfollicular route would likely involve permeation through the highly lipophilic, cylindrical expanse of sebum present in the upper follicle. In this case, drug solubility, partitioning, and diffusion in sebum would primarily determine the localization of the molecules deeper in the gland. However, after reaching the far edge of the sebum-rich field, the next 500–4000 µm would have to be molecularly breached through a transport field to reach the lower bulb. The most likely conduit of lipophilic molecules would be the junction between the inner and outer root sheath, particularly Henle's and Huxley's layers of the follicle. We have precious little appreciation concerning how molecules might transport through these tissues.

If we are interested in regulating the growth of hair, we have to concentrate on getting drug into the lower, proliferative territory of follicles, that is, the bulge region. The bulge region of the follicle (the follicular bulb) is located 500–800 µm beneath the skin surface. It reportedly contains follicular stem cells and seemingly plays a critical role in regulating hair growth (13). Although nothing concerning drug delivery to this region has been conclusively established in human subjects, the bulge region nevertheless remains the prime target site, perhaps the only real target site for follicular drug delivery meant to kindle hair growth.

To support their cellular activities, both hair follicles and sebaceous glands are of necessity richly supplied with capillaries. This leads us to believe that the pilosebaceous apparatus could be reached through systemic drug delivery as well as more localized or targeted topical delivery. This also suggests follicles might even be exploited for systemic delivery. Seen the other way around, access to the deep sections of hair follicles might only be accomplished through systemic delivery.

As a bottom line, it is not clear if the transfollicular pathway is able to contribute molecules to the follicular papilla to a level of therapeutic significance. It is more than likely that distribution of drug into follicles from the systemic circulation will be the primary pathway of drug delivery to the lower follicle. The question is a difficult one to address experimentally and theoretically because transfollicularly delivered molecules permeate into the surrounding tissues and never achieve working concentrations within the lower reaches of hair follicles.

RECENT ADVANCES IN FOLLICULAR DELIVERY

Transfollicular delivery of topically applied drugs for both local and systemic effects has been an area of keen interest to dermatologists and scientists for decades. Several recently published reviews concisely capture the experience and advances in this area (16–18,26). In the latest comprehensive review, Meidan et al. (18) summarize studies associated with follicular drug delivery, including work published up to 2005. A number of recently filed patents disclose formulation and excipient effects on follicular delivery (27–29). Perusal of these literature sources suggests that delivery of small molecules to hair follicles and sebaceous glands is enhanced by incorporating surfactants and polymers such as polyethylene glycol ethers of alkyl alcohols and poloxamers in vehicles (28,29). To treat follicular diseases, the incorporation of a C_{12}–C_{16} alkyl lactate into one's topical vehicle is recommended (or claimed). In other words, it is suggested that the lactate compounds function as promoters of follicular delivery (30). Grams et al. (31) investigated the influence of permeant lipophilicity on follicular accumulation using confocal laser scanning microscopy as their research tool. These studies revealed that follicular accumulation of tested dyes increased with increased lipophilicity of the compounds. However, the study provided no information about the permeation pathway that drew the dye into the hair follicle. To address this issue, an online diffusion method using confocal laser scanning microscopy to continuously monitor the transport process of the molecules was developed, and the diffusion of the model compounds from the skin surface into hair follicles was evaluated (32). These studies demonstrated the transport time courses of the selected molecules into the hair follicles of human scalp skin. Vehicle effects on follicular drug delivery were also investigated. A lipophilic fluorophore had the highest deposition into hair follicles, again indicating the role molecular lipophilicity plays in follicular delivery.

Samples collected from the large sebaceous glands found in hamster ears have been widely used to investigate follicular drug delivery after topical applications of test vehicles to the animal's ear. Diffusion from surrounding tissues may be appreciable in this model because of the high permeability of hamster ear skin, making the estimation of actual transfollicular delivery difficult. Also uncertain is the extent to which adipose tissue surrounding the hamster ear's sebaceous glands affects drug deposition into these sebaceous glands. In an attempt to understand the correlation between hamster ear sebum and human sebum with respect to the partitioning and diffusion of drug molecules, our group has conducted a comparison study using model compounds. Our preliminary data show that differences existed in partitioning properties but that the transport rates varied appreciably. These results have been submitted for publication.

A numbers of studies have employed follicle-rich versus follicle-rare or follicle-free models to evaluate follicular drug delivery. Specific comparisons drawn in
these investigations of follicular drug delivery involved the use of hairless versus
hairy animals of the same species (15), the permeability of hair follicle-free skin (33),
and the permeability of human scalp or facial skin versus body skin (34). These
approaches are obviously primarily aimed at the effect of follicle density on percutaneous drug transport. However, inherent differences in the anatomical features of
the different skins used in this comparison (i.e., variation in respective thicknesses
and actual permeability of respective stratum cornea), and the effects these may
have with respect to drug delivery have never been characterized. One has to consider that differences in follicular count may not be the only reason for permeability
variation in these studies. Ogiso et al. (34) demonstrated a correlation ($r = 0.65$–0.67)
between hair density and skin flux of tested compounds through human scalp skin.
Measured fluxes as well as calculated permeation and diffusion coefficients through
scalp skin were substantially higher than those measured on abdominal skin. These
results were interpreted to mean that follicular delivery contributes appreciably
to transport across the skin membrane. Furthermore, using histological methods,
these investigators showed that fluorescent probes (both lipophilic and hydrophilic)
quickly penetrated into the junction between the follicle's internal and external root
sheaths and eventually permeated into surrounding skin tissue.

Skin sandwiches have been used to measure transepidermal drug permeation
in the absence of a transfollicular pathway (19,35). In the sandwich procedure, a
layer of isolated stratum corneum is placed over a layer of isolated epidermis. This
is done in such a way that the pores (follicles and sweat ducts) through each layer
do not overlap and thus are blocked by the companion layer. It is reasoned that the
first half of the distance a molecule has to travel through the skin sandwich has its
pore route, but the second half is functionally pore-free. The flux or permeability
obtained from the overlays is then compared with the result from a single layer of
epidermis with pores. Such data could be used to estimate the effect of the shunt
pathway as long as the isolated layers make intimate contact over the whole of their
surfaces. Although quite an innovative approach, more studies are needed to evaluate the correlation between experimental data and theoretic assumptions as well as
to establish the reproducibility of the method and its effectiveness in measuring the
skin permeability of various compounds.

IDENTIFICATION OF MOLECULES SUITABLE FOR FOLLICULAR DELIVERY

In addition to exploring transepidermal absorption as a route of drug administration, scientists and physicians have long been interested in delivering medicine
through hair follicles although this passageway is not generally considered a primary route through the skin of man. It is no simple task to design a molecule that
is appropriate for follicular delivery. In addition to the criteria that must be satisfied in the conventional selection of drug candidates (i.e., desirable physiochemical
properties, local efficacy, lack of dermal and systemic adverse effects, and phar-
macokinetic/pharmacodynamic profiles), follicular accumulation is an additional
parameter that has to be added into what is already a complicated equation. There
is always the chance that changes in molecular structure to improve follicular deliv-
erability could adversely affect other properties of the drug candidate. It could alter
accumulations in ways and amounts that would change the pharmacological and
toxicological aspects of the medicine. Therefore, enhancing or targeting follicular

drug delivery remains a complicated yet important challenge to researchers in the discovery phases of new drug design.

Drug Partitioning Into and Diffusion Through Sebum

Other than for the stratum corneum itself, pilosebaceous glands are the most accessible anatomical feature found on the surface of the skin. As mentioned earlier, the sebaceous glands reach to depths between 0.2 and 0.5 mm in the skin surface; they are functionally connected to hair follicles. Sebum produced in the sebaceous glands vents through the upper third of the hair follicle to get to the skin surface. It has been pointed out that on average, the secretion rate of sebum on to the skin surface is approximately 0.1 mg/cm^2/hr (23). To be effective, the transport rate of molecules making their way into sebum would necessarily have to be faster than the outflow of sebum onto the skin. Once the drug molecules reach their target zone, they have to reside in the sebaceous glands to accomplish their therapeutic task. Sebum flow could be counterproductive, depending on how the drug molecules distribute in the follicle. In general, based on everything we know, matching the lipophilicity of the compounds to that of the sebum is likely to direct researchers to compounds of high absolute and relative lipid solubility. Although log $K_{o/w}$, the log of the partition coefficient of a drug between *n*-octanol and water, is a valuable tool and the standard measure of compound lipophilicity, the partition coefficient between sebum and water is obviously a far more relevant measure for follicular uptake of sebum and thus the best direct indication of any drug's follicular partitioning property. Therefore, molecules having a high sebum/water partition coefficient and moderately high diffusion coefficients through the semiliquid sebum phase that exists within the follicle are most likely to be preferable for follicular delivery.

The stratum corneum of the skin folds down into the hair follicle, forming a barrier between sebum and the epidermis and dermis that reaches well below the surface of the skin. The layer thins as it approaches the embedded sebaceous glands. The trafficking of drug molecules between sebum and the thin stratum corneum that is found just above the glands (as well as the surrounding tissues) contributes to deposition of drug molecules throughout hair follicles. Therefore, at its most fundamental level, it is likely that successful sebum-targeted delivery of a drug depends on the inherent thermodynamic and kinetic behaviors of a drug molecule in sebum and the epidermis (especially the stratum corneum). Comparing the relative partitioning and diffusion of drug candidates in sebum and the ratios of these parameters to the same parameters in the stratum corneum provides valuable information about the potential of a molecule for follicle delivery. This serves as a powerful tool for drug screening.

Transfollicular and Transepidermal Analysis

The point has been made that, for a drug to be selectively transported into hair follicles and sebaceous glands, the drug should be capable of favorable, differential partitioning and diffusion in sebum. This can be understood by the following equations that consider drug transport through the skin, to a very good first approximation, to primarily be by independent, parallel transepidermal (stratum corneum is primary barrier), and follicular pathways (36,37):

$$J_{total} = J_{sebum} + J_{sc} = APC \tag{1}$$

where J_{total} is the total flux, J_{sebum} and J_{sc} are fluxes through the independent pathways, A is the total area of application, and C is the concentration of drug in the application. It follows that

$$J_{\text{total}} = A\left[f_{\text{sebum}} \frac{D_{\text{sebum}}K_{\text{sebum}}}{h_{\text{sebum}}} + f_{\text{sc}} \frac{D_{\text{sc}}K_{\text{sc}}}{h_{\text{sc}}} \right]C = \left[A_{\text{sebum}} \frac{D_{\text{sebum}}K_{\text{sebum}}C}{h_{\text{sebum}}} \right] + \left[A_{\text{sc}} \frac{D_{\text{sc}}K_{\text{sc}}C}{h_{\text{sc}}} \right] \quad (2)$$

In these equations, f_{sebum} and f_{sc} are the fractional areas of the transfollicular and transepidermal routes, respectively, making A_{sebum} and A_{sc} the actual areas of the sebum and stratum corneum routes, respectively. D_{sebum} and D_{sc} are the functional diffusion coefficients for the drug in question through sebum and the stratum corneum, whereas K_{sebum} and K_{sc} are the drug's partition coefficients in sebum and stratum corneum, respectively. The terms, h_{sebum} and h_{sc} are the functional thicknesses of the sebum and stratum corneum, respectively. In these equations, the partition coefficients exhibit the greatest variability between compounds within a family and thus are the parameters most likely differentiate the mechanism (36). Therefore, when $K_{\text{sebum}} \gg K_{\text{sc}}$, drug molecules will be preferably transported through sebaceous and hair follicles. When the reverse is true, that is, when $K_{\text{sebum}} \ll K_{\text{sc}}$, the principal pathway for diffusion and accumulation with be that through the stratum corneum (the transepidermal pathway). The ratios of $K_{\text{sebum}}/K_{\text{sc}}$ and $D_{\text{sebum}}/D_{\text{sc}}$ reflect the potential for follicular drug delivery.

Drug Partitioning and Diffusion Through Facsimile Sebum

The pilosebaceous glands (hair follicles) are potential therapeutic target sites for treating both androgenetic alopecia and acne (18,38). Significant effort has been directed toward enhancing the accumulation of molecules in these structures (4,39–42) to treat each of these conditions. However, rarely, if ever, have the investigators addressed the role sebum plays in the delivery of drugs into the hair follicles and their associated sebaceous glands. We have made the case that effective drug delivery to the hair follicle depends on partitioning and diffusion of a therapeutic agent into and within sebum at the same time balancing and counteracting the outward flow of sebum and accounting for drug elimination from hair follicles to surrounding tissues, including the local circulation. Hence, it is imperative that scientists in this field better understand drug partitioning and diffusion properties in sebum if they are really going to target therapeutic agents to the sebum-filled hair follicle. Partition coefficients are thermodynamic parameters best measured under equilibrium conditions. That said, they obviously appear in physical kinetic statements describing permeability. It is important to know that partition coefficients actually have the same numerical value in mass transport equations that they would have if measured at equilibrium (or if they could actually be measured at equilibrium[a]). This is so because concentrations across interfaces in transport scenarios only involve one or two molecular depths on each side of the interfaces. Over such limited distances (a few angstroms), the prevailing thermodynamic activities of a permeating substance

---

[a] It is easy to show that equilibrium and kinetic partition coefficients are the same in the case of permeation of an isotropic membrane. However, when a membrane is complex (i.e., it has more than one phase), the permeant is distributed into more than one phase, at least one of which is a diffusion conduit. In this case, equilibrium measurement reflects accumulations in all membrane phases, not just the kinetically meaningful one.

are, for all practical purposes, equal. By way of contrast, permeability coefficients reflect both thermodynamic and kinetic properties in that they contain elements of partitioning and molecular mobility (Eqs. 1 and 2). Diffusion coefficients evidence the kinetic (point to point mobility) properties of diffusing molecules.

Partitioning and diffusion of molecules of topical drug delivery interest within human sebum have not been investigated. This situation is likely because of the difficulty in collecting sebum samples from human subjects. With these facts in mind, we considered it desirable to develop an artificial sebum that would act as a good substitute for the real thing in investigations of follicular drug delivery. We were not the first to have this thought. A number of published studies have demonstrated the usefulness of artificial sebum in the evaluation of formulation effects of topical dosage forms (11,14,43–45). However, the compositions of literature-reported sebum facsimiles have varied substantially, and it is hard to tell which might act best as a sebum substitute. Therefore, we found it necessary to evaluate the differences and similarities of the artificial forms of sebum relative to human sebum (46). We carefully compared the sebum reproductions with human sebum. The artificial sebum we chose correlates well with human sebum with respect to its chemical composition and physicochemical properties. These deductions are based on measurements of both partition coefficients and sebum fluxes of model compounds. Hence, the use of artificial sebum to mimic human sebum seems well justified for in vitro studies.

Valiveti et al. (37) evaluated drug partitioning between artificial sebum (K_{sebum}) and water and human stratum corneum and water (K_{sc}). They also evaluated the relationships of these partition coefficients to octanol–water partition coefficients ($K_{o/w}$). K_{sebum} and K_{sc} values were determined for a diverse set of chemical structures, including a homologous series of 4-hydroxybenzoic esters, all at 37°C. The K_{sebum} values of some drugs were significantly higher than the corresponding K_{sc} values. However, some of the test compounds exhibited lower or similar K_{sebum} values in comparison with the respective K_{sc} measurements. Importantly, the correlations among log K_{sebum}, log K_{sc}, and log $K_{o/w}$ for the diverse test compounds were generally poor. However and not unexpectedly, a linear relationship was observed between log K_{sebum} and log $K_{o/w}$ for the compounds in the 4-hydroxybenzoic ester homologous series, a sure sign that K_{sebum} directly depends on the lipophilicity of compounds. These studies demonstrate that K_{sebum} is different from K_{sc} and also $K_{o/w}$, attesting to the fact that these three media have fundamentally different capacities to dissolve organic compounds. From the standpoints of modeling and eventual compound selection, K_{sc} is likely to be the parameter that best reflects drug delivery into hair follicles and sebaceous glands.

In another study, these investigators (47) studied the diffusion of their diverse test compounds through sebum itself. Members of the 4-hydroxybenzoate ester homologous series were included. They used the sebum loaded onto a 24-well plate (Transwell®; Cole-Palmer, Vernon Hill, Illinois, U.S.A.), with polycarobonate support as a model. Drug diffusion into and through artificial sebum gives information about the transferability and mobility of substances in and out of the sebum that are applied in aqueous solution or suspensions. These drug transport studies indicate that the fluxes of substances through artificial sebum (J_{sebum}) is primarily a function of lipophilicity and solubility, whereas acidity, charge, molecular weight (or volume), and molecular orientation also contribute to the transport across artificial sebum. Interestingly, a bell-shaped curve was observed upon plotting log J_{sebum} versus the alkyl chain length of the tested homologous series of compounds that proved to be different from the curve obtained upon plotting log J_{skin} versus log $K_{o/w}$ for the same compounds. This indicated that selection of appropriate compounds for sebum-targeted delivery was possible, based on the differences in the skin flux and sebum transport profiles of the molecules.

For a sebum-targeted molecule, a relatively high partition coefficient and probably a high ratio of sebum–water partition coefficient to stratum corneum–water partition coefficient are desirable. However, for a molecule intended to regulate hair growth, the sebum flux and the ratio of sebum flux to total skin flux may even be more relevant. As mentioned, follicular delivery of a molecule is only one of the variables in any drug discovery scheme. It is not uncommon for an added methyelene (CH_2) group or two to change the pharmacokinetic/pharmacodynamic profile of a drug, reduce its efficacy, and/or potentially increase its adverse effects. A simple, but nevertheless enlightening, example of this kind of structural dependency is found in the use of short-chain alcohols as topical excipients. Ethanol and isopropanol are considered as safe topical excipients and are, therefore, widely used as such. Methanol and *n*-butanol, by way of contrast, are not acceptable for topical application because they are frankly toxic.[b] Therefore, any efforts to develop a new drug molecule or to modify an existing drug molecule for follicular delivery cannot be based solely on structural influences on permeation but also have to be carefully integrated into the whole drug discovery process. Seemingly, a less risky approach is, therefore, to modify the formulation to achieve follicular delivery because this presumably focuses on the deposition of a drug of known pharmacological properties.

FORMULATIONS FOR FOLLICULAR DELIVERY
Emulsions and Liposomes

Liposomal formulations have proven useful for the delivery of drugs into follicles (7,48–51). Just as with cell membranes, liposomes mainly consist of phospholipids having two long alkyl chains. As such, these molecules form closed vesicular structures having one or more bilayers wrapped about an aqueous core (52). The bilayer (unilamellar liposomes) or bilayers (multilamellar liposomes) provide the liposome with a hydrophobic "compartment." Liposomes form spontaneously when natural or synthetic amphiphatic phospolipids are mixed into an aqueous medium.

It has been shown that the encasement of vaccines in liposomes raises humoral and/or cellular immune responses (53–57). More to the point, it has also been shown that liposomes penetrate deeper into the hair follicle than standard formulations. The topical application of a liposome-entrapped monoclonal antibody to doxorubicin completed suppressed doxorubicin-induced alopecia in rats (58). Li et al. (51) determined that liposomal entrapment of calcein, melanin, and high-molecular weight DNA resulted in the accumulation of each these compounds in hair follicles of histocultured mouse skin. Jung et al. (59) showed the application of cationic and amphoteric liposomes gave high follicular penetration of the model compounds compared with more standard solution formulations. Either of these types of liposomes might be more suitable for follicular drug delivery than anionic liposomes having a constant surface charge. Niemiec et al. (60) experimented with topical applications of nonionic liposomes that were loaded with the hydrophilic protein, α-interferon, and separately with the hydrophobic peptide, cyclosporine A. These

---

[b] Methanol is metabolized to formaldehyde; systemic formaldehyde causes blindness. *N*-Butanol and somewhat higher alkanols are powerful central nervous system depressants and relatively good skin penetrants and, thus, cannot be used as vehicles.

authors reported that appreciable follicular accumulations of both drugs could be achieved in hamster ear follicles. Ciotti and Weiner (61) investigated follicular delivery in vivo in mice and found that nonionic liposomes facilitated the follicular delivery of both minoxidil and plasmid DNA. Han et al. (62) demonstrated that the coupling of cationic liposomes containing adriamycin with iontophoresis had a synergistic effect on the transfollicular deposition of adriamycin. In a recent study, Tabbakhian et al. (63) showed that both liposomes and niosomes could successfully deliver finasteride into the follicles of hamster ear. Because the formulations they employed contained surfactants and phospholipids, it is possible that they may enhance transepidermal delivery in addition to transfollicular delivery.

Solid Dispersions

Several studies have demonstrated that solid particulate systems have potential for follicular drug delivery. Rolland et al. (4) reported that adapalene-loaded poly(lactic-*co*-glycolic acid) microspheres penetrated into mouse and human hair follicles. In the course of investigating poly(lactic-*co*-glycolic acid) particle size dependency, they observed that 5-μm particles penetrated into hair follicles and 1-μm particles scattered in the stratum corneum and the hair follicles, but the 20-μm microspheres did not penetrate either the dermis or the follicles. In these studies, topical application of formulations (in both in vitro and in vivo studies) was followed by a 3-minute massage with a glass spatula. One cannot escape wondering if these small objects were actually kneaded into the tissue. If so, physical manipulation may play a large role in the follicular delivery of drug-containing particles, particularly for the initial localization of 5-μm microspheres in the openings of hair follicles. Toll et al. (13) further studied follicular delivery of polystyrene microspheres by applying them to human scalp and axillary and pubic skin. Using particles ranging in size from 0.75 to 6 μm and an application method similar to that of Rolland et al. (4) (i.e., massaging after application), the investigators demonstrated that optimal follicular delivery was obtained with 1.5-μm microspheres. Contrastingly, Alvarez-Roman et al. (64) found that a much smaller polystyrene particle size, namely, 20 nm, favored delivery of the particles into hair follicles of porcine ear skin as compared with a particles 10 times as large (200 nm). Shim et al. (65) reported that in guinea pig skin, drug permeation from 40-nm minoxidil-loaded poly(ε-caprolactone)-block-poly(ethylene glycol) nanoparticles was faster than it is from 130-nm nanospheres. Significantly, a comparable particle size effect was not seen with hairless guinea pig skin. These studies are so dissimilar that it is hard to generalize concerning them. They do suggest that the smaller the nanoparticles are, the more they are likely to contribute to follicular delivery (65).

Along similar lines, Chen et al. (66) got better drug deposition of podophyllotoxin in porcine skin after application of 73-nm-diameter podophyllotoxin-loaded solid-lipid nanoparticles in comparison with 123-nm-diameter nanoparticles. Again, this indicates that smaller particle size favors follicular penetration by particles. Interestingly, Vogt et al. (67) recently demonstrated that 40-nm nanopaticles, but not 750- or 1500-nm particles, were internalized by Langerhans cells found around hair follicles of human skin (67).

In general, the wide-ranging results of these studies point to differences in the animal skins used but even more to the fact that the use of solid particulate systems for follicular drug delivery is far from fully understood. The choice of animal for the research, the effect of particle size, the influence of surface properties of the particles, the influence of drug release from the particles, and the nature of sebum and its secretion need to be further investigated.

METHODS FOR INVESTIGATION AND QUANTITATION
Drug Delivery to Hair Follicles: Methodology
There have been several diverse approaches to the qualitative and quantitative measurement of drug disposition into follicular structures (Fig. 2). In vitro methodologies fall into the general categories of (1) comparative skin models (skin plus follicles permeability versus skin without follicles permeability), (2) differential biopsy techniques (skin plus follicle content versus skin without follicle content), and (3) direct visualization techniques (microscopy, histochemistry, autoradiography). On the other hand, in vivo techniques utilize (1) pharmacodynamic responses, such as hair regrowth rates, (2) differential biopsy techniques, and (3) absorption characteristics in the presence and absence of follicles achieved by plugging follicle openings on test sites.

In Vitro Follicular Penetration Measurement
Comparative Skin Models
Two rat models of comparative skin permeation have been used to estimate the contribution of follicular delivery to drug penetration through full-thickness skin. In the first model reported by Illel et al. (68), rat skin was scalded under anesthesia, and the epidermis was removed from the treated area and allowed to repair. After 9–10 weeks, the stratum corneum regrew across the defect as a continuous membrane, and there was a noticeable absence of pilosebaceous units. Using this model, the authors showed around a threefold decrease in the steady-state flux of hydrocortisone, caffeine, niflumic acid, and p-aminobenzoic acid through the regrown skin compared with equivalent intact rat skin. The advantage of this model is that permeation can be studied through skin harvested from adjacent sites on the same animal, minimizing variability. However, the disadvantage of this technique is that no consideration is given to other physiological changes that may have occurred within the membrane during healing, such as changes in the amount and deposi-

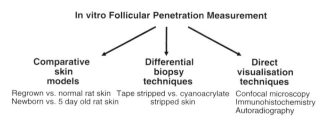

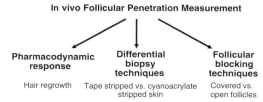

FIGURE 2 Methods used for the qualitative and quantitative determination of follicular penetration in in vitro and in vivo systems.

tion of specific collagen types within the dermis and transient changes in structure of the regrown stratum corneum before full maturity.

In the second model (15), the permeation of molecules through the skin of newborn rats, devoid of follicle structures, was compared with that from 5-day old rats, with full functional follicle development. The concept behind this model was that the difference in permeation between the two skin types would be attributable to the contribution of the follicular route of penetration. There was a fivefold increase in skin permeability to hydrocortisone in 5-day-old rat skin compared with newborn skin samples. Although it can be argued that the barrier function of the stratum corneum may not be fully developed within the first few hours after birth and, therefore, expected to be more permeable, the results of this study suggested that this potential effect was of minor importance compared with the contribution of the presence of pilosebaceous structures.

Differential Biopsy Techniques

Differential biopsy techniques involve the comparison of drug recovery using tape stripping with that using cyanoacrylate stripping to remove the stratum corneum. Tape stripping removes sequential layers of stratum corneum, allowing quantification of material deposited within these layers without removing follicular contents. On the other hand, cyanoacrylate stripping removes both a significant proportion of the stratum corneum and a large proportion of the follicular contents (Fig. 3) (15). The difference between amounts of material collected using the two methods is then attributed to that present in the follicles.

The cyanoacrylate skin surface biopsy technique itself is not new, being originally introduced in 1971 (69) to remove samples of stratum corneum from patients with various skin diseases to examine them for morphological changes. The technique was later modified to include separation of the strands of follicular contents from the cast under a magnifying glass to allow examination of isolated follicular contents (70). This separation technique is quite challenging however, and technically, separation of the casts requires concentration and reasonable operator dexterity.

The removal of surface material that may contaminate the sample is extremely important when using cyanoacrylate casts, in a similar way to the discarding of the first tape in stripping methodologies because they are likely to contain unpenetrated surface material associated with creases in the skins surface.

Direct Visualization Techniques

Immunohistochemistry

This technique enables the detection of antigens within tissues. The basic requirement is an antibody, which may be polyclonal or monoclonal, against the antigen of interest. Detection of the antigen-antibody complex may be done directly if the primary antibody is labeled with an enzyme (e.g., horseradish peroxidase, alkaline phosphatase) or a fluorophore (e.g., fluorescein, rhodamine, Texas red). More commonly, a second antibody, usually incorporating a fluorescent label, is used for detection. Quantitation may also be performed by digital image analysis, and sophisticated software is readily available for this purpose (for a recent example of the techniques involved, see Reference 71). Most applications of the technique reported in the literature, including those dealing with skin and appendages such as follicles, involve in situ detection of endogenous species such as receptor and other proteins or peptides. However, this is outside the scope of this chapter, and the following

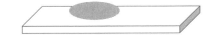

1. Drop of "supaglue" on microscope slide

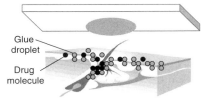

Glue droplet

Drug molecule

**2. Press on to skin; glue spreads across
skin surface and into follicle openings
and then dries**

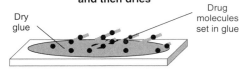

Dry glue

Drug molecules set in glue

**3. Pull off to harvest stratum corneum
and contents of the follicle where glue
has penetrated**

FIGURE 3 Use of cyanoacrylate stripping technique to biopsy stratum corneum and follicular contents.

will be concerned with the detection of exogenous, topically applied substances within skin and hair follicles.

Although this technique should be an attractive proposition for the visualization and possible quantitation of topically applied substances within skin structures, few examples have appeared in the literature. An early study attempted unsuccessfully to identify minoxidil in epidermis, dermis, or pelage follicles of skin from mice treated in vivo with topical minoxidil formulations. Although they did show clear evidence for minoxidil immunoreactivity in various structures of cultured vibrissa follicles incubated with minoxidil (72), this was regarded as nonspecific. A novel application used an antibody raised against partial sequences of keratins adducted to a 2-hydroxythioethyl group for fluorescent detection of sulfur mustard in exposed human skin (73). More recently, the technique was used to show that topically applied antisense oligonucleotides penetrated mouse skin via a follicular route (74).

Specific protocols for immunohistochemical visualization of particular antigens must be developed for each individual case. There is a wealth of information regarding basic techniques, antibody selection and preparation, choice of detection methods, and others available on the World Wide Web from proprietary and other sources, but some specific factors relating to the visualization of topically applied substances should be mentioned. Because these compounds are generally of low molecular weight, successful raising of polyclonal antibodies requires conjugation to carrier proteins such as keyhole limpet hemocyanin, bovine serum albumin, or ovalbumin. Another important consideration is to ensure that antigens remain in situ throughout the various processes leading to visualization. To this end, it may be preferable to prepare frozen sections without chemical fixatives, although paraffin sections, for example, would be expected to give greater sensitivity and deteriorate less over time.

Autoradiography

In transdermal studies, the technique of autoradiography applied to thin vertical sections allows the distribution of topically applied substances to be visualized, with resolution to the cellular level. Quantitation may be performed by optical densitometry, and commercial systems are available. A major advantage is that images obtained represent true in vivo or in vitro experimental conditions, provided appropriate fixation procedures are carried out. A disadvantage, however, is the long exposure times that may be required (e.g., 8 months in a recent study using [³H]maxacalcitol) (75). Exposure times are generally empirically determined but are influenced by the half-life of the particular nuclide used. Appropriate choice of modern films may assist in reducing exposure time. Another disadvantage is that autoradiographic imaging of in vivo penetration is limited to animal models or human skin xenografts. The technique has been regarded by some as a gold standard for visualization (and quantitation) of the spatial distribution of topically applied substances (75,76), but since a major review of this and other techniques in 1998 (76), relatively little has been published.

In Vivo Follicular Penetration Measurement

Cyanoacrylate Casting and Differential Stripping Techniques

As outlined previously for use in in vitro sampling of follicular contents, the techniques of tape stripping and cyanoacrylate casting are easily applicable to in vivo studies. However, various approaches to discriminating follicle-penetrated from other material have been taken.

Cyanoacrylate casting was used to determine the amount of azelaic acid recovered from the forehead and backs of young adult volunteers after the application of a topical cream formulation (77). In this study, the surface of the skin was carefully wiped with acetone to remove any formulation remaining on the surface of the skin, which could potentially contaminate the casts.

Other workers (78) employed follicular casting to study changes in the lipid composition of sebaceous secretions residing in the upper follicle on the foreheads of volunteers treated with different topical antiacne agents. To eliminate the possibility of interference from other skin surface material, the cast projections from individual follicles were isolated by dissection under a microscope, as discussed above (70).

With the aim of directly quantitating the amount of a topically applied substance penetrating into follicles, in the absence of interference from other skin surface material, the differential stripping technique was used on back skin of human volunteers treated with a formulation containing 2% sodium fluorescein or a blue dye (79). Tape stripping was performed until all the fluorescein or blue dye was removed, after which follicular casts were taken and cast contents analyzed. Histological studies were also carried out after application of similar procedures to pig skin.

The common thread in all these stripping techniques carried out in vitro or in vivo is the need to clearly distinguish follicular contents from material on the skin surface, in skin creases, or within the stratum corneum itself. To this end, the differential stripping technique appears to be appropriate, although as the authors suggest, the penetration depth may vary according to the vehicle and physicochemical properties of the solute (79). Therefore, the number of tape strips required to eliminate surface material still requires careful evaluation. These authors have also addressed the need for strict application of standard procedures to the highly operator-dependent techniques of tape stripping and follicular casting.

Follicular Blocking Techniques

The issue of discriminating follicle-penetrated from other material has recently been taken another step further in studies where follicular openings have been selectively blocked by microparticles (80) or nail varnish (81). In the first paper (80), a sodium fluorescein-containing hydrogel was applied to skin of human volunteers, and the skin surface was stripped 10 times with adhesive tape to remove stratum corneum-deposited material, before cyanoacrylate casts were taken. The casts contained significant fluorescent material recovered from follicles after 24 hours, which had fallen fivefold by 4 days, with negligible recovery by 8 or 10 days. Most significantly, pretreatment of the skin with 5-μm microparticles resulted in almost complete blocking of hydrogel follicular penetration, measured at 24 hours. These results highlight the value of the differential stripping and follicular blocking techniques. In the hands of these workers, tape stripping effectively eliminated surface-deposited material, and cyanoacrylate casting was shown to access additional material unavailable to regular tape stripping.

In the other approach (81), nail varnish was carefully applied and pressed to ensure follicular penetration, and surface varnish was removed with two tape strips, thus selectively blocking the follicular openings. Analysis of penetration profiles of a topically applied UV-filter compound, determined from 20 tape strips, showed differences between treated and untreated skin, which were attributed to the effect of blocking follicular openings.

Both of these blocking techniques could also be exploited to discriminate the contribution of follicular transport to transdermal drug permeation from that of other routes in an approach analogous to that of the skin sandwich technique discussed above (18,19,35).

REFERENCES

1. Lauer AC, Lieb LM, Ramachandran C, et al. Transfollicular drug delivery. Pharm Res 1995; 12:179–186.
2. Turner NG, Guy RH. Visualization and quantitation of iontophoretic pathways using confocal microscopy. J Invest Dermatol Symp Proc 1998; 3:136–142.
3. Schaefer H, Watts F, Brod J, et al. Follicular penetration. In: Scott RC, Guy RH, Hadgraft J, eds. Prediction of Percutaneous Penetration. Methods, Measurements, Modelling. London: IBC Technical Services, 1989:163–173.
4. Rolland A, Wagner N, Chatelus A, et al. Site-specific drug delivery to pilosebaceous structures using polymeric microspheres. Pharm Res 1993; 10:1738–1744.
5. Sumian CC, Pitre FB, Gauthier BE, et al. A new method to improve penetration depth of dyes into the follicular duct: potential application for laser hair removal. J Am Acad Dermatol 1999; 41:172–175.
6. Lademann J, Weigmann HJ, Rickmeyer C, et al. Penetration of titanium dioxide microparticles in a sunscreen formulation into the horny layer and the follicular orifice. Skin Pharmacol Appl Skin Physiol 1999; 12:247–256.
7. Lieb LM, Ramachandran C, Egbaria K, et al. Topical delivery enhancement with multilamellar liposomes into pilosebaceous units. I. In vitro evaluation using fluorescent techniques with the hamster ear model. J Invest Dermatol 1992; 99:108–113.
8. Tata S, Weiner N, Flynn G. Relative influence of ethanol and propylene glycol cosolvents on deposition of minoxidil into the skin. J Pharm Sci 1994; 83:1508–1510.

9.   Touitou E, Godin B, Weiss C. Enhanced delivery of drugs into and across the skin by ethosomal carriers. Drug Develop Res 2000; 50:405–415.
10. Bamba FL, Wepierre J. Role of the appendageal pathway in the percutaneous absorption of pyridostigmine bromide in various vehicles. Eur J Drug Metab Pharmacokinet 1993; 18:339–348.
11. Motwani MR, Rhein LD, Zatz JL. Deposition of salicylic acid into hamster sebaceous. J Cosmet Sci 2004; 55:519–531.
12. Mordon S, Sumina C, Devoiselle JM. Site specific methylene blue delivery to pilosebaceous structure using highly porous nylon microspheres: an experimental evaluation. Laser Surg Med 2003; 33:119–125.
13. Toll R, Jacobi U, Ritcher H, et al. Penetration profile of microspheres in follicular targeting of terminal hair follicles. J Invest Dermatol 2004; 123:168–176.
14. Pena L. Topical pharmaceutical compositions. WO/1994/07478, A1.
15. Illel B. Formulations for transfollicular drug administration: some recent advances. Crit Rev Ther Drug Carrier Syst 1997; 14:207–217.
16. Agarwal R, Katara OP, Vyas SP. The pilosebaceous unit: a pivotal route for topical drug delivery. Method Find Exp Clin Pharmacol 2000; 22:129–133.
17. Lauer AC. Percutaneous drug delivery to the hair follicle. Drugs Pharm Sci 1999; 97:427–449.
18. Meidan VM, Bonner MC, Michniak B. Transfollicular drug delivery – is it a reality? Int J Pharm 2005; 306:1–14.
19. Barry BW. Drug delivery routes in skin: a novel approach. Adv Drug Deliver Rev 2002; 54:S31–S40.
20. Whiting DA. Histology of normal hair. In: Hordinsky MK, Sawaya ME, Scher RK, eds. Atlas of Hair and Nails. Philadelphia, Pa: Churchill Livingstone, 2000:918.
21. Bertolino AP, Klein LM, Freedberg IM. Biology of hair follicles. In: Fitzpatrick TB, Eisen AZ, Wolff K, et al., eds. Dermatology in General Medicine. New York: McGraw-Hill, 1993:289–293.
22. Greene RS, Downing DT, Pochi PE, et al. Anatomical variation in the amount and composition of human skin surface lipid. J Invest Dermatol 1970; 54:240–247.
23. Downing DT, Stewart ME, Strauss JS. Changes in sebum secretion and the sebaceous gland. Dermatol Clin 1986; 4:419–423.
24. Downing DT, Strauss JS. On the mechanism of sebaceous secretion. Arch Dermatol Res 1982; 272:343–349.
25. Cullander C, Guy RH. Routes of delivery: case studies; transdermal delivery of peptides and proteins. Adv Drug Deliver Rev 1992; 8:291–329.
26. Grams YY, Bouwstra JA. Penetration and distribution of three lipophilic probes in vitro in human skin focusing on the hair follicle. J Control Release 2002; 83(2):253–262.
27. Weiner ND, Roessler B, Niemiec S. Hair follicle DNA delivery system. WO/1998/046208, A1.
28. Niemiec SM, Wang JCT, Wisniewski SJ, et al. Topical delivery systems for active agents. WO/2000/007627, A2.
29. Chou JT, Parab P. Topical composition for follicular delivery of an ornithine decarboxylase inhibitor as hair growth inhibitors. WO/2003/015729, A1.
30. Wu J et al. Compositions useful for the treatment of follicular diseases. U.S. Patent 20060009499, A1.
31. Grams YY, Alaruikka S, Lashley L, et al. Permeant lipophilicity and vehicle composition influence accumulation of dyes in hair follicles of human skin. Eur J Pharm Sci 2003; 18(5):329–336.
32. Grams YY, Whitehead L, Lamers G, et al. On-line diffusion profile of a lipophilic model dye in different depths of a hair follicle in human scalp skin. J Invest Dermatol 2005; 125:775–782.
33. Behl C, Wittkowsky A, Barrett M, et al. Technique for preparing appendage-free skin (scar) on hairless mouse. J Pharm Sci 1981; 70:835–837.
34. Ogiso T, Shiraki T, Okajima K, et al. Transfollicular drug delivery: penetration of drugs through human scalp skin and comparison of penetration between scalp and abdominal skin in vitro. J Drug Target 2002; 10:369–378.

35. El Maghraby GMM, Williams AC, Barry BW. Skin hydration and possible shunt route penetration in controlled oestradiol delivery from ultradeformable liposomes. J Pharm Pharmacol 2001; 53:1311–1322.

36. Flynn G. Cutaneous and transdermal delivery. In: Banker GS, Rhodes CT, eds. Modern Pharmaceutics. 3rd ed. New York: Marcel Dekker, 1996:262–269.

37. Valiveti S, Wesley J, Lu GW. Investigation of drug partition property in artificial sebum for follicular delivery. AAPS J 2005; 7(Suppl. 2):W5108.

38. Thiboutot D. Regulation of human sebaceous glands. J Invest Dermatol 2004; 123:1–12.

39. Morgan AJ, Lewis G, van den Hoden WE, et al. The effect of zinc in the form of erythromycin–zinc complex (Zineryt lotion) and zinc acetate on metallothionein expression and distribution in hamster skin. Br J Dermatol 1993; 129:563–570.

40. Tschan T, Steffen H, Supersaxo A. Sebaceous-gland deposition of isotretinoin after topical application: an in vitro study using human facial skin. Skin Pharmacol 1997; 10:126–134.

41. Bernard E, Dubois J, Wepierre J. Importance of sebaceous glands in cutaneous penetration of an antiandrogen: target effect of liposomes. J Pharm Sci 1997; 86:573–578.

42. Munster U, Nakamura C, Haberland A, et al. RU 58841-myristate-prodrug development for topical treatment of acne and androgenetic alopecia. Pharmazie 2005; 60:8–12.

43. Motwani MR, Rhein LD, Zatz JL. Influence of vehicles on the phase transitions of model sebum. J Cosmet Sci 2002; 53:35–42.

44. Friberg SE, Osborne DW. Interaction of a model skin surface lipid with a modified triglyceride. J Am Oil Chem Soc 1986; 63:123.

45. Motwani MR, Rhein LD, Zatz JL. Differential scanning calorimetry studies of sebum models. J Cosmet Sci 2001; 52:211–224.

46. Valiveti S, Lu GW, Spence J, et al. Comparison of partition and diffusion properties of model compounds in various artificial sebums with human sebum. AAPS J 2006; 8(Suppl. 2):M1138.

47. Valiveti S, Lu GW. Diffusion properties of model compounds in artificial sebum. Int. J. Pharm (in press). doi:10.1016/j.ijpharm.2007.05.043.

48. Li L, Hoffman RM. Topical liposome delivery of molecules to hair follicles in mice. J Dermatol Sci 1997; 14:101–108.

49. Hoffman RM. Topical liposome targeting of dyes, melanins, genes, and proteins selectively to hair follicles. J Drug Target 1998; 5:67–74.

50. Lieb LM, Flynn G, Weiner N. Follicular (pilosebaceous unit) deposition and pharmacological behavior of cimetidine as a function of formulation. Pharm Res 1994; 11: 419–1423.

51. Li L, Lishko V, Hoffman RM. Liposomes can specifically target entrapped melanin to hair follicles in histocultured skin. In Vitro Cell Dev Biol 1993; 29A:192–194.

52. Bouwstra JA, Honeywell-Nguyen PL. Skin structure and mode of action of vesicles. Adv Drug Deliver Rev 2002; 54:S41-S55.

53. Yu WH, Kashani-Sabet M, Liggitt D, et al. Topical gene delivery to murine skin. J Invest Dermatol 1999; 112:370–375.

54. Niemiec SM, Ramachandran C, Weiner N. Perifollicular transgenic expression of human interlukin-1 receptor antagonist protein following topical application. J Pharm Sci 1997; 86:701–708.

55. Adamina M, Bolli M, Albo F, et al. Encapsulation into sterically stabilised liposomes enhances the immunogenicity of melanoma-associated Melan-A/MART-1 epitopes. Br J Cancer 2004; 90:263–269.

56. Gupta PN, Mishra V, Rawat A, et al. Non-invasive vaccine delivery in transfersomes, niosomes and liposomes: a comparative study. Int J Pharm 2005; 293:73–82.

57. Weiner N. Targeted follicular delivery of macromolecular via liposomes. Int J Pharm 1998; 162:29–38.

58. Balsari AL, Morelli D, Menard S, et al. Protection against doxorubicin-induced alopecia in rats by liposome-entrapped monoclonal antibodies. FASEB J 1994; 8:226–230.

59. Jung S, Otberg N, Thiede G, et al.. Innovative liposomes as a transfollicular drug delivery system: penetration into porcine hair follicles. J Invest Dermatol 2006; 126(8): 1728–1732.

60. Niemiec SM, Ramachandran C, Weiner N. Influence of nonionic liposomal composition on topical delivery of peptide drug into pilosebaceous units: an *in vivo* study using the hamster ear model. Pharm Res 1995; 12:1184–1188.
61. Ciotti SN, Weiner N. Follicular liposomal delivery systems. J Liposome Res 2002; 12:143–148.
62. Han I, Kim M, Kim J. Enhanced transfollicular delivery of adriamycin with a liposome and iontophoresis. Exp Dermatol 2004; 13:86–92.
63. Tabbakhian M, Tavakoli N, Jaafari MR, et al. Enhancement of follicular delivery of finasteride by liposomes and niosomes 1. In vitro permeation and in vivo deposition studies using hamster flank and ear models. Int J Pharm. 2006; 323(1–2):1–10.
64. Alvarez-Roman R, Naik A, Kalia YN, et al. Skin penetration and distribution of polymeric nanoparticles. J Control Release 2004; 99(1):53–62.
65. Shim J, Seok Kang H, Park WS, et al. Transdermal delivery of minoxidil with block copolymer nanoparticles. J Control Release 2004; 97(3):477–484.
66. Chen H, Chang X, Du D, et al. Podophyllotoxin - loaded solid lipid nanoparticles for epidermal targeting. J Control Release 2006; 110:296–306.
67. Vogt A, Combadiere B, Hadam S, et al. 40 nm, but not 750 or 1,500 nm, nanoparticles enter epidermal CD1a+ cells after transcutaneous application on human skin. J Invest Dermatol 2006; 126:1316–1322.
68. Illel B, Schaefer H, Wepierre J, et al. Follicles play an important role in percutaneous absorption. J Pharm Sci 1991; 80(5):424–427.
69. Marks R, Dawber RP. Skin surface biopsy: an improved technique for the examination of the horny layer. Br J Dermatol 1971; 84:117–123.
70. Mills OH Jr., Kligman AM. The follicular biopsy. Dermatologica 1983; 167:57–63.
71. Zippel R, Hoene A, Walschus U, et al. Digital image analysis for morphometric evaluation of tissue response after implanting alloplastic vascular prostheses. Microsc Microanal 2006; 12:366–375.
72. Zelei BV, Walker CJ, Sawada GA, et al. Immunohistochemical and autoradiographic findings suggest that minoxidil is not localized in specific cells of vibrissa, pelage, or scalp follicles. Cell Tissue Res 1990; 262(3):407–413.
73. van der Schans GP, Noort D, Mars-Groenendijk RH, et al. Immunochemical detection of sulfur mustard adducts with keratins in the stratum corneum of human skin. Chem Res Toxicol 2002; 15:21–25.
74. Dokka S, Cooper SR, Kelly S, et al. Dermal delivery of topically applied oligonucleotides via follicular transport in mouse skin. J Invest Dermatol 2005; 124(5):971–975.
75. Hayakawa N, Kubota N, Imai N, et al. Receptor microscopic autoradiography for the study of percutaneous absorption, in vivo skin penetration, and cellular-intercellular deposition. J Pharmacol Toxicol Methods 2004; 50:131–137.
76. Touitou E, Meidan VM, Horwitz E. Methods for quantitative determination of drug localized in the skin. J Control Release 1998; 56(1–3):7–21.
77. Bojar RA, Cutcliffe AG, Graupe K, et al. Follicular concentrations of azelaic acid after a single topical application. Br J Dermatol 1993; 129:399–402.
78. Thielitz A, Helmdach M, Ropke E-M, et al. Lipid analysis of follicular casts from cyanoacrylate strips as a new method for studying therapeutic effects of antiacne agents. Br J Dermatol 2001; 145:19–27.
79. Teichmann A, Jacobi U, Ossadnik M, et al. Differential stripping: determination of the amount of topically applied substances penetrated into the hair follicles. J Invest Dermatol 2005; 125:264–269.
80. Teichmann A, Ossadnik M, Richter H, et al. Semiquantitative determination of the penetration of a fluorescent hydrogel formulation into the hair follicle with and without follicular closure by microparticles by means of differential stripping. Skin Pharmacol Physiol 2006; 19:101–105.
81. Teichmann A, Otberg N, Jacobi U, et al. Follicular penetration: development of a method to block the follicles selectively against the penetration of topically applied substances. Skin Pharmacol Physiol 2006; 19:216–223.

Drug Penetration Enhancement Through Human Nail and Skin

Thomas C. K. Chan
ArQule Inc., Woburn, Massachusetts, U.S.A.

Kenneth A. Walters
An-eX Analytical Services Ltd., Cardiff, U.K.

Xiaoying Hui and Howard I. Maibach
University of California, San Francisco, San Francisco, California, U.S.A.

INTRODUCTION

Although they only constitute a small proportion of the body and are somewhat vestigial in man, the nails, especially those of the hand, are highly visible and often cosmetically decorated. Diseases of the nail plate and surrounding area are rarely life threatening but always generate a high degree of self-consciousness that can lead to psychological stress and physical discomfort. The most common nail plate diseases are the result of fungal infections, onychomycoses, which may invade the nail bed, the periungual area or the nail plate itself. The prevalence of onychomycoses may be as high as ~27% in Europe (1) and 10% in the United States (2). There are many treatment regimens for onychomycoses, the most common of which involves oral dosing with one or more of the available antifungal agents. The past 15 years have seen the emergence of new experimental techniques to investigate the penetration, permeation, and distribution of topically applied chemicals into and through the nail plate, and this has led to a deeper understanding of the movement of drugs within the nail plate. Furthermore, this understanding has resulted in the development of newer, more effective topical products for the treatment of onychomycoses and other nail diseases (3–6).

This chapter briefly describes nail structure and chemical composition, and provides an overview of the studies that enhanced our knowledge on the nature of chemical permeation through the nail plate. This is followed by a discussion of the penetration of various antifungal agents in the nail. We also contrast the differences between drug permeation in the nail plate and the stratum corneum.

NAIL STRUCTURE

Although for the most part the nail plate may be vestigial, there is possibly some protective function for this hard keratinous tissue. Certainly, nail plate composition, layers of flattened keratinized cells fused into a dense but somewhat elastic mass, will afford a measure of protection to the highly sensitive terminal phalanx. The cells of the nail plate grow distally from the nail matrix at a rate of about 0.1 mm/ day. In the keratinization process, the cells undergo shape and other changes similar to those experienced by the epidermal cells that form the stratum corneum. The structure of the keratinized layers is tightly knit and comprises three strata: a thin dorsal lamina, the thicker intermediate lamina, and a ventral layer from the nail bed

(7). The keratins in hair and nail are classified as "hard" trichocyte keratins. Unlike the stratum corneum, in the nail plate no exfoliation of cells occurs.

Given that it is a cornified epithelial structure, the chemical composition of the nail plate is not remarkable, and there are many similarities to that of the hair (8). Thus the major components are keratin proteins with small amounts (0.1–1.0%) of lipid, the latter presumably located in the intercellular spaces. The nail contains significant amounts of phospholipid, mainly in the dorsal and intermediate layers, which contribute to its flexibility. The principal plasticizer of the nail plate is water, which is normally present at a concentration of 7% to 12%.

NAIL PLATE PERMEABILITY

Early studies on nail plate permeation were extensions of experiments designed to investigate water permeability across the skin. Walters et al (9–12) indicated that there is a marked difference between the permeability characteristics of the nail plate and the epidermis. These observed differences were attributed to the relative amounts of lipid and protein regimes within the structures (9) and the possible differences in the physicochemical nature of the respective phases. The nail plate was shown to be permeable to dilute aqueous solutions of a series of low-molecular-weight homologous alcohols. However, it has a unique ability to increasingly restrict the diffusive passage with increase in alkyl chain length. Interestingly, the applied concentration of alcohols was shown to be a determinant of their penetration velocities, with pure liquid forms of the alcohols giving a five-fold decrease in permeation (10). It was suggested that the nail plate possesses a highly "polar" penetration route that was capable of excluding permeants on the basis of their hydrophobicity. The existence of a minor "lipid" pathway through the nail matrix, which could become rate-controlling for hydrophobic solutes, was suggested based on the significant decrease in the permeation of the hydrophobic entity *n*-decanol after delipidization of the nail plate by chloroform/methanol (10).

Mertin and Lippold (13–15) have performed extensive work on nail and hoof penetration in vitro. Most of the work was done by using a hoof membrane, and this was used to examine permeation of chemicals from different formulations. They noticed that the permeability coefficient for compounds through the nail plate as well as the hoof membrane did not increase with increasing partition coefficient (range, 7 to >51,000) or lipophilicity, indicating that these barriers behaved like hydrophilic gel membranes rather than lipophilic partition membranes as is the case for the stratum corneum. Further penetration studies with paracetamol and phenacetin showed that maximum flux was first a function of drug solubility in water or in the swollen keratin. Mertin and Lippold were also able to predict the maximum flux of 10 antimycotics through the nail plate on the basis of their penetration rates through the hoof membrane, their water solubilities, and their molecular weights. Although this was a speculative extrapolation, the authors' prediction for the permeation of the antimycotic amorolfine was in remarkably close agreement with the value obtained by Franz (16) using human nail plate.

Investigators have evaluated the nail plate penetration of drugs after topical application in vivo (17–19). After application to the nail surface, the nails are allowed to grow and clippings are taken from the free distal ends for drug analysis. Although this method provides reasonably reliable data, it is time-consuming and cannot be considered a rapid screening test for formulations because of the lengthy interval required to obtain data and the environmental variability imparted on nails.

The composition of the nail plate suggests that it would be comparatively less sensitive to the effects of stratum corneum penetration enhancers that, for the most part, produce their effects by delipidization or fluidization of matrix lipids of the stratum corneum. For example, although many studies using dimethylsulphoxide (DMSO) have shown that this compound can penetrate and has a significant effect on the stratum corneum, the nail plate is incapable of absorbing much of the applied DMSO (20). The strategy of delipidizing the nail plate before drug application has yielded mixed results. Increases in nail plate absorption of the antifungal amorolfine after pretreatment with DMSO have been demonstrated by Franz (16); however, a decrease in the absorption of methanol and hexanol applied with DMSO was noted by Walters and colleagues (12). Another strategy for enhancing permeability across the nail plate that has demonstrated some promise is the use of keratolytic agents (21–23) within the formulation. It is postulated that partial disruption of the keratin matrix will reduce the barrier properties. A third strategy is to provide a delivery matrix capable of maintaining high concentrations of selected drugs that have good inherent nail penetration against the nail surface to create a large chemical gradient to drive drugs into the nail plate. This strategy is technically difficult because most delivery vehicles such as solutions, gels, lotions, and tinctures do not have adequate persistence on the nail surface to maintain a chemical gradient for any significant period, whereas lacquer formulations tend to retain drugs within the dried lacquer matrix instead of delivering them to the nail surface. However, the report by Hui et al (24) showing that the addition of 2-n-nonyl-1,3-dioxolane (SEPA, also used as a skin penetration enhancer) to an econazole nail lacquer dramatically increased econazole penetration through human cadaver nails clearly illustrates the feasibility of this strategy. In the same study, radiolabeled SEPA failed to penetrate the nail plate to a significant degree; therefore, it is unlikely to work by disrupting nail structure. In addition, this finding confirms earlier data showing that molecules with long alkyl chains in general penetrate the nail poorly (10). The major difference noted between econazole lacquers with and without SEPA is the amount of econazole released per unit time into an aqueous environment (Figure 1). Addition of SEPA to the econazole lacquer resulted in a softer film that allowed the release of the active ingredient into the lacquer-nail interface.

MEASUREMENT OF DRUG PENETRATION THROUGH HUMAN NAILS

The application of static diffusion cells to measure drug penetration across full-thickness human skin and across intact human nail has generated important new

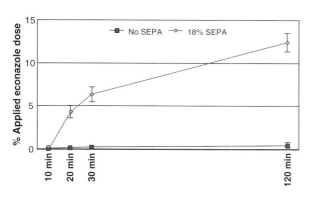

FIGURE 1 Drug release from lacquer formulations. Lacquers were painted on ceramic tiles with comparable porosity to human nail, allowed to air-dry, then submerged in a known volume of normal saline. The concentrations of econazole in the saline were monitored over a period of two hours by high-performance liquid chromatography. Values are mean ± SE of six experiments. *Source*: From Ref. 25.

data in this field. In our studies, human cadaver fingernails were mounted onto PermeGear static diffusion cells (PermeGear Inc., Bethlehem, Pennsylvania, U.S.) with a saline-soaked cotton ball serving as the receptor phase. Nail lacquers containing radiolabeled drugs were painted onto the dorsal surface of each nail. After 14 days, the nail was removed and turned upside down (ventral surface facing up), and pulverized nail powder was harvested from the ventral surface by using a Dremel® tool (Dremel International, Racine, Wisconsin, U.S.) mounted on a micromanipulator (24). Radioactivity per unit mass of nail was compared after application of the SEPA-containing lacquer and the non-SEPA lacquer. Table 1 shows the measured radioactive econazole concentration in the nail plate and in the nail bed (saline-saturated cotton ball) after 14 days of lacquer application. It is interesting to note that the calculated flux across the nail plate for the SEPA containing lacquer was 1.58 ± 0.32 µg/cm²/hr, whereas the flux for the lacquer without SEPA was 0.21 ± 0.04 µg/cm²/hr (24).

MEASUREMENT OF DRUG PENETRATION THROUGH HUMAN SKIN

Static Franz diffusion cells were used to evaluate drug penetration through human cadaver skin by using the same lacquer formulations as described earlier. Because of the relatively slow penetration of econazole through human skin, these experiments were run for 48 hours to allow for adequate data collection. Human cadaver skin specimens were mounted onto diffusion cells and allowed to equilibrate for two hours at 37°C. After checking for leakage and physical damage of each skin specimen, we randomly assigned blocks of six Franz cells to a lacquer formulation (with or without SEPA). After the application of test lacquers to the donor compartments of the cell, the receptor phases were removed at timed interval and assayed for econazole by using reverse-phase, high-performance liquid chromatography with UV detection.

Figure 2 shows that the transdermal flux of econazole from the lacquer containing SEPA (10% or 18% by weight) was significantly increased from six hours after application and was maintained at 4-times higher flux level compared to a similar lacquer without SEPA throughout the experimental period. As expected from published reports, transdermal econazole penetration was slow. The peak flux measured was less than 0.05 µg/cm²/hr. The addition of SEPA to the lacquer resulted in four-fold increase in econazole flux across full-thickness human skin. These data served to illustrate the difference of econazole flux across skin and nail. It is noteworthy that in the absence of SEPA, the net flux of econazole was four-fold higher in human nails compared to human skin (0.21 vs. 0.05 µg/cm²/hr). The difference was further accentuated when optimal amounts of SEPA were used to enhance penetration. The net flux of econazole across human nail was 1.58 µg/cm²/hr when 18% SEPA was

TABLE 1 Econazole Penetration into and Through Human Nail: Effect of SEPA

	Normalized econazole concentrations (µg equivalent/mg nail)[a]		P
	Lacquer containing SEPA	Lacquer without SEPA	
Ventral nail	11.15	1.78	0.0079
Dorsal nail	0.25	0.37	0.0038
Nail bed (cotton ball), µg/ball	47.55	0.24	0.0079

[a]Values represent the mean of five experiments.
Source: From Ref. 24.

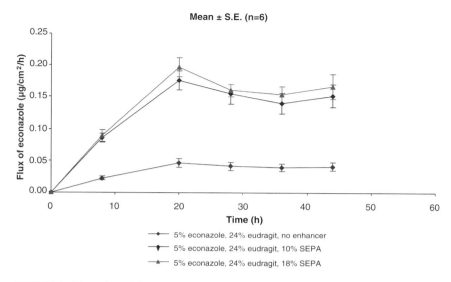

FIGURE 2 Transdermal flux of econazole in full-thickness human skin. Values are the mean from six diffusion cells with skin specimens from different donors. Econazole penetrated skin slowly and sparingly, so a longer time course (48 hours) was used in these experiments. Drug fluxes are typically measured for 24 hours or less.

added to the lacquer. In comparison, the net flux of econazole across human skin was about 0.19 $\mu g/cm^2/hr$ when delivered by lacquer containing 10% or 18% SEPA. It is interesting to note that although 10% SEPA offered maximal penetration enhancement of econazole in human skin, 18% SEPA was required to maximize drug penetration across human nail. This is likely the result of two separate mechanisms of action of SEPA in drug penetration enhancement. In the skin, SEPA penetrates the stratum corneum readily and promotes penetration of co-formulated drugs. In nail, especially in lacquer formulations, SEPA at a higher concentration acts as a biphasic plasticizer of lacquer films to allow high concentrations of drug to be present at the nail-lacquer interface. In the example of econazole, the natural ability of the drug to permeate nail (15) was responsible for the high level of drug penetration.

CONCLUSIONS

The addition of SEPA to lacquers containing econazole resulted in a softer lacquer film (physical testing, data not shown), which in turn led to more rapid and sustained release of econazole into the aqueous fluid bathing the lacquer films. The increase in cumulative drug release over a two-hour period was greater than 200-fold between a lacquer containing no SEPA and a lacquer that contained 18% SEPA. In a transdermal drug penetration assay involving human cadaver skin, SEPA-containing lacquers typically delivered significantly more econazole through human skin over a 48-hour study period, although the magnitude of enhancement did not approach that measured in the nail. This difference in econazole penetration highlights the fact that the lipid-rich stratum corneum represents a more substantial barrier for a drug such as econazole, whereas the aqueous porosity of the human nail will allow small, water-soluble molecules to diffuse into the nail plate. The penetration enhancer SEPA increases drug penetration through the nail via a mechanism different to its action on the stratum corneum.

REFERENCES

1. Hay R. Literature review. Onychomycosis. J Eur Acad Dermatol Venereol 2005; 19(Suppl 1): 1–7.
2. Elewski E. Onychomycosis: pathogenesis, diagnosis, and management. Clin Microbiol Rev 1998; 11:415–429.
3. Hui X, Wester RC, Barbadillo S, et al. Ciclopirox delivery into the human nail plate. J Pharm Sci 2004; 93:2545–2548.
4. Monti D, Saccomani L, Chetoni P, et al. In vitro transungual permeation of ciclopirox from a hydroxypropoyl chitosan-based, water-soluble nail lacquer. Drug Dev Ind Pharm 2005; 31:11–17.
5. Donnelly RF, McCarron PA, Lightowler JM, et al. Bioadhesive patch-based delivery of 5-aminolevulinic acid to the nail for photodynamic therapy of onychomycosis. J Contr Rel 2005; 103:381–392.
6. Sanchez Regana M, Martin Ezquerra G, Umbert Millet P, et al. Treatment of nail psoriasis with 8% clobetasol nail lacquer: positive experience in 10 patients. J Eur Acad Dermatol Venereol 2005; 19:573–577.
7. Runne U, Orfanos CE. The human nail—structure, growth and pathological changes. Curr Probl Dermatol 1981; 9:102–149.
8. Baden HP, Goldsmith LA, Fleming B. A comparative study of the physicochemical properties of human keratinized tissues. Biochim Biophys Acta 1973, 322: 269–278.
9. Walters KA, Flynn GL, Marvel JR. Physicochemical characterization of the human nail: I. Pressure sealed apparatus for measuring nail plate permeabilities. J Invest Dermatol 1981; 76:76–79.
10. Walters KA, Flynn GL, Marvel JR. Physicochemical characterization of the human nail: permeation pattern for water and the homologous alcohols and differences with respect to the stratum corneum. J Pharm Pharmacol 1983; 35:28–33.
11. Walters KA, Flynn GL, Marvel JR. Penetration of the human nail: the effects of vehicle pH on the permeation of miconazole. J Pharm Pharmacol 1985; 37:498–499.
12. Walters KA, Flynn GL, Marvel JR. Physicochemical characterization of the human nail: solvent effects on the permeation of homologous alcohols. J Pharm Pharmacol 1985; 37:771–775.
13. Mertin D, Lippold BC. In vitro permeability of the human nail and of a keratin membrane from bovine hooves: influence of the partition coefficient octanol/water and the water solubility of drugs on their permeability and maximum flux. J Pharm Pharmacol 1997; 49:30–34.
14. Mertin D, Lippold BC. In vitro permeability of the human nail and of a keratin membrane from bovine hooves: penetration of chloramphenicol from lipophilic vehicles and a nail lacquer. J Pharm Pharmacol 1997; 49:241–245.
15. Mertin D, Lippold BC. In vitro permeability of the human nail and of a keratin membrane from bovine hooves: prediction of the penetration rate of antimycotics through the nail plate and their efficacy. J Pharm Pharmacol 1997; 49:866–872.
16. Franz TJ. Absorption of amorolfine through human nail. Dermatology 1992;184(Suppl 1): 18–20.
17. Ceschin-Roques CG, Hanel H, Pruja-Bougaret SM, et al. Ciclopirox nail lacquer 8%: in vivo penetration into and through nails and in vitro effect on pig skin. Skin Pharmacol 1991; 4:89–94.
18. Schatz F, Brautigam M, Dobrowolski E, et al. Nail incorporation kinetics of terbinafine in onychomycosis patients. Clin Exp Dermatol 1995; 20:377–383.
19. van Hoogdalem EJ, van den Hoven WE, Terpstra IJ, et al. Nail penetration of the antifungals oxiconazole after repeated topical application in healthy volunteers, and the effect of acetylcystein. Eur J Pharm Sci 1997; 5:119–127.

20. Kligman AM. Topical pharmacology and toxicology of dimethyl sulfoxide. J Am Med Assoc 1965; 193:796–804.
21. Sun Y, Liu JC, Kimbleton E, Wang J. Antifungal treatment of nails. US Patent 5,696,164, 1977.
22. Quintanar-Guerrero D, Ganem-Quintanar A, Tapis-Olgium P, et al. The effect of keratolytic agents on the permeability of three imidazole antimycotic drugs through the human nail. Drug Dev Ind Pharm 1998; 24:685–690.
23. Mohorcic M, Torkar A, Friedrich J. Actions of a fungal keratinase and reducing agents on the nail plate. Int J Pharm 2007; 332:196–201.
24. Hui X, Chan TCK, Barbadillo S, et al. Enhanced econazole penetration into human nail by 2-N-nonyl-1,3-dioxolane. J Pharm Sci 2003; 92:142–148.
25. Chan et al, Development of EcoNail™—an antifungal nail lacquer. Presented at 9th Biennial International Conference of Perspectives in Percutaneous Penetration, 2004.

12	# Getting the Dose Right in Dermatological Therapy

Adrian F. Davis
Limeway Consultancy, Dorking, Surrey, U.K.

INTRODUCTION

Dosing strategies for topical and regional products applied to the skin are poorly defined and developed. For example, dose is usually expressed as the percentage concentration of the drug in a topical formulation. In fact, clearly, the dose applied is a multiple of the concentration of drug in the formulation, times the amount of formulation applied per area of skin. Also topical bioavailability, the ratio of dose absorbed to dose applied, is most usually in the range of 0.01 of 0.02 (1–2%), exceptionally up to 0.10 (10%), and, not infrequently, as little as 0.001 (0.1%). Thus, percentage dose absorbed is low, "99% is wasted" (1), and dose absorbed is poorly correlated to dose applied. Finally, dose intervals are based on consumer habits, which are derived from oral drug usage, and in general have little basis in science.

Although formulation can have significant effects, in clinical practice, for the majority of topical formulations, the skin, and not the formulation, controls the dose absorbed. This lack of formulation control leads to skin site and skin condition being the major control factors in the potential for local and systemic adverse effects. For example, topical corticosteroid warnings include avoidance of use on the face and anogential regions, at which permeable skin sites local adverse effects are much more common. Similarly, topical corticosteroid use in children with extensive, severe eczema, where the skin barrier is damaged, can lead to systemic adverse effects on adrenal function (2).

As dose applied is increased, either by increase in drug concentration or amount of product applied, it is common for dose absorbed to remain relatively constant. Thus dose titration, which is essential to optimise clinical response where there is large variation between subjects in skin pharmacodynamics and/or skin clearance pharmacokinetics, may be difficult or impossible.

In the almost 60 years since the beginning of modern dermatology, that is, from the introduction of topical corticosteroids (3), there have been repeated calls for rationalization of dosage. In 1967, Keczkes et al. (4) urged that we "try to determine a suitable therapeutic regimen made up of minimally effective doses (*of topical corticosteroids*) which are known not to affect the function of the adrenal and pituitary glands." Marples and Kligman, in 1974, noted that "concentrations of active substances in practically all topicals are in the range 1% to 3% suggesting the influence of fashion rather than of a rigorous appraisal" (5). More recently, Langford and Benrimoj (6) argued that "The arbitrary and empirical selection of antimicrobial concentration would be unacceptable for systemically administered drugs, and should also be so for topical therapies." Yet, still today, irrational dosing is the norm and clinical performance is adversely affected. This chapter aims to bring together principles and processes that may form the basis for future rational dosing of topical dermatological products.

DOSE RESPONSE AND ITS VARIATION

The concepts of dose and dose response were first introduced into medicine by Paracelus (1493–1541) "Alle Ding sind Gift und nichts ohn Gift; alein die Dosis macht das ein Ding kein Gift ist," roughly "all things are poison and not without poison; only the dose makes a thing not a poison." Dose response is the fundamental concept underlying rational dosing.

Figure 1 shows the in vitro dose response of SDZ ASM 981 (pimecrolimus) to human cloned T cells and human keratinocytes and dermal fibroblasts (7). T cells are implicated in a variety of inflammatory skin disorders and the high potency of SDZ ASM 981 on T cell response is one predictor of its potential topical efficacy in these inflammatory conditions. Also shown are the 50% inhibitory concentration (IC_{50}) values for effects of SDZ ASM 981 on human keratinocytes and dermal fibroblasts. Effects on these cells may predict the potential for skin thinning, for example, as found with potent corticosteroids. The potential to provide anti-inflammatory activity, but without skin thinning, is clear from the 1000-fold difference in in vitro IC50 between the cell types. For example, a suitable dosing strategy might be to achieve free drug levels at the target site in the skin of about 10 nmol/L. Studies on topical dosing of SDZ ASM 981 in patients with eczema confirm efficacy yet lack of skin thinning (8,9).

SDZ ASM 981 is an extreme case with high specificity between cell types. In vitro, newer corticosteroids such as mometasone furoate show 10- to 100-fold less effect on human keratinocytes and fibroblasts than fluorinated corticosteroids, such as betamethasone valerate (10). Because mometasone furoate has similar potency to betamethasone valerate, this may predict the potential for topical dosing to provide equivalent anti-inflammatory activity but without skin thinning. However, such differential effects are not seen when mometasone furoate and betamethasone valerate are compared topically in vivo in man (11,12). Similarly, novel retinoids such as tazarotene and adapalene, with clear in vitro specificity for RAR over RXR (13), which specificity may predict efficacy but low irritation, are as irritant as retinoic acid when applied topically to man (14).

Clearly, especially with the development of newer compounds with high specificity, there is potential for local efficacy within the skin, but without local adverse

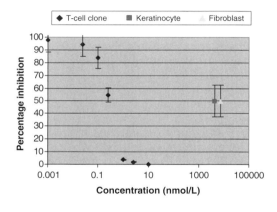

FIGURE 1   Dose response of SDZ ASM 981 (pimecrolimus) to human cloned T cells and human keratinocytes and dermal fibroblasts. Inhibition of T cell function, associated with anti-inflammatory effects, occurs at approximately 1000-fold lower concentrations than effects on keratinocytes and fibroblasts, which are associated with skin thinning. *Source*: Adapted from Ref. 7.

effects. However, when formulated as topical products, this potential may not be realized. Equally clearly, a major contributor to this failure is the inability to control dose and thus dose response. Thus, an optimized dosing strategy requires that the input rate of drug penetration into the skin is controlled in order to achieve and sustain biologically active free drug levels at the target site within defined limits. Also, ideally, these conditions should be met independent of skin site and skin condition, which is a considerable challenge, as these vary by 10- to 50-fold or more (15,16).

If the input rate is lower than the optimum value, efficacy will be poor and may only be achievable on permeable skin sites. For example, SDZ ASM 981 (pimecrolimus) is only effective in psoriasis when used on the permeable skin sites of the face, genital, or intertriginous areas (17), or under occlusion (18). This general problem of subtherapeutic input rates has led to the development of many and varied enhancer technologies, beyond the scope of this chapter. As shown earlier, if the input rate is substantially higher the target, unwanted and unnecessary local adverse effects may occur.

Even if such conditions are met with the innovator product, the product that establishes the clinical utility of the drug based on clinical efficacy and safety, there is no guarantee that generic copies will maintain these. For example, generic copies of topical ibuprofen and aciclovir on the European market have been shown to have an approximately 6- and 30-fold (19,20) variation in dose absorbed.

Similar thinking is appropriate in consideration of systemic adverse effects potential, although the control factors are different. For some compounds, there may be biological specificity for the local skin site as opposed to systemic sites, as is the case with site-specific enzyme isoforms with third-generation PDE4 inhibitors (21,22). However, even if drug potency is the same at local and systemic sites, pharmacokinetic factors may provide specificity of action. Depending on the area of topical application, the drug input rate per area of skin, and systemic drug clearance, steady-state free drug levels in systemic plasma may be much lower than therapeutic levels, whereas those in the skin are at, or above these levels. For example, Muller et al. (23) used cutaneous microdialysis and systemic plasma sampling to show that local free skin tissue levels of diclofenac were 110 ng/mL compared with free drug plasma levels of 0.009 ng/mL at steady state, after topical application to 200 cm^2 of human skin in vivo. Similarly, Dehghanyar et al. (24) found 24 ng/mL diclofenac locally and 0.0008 ng/mL diclofenac systemically at steady state after topical application to 100 cm^2. The IC_{50} anti-inflammatory potency for free diclofenac is approximately 0.6 ng/M1 (25,26), and thus these data predict local efficacy but without systemic adverse effects potential. However, despite this potential for pharmacokinetic specificity, topical administration for local therapy does result in systemic effects for several drug classes including corticosteroids (2,27), vitamin D derivatives (28,29), retinoids (30), PDE4 compounds (31), and antihistamines (32). Even where the balance of pharmacokinetic factors provides the potential for pharmacokinetic selectivity, significant increases in dose absorbed, for example, in severe disease with large areas of permeable skin, will lead to the occurrence of unwanted and unnecessary systemic adverse effects. Of course, with transdermal delivery, the objective is to achieve therapeutic drug levels systemically via topical delivery.

Thus far, only variation around a single target free tissue concentration, thus single target drug input rate, has been considered; for example, the free drug levels at the target site in the skin of about 10 nmol/L proposed for SDZ ASM 981. In humans, especially humans with skin disease, IC_{50} values vary considerably within a target cell type (33). Also, skin metabolism, particularly P450 metabolism, varies considerably between subjects and is induced with time (34,35). Thus, drug input

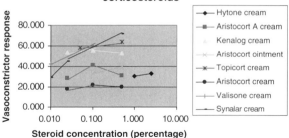

Dose response to U.S. commercial topical corticosteroids

Legend:
- Hytone cream
- Aristocort A cream
- Kenalog cream
- Aristocort ointment
- Topicort cream
- Aristocort cream
- Valisone cream
- Synalar cream

FIGURE 2 Vasoconstrictor dose response to U.S. commercial topical corticosteroids. Topical corticosteroids indicated for mild-moderate-severe dermatoses give similar pharmacokinetically controlled dose response. *Source*: Adapted from Ref. 36.

rate has to be modified to match the relevant IC_{50}, or to account for difference in local metabolic clearance to sustain an IC_{50} value, or both. Drug titration is common in clinical practice, for example, in the administration of narcotic analgesics. In topical dermatological therapy, drug titration is often impossible. Figure 2 shows the vasoconstrictor response to increasing concentrations of a number of topical corticosteroids on the U.S. market (36). For the majority of these formulations, there is little increase in vasoconstrictor activity as dose applied is increased. It has been argued that these embarrassing dose responses are an artifact of the vasoconstrictor assay; for example, caused by saturation of the vasoconstrictor response, although saturation would have to occur at different responses for different corticosteroids. There is a strong scientific argument that the flat dose response is under pharmacokinetic control, thus, as dose applied is increased by drug concentration, dose absorbed remains constant. For example, Barry et al. (37) found no difference in the vasoconstrictor or clinical responses of 0.05% and 0.1% desonide creams, and argued that this was attributable to pharmacokinetic control. It is clear that, independent of drug concentration, if drug is saturated in the formulation, thus at unit thermodynamic activity, dose absorbed is constant, and there is no difference in vasoconstrictor or clinical effect (38–40). In these studies, dose applied was varied by drug concentration. Also, variation in dose applied by amount of formulation per area of skin does not increase dose absorbed or vasoconstrictor activity (41). The biopharmaceutical basis for this, that all saturated solutions and suspensions are at unit thermodynamic activity and give the same skin penetration, is very well established in the relevant scientific literature (36–52).

However, what has not been fully appreciated is the importance of lack of depletion (of saturated systems or systems at the same thermodynamic activity) in the flat dose applied–dose absorbed relationship. Saturated systems applied to the skin remain essentially saturated over the absorption period, when bioavailability is in the typical range of 1% to 2%. Only when the dose absorbed becomes a significant fraction of the dose applied, does depletion occur. This depletion reduces thermodynamic activity and input rate to drive dose response. Dose-response curves from high bioavailability, low-dose formulations will be described later.

Thus, in conclusion, rational dose design of topical dermatological products requires that:

- the input rate (flux) of drug penetration into the skin is controlled so as to achieve and sustain appropriately biologically active free drug levels at the target site, within defined limits;

- from this (and from dose definitions in the transdermal patch area), dose should be defined as an amount of drug absorbed per area per time;
- this control should, ideally, be independent of skin site and condition;
- this control should exist in therapeutically equivalent generic copies;
- the input rate should be capable of modification to allow dose titration to individual patient requirements.

The following sections outline progress towards this objective and also point to areas for further development.

POTENCY AND SKIN PENETRATION ARE EQUALLY IMPORTANT IN PREDICTING EFFICACY POTENTIAL

Depending on our training, or experience, or prejudice, we may believe one or other of these is the dominant factor in deciding therapeutic efficacy potential. For topical dermatological products, the two are equally and essentially important. In the style of the football pundits, all you have to do is achieve and sustain appropriately biologically active free drug levels at the target site, within defined limits. From this, it is intuitive that potency and skin penetration are equally important. The first application of this concept may have been in the selection of topical antiviral agents (53–55). Certainly, the C star concept of Higuchi et al. (56–59) introduced the idea of free drug concentration at the target site in the skin. Also, in their work, Lee et al. (57) described the relationship between flux and free drug concentration at the target site, and defined dose (as flux) as micrograms of drug per square centimeter of skin per day.

DOSE SELECTION BEGINS WITH DRUG SELECTION

In the industrial drug development process, at the discovery stage, dose selection begins with drug selection. Clearly, penetration and potency are important. Lippold et al. (60,61) used the efficacy coefficient (60), the numerical ratio of membrane flux from saturated solutions, divided by numerical value of the drug potency, in drug selection. Thus, the higher the membrane flux and the lower the potency (in concentration units), the higher the efficacy coefficient and the higher the probability of a topical therapeutic effect. Table 1 shows the predicted nail penetration, antifungal potency, and efficacy coefficient for a series of drug candidates for treatment of onychomycosis. The first point to note is that the efficacy coefficient varies over the range approximately 1×10^{-2} to 1×10^{-9}, a 10-million-fold range. Clearly, drug candidates at the top of this range are preferred in terms of therapeutic efficacy potential. The second is that the efficacy coefficient is a ranking only; thus all, unlikely, some, or none of the candidates may have true therapeutic potential based on this data alone. However, both ciclopirox and amorolfine topical nail lacquers are marketed for the treatment of onychomycosis, which may thus be used as benchmarks for clinical activity.

Cordero et al. (62) used the same concept of ratio of penetration from saturated solutions (63) to potency for a range of nonsteroidal drugs. Table 2, column 4, shows the efficacy coefficient derived from their data. Again, there is more than a 20,000-fold range in the efficacy coefficient, and drug candidates at the top of this range are preferred in terms of therapeutic efficacy potential. Recent clinical studies clearly show the efficacy of topical diclofenac (64–66) and ketoprofen (67,68), and thus help validate and benchmark the ranking.

TABLE 1 Predicted Nail Penetration from Saturated Solutions, Antifungal Potency, and the Ratio of These Two (Efficacy Coefficient) for a Series of Drug Candidates for Treatment of Onychomycosis

Antifungal	Flux saturated, mg/cm^2/sec (A)	MIC potency, mg/L (B)	Efficacy coefficient, (A)/(B)
Amorolfine	2.15×10^{-4}	0.01	2.15×10^{-2}
Naftifine	5.38×10^{-4}	0.55	9.78×10^{-4}
Econazole	4.74×10^{-5}	0.35	1.35×10^{-4}
Ciclopirox	1.98×10^{-4}	2.0	9.87×10^{-5}
Bifonazole	1.39×10^{-8}	0.1	1.39×10^{-7}
Clotrimazole	7.77×10^{-8}	2.3	3.38×10^{-8}
Ketoconazole	5.85×10^{-8}	2.2	2.62×10^{-8}
Griseofulvin	7.56×10^{-8}	3.1	2.44×10^{-8}
Tolnaftate	3.36×10^{-9}	0.6	6.11×10^{-9}
Nystatin	4.02×10^{-9}	4.5	8.93×10^{-10}

Abbreviation: MIC, minimum inhibitory concentration.
Source: Adapted from Ref. 60.

Thus, a simple process is available using readily obtained experimental or predicted data (69,70) to enable topical dermatological drug candidate selection.

EXACT EQUATIONS RELATING PENETRATION AND POTENCY

This section is not going to be a mathematical fest, and for various reasons. Earlier, implicitly, the general equation between penetration and potency and efficacy was assumed as,

$$\text{Penetration (flux)/Potency} = \text{Efficacy} \times \{\text{pharmacokinetic black box}\} \qquad (1)$$

For example, the well-known equation to predict steady-state plasma levels after transdermal delivery is shown in Equation (2) below but rearranges to be in the form of Equation (1), as in Equation (3), below.

$$\text{Flux} \times \text{Area} = C_{\text{plasma steady state}} \times Cl \qquad (2)$$

$$\text{Flux}/C_{\text{plasma effective}} = \text{Efficacy (Index)} \times \{Cl/A\} \qquad (3)$$

TABLE 2 Skin Penetration from Saturated Solutions, Anti-inflammatory Potency, and the Ratio of These Two (Efficacy Coefficient) and ITAA for a Series of Drug Candidates.

Nonsteroidal drug	Flux saturated, μg/cm^2/hr (A)	MIC potency, μg/cm^3 (B)	Efficacy coefficient, (A)/(B) = (C)	ITAA (C)/3.6 from Eq. (6)
Diclofenac	1.4	0.009	157.7	43.8
Ketorolac	13	0.097	134.2	37.3
Ketoprofen	16	0.188	85.1	23.7
Indomethacin	0.7	0.057	12.2	3.4
Tenoxicam	0.7	18.62	0.04	0.01
Piroxicam	0.08	11.55	0.007	0.0019

Abbreviation: ITAA, index of topical anti-inflammatory activity.
Source: Adapted from Ref. 62.

where A is area of application, Cl is systemic clearance in volume/time, and Efficacy (Index) is $C_{plasma}/C_{plasma\ effective}$.

Recently, independently, Cordero et al. (62) and Trottet (71) published the exact equation in the form of Equation (1), which describes the relationship between penetration, potency, and dermal efficacy, as shown in Equation (4) below.

$$\text{Flux/IC}_{50} \text{ potency} = \text{Efficacy} \times \{2D_d/h_d\} \tag{4}$$

where D_d is the dermal diffusion coefficient and h_d is the thickness of the dermis.

Equation (4) now allows an exact form for efficacy, called index of topical anti-inflammatory activity (ITAA) by Cordero et al. (62) and efficacy index (EI) by Trottet (71), to be expressed as in Equation (5) below.

$$\text{Efficacy (ITAA/EI)} = \text{Flux/IC}_{50} \times h_d/2D_d \tag{5}$$

From Equation (5), Efficacy has no units because $m \times t^{-1} \times cm^{-2}/m \times cm^{-3} \times cm/cm^2 \times t^{-1}$ is dimensionless. It is also important that units are consistent, for example, flux is expressed in $\mu g/cm^2/hr$, IC_{50} is in $\mu g/cm^3$, h_d is in cm, and D_d is in cm^2/hr. Cordero et al. (62) used a value of 0.02 cm (200 μm) for h_d, 0.036 cm^2/hr (1×10^{-5} cm^2/sec) for D_d, and thus, for diclofenac where flux is1.4 $\mu g/cm^2/hr$ and IC_{50} is ~0.009 $\mu g/cm^3$ (0.03 μM) then,

$$\text{Efficacy Index (ITAA)} = 1.4/0.009 \times 0.02/2 \times 0.036,$$

which is equal to 43.8 as shown in Table 2 (column 5).

Cordero et al. (62) and Trottet (71) use slightly different assumptions for values of D_d and h_d, and assume that D_d is constant for molecules over a certain size range. Despite these approximations, Equations (4) and (5) are valuable, not only to rank drug candidates, but also to give some absolute measure of efficacy prediction, within the limits of the assumptions. For example, compounds with an EI between 1 and 10 and higher can be considered candidates for topical development. Those with an EI between 0.1 and 1 may have therapeutic efficacy potential but will likely require enhancer technology, and those lower than 0.1 should be rejected. Cordero et al. (62) calculate the ITAA for diclofenac and ketoprofen to be 44 and 24, respectively, consistent with their strong topical anti-inflammatory activity. Trottet (71) calculates the EI of the topical immunomodulators tacrolimus and pimecrolimus to be six and two, respectively, compared with 0.04 for topical cyclosporin, again consistent with the clinical efficacy of tacrolimus (72) and pimecrolimus (73) and the lack of efficacy with topical cyclopsorin (74,75). It may be useful to refine predictions by determination of D_d for a compound of particular interest, and also to compare ITAA-EI for this compound with compounds of known efficacy in the indication of interest.

Equations (4) and (5) are concerned with the dermis as the target site. Trottet has suggested adjustments to the basic equations to account for other target sites within the skin, and for skin metabolism and disease-induced changes in blood flow (71).

Finally, from Equations (4) and (5), and assuming an EI of 1, the relationship between flux and free drug levels at the target site at steady state can be established, as in Equation (6) below.

$$\text{Flux} = C_{free\ drug\ target\ site} \times 2D_d/h_d \tag{6}$$

As noted earlier, this equation and the underlying concepts are based on an early work by Higuchi et al. (56–59). This equation forms the basis for rational dosing, as will be described in the next section.

ESTIMATES OF MINIMUM THERAPEUTIC DOSE

As discussed earlier, the constant term $2D_d/h_d$, as used in Equation (6), is subject to some assumptions. In illustrating the application of Equation (6) to estimates of minimum dose, a value of $2D_d/h_d$ of 2 will be used to make the calculations transparent. For example, using values of 0.04 cm for h_d and 0.036 cm^2/hr for D_d makes the constant term $2D_d/h_d$ equal to 2 × 0.036/0.04, thus 1.8, ~2.0. Clearly, from Equation (6), the higher this value, the higher the flux needed, and thus the higher the drug dose to sustain the flux.

Using ibuprofen as an example, the IC50 free drug potency is 0.25 µg/cm^3 and thus a flux of 0.50 µg/cm^2/hr [0.25 × 2 (2D_d/h_d) = 0.5] is needed at steady state to sustain this therapeutic target concentration in the dermis. Again, for simplicity and transparency of calculation, if we assume a 20-hour day and twice-a-day dosing, then a minimum (theoretical) dose of 5.0 µg/cm^2 per 10 hours is needed. Finally, if we assume a dose of product applied per area of skin of 2 mg/cm^2, then the minimum concentration of ibuprofen needed is given by 5.0/2000 × 100 = 0.25%. Of course, this is the very minimum dose and assumes 100% bioavailability and a square-wave input profile, and so, is a theoretical figure. Even so, the minimum dose of 0.25% applied at 2 mg/cm^2 of product is considerably lower than the concentration of 5%, which is found in most commercial ibuprofen products (19). As discussed earlier, topical bioavailability is low and can be estimated for ibuprofen to be at approximately 5% over a 10-hour period (19), exactly the same as that predicted (0.25/5.0 × 100 = 5%). Thus, for ibuprofen, there is excellent agreement for the minimum therapeutic dose estimated from Equation (6) and that predicted on the basis of the known extent of absorption of current products of known therapeutic activity.

In Table 3, this calculation is repeated for compounds whose potency is typical of the range found in topical dermatological products, thus, from potent corticosteroids, through the retinoids, Vitamin D3 derivates, and topical immunomodulators to the relatively low-potent nonsteroidal ibuprofen. Again, there is a good agreement for the minimum therapeutic dose estimated from Equation (6) and that predicted on the basis of the known extent of absorption of current products of known therapeutic activity (1,19,71).

The low topical bioavailability of the vast majority of current products is well established and undisputed. What is much more interesting is that a rationally based process gives predictions of dose absorbed, thus minimum dose required, in very close agreement. Thus, this process may provide the basis for rational dose-formulation development.

RATIONAL DOSE-FORMULATION DEVELOPMENT

Review of the biopharmaceutically driven formulation of topical dermatological products is beyond the scope of this chapter, but several points for guidance are clear.

TABLE 3 Prediction of Minimum Therapeutic Dose and Topical Bioavailability Based on Equation (6)

Drug IC_{50}, ng/cm^3	Flux, ng/ cm^2/hr, from Eq. (6)	Drug dose, $ng/cm^2/10$ hr	Percentage in product at 2 mg/cm^2 (A)	Typical percentage drug in commercial product (B)	Estimate of topical bioavailability $(A)/(B) \times 100$	Typical drug example and brand
0.05	0.10	1.0	0.00005%	0.005–0.05%	1.0–0.1%	Fluticasone propionate (Cutivate)
0.1	0.20	2.0	0.0001%	0.025–0.1%	0.4–0.1%	Retinoic acid (Retin-A)
0.1	0.20	2.0	0.0001%	0.005%	2.0%	Calcipotriol (Dovonex)
0.25	0.50	5.0	0.00025%	1.0%	0.025%	Diclofenac (Voltaren)
0.50	1.00	10.0	0.0005%	0.3–1.0%	1.67–0.5%	Tacrolimus (Elidel)
0.50	1.00	10.0	0.0005%	1.0%	0.05%	Pimecrolimus (Protopic)
5.0	10.0	100.0	0.005%	0.5–1.0%	1.0–0.5%	Hydrocortisone (Generic)
5.0	10.0	100.0	0.005%	1%	0.5%	Terbinafine (Lamasil)
250	500.0	5,000	0.25%	5%	5%	Ibuprofen (Generic)

Note: Column 1 is the potency of a typical drug shown in column 7. Columns 2, 3, and 4 show drug flux, dose, and drug percentage (at 2 mg/cm^2 of product) based on Equation (6). Columns 5 and 6 show actual dose in typical current products and estimate of topical bioavailability based on columns 4 and 5. Predicted topical bioavailability is highly consistent with that found from in vitro skin permeation studies.

- Drug selection, including drug form selection (salt, free base, acid, etc.) should be based on efficacy coefficient (ratio of penetration to potency). As an early screen use of predicted flux (69,70) may be appropriate, but this should be confirmed experimentally.
- Efficacy prediction should be based on Equation (5), and may be refined by using an experimentally determined value of D_d and by comparing values of the EI obtained with those obtained for relevant compounds. For example, for an anti-proliferative compound with potential in psoriasis, comparison with calcipotriol, retinoids, and appropriate corticosteroids may be appropriate.
- Dose selection should be based on Equation (6), but only as a guide. Even doses at 2 to 4 times the minimum (50–25% bioavailability) are much preferred over 100- to 1000-fold excesses.
- Preformulation work should then be conducted and suitable solvents selected on the basis of appropriate solubility for the drug dose. To be clear, it is important that the thermodynamic activity of the drug is at, or greater than, saturation level. Also, this should be with respect to the residual phase formed, for example, on loss of volatiles.

After such a formulation development process, a natural further step would be to measure drug levels at the target site in vivo in man. This is briefly discussed in the next section.

IN VIVO HUMAN DERMATOPHARMACOKINETICS

First, because of the reduced dermal clearance of drugs applied in vitro, in vitro measurements of skin tissue concentration greatly overestimate in vivo concentrations (76).

Also, and somewhat churlishly, it may be appropriate to mention the role of the vasoconstrictor assay in the state of current dermatopharmacokinetics. Although this assay was a wonderful innovation and brought many new products and companies into dermatology, its introduction coincided with a decline in in vivo dermatopharmacokinetics pioneered in the 1950s and 1960s (15,16,77–80). The vasoconstrictor, pharmacological, measure bypassed the dermatopharmacokinetic black box.

Briefly, two major dermatopharmacokinetic techniques, cutaneous microdialysis and stratum corneum tape stripping, are being developed which have the potential to greatly improve the dose-formulation development process. Cutaneous microdialysis samples free drug concentrations in the dermis, and so is particularly relevant to confirmation of prediction of efficacy, based on Equations (5) and (6). Several recent reports are of interest (81–87). In the case of stratum corneum tape stripping, the skin site measured is not the target site for the majority of drugs. However, Guy et al. (88–91) have greatly advanced and validated the technique in recent years so that prediction of drug concentration in the lower layers of the skin may be possible. Tape stripping is being developed for comparison of bioavailability of topical dermatological products and thus is important at the later stages of drug life cycle in the development of generics.

EXAMPLES OF RATIONALLY DOSED TOPICAL DERMATOLOGICAL PRODUCTS

First, there are a few examples of marketed topical dermatological products where dose has been carefully considered. Barry and Woodford (91) showed that Dioderm hydrocortisone cream 0.1% (Dermal Laboratories, Ltd., Hitchin, U.K.) was superior in the vasoconstrictor test compared to a range of 1% hydrocortisone creams and ointments. Cutivate ointment, 0.005%, contains 1/10th of the dose of fluticasone propionate compared with that in Cutivate cream, 0.05% (GlaxoSmithKline Uxbridge, U.K.), yet is two potency grades higher because of a higher dose absorbed at approximately 10% to 20% absolute bioavailability (70). It is interesting that fluticasone ointment 0.005% appears to be without local and systemic adverse effects (92,93). Because of its action on the vitamin D receptor, calcipotriol has the potential to cause effects on systemic calcium metabolism. Dovonex (Leo Laboratories Limited, Princes Risborough, U.K.) is 0.005% calcipotriol, and the dose applied of the ointment, cream, or scalp solution is limited to 100 g/wk, equivalent to 5 mg of calcipotriol. Various data converge to suggest that topical bioavailability is up to 5%, equivalent to 250 µg absorbed per week and that this is near the estimated minimum no-systemic-effect dose of 50 µg/day or 350 µg/wk. Although it is clear that great care was taken in dose selection, there is potential to increase systemic safety with further dose reduction, as shown in Table 3.

As in Figure 3, Davis (94) showed in the vasoconstrictor assay, that low dose, 0.02% hydrocortisone acetate was bioequivalent to 1.0% hydrocortisone acetate, despite the 50-fold reduction in dose. Marks et al (95) showed very similar results with these same formulations, using a surfactant-induced erythema model in hu-

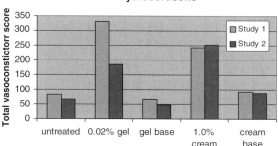

FIGURE 3 Bioequivalence of 0.02% hydrocortisone acetate gel with 1.0% hydrocortisone acetate cream, mean results from two studies. The 0.02% and 1.0% hydrocortisone products are not significantly different from each other, but are so from control treatments (Wilcoxon matched-pairs signed ranks, $P < 0.05$). *Source:* Adapted from Ref. 95.

man volunteers. It can be estimated that the absolute bioavailability of the low dose formulations is in the order of 25% to 50%. Clearly, if these were put onto permeable skin sites, the absolute bioavailability could not exceed 100%, so a 2- to 4-fold increase, despite a 10- to 50-fold or higher (15,16) increase in skin permeability. Thus, low dose, bioequivalent-to-clinically proven–conventional doses limit the potential for local and systemic adverse effects.

Figure 4 compares the 10-day cumulative irritancy with time of conventional and low-dose retinoic acid formulations in humans (95). Irritancy is used as a surrogate measure for retinoic acid percutaneous absorption. The left panel shows lack of dose response from 0.025% and 0.05% conventional cream formulations. Comparison with the right panel shows that the low dose 0.00125% gel formulation is broadly bioequivalent to these, despite being at 20- and 40-fold lower dose, respectively. It can be estimated that the absolute bioavailability of the low dose formulations is in the order of 25% to 50%. Also, the right panel shows an excellent dose response

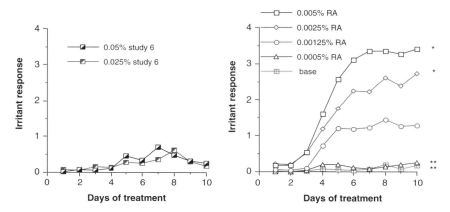

FIGURE 4 Bioequivalence of low-dose retinoic gels with conventional retinoic acid (RA) cream and dose response, and lack of, from low-dose retinoic gels and conventional retinoic acid creams in volunteers. The *left panel* shows lack of irritancy dose response from 0.025% and 0.05% retinoic acid cream applied over 10 days to volunteers. The *right panel* shows approximate bioavailability of a low dose 0.00125% retinoic acid gel to the conventional doses and dose response over the range of 0.0005% to 0.005%. *Source:* Adapted from Ref. 95.

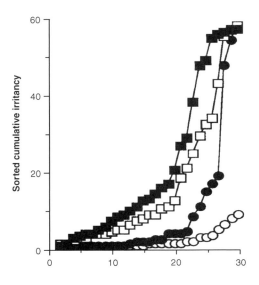

FIGURE 5 Cumulative 10-day irritancy response in 30 volunteers over the low-dose range 0.0005% to 0.005% retinoic acid (*open circle*, 0.0005%; *filled circle*, 0.00125%; *empty square*, 0.0025%, *filled square*, 0.005%). For any fixed dose of retinoic acid, there is a considerable variation in irritancy between volunteers. The variation comes from differences in local metabolic clearance, or local pharmacodynamics, or both. *Source*: Adapted from 95.

over the low-dose range 0.0005% to 0.005% retinoic acid. All of the low-dose retinoic acid gel formulations started at the same thermodynamic activity upon first application to the skin, and thus delivered initially exactly the same dose in $\mu g/cm^2/$ time. However, as this becomes a significant, yet varying, part of the dose applied, dose-related depletion occurs. This causes a relative drop in the thermodynamic activity in the lower doses and a dose response is establish, as described in the section, "Dose Response and Its Variation". Also increasing the amount of the low dose-gels applied per area of skin shows a dose-related increase in response (data not shown), which is not seen with the conventional doses. Figure 5 shows the same data as in Figure 4, right panel, but expressed as cumulative 10-day irritancy between volunteers. It is clear that there is considerable variation between volunteers and, because of the high bioavailability of the low-dose formulations, it may be inferred that this variation comes from differences in local metabolic clearance, or local pharmacodynamics, or both. Also, these factors change with time; for example, there is induction in metabolic clearance via P450 metabolism after topical dosing (97). Retinoic acid and likely other retinoids are examples of topical dermatological treatments, where dose titration, thus dose response, is required to optimise therapy. Although dose-titration concepts are established in dermatological therapy with availability of products with different drug concentrations, the technical execution has been poor; for example, as in Figure 2, and current therapy is suboptimal.

Many dermatological treatments would be improved by rationalization of dosage. One obstacle to this work is the current regulatory guidelines for bioequivalence, which will be briefly reviewed in the next section.

REGULATIONS FOR BIOEQUIVALENCE TO ALLOW DOSE RATIONALIZATION

Current regulations broadly state that pharmaceutical equivalence (same drug, same drug form, *same dose*, similar formulation) plus bioequivalence (vasoconstrictor assay or validated dermatopharmacokinetic methodology) can be assumed to assure clinical Equivalence. In the context of this chapter, the concern is that the dose must be the same, thus that dose irrationality is perpetuated, and there is no incentive for innovation. It may be just that we need to make the case with regulators and there is some precedence for this view in the position adopted for transdermal systems. For example, in the case of transdermal patches of nitroglycerin, the dose is expressed as the delivery rate in mg/hr and formulations containing different doses of nitroglycerin in total, but delivering the same rate, are considered to be bioequivalent (98). It is hoped that similar thinking can be applied to topical dermatological products, especially as we begin to express dose as amount per area per time.

CONCLUSIONS

This chapter has aimed to define a process where rational estimates of dose can be defined to help guide the topical formulation development process. It is understood that other formulation design factors may influence dose selection, not least drug stability. Also, if the drug is not a good candidate for dermal delivery, inclusion of penetration enhancers may dominate dose and also aesthetic design considerations.

However, for new drugs and rationalized doses of existing drugs, there are clear therapeutic advantages. By incorporating a rational dose-design process into dermatological formulation development, we may be more assured of drug efficacy, of realizing biological and pharmacokinetic-based drug specificity to reduce the potential for local and systemic adverse effects, and of the ability for dose titration. Thus, overall, to achieve significant improvement in topical therapy.

To paraphrase Langford and Benrimoj (6), which sums it up nicely, the arbitrary and empirical selection of drug dose would be unacceptable for systemically administered drugs, and should also be so for topical therapies.

REFERENCES

1. Maibach HI. In vivo percutaneous penetration of corticoids in man and unresolved problems in their efficacy. Dermatologica 1976;152 Suppl 1:11–25.
2. Turpeinen M, Salo OP, Leisti S. Effect of percutaneous absorption of hydrocortisone on adrenocortical responsiveness in infants with severe skin disease. Br J Dermatol 1986;115(4):475–484.
3. Sultzberger MB, Witten VH. The effect of topically applied compound F in selected dermatoses. J Invest Dermatol 1952;19(2):101–102.
4. Keczkes K, Frain-Bell W, Honeyman AL, et al. The effect of adrenal function of treatment of eczema and psoriasis with triamcinolone acetonide. Br J Dermatol 1967;79(8):475–486.
5. Marples RR, Kligman AM, Methods for evaluating topical antibacterial agents on human skin. Antimicrob Agents Chemother 1974; 5:323-379.
6. Langford JH, Benrimoj SI. Clinical rationale for topical antimicrobial preparations. J Antimicrob Chemother 1996;37(3):399–402.
7. Grassberger M, Baumruker T, Enz A, et al. A novel anti-inflammatory drug, SDZ ASM 981, for the treatment of skin diseases: in vitro pharmacology. Br J Dermatol 1999;141(2):264–73.
8. Meingassner JG, Grassberger M, Fahrngruber H, et al. A novel anti-inflammatory drug, SDZ ASM 981, for the topical and oral treatment of skin diseases: in vivo pharmacology. Br J Dermatol 1997;137(4):568–576.
9. Bos JD. Topical tacrolimus and pimecrolimus are not associated with skin atrophy. Br J Dermatol 2002;146(2):342.
10. Wach F, Bosserhoff A, Kurzidym U, et al. Effects of mometasone furoate on human keratinocytes and fibroblasts in vitro. Skin Pharmacol Appl Skin Physiol 1998;11(1):43–51.

11. Korting HC, Unholzer A, Schafer-Korting M, et al. Different skin thinning potential of equipotent medium-strength glucocorticoids. Skin Pharmacol Appl Skin Physiol 2002;15(2):85–91.

12. Koivukangas V, Karvonen J, Risteli J, et al. Topical mometasone furoate and betamethasone-17-valerate decrease collagen synthesis to a similar extent in human skin in vivo. Br J Dermatol 1995;132(1):66–68.

13. Bershad S. Developments in topical retinoid therapy for acne. Sem Cutaneous Med Surg 2001;20:154–161.

14. Kakita L. Tazarotene versus tretinoin or adapalene in the treatment of acne vulgaris. J Am Acad Dermatol 2000;43:51–54.

15. Feldmann RJ, Maibach HI. Regional variation in percutaneous penetration of 14C cortisol in man. J Invest Dermatol 1967;48(2):181–183.

16. Feldmann RJ, Maibach HI. Penetration of 14C hydrocortisone through normal skin: the effect of stripping and occlusion. Arch Dermatol 1965;91:661–666.

17. Martin EG, Sanchez RM, Herrera AE, et al. Topical tacrolimus for the treatment of psoriasis on the face, genitalia, intertriginous areas and corporal plaques. J Drugs Dermatol 2006;5(4):334–336.

18. Remitz A, Reitamo S, Erkko P, et al. Tacrolimus ointment improves psoriasis in a microplaque assay. Br J Dermatol 1999;141(1):103–107.

19. Hadgraft J, Whitefield M, Rosher PH. Skin penetration of topical formulations of ibuprofen 5%: an in vitro comparative study. Skin Pharmacol Appl Skin Physiol 2003;16(3):137–142.

20. Trottet L, Owen H, Holme P, et al. Are all aciclovir cream formulations bioequivalent? Int J Pharm 2005;304(1–2):63–71.

21. Souness JE, Rao S. Proposal for pharmacologically distinct conformers of PDE4 cyclic AMP phosphodiesterases. Cell Signal 1997;9(3-4):227–364.

22. Hoppmann J, Baumer W, Galetzka C, et al. The phosphodiesterase 4 inhibitor AWD 12-281 is active in a new guinea-pig model of allergic skin inflammation predictive of human skin penetration and suppresses both Th_1 and Th_2 cytokines in mice. J Pharm Pharmacol 2005;57(12):1609–1617.

23. Muller M, Rastelli C, Ferri P, et al. Transdermal penetration of diclofenac after multiple epicutaneous administration. J Rheumatol 1998;25(9):1833–1836.

24. Dehghanyar P, Mayer BX, Namiranian K, et al. Topical skin penetration of diclofenac after single- and multiple-dose application. Int J Clin Pharmacol Ther 2004;42(7):353–359.

25. Churchill L et al.. Selective inhibition of human cyclo-oxygenase-2 by meloxicam. Inflammopharmacology 1996; 4:135.

26. Cromlish W, Kennedy BP. Selective inhibition of cyclooxygenase-1 and -2 using intact insect cell assay. Biochem Pharmacol 1996;52:1777–1785.

27. Salde L, Lassus A. Systemic side-effects of three topical steroids in diseased skin. Curr Med Res Opin 1983;8(7):475–480.

28. Berth-Jones J, Bourke JF, Iqbal SJ, et al. Urine calcium excretion during treatment of psoriasis with topical calcipotriol. Br J Dermatol 1993;129(4):411–414.

29. Hoeck HC, Laurberg G, Laurberg P. Hypercalcaemic crisis after excessive topical use of a vitamin D derivative. J Intern Med 1994;235(3):281–282.

30. Chen C, Jensen BK, Mistry G, et al. Negligible systemic absorption of topical isotretinoin cream: implications for teratogenicity. J Clin Pharmacol 1997;37(4):279–284.

31. Baumer W, Hoppmann J, Rundfeldt C, et al. Highly selective phosphodiesterase 4 inhibitors for the treatment of allergic skin diseases and psoriasis. Inflamm Allergy Drug Targets 2007;6(1):17–26.

32. Zell-Kanter M, Toerne TS, Spiegel K, et al. Doxepin toxicity in a child following topical administration. Ann Pharmacother 2000;34(3):328–329.

33. Hanifin JM, Chan SC, Cheng JB, et al. Type 4 phosphodiesterase inhibitors have clinical and in vitro anti-inflammatory effects in atopic dermatitis. J Invest Dermatol 1996;107(1):51–56.

34. Heise R, Mey J, Neis MM, et al. Skin retinoid concentrations are modulated by CYP26AI expression restricted to basal keratinocytes in normal human skin and differentiated 3D skin models. J Invest Dermatol 2006;126(11):2473–2480.

35. Schuster I, Egger H, Bikle D, et al. Selective inhibition of vitamin D hydroxylases in human keratinocytes. Steroids 2001;66(3–5):409–422.

36. Stoughton RB, Wullich K. The same glucocorticoid in brand-name products. Does increasing the concentration result in greater topical biologic activity? Arch Dermatol 1989;125(11):1509–1511.

37. Barry BW, Fyrand O, Woodford R, et al. Control of the bioavailability of a topical steroid; comparison of desonide creams 0.05% and 0.1% by vasoconstrictor studies and clinical trials. Clin Exp Dermatol 1987;12(6):406–409.

38. Gibson JR, Kirsch J, Darley CR, et al. An attempt to evaluate the relative clinical potencies of various diluted and undiluted proprietary corticosteroid preparations. Br J Dermatol 1983;109 Suppl 25:114–116.

39. Kirsch J, Gibson JR, Darley CR, et al. A comparison of the potencies of several diluted and undiluted corticosteroid preparations using the vasoconstrictor assay. Dermatologica 1983;167(3):138–141.

40. Kirsch JM, Gibson JR, Darley C, et al. Extemporaneous dilutions of proprietary topical corticosteroid preparations. Dermatologica 1982;165(1):71–72.

41. Martin GP. The effect of dose under a hydrocolloid patch on the human bioavailability of a topical cortisosteroid. J Pharm Pharmacol 1989;41:129.

42. Ostrenga J, Steinmetz C, Poulsen B, et al. Significance of vehicle composition. II. Prediction of optimal vehicle composition. J Pharm Sci 1971;60(8):1180–1183.

43. Ostrenga J, Steinmetz C, Poulsen B. Significance of vehicle composition. I. Relationship between topical vehicle composition, skin penetrability, and clinical efficacy. J Pharm Sci 1971;60(8):1175–1179.

44. Poulsen BJ. Diffusion of drugs from topical vehicles: an analysis of vehicle effects. Adv Biol Skin 1972;12:495–509.

45. Lippold BC, Schneemann H. The influence of vehicles on the local bioavailability of betamethasone-17-benzoate from solution- and suspension-type ointments. Int J Pharmaceut 1984;22:31–43.

46. Malzfeldt E, Lehmann P, Goerz G, et al. Influence of drug solubility in the vehicle on clinical efficacy of ointments. Arch Dermatol Res 1989;281(3):193–197.

47. Bennett SL, Barry BW, Woodford R. Optimization of bioavailability of topical steroids: non-occluded penetration enhancers under thermodynamic control. J Pharm Pharmacol 1985;37(5):298–304.

48. Woodford R, Barry BW. Optimization of bioavailability of topical steroids: thermodynamic control. J Invest Dermatol 1982;79(6):388–391.

49. Hadgraft J, Hadgraft JW, Sarkany I. Proceedings: the effect of thermodynamic activity on the percutaneous absorption of methyl nicotinate from water glycerol mixtures. J Pharm Pharmacol 1973;25:Suppl:122–123.

50. Iervolino M, Raghavan SL, Hadgraft J. Membrane penetration enhancement of ibuprofen using supersaturation. Int J Pharm 2000;198(2):229–238.

51. Leichtnam ML, Rolland H, Wuthrich P, et al. Enhancement of transdermal testosterone delivery by supersaturation. J Pharm Sci 2006;95(11):2373–2379.

52. Moser K, Kriwet K, Froehlich C, et al. Permeation enhancement of a highly lipophilic drug using supersaturated systems. J Pharm Sci 2001;90(5):607–616.

53. Bach M, Lippold BC. Percutaneous penetration enhancement and its quantification. Eur J Pharm Biopharm 1998 Jul;46(1):1–13.

54. Spruance SL, McKeough M, Sugibayashi K, et al.. Effect of azone and propylene glycol on penetration of trifluorothymidine through skin and efficacy of different topical formulations against cutaneous herpes simplex virus infections in guinea pigs. Antimicrobial 1984; 26:819–823.

55. Spruance SL, McKeough MB, Cardinal JR.. Penetration of guinea pig skin by acyclovir in different vehicles and correlation with the efficacy of topical therapy of experimental cutaneous herpes simplex virus infection. Antimicrobial 1984; 25:10–15.

56. Imanidis G, Song WQ, Lee PH, et al.. Estimation of skin target site acyclovir concentrations following controlled (trans)dermal drug delivery in topical and systemic treatment of cutaneous HSV-1 infections in hairless mice. Pharm Res 1994;11:1035–1041.

57. Lee PH, Su MH, Kern ER, et al. Novel animal model for evaluating topical efficacy of antiviral agents: flux versus efficacy correlations in the acyclovir treatment of cutaneous herpes simplex virus type 1 (HSV-1) infections in hairless mice. Pharm Res 1992;9:970–989.

58. Mehta SC, Afouna MI, Ghanem AH, et al. Relationship of skin target site free drug concentration (C*) to the in vivo efficacy: an extensive evaluation of the predictive value of the C* concept using acyclovir as a model drug. J Pharm Sci 1997;86:797–801.
59. Patel PJ, Ghanem AH, Higuchi WI, et al. Correlation of in vivo topical efficacies with in vitro predictions using acyclovir formulations in the treatment of cutaneous HSV- 1 infections in hairless mice: an evaluation of the predictive value of the C* concept. Antiviral Res 1996;29:279–286.
60. Mertin D, Lippold BC. In-vitro permeability of the human nail and of a keratin membrane from bovine hooves: prediction of the penetration rate of antimycotics through the nail plate and their efficacy. J Pharm Pharmacol 1997;49(9):866–872.
61. Wenkers BP, Lippold BC. Prediction of the efficacy of cutaneously applied nonsteroidal anti-inflammatory drugs from a lipophilic vehicle. Arzneimittelforsch 2000;50(3):275–280.
62. Cordero JA, Camacho M, Obach R, et al. In vitro based index of topical anti-inflammatory activity to compare a series of NSAIDs. Eur J Pharm Biopharm 2001;51(2):135–142.
63. Cordero JA, Alarcon L, Escribano E, et al. A comparative study of the transdermal penetration of a series of nonsteroidal antiinflammatory drugs. J Pharm Sci 1997;86(4): 503–508.
64. Baer PA, Thomas LM, Shainhouse Z. Treatment of osteoarthritis of the knee with a topical diclofenac solution: a randomised controlled, 6-week trial [ISRCTN53366886]. BMC Musculoskelet Disord 2005;8;6:44.
65. Tugwell PS, Wells GA, Shainhouse JZ. Equivalence study of a topical diclofenac solution (pennsaid) compared with oral diclofenac in symptomatic treatment of osteoarthritis of the knee: a randomized controlled trial. J Rheumatol 2004;31(10):2002–2012.
66. Towheed TE. Pennsaid therapy for osteoarthritis of the knee: a systematic review and metaanalysis of randomized controlled trials. J Rheumatol 2006;33(3):567–573.
67. Esparza F, Cobian C, Jimenez JF, et al. Topical ketoprofen TDS patch versus diclofenac gel: efficacy and tolerability in benign sport related soft-tissue injuries. Br J Sports Med 2007;41(3):134–139.
68. Mazieres B, Rouanet S, Guillon Y, et al. Topical ketoprofen patch in the treatment of tendinitis: a randomized, double blind, placebo controlled study. J Rheumatol 2005;32(8):1563–1570.
69. Guy RH, Potts RO. Structure-permeability relationships in percutaneous penetration. J Pharm Sci 1992;81(6):603–604.
70. Potts RO, Guy RH. Predicting skin permeability. Pharm Res 1992;9(5):663–669.
71. Trottet T. Topical pharmacokinetics for a rational and effective topical drug development process. PhD thesis, 2005, University of Wales, Cardiff.
72. Nakagawa H. Comparison of the efficacy and safety of 0.1% tacrolimus ointment with topical corticosteroids in adult patients with atopic dermatitis: review of randomised, double-blind clinical studies conducted in Japan. Clin Drug Investig 2006;26(5):235–246.
73. Frohna JG. Efficacy and tolerability of topical pimecrolimus and tacrolimus in the treatment of atopic dermatitis: meta-analysis of randomised controlled trials. J Pediatr 2005;147(1):126.
74. Bunse T, Schulze HJ, Mahrle G. Topical administration of cyclosporin in psoriasis vulgaris. Z Hautkr 1990;65(6):538, 541–542.
75. Cole GW, Shimomaye S, Goodman M. The effect of topical cyclosporin A on the elicitation phase of allergic contact dermatitis. Contact Dermatitis 1988;19(2):129–132.
76. Ault JM, Riley CM, Meltzer NM, et al. Dermal microdialysis sampling in vivo. Pharm Res 1994;11(11):1631–1639.
77. Scott A, Kalz F. The penetration and distribution of C14-hydrocortisone in human skin after its topical application. J Invest Dermatol 1956;26(2):149–158.
78. Witten VH, Shapiro AJ, Silber RH. Attempts to demonstrate absorption of hydrocortisone by new chemical test following induction into human skin. Proc Soc Exp Biol Med 1955;88(3):419–421.
79. Malkinson FD, Kirschenbaum MB. Percutaneous absorption of C14-labelled triamcinolone acetonide. Arch Dermatol 1963;88:427–439.
80. Malkinson FD, Ferguson EH, Wang MC, Percutaneous absorption of cortisone C14 through normal human skin. J Invest Dermatol. 1957;28(3):211–216.

81. Anderson CD. Cutaneous microdialysis: is it worth the sweat? J Invest Dermatol 2006;126(6):1207–1209.
82. Ault JM, Lunte CE, Meltzer NM, et al. Microdialysis sampling for the investigation of dermal drug transport. Pharm Res 1992;9(10):1256–1261.
83. Gottlob A, Abels C, Landthaler M, et al. Cutaneous microdialysis. Use in dermatology. Hautarzt 2002;53(3):174–178.
84. Klimowicz A, Farfal S, Bielecka-Grzela S. Evaluation of skin penetration of topically applied drugs in humans by cutaneous microdialysis: acyclovir vs. salicylic acid. J Clin Pharm Ther 2007;32(2):143–148.
85. Kreilgaard M. Assessment of cutaneous drug delivery using microdialysis. Adv Drug Deliv Rev 2002;54 Suppl 1:S99–S121.
86. Kreilgaard M. Dermal pharmacokinetics of microemulsion formulations determined by in vivo microdialysis. Pharm Res 2001;18(3):367–373.
87. Morgan CJ, Renwick AG, Friedmann PS. The role of stratum corneum and dermal microvascular perfusion in penetration and tissue levels of water-soluble drugs investigated by microdialysis. Br J Dermatol 2003;148(3):434–443.
88. Alberti I, Kalia YN, Naik A, et al. Assessment and prediction of the cutaneous bioavailability of topical terbinafine, in vivo, in man. Pharm Res 2001;18(10):1472–1475.
89. Herkenne C, Naik A, Kalia YN, et al. Dermatopharmacokinetic prediction of topical drug bioavailability in vivo. J Invest Dermatol 2007;127(4):887–894.
90. Herkenne C, Naik A, Kalia YN, et al. Ibuprofen transport into and through skin from topical formulations: in vitro-in vivo comparison. J Invest Dermatol 2007;127(1):135–142.
91. Reddy MB, Stinchcomb AL, Guy RH, et al. Determining dermal absorption parameters in vivo from tape strip data. Pharm Res 2002;19(3):292–298.
92. Barry BW, Woodford R. Proprietary hydrocortisone creams. Vasoconstrictor activities and bio-availabilities of six preparations. Br J Dermatol 1976;95(4):423–425.
93. Cornell R. Fluticasone propionate ointment 0.005%: its lack of suppression of the HPA axis when used for the treatment of psoriasis or eczema. Abstract presented at the Annual AAD meeting, Washington, 1996, 10–15 ed.
94. Tan MH, Meador SL, SingerG, et al. An open-label study of the safety and efficacy of limited application of fluticasone propionate ointment, 0.005%, in patients with atopic dermatitis of the face and intertriginous areas. Int J Dermatol.2002;41(11):804–809.
95. Davis AF. Novel formulations for improved therapy. PhD thesis 1995. University of Wales, Cardiff.
96. Marks R, Dykes PJ, Gordon J, et al. Percutaneous penetration from a low-dose supersaturated hydrocortisone acetate formulation. Society of Investigative Dermatology Annual Meeting, Sheffield, September 1992.
97. Duell EA, Astrom A, Griffiths CE, et al. Human skin levels of retinoic acid and cytochrome P-450-derived 4-hydroxyretinoic acid after topical application of retinoic acid in vivo compared to concentrations required to stimulate retinoic acid receptor-mediated transcription in vitro. J Clin Invest 1992;90(4):1269–1274.
98. Shah VP. Transdermal drug delivery system regulatory issues. In: Guy RH, Hadgraft, J eds. Transdermal Drug Delivery, Drugs and the Pharmaceutical Sciences Series 2003, volume 123, Chapter 11. Basal, New York: Marcel Dekker, Inc., pp 361–367.

13 | Drugs for Pain and Inflammation

Michael W. Whitehouse, Mantu Sarkar, and Michael S. Roberts

School of Medicine, University of Queensland, Princess Alexandra Hospital, Woolloongabba, Queensland, Australia

INTRODUCTION

Topical analgesic and anti-inflammatory therapy aims to (1) relieve pain; (2) reduce the clinical signs of inflammation (edema, loss of function, etc.) whether local (e.g., dermatitis) or distal (e.g., synovitis); and (3) facilitate healing. A drug (or placebo) is accepted as useful if symptoms are controlled without impairing healing or inducing other toxicities.

In this chapter, we consider the topical absorption and efficacy of drugs applied to the skin for either a local or systemic effect (Table 1, Fig. 1). Local delivery can help minimize pain and inflammation from superficial injury or due to ongoing skin disorders (e.g., psoriasis, persistent itch). Systemic delivery uses the skin as a portal of entry (rather than site of action) for appropriately formulated drugs or their metabolic precursors (prodrugs). The effects of the drug are then exerted in distal (i.e., nondermal, tissues). This stratagem relies on efficient transdermal (percutaneous) delivery of the drugs and is used when oral drug delivery is either contraindicated (e.g., predisposition to stomach ulcers) or inefficient (e.g., poor absorption, high hepatic first-pass-clearance). Systemic transdermal delivery is most often used with lipophilic potent drugs.

Historically, there is considerable precedent for topical/transdermal therapy to treat both pain and inflammation. Compendia of traditional folklore remedies repeatedly cite the dermal application of ointments, salves, liniments, poultices, medicated plasters, and others, with many whose composition was carefully specified to ensure probable benefit. Some of these undoubtedly contained known pharmacoactive principles (e.g., methyl salicylate, the so-called oil of wintergreen) from

TABLE 1 Usage of (Trans)Dermal Analgesic/Anti-Inflammatory Drugs

Aim	Context
Superficial local action	Prevent sunburn
	Antidote for stings
	Antiseptic /assist healing
Penetrant local action	Analgesia
	Sports injuries
	Antimitotic (psoriasis)
	Antipruritus
	Antiseptic (acne)
Systemic relief at mainly distal sites	Pain
	Inflammation
	Antithrombotic
	Nutritional reinforcement

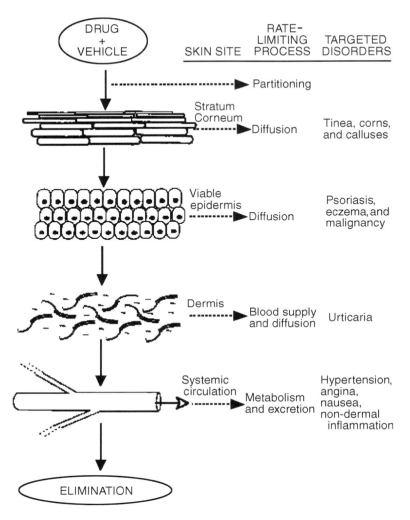

FIGURE 1   Sites of drug action below the skin after topical application.

various plant sources. It was certainly known to the early Greek physicians being cited by Dioscorides of Anazarbos, 1st century CE, the noted botanist whose encyclopedia of materia medica was widely used for centuries after his death [e.g., a Latin edition published at Caesarea, Asia Minor, in 1598, and an English edition in 1655 (1)].

Folk medicines also include many examples of counterirritation/revulsion being used to reduce nagging pains such as toothache. This occurs when substances such as turpentine or methyl salicylate are deliberately applied to the skin to produce not only some degree of superficial inflammation (erythema, vesication, or pustulation) but also induce the desired hyperstimulation analgesia and other counter-

TABLE 2 Formulations for Dermal Application

Format
Dab on: solid, liquid
Spray on: liquid, gel
Rub on/in: liquid, gel, cream, paste
Stick on: Patch
Designed for
Stability
Control/promote penetration
Minimal drug solubility in vehicle/maximal transfer onto skin
Facilitated entry into/through skin
Slow release
Ease of repeated application
Safety, acceptability, etc.
Composed of
Steroids with anti-inflammatory action
Nonsteroidal anti-inflammatory drugs
Analgesics/anesthetics
Adjuncts
Skin penetrants
Preservatives
Antidesiccants
Vehicle reservoir

irritant phenomena (2–4). These can subsequently relieve pain and other symptoms of a deep-seated/distal inflammatory process. The long-standing controversy over the acceptability of applying dimethyl sulfoxide (DMSO) externally was launched by its attested efficacy in relieving systemic inflammatory symptoms (5).

Orally administered nonsteroidal anti-inflammatory drugs (NSAIDs) may adversely affect the gastrointestinal tract (6) and even reduce the life expectancy of patients with rheumatoid arthritis (7). Concerns about NSAID use apply particularly to elderly patients, the main consumers of these drugs (8,9). Most topically applied anti-inflammatory drugs do not cause serious upper gastrointestinal bleeding (10) but may still impair renal function (11).

Table 2 surveys the range of topical products and types of physical formulations used to relieve pain and inflammation.

PHARMACOMETRICS

The bioavailability of a topical/transdermal formation of a pharmacoactive agent is most frequently sought/proven by measuring its physical penetration into/through the skin (either in vivo or in vitro). This requires sensitive microanalytical procedures to identify and quantitate the drug or its prime metabolites after they appear in skin perfusates or the blood or urine whenever direct analysis of transverse dermal sections is not feasible. This type of analysis permits detailed pharmacokinetic studies and rapid comparison between different formulations (see "Dermatopharmacokinetics").

The alternative approach of measuring drug efficacy (i.e., therapeutic responses to a dermally applied formulation) may often provide a more realistic evaluation of drug availability. Efficacy is assessed by physiological or pathometric assays, related to the amount of active drug present at local/distal sites (e.g., reducing an induced inflammation). Vasoconstrictor and blood flow assays are well established for assessing corticosteroid penetration. The major limitation of such assays is saturation of the dose-response curve.

Models of Analgesia
Traditionally, the methods used to evaluate nonsteroid systemic analgesics (as opposed to local anesthetics) (12) in rodents have largely centered on reducing (1) the prostaglandin-mediated "writhing" response to intraperitoneally injected irritants (e.g., acetic acid); (2) nociception (i.e., the expression of a response usually vocal) to pain as induced by pressure on preinflamed tissue; or (3) avoidance response to applied noxia (e.g., tail flick after focused heat irradiation). Most of the analgesics found with these methods are either (1) relatively feeble (e.g., paracetamol) or (2) more readily detected and quantified by other assays (e.g., those for NSAID activity) (13). Topical opioids can be detected by changes in the "licking" response after injecting 20% formalin into tails of mice (14).

Models of Local Inflammation
These have direct relevance in assessing the likely benefits from topically applied analgesics and anti-inflammatory drugs for treating a number of ophthalmic, periodontal, and dermal disorders or the trauma (and pain) associated with surgery upon these tissues (eye, gums, skin).

Ocular Inflammation
Considerable effort has been expended in trying to develop alternative procedures to screen potential corneal irritants that were formerly assessed in the Draize test. However, as a test of both corneal penetration and local efficacy, it is still necessary to have a model of keratitis (corneal inflammation), particularly when it can be shown, for example, that a steroid, dexamethasone, can show much greater drug efficacy in one esterified form (acetate) than another (phosphate) (15).

To elicit corneal inflammation, chemicals such as alkalis or clove oil or physical procedures (laser, scalpel) are applied either to the underlying stroma or to the epithelium. The anti-inflammatory effect is quantified by reduction in corneal radioactivity after drug treatment of one eye versus an untreated eye when the animal's polymorphonuclear leukocytes have been radiolabeled in advance (16). More long-term assays involve photographic recording of induced ulceration or the corneal "haze"—the vision-impairing fibrosis that may occur because of an excessive healing response after ophthalmic surgery (17). Even less exact measurements have to be used when assessing availability/efficacy of topically applied anti-inflammatory drugs to treat postoperative ocular pain (e.g., flurbiprofen) or itching associated with seasonal allergic conjunctivitis (e.g., ketorolac).

Periodontal Disease
Oral bacterial residues can initiate chronic inflammation leading to destruction of the gingival tissue (gum) and resorption of underlying alveolar bone (tooth socket) (18–21). Much of the experimental evaluation of analgesic/anti-inflammatory drugs has been carried out using dogs, nonhuman primates, or, more directly, in dental clinics. The progression of periodontitis is measured by radiographic records of bone loss, changes in levels of proinflammatory agents such as prostaglandin

E2, or elastase in the gingival cervicular fluid and by other clinical parameters. Test drugs are routinely applied in toothpastes (e.g., flurbiprofen) or mouthwashes (e.g., ketorolac)—rarely by direct inunction.

Dermal Inflammation

Various irritants are applied to mouse ears usually as solutions in acetone, ethanol, or DMSO. Drugs are also applied to one treated ear (usually in 5–10 µL acetone, DMSO, etc.) but not to the other (treated with solvent only). Differences between the untreated/treatment edemas are directly measured with calipers or by weighing excised ears after sacrifice. The edemic response can also be quantified by measuring extravasation of serum albumin (usually prelabeled with ^{125}I) into the irritant-treated ears.

Arachidonic acid induces a rapid and severe inflammation peaking within one hour that responds to both indomethacin and dexamethasone. By contrast, the local edema triggered by a phorbol ester develops more slowly and is measured after three to five hours. The later influx of inflammatory cells (peak at 24 hours), mainly PMN leukocytes, is quantified by measuring myeloperoxidase activity in biopsies from the ears (22). These two markers of inflammation, edema and cell infiltration, are temporally separated and may respond differentially to applied drugs (23).

For human studies, the rubefacient action of topically applied nicotinate esters has been often used to evoke transient dermal inflammation (mainly an erythema) by which to evaluate the availability of aspirin and NSAIDs. It is possible to compare several drugs or several formulations of one drug with relatively few experimental subjects (24) by first applying an NSAID to the skin under occlusion, followed by application of a methyl nicotinate solution, and then measuring cutaneous blood flow by laser Doppler velocimetry, The whole technique is essentially noninvasive.

Anti-inflammatory steroids have a vasoconstrictive effect on capillaries, decreasing leakage of cells and fluid into an inflammatory site. This is the basis of the McKenzie-Stoughton skin "blanching" test. Serial dilutions of an alcoholic solution of a test corticosteroid and a standard reference steroid are applied to the forearm. The endpoint is subjective, being the weakest dilution that produces vasoconstriction (25). More objectivity is obtained by using laser Doppler velocimetry to measure the number and velocity of erythrocytes moving through the superficial dermal vasculature before and after blanching by the steroid being evaluated (26). Other, more objective tests of steroid potency include measuring antimitotic activity in hairless mouse dorsal skin, stripped of the stratum corneum (with sticky tape), or the atrophy/thinning induced in mouse ear or human skin, measured with a micrometer (27). These latter measurements may be construed as toxicity, rather than therapeutic assays. A few reports have compared dose-response data from in vivo skin stripping and blanching of human skin (28).

Such dermal-response assays of this type are particularly important for establishing local bioefficacy when corticosteroids are presented as more lipophilic prodrugs (e.g., esters). These are usually less potent than the parent steroid and may require metabolic activation by intradermal esterases.

By contrast, metabolic inactivation in the skin has been rarely used in designing prodrugs. One example is fluocortin butyl ester, with a 21-COOButyl group replacing the usual 21-CH$_2$OH of an active steroid, which shows topical anti-inflammatory activity but is intradermally transformed to the inactive 21-carboxylate which then passes into the general circulation. This enormously enhances the safety margin for its extended use in patients at risk from systemic (i.e., extradermal) side effects of steroid drugs (e.g., children, pregnant women, or the elderly) (29).

Models of Systemic (Nondermal) Inflammation

In these models, an inflammation is experimentally established in nondermal tissues; the assays then disclose the bioavailability of active drug at the site of inflammation after its dermal application.

In small rodents, it is important that the drug application site is chosen so that minimal amounts of the active drug will be removed in the normal course of grooming, lest the experiment be inadvertently transformed into one in which the drug is ingested orally as well as transdermally. Some experimentalists use restraint collars (so-called Elizabethan ruffs) to prevent autogrooming of the shaved upper dorsum; one of the more convenient sites to apply a transdermal formulation. Animals must then be isolated from each other (to prevent "cross-licking"), but this can be stressful to them. Occlusive dressings on small rodents may be chewed, but may be more useful on guinea pigs and large animals. Adding a bitter principle in the test formulation may reduce its removal by licking. Thus penetrant enhancers with a bitter taste such as cineole (eucalyptol) and DMSO often seem more effective than bland-tasting alternatives (e.g., isopropanol) for increasing the apparent potency of a neutral-tasting formulation.

Acute Inflammation

These models detect acute-acting drugs such as aspirin and the NSAIDs, rather than corticosteroids. They are based on inducing a superficial irritation readily assessed by physical measurements, rather than detailed biochemical analyses. Examples are the initiation of a fast-developing edema (over 2–5 hours) by injection of a carrageenan solution or a dispersion of kaolin, to increase vascular permeability, activate complement, and attract leukocytes.

When irritants are injected into the rear paws of rodents, the consequent edema is measured by increase in paw volume. Alternatively, they can be inoculated subdermally into shaved skin of rats, guinea pigs, or rabbits, previously injected intravenously with a reagent to label intravascular proteins (e.g., Evans blue or [^{125}I] albumin). The dermal inflammation is then quantified by measuring the blue dye or the accumulation of ^{125}I, both within the site of irritation and (as a control) in an equal area of adjacent nonirritated skin.

Another assay for dermal inflammation, rather more difficult to quantify but still useful for clinical investigations, is based on inducing an erythema (rather than a measurable edema) by UV irradiation or rubbing in a rubefacient (e.g., a nicotinate ester).

Chronic Inflammation

These assays are more relevant for assessing the suitability of drug formulations to treat established arthritis, inflammatory bowel disease, asthma, and some syndromes involving neurogenic inflammation, etc.

In rodents, two good models of periarticular inflammation are the autoimmune disorders caused either by sensitization to collagen type II (mice, rats) (30) or the more severe polyarthritis that develops in some (not all) strains of rats inoculated intralymphatically with a mycobacterial adjuvant (31). Rather less drug developmental work has been undertaken using the collagen-induced arthritis partly because it is a "fickle" disease, not being expressed fully in all animals challenged with this autoantigen (usually chick or bovine collagen type II) and also being difficult to quantify. By contrast, the adjuvant arthritis is expressed in a susceptible rat strain by gross, readily measured swelling of ankle, tail, and all four paws.

After dermal application, it is possible to recognize the "worth" of certain anti-inflammatory agents or antoxidants, which—if given orally—do not adequately survive first-pass metabolism (32) or are inadequately absorbed from the gut (e.g., prostanoids) (33) or metal-containing drugs (34–36).

SURVEY OF SOME TRANSDERMAL DRUGS

In this section, the emphasis is mainly on the pharmacoefficacy of each active agent rather than the technology of formulation. Table 3 illustrates several various modalities for effective delivery through the skin.

Placebos

A placebo is defined by its "effect," namely, the improvement that many patients exhibit, or feel, after receiving something that they believe will provide some benefit (41–44). Implicit in this definition is the lack of a specific effect—i.e., one that is supported by some theory about its precise mechanism of action.

In the present context, we must recognize the potentially extensive placebo component associated with the dermal application of agents that seem therapeutic (camphor, eucalyptus oil, menthol, etc.); give the sensation of warmth (methyl salicylate, DMSO); have a pseudoanesthetic effect after an initial painful stimulus (mustard oil, capsaicin); or just smell pleasant (many tinctures). Some of these topically applied placebos, although lacking intrinsic analgesic/anti-inflammatory activity per se, may still be useful adjuncts to other modes of therapy—not least by reducing the requirement for more noxious drugs (e.g., gastroirritant NSAIDs).

TABLE 3 Various Modalities for Delivery of Transdermal Drugs

Characteristic/method	Drug	Potency amplification	Reference
Elastic liposomes	Diclofenac	2-fold	13
DMSO as solvent	Metal drugs		34,36, many patents
Solid lipid nanoparticles	Prednicarbate	Great potential of SLN to improve drug absorption by the skin	37
Diethylamine salts	Rubisal (salicylate), Emulgel (diclofenac)		
Di-isopropanolamine salt	Piroxicam (Feldene gel)		
Inclusion of Anesthetics	Lidocaine ocular formulation		38
Vasoconstrictors	Salicylic acid, diclofenac	Extensive	39, several patents
Penetration enhancer (e.g., 1% limonene and 1% cineole)	Ibuprofen, flufenamic acid	Significant (5-fold)	40, many patents

These "properties" of placebos must be considered when objectively evaluating any transdermal (or indeed many other) therapies. In working with animals, it is relatively simple to apply mock placebos in the form of "dummy formulations," such as vehicle/excipient mixtures, to control groups. This is essential to determine the contribution of (1) the act of rubbing into the skin, and (2) components of these placebos/"negative controls" to the overall pharmacological actions of "active" formulations. It is, however, quite another problem to disentangle placebo effects from specific pharmacological effects in the true clinical context, particularly when the "placebo effect" may actually be negative(!) or (the attention given by) the doctor/prescriber is actually a significant placebo.

Data suggest that some 40% to 60% of patients with soft-tissue and local joint disorders respond to placebo and that 60% to 80% respond to active NSAIDs (8). The placebo effect is more dramatic than with oral preparations—so that it has been suggested that patients should first use the cheapest embrocations; only when this is inadequate should a more expensive transdermal NSAID be prescribed (45).

Local Irritants

These are agents that have a nonspecific effect on the cells of the skin, mucous membranes, or superficial wounds. They release inflammatory amines from mast cells, induce hyperemia (so-called rubefacient action), and/or trigger counterirritant phenomena so providing useful analgesia. Irritants that are not considered placebos include turpentine oil (from several species of *Pinus*, Pinaceae) and various plant essences (oils) such as clove, wintergreen, cajeput, origanum, camphor, and mustard oil, provided they reduce sensations of pain. This can be partly by specific effects, as discussed below, and also by blunting the sensation of pain with other perceptions associated with applying the (counter) irritant, e.g., warmth, massage, penetrating odor, etc. The variable composition of some of these irritants, as harvested from natural sources, raises doubts about their reliability. They are increasingly being replaced by defined chemical entities such as capsaicin and methyl salicylate, much diluted and blended into liniments/creams/ointments, for more reproducible action.

Rubefacients increase skin capillary blood flow by acting as local peripheral vasodilators. As such, they may have some role in enhancing dermal absorption. Well-characterized rubefacients include tetrahydrofurfuryl(thurfyl) alcohol and various esters of nicotinic acid.

Refrigerants are agents that induce a strong cooling sensation when applied to the skin and "numb" the sensation of pain. Besides ice, two examples with long-standing usage are menthol from various mint oils and camphor (ketone), extracted from plants or produced synthetically. They are usually administered at concentrations of 0.1% to 3% (w/w) in the topical formulation.

Some skin "irritants" may stimulate immunoreactivity within the skin mediated by epidermal Langerhans cells, keratinocytes, and other specialist cells residing in the dermis (46, 47). These immunoactive skin cells produce a range of cytokines—some that are proinflammatory and others that are certainly anti-inflammatory [e.g., interleukin (IL)-4, IL-l0). If these pass into the general circulation, they might provide a further, nonneural link between the skin "irritant" and a distal responsive target organ.

Capsaicin

Capsaicin (*trans*-8-methyl-*N*-vanillyl-6-nonene-amide) is the pungent principle in the fruits of various species of *Capsicum solanaceae* (e.g., paprika, cayenne, other red peppers). Paradoxically, it is both a powerful irritant, causing intense pain, and also a pain-desensitizing agent. It is incorporated into a number of commercial topical formulations to provide temporary relief of pain of rheumatism, arthritis, lumbago, muscular aches, sprains, sporting injuries, and postherpes neuralgia. It is used either alone or in combination with various rubefacients that cause peripheral vasodilatation and give an added local warming effect.

Capsaicin itself is not a vasodilator but will inhibit irritant-induced vasodilation (48). There is a sustained neurogenic component contributing to both the pain and the inflammation in many forms of arthritis through the release of substance P and other neurokinins (49). Thus, any effects of capsaicin that locally deplete these neuropeptides (50, 51) may be anti-inflammatory per se, in addition to its analgesic/counterirritant action. In clinical studies, capsaicin creams (0.025–0.075%) seemed more effective for treating painful joints in osteoarthritis than rheumatoid arthritis (52,53).

The undesirable sensations of burning and pain with the first application of capsaicin are largely caused by the massive release of neuropeptides. The analgesic/anti-inflammatory effects are obtained only after repeated application of sufficient capsaicin to totally deplete, and then prevent reaccumulation of, pro-inflammatory neuropeptides within the sensory nerve fibers. This transition from (hyper)sensitivity to desensitization provides another example of the depletion mechanism of counterirritancy (discussed in Reference 3) that can be evoked by topically applied agents. Their potency usually precludes systemic administration.

Pure capsaicin should not be confused with capsicum oleoresin, a by-product of purified capsaicin containing 80 or more components. Although this resin may elicit counterirritation with vasodilation, in contrast to capsaicin, some resin components may antagonize capsaicin itself (54). Capsaicin may have other pharmacological effects unrelated to its actions on sensory afferent neurons (e.g., inhibition of platelet aggregation) (55). This is also a property of aspirin and many NSAIDs.

Narcotic Analgesics

Fentanyl is a lipophilic semisynthetic opioid with a short half-life after bolus administration (l–2 hours). A transdermal administration system that delivers 25 to 100 μg/hr is commercially available for management of cancer pain and others. Serum fentanyl levels increase gradually, plateauing after 12 hours, and decline slowly after 24 hours, as would be expected if the drug enters into a transcutaneous depot that then maintains the plasma concentration (56). The dosage interval is 48 to 72 hours with the 100 μg/hr fentanyl patch providing a level of analgesia approximately that attained with 2 to 4 mg/hr IV morphine (57).

Buprenorphine is also available in a transdermal matrix patch formulation (NORSPAN®) for managing pain unresponsive to nonopioid analgesics (58). Patches are available to deliver 5 to 20 μg/hr or for an entire week to treat moderate to severe arthritis and back pain.

The limitations of this transdermal system include cost, need for an alternative short-acting opioid to suppress breakthrough pain, and poor adhesion to the skin in some patients. The U.S. Food and Drug Administration has issued an alert for overdose of fentanyl concerning side effects including death.

Other analgesics are still being developed for transdermal delivery. There are continuing problems of possible interactions with a range of central acting drugs (e.g., other narcotic analgesics, phenothiazines, tranquilizers, MAO inhibitors, tricyclic antidepressants, even alcohol).

Dimethyl Sulfoxide

Topical use of this drug is still largely restricted to treating inflammation in horses and dogs. It can behave as a "sacrificial substrate" to neutralize oxidative reactants generated by activated inflammatory cells. Thus the reaction of hydroxyl radicals (OH˙) with DMSO generates methane or formaldehyde, among other products (59).

In view of these potential transformations, DMSO should not be considered an inert solvent after transdermal absorption.

Diluting DMSO with water generates considerable heat. The perceived warming of the subcutaneous tissues after topical application provides a very positive placebo effect. When applied to the skin, it is almost instantly bioavailable because of the rapid permeation of the dermal barriers. Consequently, it has been used as a reagent/probe to crudely assess the rate of blood return from (sites of application in) peripheral tissues to the taste receptors in the palate. The taste is not of the sulfoxide but traces of sulfide impurity, which is also formed by bioreduction in vivo.

The remarkable potency of DMSO, used at high concentrations ($\geq 0:60\%$), as a penetration enhancer for corticosteroids and other topical drugs is probably attributable to its effects on the barrier lipids (60).

Topical Aspirin

> "Pain is the raison d'être for aspirin in the marketplace." –N. Varey

Aspirin is an effective analgesic at lower doses than what is required for anti-inflammatory activity. Analgesics were formerly believed to relieve only nociceptive pain, acting peripherally. However, there is now evidence from experimental studies with topical aspirin therapy that even aspirin may alleviate neurogenic pain.

The direct application of crushed aspirin in chloroform (61) or diethyl ether (62) to affected hyperpathic areas of skin in patients with shingles provides significant pain relief within 20 minutes and lasting four to eight hours. These solvents prove to be superior suspending vehicles partly by acting as cleansing agents to remove cutaneous lipids, but also by delivering the aspirin as a fine powder adhering to the skin close to cutaneous nociceptors.

Patches containing aspirin, applied to the upper arm, chest, or thigh have been shown to suppress platelet thromboxane production in normal volunteers. Analyses of residual aspirin showed that the patches could deliver more than 30 mg of aspirin daily when they contained added limonene as a penetration enhancer (63). Applying aspirin in this patch format conferred stability, whereas application of the aspirin in alcoholic vehicles required much larger doses (≥ 750 mg) to attain similar antithrombotic efficacy, because of spontaneous hydrolysis of the aspirin in these vehicles. This antiplatelet effect of aspirin would retard local liberation of inflammagenic agents (e.g., serotonin, PAF, thromboxane itself) when platelets are destroyed (as innocent bystanders) within an inflammatory locus. Topical aspirin may also inhibit skin carcinogenesis caused by UVB radiation by inhibiting various UVB signalling pathways (64).

Topical Salicylates

Methyl salicylate is the active principle of wintergreen and sweet birch oils, historically obtained by distilling *Gaultheria* leaves or *Betula* bark. It is included, often as principal component, in many traditional topical remedies for muscle pain and rheumatism. Today, the main source is esterification of synthetic salicylic acid.

Being liquid and a phenol, it is considered a counterirritant and applied in various liniments, gels, lotions, or ointments in concentrations ranging from 10%

to 60%. Because strenuous physical exercise and heat increase its transdermal absorption, athletes who use it prophylactically may be at risk for salicylate intoxication. Its use is declining among nonathletes who seem to prefer the nonodorous and less irritating lipophilic salicylate salts. These are also more potent than the methyl ester (65) as anti-inflammatory agents. This is partly attributable to the low plasma salicylate concentrations likely to be achieved after the topical application of commercially available ester formulations (66). A particular problem with the methyl ester is the risk of (subclinical) poisoning by the methanol and formaldehyde formed as principal metabolites after dermal absorption. Unfortunately, some of the less toxic salicylate esters (isopropyl, menthyl) show even less anti-inflammatory activity after dermal application, probably due to lower rates of hydrolysis in vivo.

Another potentially toxic ester is 2-hydroxyethyl (glycol) salicylate, still being used in many topical analgesic formulations because it is less hydrophobic than methyl salicylate and more readily absorbed (67). Its main metabolite, ethylene glycol (ethane-1,2-diol), formed by various esterases, is now proscribed for human consumption because it can generate nephrotoxic oxalic acid in vivo.

By contrast, the salicylate salts have been developed as alternative analgesics because their counterions (e.g., diethylamine, triethanolamine) provide the requisite lipophilicity to promote dermal uptake and are considered potentially less noxious (68). Triethanolamine itself is classed as an analgesic [see *Merck Index* (69)]. These salts are used in topical formulations at concentrations up to 15%. Unlike the esters, they are not rubefacient, odiferous, or greasy. In contrast to salicylic acid, they are not keratolytic. Although widely used in over-the-counter topical "rubs," their pharmacological activity is as yet poorly documented (70). Their systemic toxicity is assumed to be less than that of salicylic acid (71).

Topical NSAIDS

Several reviews are available that discuss the formulation of these drugs for dermal application (72) and their pharmacological evaluation after transdermal delivery in both animal models (73,74) and clinical studies (Fig. 2) (8,75,76,77). These drugs are applied dermally in formulations containing the free acid (e.g., biphenylacetic acid, 3% w/w; piroxicam, 0.5–1.5%; indomethacin, 1–5%; ketoprofen, 2.5%), a lipophilic counterion (e.g., diethylammonium diclofenac, 1%; ketorolac tromethamine, 2%), or, more rarely, as an ester (e.g., etofenamate, 5%) (Table 4).

An interesting role reversal is the use of salicylic acid/NSAIDs as acidic counterions (anion) to facilitate the dermal uptake of basic drugs/cations such as pharmacoactive transition metal ions or nitrogenous bases (see "Benzydamine" and "Metal-Based Drugs").

The pH of the skin usually affects penetration (and bioavailability) of the free acids to a greater degree than the ionic (salt) or ester forms.

A peculiar feature of NSAIDs as used to treat rheumatic diseases is that there is often no direct relationship between drug concentration in either the blood or synovial fluid and the clinical efficacy (84). This means that transdermal NSAIDs will ultimately have to be assessed by beneficial effects on clinical parameters, rather than more readily obtained comparator indices such as bioavailability, tissue levels, etc.

These topical formulations were introduced largely to mitigate adverse reactions of NSAIDs expressed within the gastrointestinal tract. However, even the currently available parenteral NSAIDs (especially acids) may cause gastrotoxic effects, being secreted into the stomach in the gastric juices after transdermal absorption.

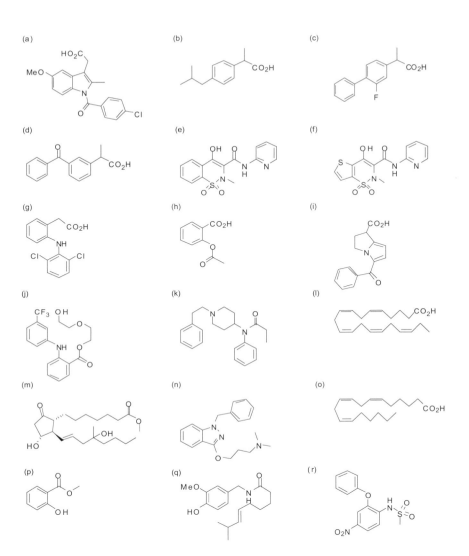

FIGURE 2 NSAIDs for dermal use: (**A**) indomethacin, (**B**) ibuprofen, (**C**) flurbiprofen, (**D**) keto-profen, (**E**) piroxicam, (**F**) tenoxicam, (**G**) diclofenac, (**H**) aspirin, (**I**) ketorolac, (**J**) etofenamate, (**K**) fentanyl, (**L**) eicosapentanenoic acid, (**M**) misoprostol, (**N**) benzydamine, (**O**) gamma-linolenic acid, (**P**) methyl salicylate, (**Q**) capsaicin, (**R**) nimesulide.

TABLE 4 Some Transdermal NSAID Formulations

Drug name (trade name)	Formulation
Benzydamine[a] (Difflam)	3% and 5% w/w
Diclofenac sodium (Voltaren Ophtha)	0.1% w/v eye drops, ampoule
	Also contains boric acid, polyoxyl 35 castor oil, trometamol, water. Multidose bottle also contains thimerosal
Diclofenac sodium (Dencorub)[a]	1% w/w tube
Diclofenac (Emulgel)	DF diethylammonium gel 1.16% w/w
Diclofenac hydroxyethyl-pyrrolidone[a] (Dicloreum tissugel)	180 mg plaster
Etofenamate (Etofen gel)[a]	5–10% w/w
Felbinac (Traxam)[a]	1–3% w/w
Flurbiprofen Na (Ocufen solution)	0.03% eye drops, bottle
Ibuprofen (Nurofen gel)[a]	5% w/w tube
Indomethacin (Elmetacin)[a]	1% w/w solution aerosol pump actuated
Ketoprofen (Orudis gel)[a]	1–5% w/w gel/ointment
Naproxen (Naprossene)[a]	10–12% w/w
Nifumic acid (Niflugel R)	2.5% w/w
Oxyphenbutazone (Tanderil)	10% w/w
Piroxicam (Feldene gel)[a]	0.5–2% w/w
Nimesulide (Sulidin gel)	1% (80,81,82)
Triethanolamine salicylate (Dencorub)	10% w/w Triethanolamine salicylate
Tenoxicam	Oleic acid, propylene glycol (83)

[a]Many trade names are available in Reference (8) and some overlap more than one product. For example, "Dencorub" for both diclofenac or methyl salicylate. *Source*: From Refs. 8, 78, 79.

It is still one of the ironies of contemporary medicine that the NSAIDs are, with some exceptions, largely ineffective in controlling inflammatory diseases of the skin. Moreover, to the dermatologist, they present themselves more often as agents inciting dermal inflammation(!) after their oral/rectal administration (85). Some of these NSAIDs are potentially fatal (e.g., causing Lyell's or Steven-Johnson syndromes involving the skin). The "casualty list" of NSAIDs that have been withdrawn from the clinic for, among other reasons, their adverse effects on the skin after oral administration includes alclofenac, fenclofenac, indoprofen, isoxicam, myalex, pirprofen, phenylbutazone, and zomepirac.

Among the fenamates, only meclofenamate containing two chlorine atoms on one benzene ring seems to cause these problems. It is unfortunate that it is only rarely possible to anticipate likely skin/systemic problems that may be idiosyncratic to man, after exposing experimental animals to dermally applied drugs, beyond recognizing immediate local (irritancy, antimitotic action, etc.) or overall percutaneous toxicity (86). Despite these problems, new topical NSAIDs have been developed, notably in Spain and Japan, such as amides of ketoprofen (piketoprofen) and ibuprofen (aminoprofen) and esters of ibuprofen (pimaprofen) (87).

Benzydamine

This is a basic drug, in contrast to most NSAIDs. Interest in this drug for both topical and transdermal use largely predated the development of topical NSAIDs (88,89). In laboratory animals, it mimics the NSAID acids in controlling the pain, edema, fever, and granuloma formations caused by various inflammatory stimuli (90). Like the acidic NSAIDs, it also inhibits platelet aggregation (91) and shows a local anesthetic action when used topically. The hydrochloride salt is used locally (a) in creams or gels (3–5%) to relieve traumatic conditions such as sprains and contusions and some inflammatory disorders (myalgia, bursitis), and also (b) in solution to treat painful conditions affecting the mouth and throat.

In the adjuvant arthritis model in rats, the hydrochloride exhibits poor systemic anti-inflammatory activity after dermal application. However, its transdermal potency is much increased by coapplication of sodium salicylate. By forming an ion pair with the salicylate anion, the skin penetration and systemic bioefficacy of the benzydamine cation is substantially enhanced.

Polyunsaturated Lipids

Certain plant-sourced oils, rich in gamma-linolenic acid (GLA) and fish oils, rich in eicosapentenoic acid (EPA), show modest anti-inflammatory activity when given as dietary supplements (up to 20 g/day) (92–94). The effects of these polyunsaturated fatty acids (PUFA) derived from plant/fish oils are primarily on the polymorphonuclear leukocytes (neutrophils) and on their generation of inflammatory mediators. Clinical trials have indicated that dietary supplementation with these oils may confer some benefit in those inflammatory disorders involving neutrophilic inflammation such as rheumatoid arthritis, psoriasis, cystic fibrosis, and inflammatory bowel disease.

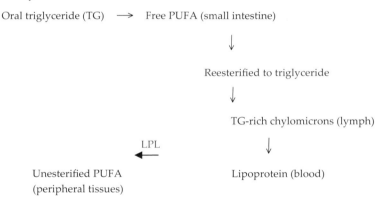

A particular problem with supplying these PUFA as dietary lipid is that they must progress through the sequence: that is, normal digestion, first liberates, then locks away the therapeutic PUFA in newly synthesized circulating lipoprotein until it is released by lipoprotein lipase (LPL). This is an enzyme bound to endothelium, particularly in striated muscle and adipose tissue, to channel newly released PUFA into these tissues.

Furthermore, some locally produced inflammatory cytokines, particularly tissue necrosis factor (95) and IL-1 (96), inhibit LPL. As a consequence, the bioavailability of dietary-sourced anti-inflammatory PUFA within an inflammatory site may be so low as to render almost useless the popular stratagem of supplementing the diet with PUFA-rich oils. One way to circumvent this problem is to ensure the PUFAs are provided by a route not involving either intestinal lipoprotein synthesis or requiring LPL function.

It is possible to demonstrate significant anti-inflammatory activity of PUFA derivatives given transdermally to polyarthritic rats (97). The same amounts of PUFA given orally were, by contrast, almost inactive. Methyl esters of active PUFAs are rather irritant to the skin, probably the consequence of local autooxidation. However, zinc salts of these PUFAs were well tolerated when applied to the skin as solutions/dispersions in DMSO glycerol (4:1, v/v). The corresponding triglycerides when mixed with various penetration enhancers (e.g., cineole, isopropanol, methyl salicylate) were almost nonirritant but considerably less active than the zinc salts, probably reflecting low lipase activity in the dermis.

The plant-derived PUFA [i.e., GLA (18:3 n-6] or its isomer, α-linolenic acid (18:3 n-3) probably requires further biotransformation in vivo, yielding either DGLA (20:3 n-6) or EPA (20:5 n-3) to manifest their anti-inflammatory effects. These 20-carbon acids can then regulate the production of inflammatory eicosanoids and cytokines by several independent mechanisms.

Arachidonic acid (20:4) has been applied topically (0.1–2%) under occlusive dressings to successfully treat psoriasis, probably by raising local prostaglandin E2 levels (98).

Prostanoids

One of the effects of DGLA or EPA is to compete with arachidonate for the cyclooxygenase enzymes (COX-I, COX-2), forming alternate prostaglandins, namely, PGE1 or PGE3 respectively, in place of PGE2 (derived from arachidonate). Both PGE1 and PGE3 are less proinflammatory than PGE2 but, like PGE2, they can down-regulate production of inflammatory cytokines. The very short half-life of these prostaglandins severely limits their potential as exogenous anti-inflammatory agents. However, relatively long-lived analogs, such as the methyl ester of a PGE1 analog, misoprostol, retain their cytokine-inhibiting action (99) and display anti-inflammatory activity in arthritic rats when delivered transdermally (33).

Misoprostol has been extensively used as a cytoprotectant to reduce the incidence of gastric bleeding from oral (and even parenteral) NSAIDs (100). Although it shows antiarthritic activity in the rat AIA model at relatively high doses applied transdermally (200 µg/kg) given alone (33), it is a very useful synergist at lower doses (50 µg/kg) for other agents, e.g., antioxidants given either orally or transdermally.

Metal-Based Drugs

The limited uptake of nonalkali metal ions from the gut is largely protective but can occasionally be pathogenic, e.g., the zinc deficiency disease acrodermatitis enteropathica caused by lack of an intestinal zinc transporter (36). Zinc itself may be made available transdermally by application of lipophilic complexes or more simply by rubbing on zinc monoglycerolate (ZMG). This alkoxide has a crystal structure resembling graphite, being two-dimensional and, like graphite, showing remarkable lubricity. This means it can be readily applied in the dry state as well as be dispersed in glycerol-containing vehicles (to retard hydrolysis to the less penetrating zinc oxide). ZMG shows useful anti-inflammatory activity (35), probably by reinforcing the supply of zinc needed to naturally combat inflammation (101).

Copper ions are also part of the body's endogenous anti-inflammatory repertoire and may likewise become insufficient to combat a severe inflammation for various reasons (dietary lack, poor absorption, excessive elimination, etc.). The traditional copper bracelet may provide a slow-release depot on and within the skin, but only if the underlying green stain (=copper salts of fatty and amino acids) is retained (i.e., by not varnishing the inside of the bracelet or excessive washing of the skin).

A complex of copper with salicylic acid is available in Australia either in alcoholic or DMSO formulations to treat inflammation. Efficacy has been proved in animals (34). A related complex formed with phenylbutazone is used to treat inflammation in horses.

Other pharmacoactive metals can be applied transdermally (e.g., Pt), showing efficacy in small animals (36). A key factor in successful transdermal delivery is ensuring intradermal lability of the complex, through a push-pull mechanism as shown by the scheme:

$$\text{Lipophilic ML}_A \rightarrow \text{Intradermal ML}_A \rightarrow \text{Plasma ML}_P$$

where LA is ligand for application of the metal M and LP is a physiological ligand that decomposes MLA at neutral pH.

The lipophilicity of the applied complex (MLA) first ensures dermal uptake ("push"), and the intradermal formation of a more water-soluble complex MLp by ligand exchange, effectively extracts the metal into the general circulation ("pull"). In the case of ZMG, these extracting ligands include albumin, citrate, and histidine (102). With copper salicylates, they include albumin and histidine and also tissue thiols.

Miscellaneous Agents
Nicotine
Ulcerative colitis, a chronic inflammatory disease of the lower bowel prevalent in 0.1% of the population, has been identified as a disease of nonsmokers or ex-smokers (sic). By contrast, the incidence of Crohn's disease, a closely related inflammatory disorder affecting any part of the gastrointestinal tract, may be higher in smokers. With the availability of transdermal nicotine delivery "patches," it has been possible to identify a likely benefit of nicotine as an adjunct for treating ulcerative colitis (103,104), notably by reducing IL-2 synthesis (105). Other diseases that might be treated with transdermal nicotine include Parkinson's, Alzheimer's, and the Tourette syndrome.

Immunoregulants/Calcineurin Inhibitors
Cyclosporin A is a natural cyclic decapeptide obtained from various fungi imperfecta and has long been a mainstay of supportive therapy for organ transplantation: the chief problem being its potential nephrotoxicity at doses required (5–12 mg/kg/day) (106). It is also used at lower doses as a "third-line agent" to treat rheumatoid arthritis and other autoimmune diseases (107).

Unlike most polypeptides, it is quite soluble in many organic solvents (acetone, chloroform, ethanol, ether). It is therefore an effective antiarthritic drug when applied dermally to rats in ethanol–propylene glycol or DMSO-glycerol (35). Given in this manner, it causes very little nephrotoxicity, in contrast to giving it orally.

Dermal formulations of pimecrolimus (Elidel®) and tacrolimus (Protopic®) have been recently introduced as safe alternatives to topical corticosteroids for treating atopic dermatitis (108–110).

Emu Oil

This is a traditional medicine of the Australian Aboriginals for treating muscular pain. The oil is derived by rendering the body fat. Its pharmacoactivity can be quite variable depending on the emu's diet/husbandry and severity of the rendering process (involving heat, bleaching agents, etc.). Animal studies have indicated it may contain systemically active antiarthritic factors, effective after dermal application particularly when admixed with 10% to 15% v/v of a penetration enhancer (cineole, methyl salicylate, 2-propanol, etc.) (32,111). Its local anti-inflammatory activity is demonstrated by the reduction of auricular edema in mice induced with topical croton oil (112,113). It also promotes wound healing after scalding.

Tea Tree Oil

This is another traditional Australian Aboriginal medication obtained from the native shrub, *Melaleuca alternifolia* (114). An essential oil, rich in terpinoids, is obtained by steam distillation of the leaves. Undiluted oil reduced histamine-induced inflammation in human skin (115,116) and mouse ears (117), and contact hypersensitivity reactions in mice (118) and human skin (119).

Removing the low boiling monoterpenes by distillation under nitrogen generates a more concentrated, nonallergenic product, Megabac®, retaining anti-inflammatory, analgesic, and anesthetic activities. It is available in Australia for pain relief by topical application (NeuMedix®) as a 5% w/w solution in soya bean oil.

Permeation of the main component terpinen-4-ol through human skin is influenced by the composition of the tea tree oil (TTO) formulations (120) .

The penetration of TTO is addressed in a separate chapter (Chapter 20).

Peppermint Oil

This provides yet another example where the natural product provides both the active drug and a permeation enhancer.

Significant analgesic effects of peppermint oil in alcohol have been described after application to the forehead and temples (121). The undiluted oil (containing 10% menthol) has been used to control post-herpetic neuralgia, involving an irritable nociceptor type of pathology (122).

D-Glucosamine

This amino sugar is a component of hyaluronan and a precursor of D-galactosamine, a component of the cartilage chondroitin sulfates A and C. Many patients are convinced glucosamine sulfate alleviates the pain of their osteoarthritis when taken orally. However, several large-scale trials have failed to establish that oral glucosamine hydrochloride, with or without chondroitin sulfate, is superior to placebo for treating knee pain (123).

Nevertheless, topical application of glucosamine sulfate, with chondroitin sulfate and camphor, in a FUSOME™ delivery system (Arthro-AID®) is reported to reduce knee pain after four weeks ($P = 0.03$) and 8 weeks ($P = 0.002$) (124).

Cartilage-Derived Antigens

Molecular fragments of cartilage, such as those present in osteoarthritis, can suppress inflammation in animal models and patients (125). A topical cream containing 30% cartilage-derived antigens (CDA) in a hydrophobic carrier (Biodermex®) proved very effective ($P < 0.002$) for reducing erythemic skin inflammation. This topical anti-inflammatory activity may involve interaction of CDA with dermal dendritic cells (126).

DERMATOPHARMACOKINETICS

Pharmacokinetic models used to describe anti-inflammatory and other drug absorption can be classified into four groups. The first group is predominately concerned with the kinetics of transport through stratum corneum or epidermis and has usually been expressed in terms of Fick's law. Much of the emphasis has been directed to better defining the relationship between the permeability coefficient of solutes and their physicochemical properties as well as alternative routes of administration. The work of Yano et al. (127) suggests that the absorption of eight salicylates and 10 NSAIDs through human skin in vivo can be related to the logarithm of the n-octanol water partition coefficient. Singh and Roberts (128) have confirmed that a similar relationship exists for excised skin.

Reigelman (129) has evaluated the early in vivo percutaneous absorption data for a range of solutes including topical steroids by using the second model type, a pharmacokinetic rate approach using plasma and urinary excretion data. He showed that the urinary excretion for cortisol after topical and intradermal administration was consistent, with the terminal urinary excretion rate-time profile being determined by the absorption rate constant of cortisol through the skin, i.e., "flip-flop," or absorption-limited, kinetics. Studies by Cooper (130) and Chandrasekan et al. (131) have developed these concepts further either to estimate in vivo skin permeability or to predict the time course of transdermal drug delivery. Cooper and Berner (132) have described the pharmacokinetics of skin penetration when a finite dose is applied.

The third pharmacokinetic model considers a combination of penetration through the stratum corneum and removal by the dermal blood supply. The models in this area include those based on diffusion (49–51) and a representation of the skin epidermis, blood supply, and systemic body as compartments (52,53).

The fourth model attempts to examine the kinetics associated with drug delivery to local subcutaneous structures after topical administration (54), where the representation has predominantly been as compartments for the individual tissue levels (55). Singh and Roberts (128) showed that all NSAIDs applied dermally penetrate to a depth of 3 to 4 mm below the applied site, distribution to deeper tissues being mainly by the systemic blood supply. This model accounts for findings that synovial tissue levels of topical applied diclofenac (56) and biphenyl acetic acid (57) can be attributed to the systemic blood supply.

Subsequent work (58) suggests that deep tissue concentrations for disparate solutes are difficult to predict directly from solute structures with any certainty in vivo. Using an isolated perfused limb preparation, Cross et al. (143) showed that the depth of penetration of solutes was decreased as blood flow increased. This finding is consistent with that of Singh and Roberts (144), in which it was shown that the depth of penetration of solutes could be increased if coadministered with a vasoconstrictor. Cross et al. (145) showed that the protein binding of solutes also affected the depth of penetration. Diffusion of solutes between tissues is not the only mechanism by which drugs are transported to deeper tissues. In some subcutaneous structures, drug delivery to deeper tissues occurs via the presence of a local blood supply (62).

In general, absorption of many solutes into the skin can be approximated to zero-order kinetics, as the loss of the applied substance is often relatively small over the time period of application. Guy et al. (147) have suggested that the systemic delivery of scopolamine, nitroglycerin, clonidine, and estradiol follows zero-order kinetics for between 1 and 7 days after application. They point out that one area which has been relatively poorly studied in terms of dermatopharmacokinetics is the first-pass effect. The limited in vivo data suggest that nitroglycerin has a first pass of between 10% and 50% through skin. A substantially higher first pass is evident for methyl salicylate, as shown in the work of Megwa et al. (148). With repeated application, the epidermal penetration of salicylic acid changes with time as a consequence of the keratoplastic and keratolytic properties of the agent (65).

A number of more recent studies have used microdialysis to examine the penetration of topically applied solutes into deeper tissues in both animals and in man. Early n studies showed dermal nicotine concentration time profiles after transdermal nicotine application (150). Cross et al. (151) showed significant direct penetration of salicylate from topically applied methyl salicylate in human volunteers. Significant levels of salicylate was detected in the dermis and subcutaneous tissue of volunteers treated with a methyl salicylate formulation were much higher than those seen with application of a triethanolamine salicylate formulation and about 30-fold higher than the plasma concentrations (152).

Muller et al. (153) measured diclofenac concentrations in the superficial and deep dermis directly below the site of topical diclofenac application to 20 healthy volunteers by in vivo microdialysis over five hours. No correlation between area under the concentration-time curve in a defined layer and the depth of probe insertion. A later work showed diclofenac penetration into underlying muscle (154) and used microdialysis to measure ibuprofen muscle and subcutaneous tissue concentrations after oral and topical applications (155). Substance penetration into such layers can be affected by skin integrity as shown for salicylic acid (156). The effectiveness of iontophoretic delivery of propranolol to human skin in vivo has also been studied using cutaneous microdialysis (157). Boelsma et al. (158) also applied microdialysis to study the percutaneous penetration of methyl nicotinate into human skin in vivo. The concentration-time courses of 8-methoxypsoralen

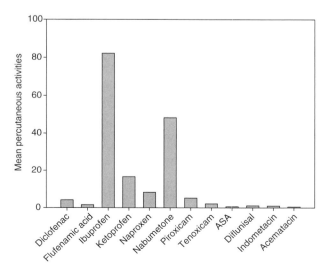

FIGURE 3 Percutaneous activities as defined by the product of maximum flux and intrinsic activities in tissues.

in the skin after oral, bath, and cream administration of 8-methoxypsoralen have been studied in a three-way crossover microdialysis study of eight healthy subjects (159). Tissue concentrations after oral administration of 0.6 or 1 mg/kg 8-methoxypsoralen had a peak plasma concentration (1.7–6.6 ng/mL) that was much lower than the peak concentrations found with 0.1% 8-methoxypsoralen cream (200–520 ng/mL) and 3 mg/L 8-methoxypsoralen bath (720–970 ng/mL), respectively. Peak tissue concentrations occurred in the first 20 minutes with both topical applications compared to 1 to 4 hours after oral administration. Cutaneous blood flow is a major determinant of dermal concentrations of penciclovir and aciclovir after topical application with significant levels for normal skin only being measurable after noradrenaline-induced local vasoconstriction (160). A close correlation was also shown between penciclovir concentration absorbed per hour and tape stripping barrier disruption measured by transepidermal water loss. As highlighted by the work on transdermal penetration of diclofenac after multiple as well as after single application, the rate and extent of absorption into deeper tissues is highly variable (161). Good agreement has been found for dermal microdialysis sampling and the dermatopharmacokinetic method when used in the bioequivalence investigation of a topical formulation of lidocaine (162).

In a far-reaching evaluation, the likely activity of topical NSAIDs was defined by the product of maximum cutaneous fluxes for an NSAID from a (lipophilic) formulation and their intrinsic activity in the underlying tissue (163). They suggested that the percutaneous activities of ibuprofen (CAS 15687-27-1) and nabumetone (CAS 42924-53-8) were good because they had high maximum fluxes. Apparently unaware of this work, a similar proposition was expressed by Cordero et al. (164). They reported that the percutaneous activities for a series of NSAIDs were in the order: ketorolac > diclofenac > indomethacin, ketoprofen >> piroxicam, tenoxicam—the almost identical to results of Wenkers and Lippold (Fig. 3) (163).

In conclusion, selective targeting of underlying tissues below the stratum corneum after topical application is possible but is associated with much variability. Optimal activity is determined by a combination of percutaneous penetration and intrinsic activity of the compounds of interest.

ACKNOWLEDGEMENT

We thank Desley Butters and Narelle Walker for their assistance in preparing this manuscript.

REFERENCES

1. Gunther RT. The Greek Herbal of Dioscorides. Oxford, UK: Oxford University Press, 1934.
2. Wall PD, Melzack R, eds. Textbook of Pain. 3rd ed. Edinburgh, UK: Churchill Livingstone, 1994.
3. Atkinson DC, Hicks R. The anti-inflammatory activity of irritants. Agents Actions 1975; 5:239.
4. Norrnann S, Besedovsky H, Schardt M, del Rey A. Mechanisms of anti-inflammation induced by tumour transplantation, surgery and irritant injection. J Leukoc Biol 1991; 49:455.
5. Jacob SW, Bischel M, Herschler RJ. Dimethylsulfoxide: a new concept in pharmacotherapy. Curr Ther Res 1964; 6:134.
6. Borda IT, Koff RS. NSAIDs: A Profile of Adverse Effects. Philadelphia, Pa: Hanley & Belfus, 1992.

7. Myllykangas-Luosujarvi R, Aho K, Isomaki H. Death attributed to antirheumatic medication. J Rheumatol 1995; 22:2214.
8. Heyneman CA, Lawless-Liday C, Wall GC. Oral versus topical NSAIDs in rheumatic diseases a comparison. Drugs (2000); 60(3):555–574.
9. Bateman DN, Kennedy JG. Non-steroidal anti-inflammatory drugs and elderly patients. The medicine may be worse than the disease. Br Med J 1995; 310:817–818.
10. Evans JM, McMahon AD, Gilchrist MM, et al. Topical non-steroidal anti-inflammatory drugs and admission to hospital for upper gastrointestinal bleeding and perforation. Br Med J 1995; 311:22.
11. O'Callaghan CA, Andrews PA, Ogg CS. Renal disease and use of topical non-steroid anti-inflammatory drugs. Br Med J 1994; 308:110.
12. Sawynok J. Topical and peripherally acting analgesics. Pharmacol Rev 2003; 55:1–21.
13. Jain S, Jain N, Bhadra D, Tiwary AK, Jain NK. Transdermal delivery of an analgesic agent using elastic liposomes: preparation, characterization and performance evaluation. Current Drug Delivery (2005); 2(3):223–233.
14. Kolesnikov Y, Cristea M, Oksman G, et al. Evaluation of the tail formalin test in mice as a new model to assess local analgesic effects. Brain Res 2004; 1029:217–223.
15. Leibowitz HM, Kupferrnan A. Anti-inflammatory medications. Int Ophthalmol Clin 1980; 20:117.
16. Leibowitz HM, Loss JH, Kupferrnan A. Quantitation of inflammation in the cornea. Arch Ophthalmol. 1974; 982:427.
17. Nassarella BA, Szerenyi K, Wang XW, et al. Effect of diclofenac on corneal haze after photorefractive keratectomy in rabbits. Ophthalmology 1995; 102:469.
18. Offenbacher S, Williams RC, Jeffcoat MK, et al. The effect of NSAIDs on beagle crevicular cyclooxygenase metabolities and periodontal bone loss. J Periodont Res 1992; 27:207.
19. Komman KS, Blodgett RP, Brunsvold M, Holt Se. Effects of topical applications of meclofenamic acid and ibuprofen on bone loss, subgingival microbiota and gingival PMN response in the primate, *Macaca fascicularis*. J Periodont Res 1990; 25:300.
20. Heasman PA, Benn DK, Kelly PJ, et al. The use of topical flurbiprofen as an adjunct to non-surgical management of periodontal disease. J Clin Peridont 1993; 20:457.
21. Jeffcoat MJ, Reddy MS, Haigh S, et al. A comparison of topical ketorolac, systemic flurbiprofen and placebo for the inhibition of bone loss in adult periodontitis. J Peridont 1995; 66:329.
22. Bradley PP, Priebat DA, Christensen RD, Rothstein G. Measurement of cutaneous inflammation: estimation of neutrophil content with an enzyme marker. J Invest Dermatol 1982; 78:206.
23. De Young LM, Kheifets JB, Ballaron SJ, Young JM. Edema and cell infiltration in the phorbol ester-treated mouse ear are temporally separate and can be differentially modulated by pharmacologic agents. Agents Actions 1989; 26:335.
24. Poelman MC, Piot B, Guyon F, et al. Assessment of topical anti-inflammatory drugs. J Pharm Pharmacol 1989; 41:720.
25. Stoughton RB. Bioassay system for formulations of topically applied glucocorticos-steroids. Arch Dermatol 1972; 106:825.
26. Smith EW, Meyer E, Hay JM, Maibach HI. The human skin blanching assay as an indicator of topical corticosteroid bioavailability. In: Bronaugh RL, Maibach HI, eds. Percutaneous Absorption. New York: Marcel Dekker, 1989:443–460.
27. Lester RS. Dermatologic pharmacology: corticosteroids. Clin Dermatol 1989; 7:80.
28. Pershing LK, Bakhtian S, Poncelet C, et al. Comparison of skin stripping, in vitro release and skin blanching response methods to measure dose response and similarity of triam-cinolide acetonide cream strengths from two sources. J Pharm Sci 2002; 91:1312–1323.
29. Taube U. Drug Metabolism in the skin: advantages and disadvantages. In: Hadgraft J, Guy RH, eds. Transdermal Drug Delivery. New York: Dekker, 1989:99–192.
30. Cremer M.Type 11 collagen-induced arthritis in rats. In: Greenwald RA, Diamond HS, eds. Handbook of Animal Models for the Rheumatic Diseases. Vol. 1. Boca Raton, Fla: CRC Press, 1988:17–27.
31. Whitehouse MW. Adjuvant-induced polyarthritis in rats. In: Greenwald RA, Diamond HS, eds. Handbook of Animal Models for the Rheumatic Diseases. Vol. 1. Boca Raton, Fla: CRC Press, 1988:3–16.

32. Whitehouse MW, Turner AG, Davis CKC, Roberts MS. Emu oil(s): a source of non-toxic transdermal anti-inflammatory agents in Aboriginal medicine. Inflammopharmacol 1998; 6:1–8.
33. Rainsford KD, Whitehouse MW. Effects of the prostaglandin-El analogue, misoprostol, on the development of adjuvant arthritis in rats. Inflammopharmacology 1995; 3:49.
34. Beveridge SJ, Whitehouse MW, Walker WR. Lipophilic copper(II). formulations: correlations between composition and anti-inflammatory / anti-arthritic activity when applied to the skin of rats. Agents Actions 1982; 12:225.
35. Whitehouse MW, Rainsford KD, Taylor RN, Vemon-Roberts B. Zinc monoglycerolate: a slow-release source of zinc with anti-arthritic activity in rats. Agents Actions 1990; 31:47.
36. Fairlie DP, Whitehouse MW. Transdermal delivery of inorganic complexes as metal drugs or nutritional supplements. Drug Des Discov 1991; 8:83.
37. Maia CS, Mehnert W, Schafer-Korting M. Solid lipid nanoparticles as drug carriers for topical glucocorticoids. Int J Pharm 2000; 196(2):165–167.
38. Shainhouse T, Cunningham BB. Topical anesthetics: physiology, formulations, and novel delivery systems. Am J Drug Deliv 2004; 2(2):89–99.
39. Higaki K, Nakayama K, Suyama T, Amnuaikit C, Ogawara K, Kimura T. Enhancement of topical delivery of drugs via direct penetration by reducing blood flow rate in skin. Int J Pharm 2005; 288(2):227–233.
40. Priborsky J, Takayama K, Obata Y, Priborska Z, Nagai T. Influence of limonene and laurocapram on percutaneous absorption of nonsteroidal anti-inflammatory drugs. Arzneim Forschung 1992; 42(2):116–19.
41. Gowdey CW. A guide to the pharmacology of placebos. Can Med Assoc J 1983; 128: 921.
42. Editorial. Shall I please? Lancet 1983; 2:1465.
43. Gotzsche Pc. The logic of the placebo effect: is there any? Lancet 1994; 334:925.
44. Buchanan WW, Bellamy N. The placebo response: clinical efficacy and toxicity. In: Rainsford KD, ed. Side Effects of Anti-Inflammatory Drugs IV. Dordrecht, the Netherlands: Kluwer Academic Publication, 1997:11–23.
45. Anon. Topical NSAIDs: a gimmick or a godsend? Lancet 1989; 4:779.
46. Bos JD. Skin Immune System. Boca Raton Fla: CRC Press, 1989.
47. Schuler G. Epidermal Langerhans Cells. Boca Raton: CRC Press, 1990.
48. Del Bianco E, Geppetti P, Zippa P, et al. The effect of repeated dermal application of capsaicin to the human skin on pain and vasodilatation induced by intradermal injection of acid and hypertonic solutions. Br J Clin Pharmacol 1996; 41:1.
49. Kidd BL, Mapp PI, Blake DR, et al. Neurogenic influences in arthritis. Ann Rheum Dis 1990; 49:649.
50. Holtzer P, Capsaicin: cellular targets, mechanisms of actions and selectivity for thin sensory neurons. Pharmacol Rev 1991; 43:143.
51. Rumsfield JA, West DP. Topical capsaicin in dermatologic and peripheral pain disorders. Ann Pharmacother 1991; 25:381.
52. Schnitzer G. Neuropeptides, capsaicin and musculoskeletal pain. Semin Arth Rheum 1994; 23(Suppl. 6):1–2.
53. Cerinic MM, McCarthy G, Lombardi A, et al. Neurogenic influences in arthritis: potential modification by capsaicin. J Rheumatol 1995; 22: 1447.
54. Cordell GA, Aranjo OE. Capsaicin: identification, nomenclature and pharmacotherapy. Ann Pharmacother 1993; 27:330.
55. Hogaboam CM, Wallace JL. Inhibition of platelet aggregation by capsaicin. Eur J Pharmacol 1991; 202:129.
56. Varvel JR, Schafter SL, Hwang SS. et al. Absorption characteristics of transdermally administered fentanyl. Anesthiology 1989; 40:21.
57. Herrero-Beaumont G, Bjorneboe O, Richarz, U. Transdermal fentanyl for the treatment of pain caused by rheumatoid arthritis. Rheumatol Int 2004; 24(6):325–332.
58. Sittl R, Transdermal buprenorphine in the treatment of chronic pain. Exp Rev Neurother 2005; 5(3):315–323.
59. Klein SM, Cohen G, Cedarbaum AI. Production of formaldehyde during metabolism of DMSO by hydroxyl radical generating systems. Biochemistry 1981; 20:6006.

60. Franz TJ, Lehman PA, Kagy MK. Dimethylsulfoxide. In: Smith EW, Maibach HI, eds. Percutaneous Penetration Enhancers. Boca Raton Fla: CRC Press, 115–127.
61. King RB. Concerning the management of pain associated with herpes zoster and of post-herpetic neuralgia. Pain 1988; 33:73.
62. De Benedittis G, Besana F, Lorenzetti A. A new topical treatment for acute herpetic neuralgia and post-herpetic neuralgia: the aspirin/diethyl ether mixture. Pain 1992; 48:383.
63. McAdam B, Keimowitz RM, Maher M, Fitzgerald D. Transdermal modification of platelet function: an aspirin patch system results in marked suppression of platelet cyclooxygenase. J Pharmacol Exp Ther 1996; 277:559.
64. Bair WB III, Hart N, Einspahr J, Liu G, Dong Z, Alberts D, Bowden GT. Inhibitory effects of sodium salicylate and acetylsalicylic acid on UVB-induced mouse skin carcinogenesis. Cancer Epidemiol Biomark Prev 2002; 11(12):1645–1652.
65. Rainsford KD. ed. Aspirin and Related Drugs. London, U.K.: Taylor & Francis, 2004.
66. Roberts MS, Favretto WA, Meyer A, et al. Topical bioavailability of methyl salicylate. Aust NZ J Med 1982; 12:303.
67. Brown EW, Scott WO. The comparative absorption of certain salicylate esters by the human skin. J Pharmacol 1934; 50:373.
68. Megwa SA, Benson HAE, Roberts MS. Percutaneous absorption of salicylates from some commercially available topical products containing methyl salicylate or salicylate salts in rats. J Pharm Pharmacol 1995; 47:891.
69. Merck Index. 13th ed. Rahway, NJ: Merck, 2001.
70. Halpern BN, Gaudin 0, Stiffel M. Etude de l'influence des cations sur la permeabilite cutanee et cellulaire vis-a-vis de certains derives salicyles. CR Acad Sci (Paris), 1948; 142:819.
71. Davies MG, Briffa DV, Grieves MW. Systemic toxicity from topically applied salicylic acid. Br Med J 1979; 100:661.
72. Hadgraft J. Formulation of anti-inflammatory compounds. In: Lowe NJ, Hensby CN, eds.
73. Wada Y, Etoh Y, Ohira A, et al. Percutaneous absorption and anti-inflammatory activity of indomethicin in ointment. J Pharm Pharmacol 1982; 34:467.
74. Hiramatsu Y, Akita S, Salamin PA, Maier Rs. Assessment of topical non-steroidal anti-inflammatory drugs in animal models. Arzneim Forsch 1990; 40:1117.
75. Wildfang I, Maibach HI. Topical application of NSAIDs. In: Famaey JP, Paulus HE, eds. Therapeutic Application of NSAIDs. New York: Marcel Dekker, 1992:461–490.
76. White S. Topical NSAIDs in the treatment of inflammatory musculoskeletal disorders. Prostaglandins Leukotriene and Essential Fatty Acids. 1991; 43:209.
77. Moore RA, Tramer MR, Carroll D, Wiffen PJ, Mcquay HJ. Quantitive systematic review of topically applied non-steroidal anti-inflammatory drugs. Br Med J 1998; 316(7128):333–338.
78. Beetge E, du Plessis J, Muller DG, Goosen C, van Rensburg FJ. The influence of the physicochemical characteristics and pharmacokinetic properties of selected NSAID's on their transdermal absorption. Int J Pharm (2000); 193(2):261–264.
79. Cordero JA, Camacho M, Obach R, Domenech J, Vila L. In vitro based index of topical anti-inflammatory activity to compare a series of NSAIDs. Euro J Pharm Biopharm 2001; 51(2):135–142.
80. Erdogan F, Ergun H, Gokay NS, Gulmez SE, Bolay B, Tulunay FC. The diffusion of nimesulide gel into synovial fluid: a comparison between administration routes. Int J Clin Pharmacol Ther 2006; 44(6):270–275
81. Sengupta S, Velpandian T, Kabir SR, Gupta SK. Analgesic efficacy and pharmacokinetics of topical nimesulide gel in healthy human volunteers: double-blind comparison with piroxicam, diclofenac and placebo. Eur J Clin Pharmacol 1998; 54(7):541–547.
82. Sengupta S, Velpandian T, Sapra P, Mathur P, Gupta SK. Comparative analgesic efficacy of nimesulide and diclofenac gels after topical application on the skin. Skin Pharmacol Appl Skin Physiol 1998; 11(4-5):273–278.
83. Larrucea E, Arellano A, Santoyo S, Ygartua P. Combined effect of oleic acid and propylene glycol on the percutaneous penetration of tenoxicam and its retention in the skin. Eur J Pharm Biopharm 2001; 52(2):113–119.
84. Brooks PM, Day RO. Plasma concentration and therapeutic effects of antiinflammatory and antirheumatic drugs. In: Lewis AJ, Furst DE, eds. Non-Steroidal Anti-Inflammatory Drugs-Mechanism and Clinical Use. New York: Marcel Dekker, 1987:189–199.

85. Albers HI. Dermatological aspects of nonsteroid anti-inflammatory drugs. In: Borda IT, Koff RS. NSAIDs: A Profile of Adverse Effects. Philadelphia, Pa: Hanley & Belfus, 1992: 185–217.
86. Grandjean P. Skin Penetration: Hazardous Chemicals at Work. London, U.K.: Taylor & Francis, 1990.
87. Anon. Annual Reports Medical Chemistry 1985; 20:332, and 1990; 26:298.
88. Andersson K, Larsson H. Percutaneous absorption of benzydamine in guinea pig and man. Arzneim Forsch 1974; 24:1686.
89. Fantato S, De Gregorio M. Clinical evaluation of topical benzydamine in traumatology. Arzneim Forsch 1971; 21:1530.
90. Silvestrini B, Garau A, Pozzati D, and Cioli V. Pharmacological research on benzydamine-a new analgesic-anti-inflammatory drug. Arzneim Forsch 1966; 16:39.
91. Jansen JWCM. Antithrombotische. Wirkung Benzydamin Arzneim Forsch 1987; 37:626.
92. McCarthy GM, Kenny D. Dietary fish oils and rheumatic diseases. Semin Arthritis Rheum 1992; 21:368.
93. Rothman D, DeLuca P, Zurier RB. Botanical lipids: effects on inflammation, immune responses, and rheumatoid arthritis. Semin Arthritis Rheum 1995; 25:87.
94. Nettleton lA. Omega-3 Fatty Acids and Health. New York: Chapman & Hall, 1995.
95. Gouni I, Oka K, Etienne J, Chan L. Endotoxin-induced hypertriglyceridemia is mediated by suppression of lipoprotein lipase at a posttranscriptional level. J Lipid Res 1993; 34:139.
96. Beutler BA, Cerami 1. Recombinant IL-1 suppresses liproprotein lipase activity in 3T3-Ll cells. I Immunol 1985; 135:3969.
97. Whitehouse M, Bolt AG, Ford GL, Vernon-Roberts B. Anti-arthritic activity of poly-unsaturated fatty acid derivatives in adjuvant arthritic rats. In: McLean AJ, Wahlqvist ML, eds. Current Problems in Nutrition Pharmacology & Toxicology. London, U.K.: Libbey, 1988:101–103.
98. Hebbom P, Jablonska S, Beutner EH, et al. Action of topically applied arachidonic acid on the skin of patients with psoriasis. Arch Dermatol 1988; 124:387.
99. Haynes DR, Whitehouse MW, Vemon-Roberts B. Misoprostol regulates inflammatory cytokines and immune functions in vitro like the natural prostaglandins. Immunology 1992; 76:251.
100. Graham DY, Agrawal NM, Roth SH. Prevention of NSAID-induced gastric ulcer with misoprostol. Lancet 1988; 2:1277.
101. Whitehouse MW. Trace element supplements. In: Dixon JS, Furst DE, eds. Second-Line Agents in the Treatment of Rheumatic Diseases. New York: Marcel Dekker, 1992:549–578.
102. Fairlie DP, Whitehouse MW, Taylor RM. Zinc monoglycerolate-solubilization by endogenous ligands. Agents Actions 1992; 36:152.
103. Rhodes J, Thomas G. Nicotine treatment in ulcerative colitis. Drugs 1995; 49:157.
104. Zijlstra FJ. Smoking and nicotine in inflammatory bowel disease: good or bad for cytokines? Mediat Inflam 1998:7:153–155.
105. Van Dijk APM, Meijssen MAC, Brower AJB, et al. Transdermal nicotine inhibits interleukin-2 synthesis by mononuclear cells derived from healthy volunteers. Eur J Clin Invest 1998; 28:664–671.
106. Pei Y. Chronic cyclosporin nephrotoxicity in rheumatoid arthritis. J Rheumatol 1996; 23:4.
107. Lugmani R, Gordon C, Bacon P. Clinical pharmacology and modification of autoimmunity and inflammation in rheumatoid disease. Drugs 1994; 47:259.
108. Billich A, Aschauer H, Aszodi A, Stuetz A. Percutaneous absorption of drugs used in atopic eczema: pimecrolimus permeates less through skin than corticosteroids and tacrolimus. Int J Pharm 2004; 269:29–35.
109. Draelos Z, Nayak A, Pariser D, et al. Pharmacokinetics of topical calcineurin inhibitors in adult atopic dermatitis. J Am Acad Dermatol 2005; 53:602–609.
110. Hultsch T, Kapp A, Spergel J. Immunomodulation and safety of topical calcineurin inhibitors for the treatment of atopic dermatitis. Dermatology 2005; 211:174–187.
111. Ghosh P, Whitehouse MW, Dawson M, Turner AG. Anti-inflammatory composition derived from emu oil. U.S. Patent 5431922, 1995.
112. Lopez A, Sims DE, Ablett RD, et al. Effect of emu oil on auricular inflammation induced with croton oil in mice. Am J Vet Res 1999; 60:1558–1561.
113. Yoganathan S, Nicolosi R, Wilson T, et al. Antagonism of croton oil inflammation by topical emu oil in CD-1 mice. Lipids 2003; 38:603–607.

114. Carson SF, Hammer Ka, Riley TV. Melaleuca alternifolia (tea tree) oil: a review of antimicrobial and other medicinal properties. Clin Microbiol Rev 2006; 19:50–62.
115. Koh KJ, Pearch Al, Marshaman G, Finlay-Jones JJ, Hart, PH. Tea tree oil reduces histamine-induced skin inflammation. Brit J Dermatol 2000; 147:1212–1217.
116. Khalil Z, Pearce AL, Satkunanathan N, Storer E, Finlay-Jones JJ, Hart PH. Regulation of wheal and flare by tea tree oil: Complementary human and rodent studies. J Invest Dermatol (2004); 123(4):683–690.
117. Brand C, Townley SL, Finlay-Jones JJ, Hart PH. Tea tree oil reduces histamine-induced oedema in murine ears. Inflamm Res 2002; 51:283–289.
118. Brand C, Grimbaldeston MA, Gamble JR, Drew J, Finlay-Jones JJ, Hart PH. Tea tree oil reduces the swelling associated with the efferant phase of a contact hypersensitivity response. Inflamm Res 2002; 51:236–244.
119. Pearce AL, Finlay-Jones JJ, Hart PH. Reduction of nickel-induced contact hypersensitivity reactions by topical tea tree oil in humans. Inflamm Res 2005; 54:22–30.
120. Reichling J, Landvatter U, Wagner H, Kostka K-H, Schaefer UF. In vitro studies on release and human skin permeation of Australian tea tree oil (TTO) from topical formulations. Eur J Pharm Biopharm 2006; 64:222–228.
121. Gobel H, Schmidt G, Soyka D. Effect of peppermint and eucalyptus oil preparations on neurophysiological and experimental algesimetric headache parameters. Cephalalgia 1994; 14:228–234.
122. Davies SJ, Harding LM, Baranowski AP. A novel treatment of postherpetic neuralgia using peppermint oil. Clin J Pain 2002; 18:200–202.
123. Hochberg MC. Nutritional supplements for knee osteoarthritis – still no resolution. N Engl J Med 2006; 354:858–860.
124. Cohen M, Wolfe R, Mai T, Lewis D. A randomized, double blind, placebo controlled trial of a topical cream containing glucosamine sulfate, chondroitin sulfate, and camphor for osteoarthritis of the knee. J Rheumatol 2003; 30:523-528, 826–827.
125. Ghosh P, Shimmon S, Whitehouse MW. Arthritic disease suppression and cartilage protection with glycosaminoglycan polypeptide complexes (Peptacan) derived from the cartilage extracellular matrix: a novel approach to therapy. Inflammopharmacol 2006; 14:155–162.
126. Ghosh P, Shimmon S, Wilson-Ghosh N. A novel cartilage matrix derived preparation (Biodermex®) suppresses experimentally induced dermal inflammation in human subjects under double blind clinical conditions. 5th Int Congress on Autoimmunity, Sorrento, Italy, 2006.
127. Yano T, Nakagawa A, Tsuji M, Noda K. Skin permeability of various nonsteroidal anti-inflammatory drugs in man. Life Sci 1986; 39:1043.
128. Singh P, Roberts MS. Skin permeability and local tissue concentrations of non steroidal antinflammatory drugs (NSAIDs) after topical application. J Pharmacol ExpTher 1994; 268:144.
129. Riegelman S. Pharmacokinetics. Pharmacokinetic factors affecting epidermal penetration and percutaneous adsorption. Clin Pharmacol Ther 1974; 16:873.
130. Cooper ER. Pharmacokinetics of skin penetration. J Pharm Sci 1976; 65:1396.
131. Chandrasekaran SK, Bayene W, Shaw JE. Pharmacokinetics of drug permeation through human skin. J Pharm Sci 1978; 67:1370.
132. Cooper ER, Bemer B. Finite dose of pharmacokinetics of skin penetration. J Pharm Sci 1985; 74:1100.
133. Guy RH, Hadgraft 1. Physicochemical interpretation of the pharmacokinetics of percutaneous absorption. J Pharm Biopharm 1983; 11:189.
134. Kubota K, Ishizaki T. A diffusion-diffusion model for percutaneous drug absorption. J Pharm Biopharm 1986; 14:404.
135. Siddiqui O, Roberts MS, Po lack AE. Percutaneous absorption of steroids, relative contributions of epidermal penetration and dermal clearance. J Pharm Biopharm 1989; 17:405.
136. Guy RH, Hadgraft J, Maibach HI. Percutaneous absorption in man: a kinetic approach. Toxicol Appl Pharmacol 1985; 78:123.
137. Williams PL, Riviere JE. A biophysically based dermato pharmacokinetic compartment model for quantifying percutaneous penetration and absorption of topically applied agents. 1. Theory. J Pharm Sci 1995; 84:599.

138. Guy RH, Maibach HI. Drug delivery to local subcutaneous structures following topical administration. J Pharm Sci 1983; 72:1375.
139. Singh P, Roberts MS. Dermal and underlying tissue pharmacokinetics of salicylic acid after topical application. J Pharm Biopharm 1993; 21:337.
140. Radermacher J, Jentsck D, Sholl MA, Lustinetz T, Frolich JC Diclofenac concentrations in synovial fluid and plasma after cutaneous application in inflammatory and degenerative joint disease. Br J Clin Pharmacol 1991; 31:537.
141. Dawson M, McGee CM, Vine JH, Nash P, Watson TR, Brooks PM. The disposition of biphenyl acetic acid following topical application. Eur J Clin Pharmacol 1988; 33:639.
142. Singh P, Roberts MS. Local deep tissue penetration of compounds after dermal application: Structure-tissue penetration relationships. J Pharmacol Exp Ther (in press).
143. Cross SE, Wu ZY, Roberts MS. Effect of perfusion flow rate on the tissue uptake of solutes after dermal application using the rat isolated perfused limb preparation. J Pharm Pharmacol 1994; 46:844.
144. Singh P, Roberts MS. Effects of vasoconstriction on dermal pharmacokinetics and local tissue distribution of compounds. J Pharm Sci 1994; 83:783.
145. Cross SE, Wu ZY, Roberts MS. The effect of protein binding on the deep tissue penetration and efflux of dermally applied salicylic acid, lidocaine and diazepam in the perfused rat hindlimb. J Pharmacol Exper Ther 1996; 277:366.
146. McNeill SC, Potts RO, Francoeur ML. Local enhanced topical delivery (LETD) of drugs. Does it truly exist? Pharm Res 1992; 9:1422.
147. Guy RH, Hadgraft J, Bucks DA. Transdermal drug delivery and cutaneous metabolism. Xenobiotica 1987; 17:325.
148. Megwa SA, Benson HAE, Roberts MS. Percutaneous absorption of salicylates from some commercially available topical products containing methyl salicylate or salicylate salts in rats. J Pharm Pharmacol 1995; 47:891.
149. Roberts MS, Horlock E. Effect of repeated application of salicylic acid to the skin on its percutaneous absorption. J Pharm Sci 1978; 67:1685.
150. Hegemann L, Forstinger C, Partsch B, Lagler I, Krotz S, Wolff K. Microdialysis in cutaneous pharmacology: kinetic analysis of transdermally delivered nicotine. J Invest Dermatol. 1995; 104:839–843.
151. Cross SE, Anderson C, Thompson MJ, Roberts MS. Is there tissue penetration after application of topical salicylate formulations? Lancet 1997; 350:636.
152. Cross SE, Anderson C, Roberts MS. Topical penetration of commercial salicylate esters and salts using human isolated skin and clinical microdialysis studies. Br J Clin Pharmacol. 1998; 46:29–35.
153. Muller M, Mascher H, Kikuta C, Schafer S, Brunner M, Dorner G, Eichler HG. Diclofenac concentrations in defined tissue layers after topical administration. Clin Pharmacol Ther 1997; 62:293–292.
154. Muller M, Rastelli C, Ferri P, Jansen B, Breiteneder H, Eichler HG. Transdermal penetration of diclofenac after multiple epicutaneous administration. J Rheumatol 1998; 25:1833–6.
155. Tegeder I, Muth-Selbach U, Lotsch J, Rusing G, Oelkers R, Brune K, Meller S, Kelm GR, Sorgel F, Geisslinger G. Application of microdialysis for the determination of muscle and subcutaneous tissue concentrations after oral and topical ibuprofen administration. Clin Pharmacol Ther 1999; 65:357–368.
156. Benfeldt E, Serup J, Menne T. Effect of barrier perturbation on cutaneous salicylic acid penetration in human skin: in vivo pharmacokinetics using microdialysis and non-invasive quantification of barrier function. Br J Dermatol 1999; 140:739–748.
157. Stagni G, O'Donnell D, Liu YJ, Kellogg DL, Morgan T, Shepherd AM. Intradermal microdialysis: kinetics of iontophoretically delivered propranolol in forearm dermis. J Control Release 2000; 63:331–339.
158. Boelsma E, Anderson C, Karlsson AM, Ponec M. Microdialysis technique as a method to study the percutaneous penetration of methyl nicotinate through excised human skin, reconstructed epidermis, and human skin in vivo. Pharm Res 2000; 17:141–7.
159. Tegeder I, Brautigam L, Podda M, Meier S, Kaufmann R, Geisslinger G, Grundmann-Kollmann M. Time course of 8-methoxypsoralen concentrations in skin and plasma after topical (bath and cream) and oral administration of 8-methoxypsoralen. Clin Pharmacol Ther. 2002; 71:153–61.

160. Morgan CJ, Renwick AG, Friedmann PS. The role of stratum corneum and dermal microvascular perfusion in penetration and tissue levels of water-soluble drugs investigated by microdialysis. Br J Dermatol 2003; 148:434–43.
161. Dehghanyar P, Mayer BX, Namiranian K, Mascher H, Muller M, Brunner M. Topical skin penetration of diclofenac after single- and multiple-dose application. Int J Clin Pharmacol Ther 2004; 42:353–9.
162. Benfeldt E, Hansen SH, Volund A, Menne T, Shah VP. Bioequivalence of topical formulations in humans: evaluation by dermal microdialysis sampling and the dermatopharmacokinetic method. J Invest Dermatol 2007; 127:170–8.
163. Wenkers BP, Lippold BC. Prediction of the efficacy of cutaneously applied nonsteroidal anti-inflammatory drugs from a lipophilic vehicle. Arzneim Forsch 2000; 50:275–80.
164. Cordero JA, Camacho M, Obach R, Domenech J, Vila L. In vitro based index of topical anti-inflammatory activity to compare a series of NSAIDs. Eur J Pharm Biopharm 2001; 51:135–42.

14 Novel Topically Active Antimicrobial and Anti-inflammatory Compounds for Acne

Joseph A. Dunn, Robert A. Coburn,
Richard T. Evans, and Robert J. Genco
Therex LLC, Buffalo, New York, U.S.A.

Kenneth A. Walters
An-eX Analytical Services Ltd., Cardiff, U.K.

INTRODUCTION

Acne vulgaris (acne) is the most common skin disease encountered, affecting over 80% of the population at some point in their lifetime. Acne not only creates relatively short-term physical and psychological effects for the sufferer, but if recalcitrant to normal treatment or left unchecked, it can also cause more permanent physical effects such as facial scarring that may produce profound psychological consequences. Acne is caused by abnormal follicular hyperkeratosis (plugging) and abnormal sebum production within pilosebaceous units (composed of a hair follicle, sebaceous glands, and a follicular canal) in the skin. Normally, sebum is secreted from the follicular canal to aid in the removal of desquamated follicular epithelial cells via the infundibulum at the top of the follicle. In acne, the dilated orifice of affected follicles can be blocked with excess sebum and/or keratin from desquamated cells, promoting proliferation of bacteria that normally reside in the pilosebaceous unit. This combination of events can result in immune reactions, inflammation, and comedone formation in the pilosebaceous unit lasting for days or weeks. Excess sebum is caused by an increase in the level of androgens, and excess keratin results from an increase in ductal keratinocytes (e.g., from hyperplasia that may also result from high androgen levels), an inadequate separation of ductal corneocytes, or a combination of both (1,2).

Acne is typically categorized into three types: comedonal, papulopustular, and nodular resulting in degrees of severity ranging from noninflammatory comedones (i.e., blackheads and whiteheads) to deep dermal inflammatory papules that appear as erythematous, raised solid lesions that can eventually coalesce and dissect under the skin producing inflamed sinus tracts which can result in scarring, sometimes severe, upon resolution.

Although one species of normal skin flora, the anaerobic diphtheroid *Propionibacterium acnes*, has been shown as the principal cause of the inflamed comedones in acne vulgaris, other dermal bacterial flora such as *Staphylococcus epidermidis* and *Staphylococcus aureus* may play a role in the etiology of this condition, particularly as secondary infections (2). *P. acnes* has also been associated with a number of other conditions such as sarcoidosis and synovitis, pustulosis, hyperostosis, and osteitis, although its precise role as a causative agent in these skin disorders remains to be determined. *P. acnes* produces a number of virulence factors and is well known for its inflammatory and immunomodulatory properties (3). The organism metabolizes excess sebaceous triglycerides, leading to expanded bacterial growth and the production of chemoattractants that recruit inflammatory cells (i.e., macrophages and neutrophils) to the infected area. The inflammatory cascade in these host cells includes stimulation of cyclooxygenases, phospholipases, and protein kinases, leading to the production of degradative enzymes and reactive chemicals intended to control or eliminate the infection. Destructive mechanisms that cause this condition involve the chronic, uncontrolled activation of proteolytic, glycolytic, and lipolytic enzymes, as well as the production of peptide mediators of inflammation such as interleukins 1β and 8 and tumor necrosis factor α, IL-8, TNF-α, and other cytokines that recruit more cells into the infected area, ultimately resulting in the breakdown of tissue and, if unattended, scarring (4,5).

CURRENT THERAPEUTIC TREATMENT OF ACNE

In treating mild acne, typically before one sees the physician, regular cleansing of the affected area, improved nutritional habits, and treatment with nonprescription topical antiseptics (e.g., benzoyl peroxide) and/or keratolytics (e.g., resorcinol, salicylic acid, sulfur) are the accepted first approaches. Therapy for moderate to severe cases of acne includes the aforementioned as well as prescription retinoids, topical or oral antibiotics, and antiandrogens (6–10). None of these approaches is intended to reduce inflammation and tissue restructuring directly.

Antibiotics that are most frequently used are minocycline (oral), tetracycline (oral), doxycycline (oral), erythromycin (oral or topical), and clindamycin (topical). In the treatment of severe cases, the same antibiotics are used but require lengthier courses of treatment before results are seen. When they are prescribed, physicians cannot expect to see maximal improvement in patients for at least six to eight weeks. In addition, there are two considerable problems with their use. The first one is a concern about the increase in bacterial resistance to antibiotics (11). In a 1993 study on 468 acne patients treated, 34% (178) carried strains of *P. acnes* resistant to one or more antibiotics (12). The second is the concern that these treatments can have dose-limiting side effects (12), including stomach complaints, skin sensitivity, and hypersensitivity syndromes ranging from urticaria to drug-induced lupus (minocyline) (13).

Another approach to the treatment of moderate to severe acne is the use of topical and systemic retinoids, analogs, and mimetics (6,7,14). Among them, oral isotretinoin is used for refractory nodulocyctic acne and functions by reducing sebum production. Topically applied tretinoin also corrects the keratinization defect in the follicle and exhibits some degree of anti-inflammatory activity. Although these products are very popular and effective for many patients, dose-dependent side effects often lead patients to reduce or eventually discontinue their use. These side effects include dry skin, atopic dermatitis (sometimes severe), epistaxis, raised triglyceride levels, thinning hair, and myalgia. Known teratogenicity is a major concern, and birth control is required for fertile women using the drug.

Finally, hormonal treatment is an option for female acne. Antiandrogenic approaches include estrogen therapy (e.g., estrogens/progestin, ethinyl estradio/cyproterone acetate, chlormadinone acetate, desogestrel, drospirenone, levonogestrel, norethindrone acetate, norgestimate), androgen receptor antagonists (e.g., flutamide), and the use of drugs that indirectly inhibit the effects of androgens (e.g., corticosteroids, spironolactone, cimetidine, ketoconazole) (15,16). However, not all individuals respond to these treatments, and those who do often require additional forms, especially when cases are moderate to severe. Antiandrogen therapies are, of course, unavailable for males.

As in most disease states, new therapeutic developments are, for the most part, modifications of existing treatment modalities. Thus we have low-dose, long-term isotretinoin regimens, new isotretinoin formulations (micronized isotretinoin), isotretinoin metabolites, combination treatments to reduce toxicity, and potential use of new retinoid analogs that also possess anti-inflammatory activity such as 0.1% adapalene. It is clear that there is an opportunity for novel, improved topical antiacne agents to compete in this marketplace.

SALICYLANILIDE DEVELOPMENT

For the past decade, our laboratory has been involved in the synthesis and evaluation of a new class of antibiotics, termed "5-substituted salicylanilides," which were originally designed to have growth-inhibitory activity against bacteria involved in initiation and progression of certain soft- and hard-tissue destructive disorders of the oral cavity, such as gingivitis and resulting periodontitis. Our early studies found that certain 5-substituted salicylanilides also possessed potent anti-inflammatory activity when topically applied, a pharmacologic effect that was independent from their antibiotic properties. All of the 5-substituted salicylanilides we synthesized were also highly lipophilic, which we expected would enhance their topical retention and consequently reduce their potential systemic effects. Therefore, we refer to those 5-substituted salicylanilides that possess both antibacterial and anti-inflammatory activities as lipophilic, antibacterial, anti-inflammatory drugs (LAADs).

Recently, we extended our investigations on the antibacterial properties of these compounds to include pathogenic dermal bacteria. We found that certain 5-substituted salicylanilide LAADs are very effective in inhibiting the growth of several species of bacteria implicated in acne, suggesting that a 5-substituted salicylanilide LAAD that could be optimized for activity against these bacteria and against dermal inflammation should be well positioned to enter the antiacne armamentarium.

The first generation of LAAD-type salicylanilides that were synthesized and tested for antigingivitis activity were the 5-acyl derivatives. The lead drug candidate from this generation, 5-(*n*-octoyl)-salicylanide-3'-trifluoromethylanilide (salifluor), was chosen for further development because of its excellent activity against a wide variety of gram-positive and gram-negative oral organisms including *Porphyromonas gingivalis*, *Actinobacillus actinomycetemcomitans*, *Prevotella intermedia*, and *Bacteroides forsythus*. Experimental oral formulations of salifluor were clinically evaluated, and it was found that oral rinses containing 0.12% salifluor were as effective as Peridex® (0.12% chlorhexidine gluconate) (Omni Prescriptive Pharmaceuticals, a division of 3M Company, St. Paul, Minnesota, U. S.) the only prescription treatment for gingivitis and periodontitis available at the time (17,18). However, difficulties in formulating salifluor into a dentifrice, along with the short patent life, discouraged its further development for this use.

Attempts to improve upon the physicochemical and pharmacologic properties of salifluor resulted in the synthesis of a second generation of LAAD-type salicylanilides, the 5-*n*-(alkylsulfonyl) derivatives (19,20). These compounds had good antibacterial potencies, but not as broad spectrum or potent as the 5-acyl derivatives. However, the 5-*n*-(alkylsulfonyl)salicylanilides did possess excellent

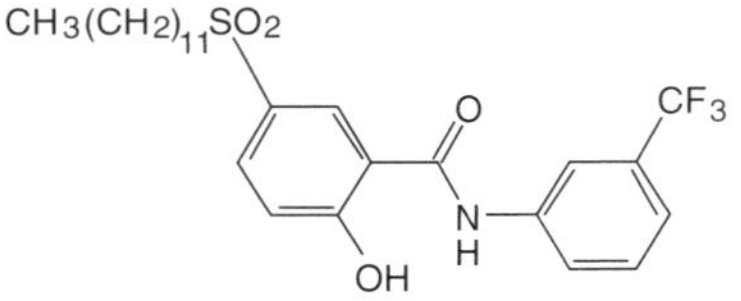

2-hydroxy-5-(dodecane-1-sulfonyl)-N-
(3-trifluoromethylphenyl)-benzamide

FIGURE 1   trifluorosal.

topical anti-inflammatory activity, presumably resulting from their effect on the prostaglandin synthetase pathways and specifically cyclooxygenases 1 and 2. An optimized 5-n-(alkylsulfonyl)salicylanilide, trifluorosal (5-(n-dodecylsulfonyl)-salicyl-3′-trifluoromethylanilide, TMF-12) (Fig. 1), underwent preclinical evaluation and early-stage pharmaceutical development as a treatment for gingivitis. Preliminary efficacy studies of a trifluorosal oral rinse formulation in both a small- and large-animal models of gingivitis were conducted producing efficacy and safety results similar to those obtained for salifluor.

Patent status, again, limited the development of trifluorosal; however, the results obtained from these studies led to the recent synthesis of a third generation of LAAD-type salicylanilides having aroyl substitutions at position 5- of the salicylate ring. Initially, two small series of 5-benzoyl- and 5-naphthoylsalicylanilides were synthesized and evaluated, and it was determined that the 5-naphthoyl derivatives had broader spectrum and more potent antibacterial activity, and one compound, naphthafluor (5-(1-naphthoyl)salicyl-3″-trifluoromethylanilide, NA1mF; Fig. 2), was more potent than salifluor while retaining trifluorosal's excellent anti-inflammatory activity.

ANTIACNE POTENTIAL OF SALICYLANILIDES

At the same time that we were investigating the utility of trifluorosal as a treatment for gingivitis, we began exploring the possibility of developing its use as a therapeutic to treat other topical bacterial infections that produce chronic inflammation and tissue destruction. This was based on the observation that several first- and second-generation anti-inflammatory salicylanilides also showed good to excellent inhibitory activity against the growth of several dermal pathogens including *P. acnes*, *S. epidermidis*, and *S. aureus*. Among a large series of 5-(alkylsulfonyl) analogs evaluated for antibacterial activity against dermal bacteria, trifluorosal proved to be the most potent, particularly against two strains of *P. acnes* where trifluorosal produced minimum inhibitory concentrations (MICs) of 0.31 and 0.15 µg/mL. This, coupled with the fact that trifluorosal was the most potent inhibitor of acute dermal inflammation in mouse skin produced by a single dose of the potent proinflammogen

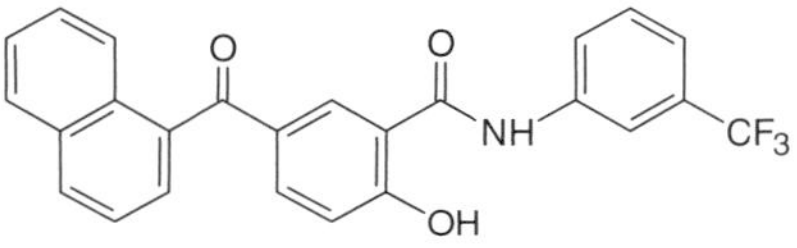

2-hydroxy-5-(naphthalene-1-carbonyl)-N-
(3-trifluoromethylphenyl)-benzamide

FIGURE 2   Naphthafluor (NA1mF).

12-*O*-tetradecanoyl phorbol-13-acetate (TPA) among all LAAD-type salicylanilides (Sigma Aldrich, St. Louis, Missouri, U.S.), led to its the further investigation as a potential antiacne treatment.

As part of this development, we conducted a more detailed study of the anti-inflammatory properties of trifluorosal compared to hydrocortisone 17-valerate (HCV) in a mouse model of chronic inflammation where tissue restructuring is produced by repeated dosing of mouse skin to TPA (21). In this study, TPA was administered to both the inner and outer surfaces of ears of female mice on alternate days for 10 days. On days 7 through 9, escalating doses of trifluorosal dissolved in acetone or of a fixed dose of HCV, also dissolved in acetone, were applied to both the outer and inner surfaces of each ear (final doses of trifluorosal were 0.5, 1.25, 2.5, or 5.0 mg/ear; final dose of HCV was 0.020 mg/ear) two or four hours after TPA dosing. Uniform punch biopsies were taken from the ears on day 10. Punch biopsies were weighed and processed for histopathologic evaluation, including measurement of cellular infiltration [polymorphonuclear leukocytes (PMNs), endothelial cells, macrophages] and epidermal thickness.

In three separate experiments, trifluorosal's maximum effective dose to inhibit TPA-stimulated ear weight gain was 1.25 mg/ear, producing responses of 27%, 37%, and 34%. Higher doses were inhibitory, but never more than 30%. The maximum inhibitory dose of HCV was 20 μg/ear, producing responses of 86%, 74%, and 92% in three separate animals. It should be noted that at higher doses, trifluorosal precipitated on the skin surface and therefore not all of the drug was bioavailable. Thus, this apparent lower efficacy of trifluorosal versus HCV may be overcome at these higher concentrations in topical formulations designed to deliver lipophilic drugs into the skin.

Histopathologic analysis of several ear biopsies showed that treatment with repetitive doses of TPA alone produced dramatic hyperplasia of the epidermis, as well as chronic inflammatory changes in the dermis (Fig. 3A and B). The more relevant changes in the dermis included hyperemia and a marked increase in the cellularity in the dermis. Surprisingly, the predominant cells were not PMNs but rather a combination of different cell types, including endothelial cells, fibroblasts, macrophages, PMNs, and mast cells. Unlike the case with a single dose of TPA, there were no clear signs of edema. Also, there were no clear indications of an increase in the thickness of the dermis. Thus, increase in weight in the biopsies of animals exposed to repetitive doses of TPA seemed to be mainly caused by hyperplasia of the epidermis, and cellular infiltration and may be secondarily contributed by an increase of density of the dermis, but not an increase of the size of the dermal compartment.

Upon histologic examination, both trifluorosal and HCV reduced epidermal thickness and the cellularity of the dermis in TPA treated tissue (Fig. 3C and D). Blood vessels were not as prominent in the samples of animals treated with either trifluorosal or HCV, and the histopathologic analysis suggested that trifluorosal and HCV may have inhibited both blood vessel dilation and angiogenesis. Control epidermis treated with the either trifluorosal or HCV did not show signs of toxicity at the microscopic levels and the ear plugs of these samples did not appear different from the samples of the control (untreated) or vehicle (acetone)-treated animals. To confirm the subjective observations, we performed quantitative determinations of three parameters (epidermal thickness, dermal thickness, and dermal cellularity) in the skin of negative controls (acetone), positive controls (TPA treatment only), and TPA-treated skin treated with three doses of trifluorosal (5.0, 1.25, and 0.5 mg/ear) and one dose of HCV (20 μg/ear). Epidermal thickness reflects the reactive proliferative activity induced by

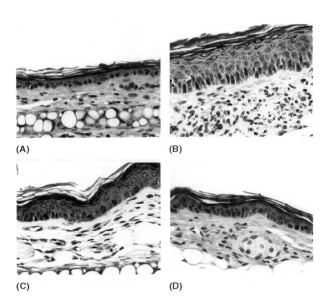

FIGURE 3 Hematotoxylin-eosin–stained vertical sections of mouse ears treated topically with TPA, TPA plus trifluorosal or TPA plus HCV (×400). (**A**) acetone control; (**B**) TPA-treated skin; (**C**) TPA- and trifluorosal-treated (1.25 mg/ear); (**D**) TPA- and HCV-treated (0.02 mg/ear). *Abbreviations*: HCV, hydrocortisone 17-valerate; TPA, 12-*O*-tetradecanoyl phorbol-13-acetate.

TPA in the dermis: dermal thickness reflects primarily edema but may also be affected by other phenomena including formation of granulation tissue, collagen synthesis, and the activity of myofibroblasts. Cellularity of the dermis is frequently used as a surrogate marker of inflammatory changes in the dermis. In the case of acute inflammation, PMN infiltration is a better determinant of inflammatory changes in the dermis. However, in these samples of chronic inflammation, the subjective information indicated that PMNs were a minor component of the cellularity of the dermis and we therefore considered a change in the number of total cells in the dermis a better indicator of dermal changes. These quantitative measurements confirmed the original subjective observations consistent with an inhibitory response of trifluorosal comparable to HCV, albeit the former at significantly higher doses. Epidermal thickness and cellularity of the dermis correlated well with the observed changes in weight, as previously observed. In contrast, the thickness of the epidermis did not appear to reflect these changes.

In separate experiments designed to understand how trifluorosal inhibited dermal inflammation, we investigated the effect of trifluorosal on TPA-stimulated prostaglandin E_2 (PGE_2) production in human keratinocytes. PGE_2 is a product of arachidonic acid metabolism resulting from the response of cells to cytokines and inflammatory mediators, and it appears that PGE_2 is critically involved in initiating and maintaining inflammation in response to infection, wounding, and other topical conditions (22,23). We found that trifluorosal by itself had no effect on PGE_2 production in these cells at doses as high as 100 µg/mL (Table 1), suggesting that this compound is not a proinflammogen. However, trifluorosal did inhibit PGE_2 pro-

TABLE 1   Effect of trifluorosal on PGE2 Production in TPA-Stimulated Human Keratinocytes

	trifluorosal (µg/mL)				
	0	1	10	30	100
PGE_2 synthesis	450 ± 50^a	620 ± 30	480 ± 80	500 ± 5	525 ± 50
PGE_2 synthesis plus TPA	2250 ± 175	1900 ± 125	1800 ± 110	1500 ± 300	1200 ± 200

[a]Values are CPM/mL media ± SEM, n = 3.
Abbreviations: PGE_2, prostaglandin E_2; TPA, 12-*O*-tetradecanoyl phorbol-13-acetate.

duction by TPA in a dose-dependent fashion. Therefore, we suggest that trifluorosal produces at least some of its anti-inflammatory effect by inhibiting enzymes in the prostaglandin synthetase pathway.

Although these studies had shown that trifluorosal had potential utility as a topical treatment for acne based on its excellent activity against *P. acnes* and inhibition of dermal inflammation produced by a very potent proinflammogen, there was an indication of potential for phototoxicity and this, coupled with its patent lifetime, removed trifluorosal from consideration for further development. Therefore, we began exploring the suitability of developing an optimized 5-aroyl-salicylanilides for this application. Initially, we determined the MICs of 17 compounds from a focused series of 5-naphthoyl-salicylanilides to inhibit the growth of 10 strains of bacteria representative of organisms routinely found in the skin (Table 2) and, more relevant to this discussion, implicated either primarily or secondarily in the pathogenesis of acne (i.e., *P. acnes*, *S. aureus*, *S. epidermidis*, and *S. pyogenes*) (24). This structure-activity study revealed that a 1-naphthoyl group substituted at the 5 position of the salicyl ring increased both the potency and spectrum of antibiotic activity when compared to compounds with 2-naphthoyl, benzoyl, 5-alkylsulfonyl (i.e., trifluorosal), or 5-acyl (i.e., salifluor) substitutions. In addition, a trifluoromethyl group substituted at the 3' position on the anilide ring appeared to be more advantageous than a cyano group at that same position. Of particular interest was the activity of naphthafluor (NA1mF) against the growth of *S. aureus*, a significant pathogenic bacteria that is unaffected by trifluorosal. In an extended MIC study, naphthafluor was shown to not only have potent activity against *P. acnes*, but also excellent activity against a clinical isolate of drug-resistant *S. aureus*, and clinical isolates of multiple drug-resistant *Staphylococcus*. species, *S. pyogenes* and *S. epidermidis*. Naphthafluor was inactive against *Escherichia coli*, *Salmonella*, and *Citrobacter* species. Against *P. acnes*, naphthafluor was found to have equivalent potency to erythromycin, clindamycin, and tetracycline.

Other structure-activity observation that came from this study revealed that electron-donating substituents on the anilide moiety such as in NA1mOPh, NA-12mOMe, and NA13BnOPh reduced antibacterial activity, whereas electron-withdrawing groups substituted on the anilide ring such as in NA1mF, NA1pF, NA1mC, NA1pC enhanced it against most tested bacterial species. Also, *meta* substitution on the anilide ring (i.e., NA1mF, NA1mC) produced compounds of higher potency than *para* substitution (NA1pF, NA1pC). With few exceptions, compounds substituted with a trifluoromethyl group on the anilide ring were more potent than those substituted with a cyano group at the same position. Both of these groups are strongly electron-withdrawing, but the trifluoromethyl group is much more lipophilic, adding another feature to the molecular interaction profile. Alternative

TABLE 2 Minimum Inhibitory Concentrations (µg/mL) for Naphthafluor (NA1mF) and a Focused Series of 17 Structurally Related Analogs Against the Growth of Two Strains of *P. acnes* and Several Other Strains of Dermal Bacterial Pathogens

Drugs	*P. acnes* 6922	*P. acnes* 11827	*S. aureus* 29213	*S. aureus* 6538	*S. aureus* 25923
NA1	25	>100	50	25	>100
NA1mF	0.39	1.56	1.56/3.12	3.12	3.12
NA1mC	6.25	6.25	12.5	6.25	12.5
NA1pC	12.5	6.25	12.5	6.25	>100
NA1pF	0.39	3.12	>100	3.12	25
NA1mF2	0.39	3.12	50	6.25	>100
NA2mF	0.39	0.19	>100	>100	>100
NA2mC	12.5	1.56	>100	>100	>100
NA2pC	3.12/6.25	1.56	12.5	25	25
NA1pBZ	>100	>100	>100	>100	>100
NA13BNoPH	>100	>100	>100	>100	>100
NA2moME	>100	>100	>100	>100	>100
NA1mopH	>100	>100	>100	>100	>100
NA1NpC	1.56	50	>100	>100	>100
NA1oHmF	3.12	12.5	>100	>100	>100
2MeNa1mF	0.78	12.5	12.5	3.12	3.12
3MeNa2mF	0.78	12.5	12.5	3.12	3.12
4MeNa1mF	0.78	25	25	6.25	12.5

	S. epidermidis 12228	*S. pyogenes* 51339	*S. pyogenes* 19615	*S. pyogenes* 49399	*S. pyogenes* 14289
NA1	>100	>100	>100	12.5	>100
NA1mF	1.56	1.56/0.39	6.25/3.12	0.39/0.78	6.25
NA1mC	12.5	12.5/12.5	25	7.8/12.5	12.5
NA1pC	6.25	12.5	>100	0.39	6.25
NA1pF	1.56	1.56	>100	1.56	3.12
NA1mF2	0.78	1.56	1.56	1.56	3.12
NA2mF	50	0.39	>100	3.12	>100
NA2mC	>100	>100	>100	>100	>100
NA2pC	25	50/50	>100	3.12	50
NA1pBZ	>100	>100	>100	>100	>100
NA13BNoPH	>100	>100	>100	>100	>100
NA12moME	>100	>100	>100	>100	>100
NA1mopH	>100	>100	>100	>100	>100
NA1NpC	>100	>100	>100	50	>100
NA1oHmF	>100	>100	>100	>100	>100
2MeNa1mF	6.25	1.56	3.12	0.78	1.56
3MeNa2mF	6.25	0.78	3.12	0.78	1.56
4MeNa1mF	6.25	0.78	1.56	0.78	1.56

electron-withdrawing groups such as -NO2, -SO2R, CONHR, etc., would likely give rise to toxicity or undesirable physical properties. Finally, salicylanilide substitution at the at the 1-naphthoyl position was spectacularly more effective than the corresponding 2-naphthoyl isomers (NA1mF vs. NA2mF) especially considering against *S. aureus* and *S. pyogenes*. Conformational preferences induced in NA1 derivatives by peri-position crowding versus the extended coplanar arrangement available for NA2s is a plausible hypothesis for these differences. This hypothesis is supported by the activity of 3MeNA2mF, which displays activity typical of a NA1 analog rather than that of an NA2 analog. The 3-position methyl group would be expected to produce a twisted conformational preference similar to that of an NA1 analog. Figure 4 demonstrates a quantitative structure-activity analysis that reveals several interesting multiple linear regression models based on common molecular descriptors, which can be calculated for these structures. Although the *S. aureus* data fail to produce useful correlations, *S. pyogenes* and *P. acnes* data give significant structural correlations with topological and electronic descriptors. Cross-validation analysis indicates the latter to be a highly predictive model, as the structure for all 5-naphthoylsalicylanilides correlated well to both *P. acnes* strain 1187 MIC values and *S. pyogenes* strain 51339 MIC values. The conclusion for both was that the training set was very well described by the regression equation, which was highly statistically relevant.

Naphthafluor and several 5-naphthoylsalicylanilides analogs that showed the best antibacterial activity were investigated for their comparative anti-inflammatory properties by using the TPA-induced mouse ear edema assay described above. Previously, naphthafluor was found to be approximately equivalent to trifluorosal and celecoxib (Celebrex) in this assay. In this study, which compared naphthafluor and several of its structural analogs to indomethacin and salifluor, all of the selected 5-naphthoylsalicylanlides inhibited dermal edema in a dose-dependent manner and over the approximately same dose range (Fig. 5), and all were more potent than indomethacin or salifluor. The dose inhibiting 50% inflammation (EC$_{50}$, Table 3) calculated from these dose-effect curves were highly reproducible and allowed us to begin to uncover structure-activity relations in this test system. EC$_{50}$ values were converted to the logarithm of the reciprocal of this value expressed in moles (pEC$_{50}$). Thus, the larger the pEC$_{50}$ value, the more potent is the agent. This representation of bioactivity is the most commonly used form in regression correlations of activity with molecular descriptors. Quantitative analysis was performed with topological and electrotopological molecular descriptors, as well as global descriptors such as log P and Clog P (measures of lipophilicity). The dataset included eight salicylanilides and indomethacin. Among the salicylanilides, six were naphthoyl analogs, one was an acyl derivative (salifluor), and one was an alkylsulfonyl derivative. In this manner, the structural diversity of the training set was enhanced. From this analysis we concluded that the training set was very well described by the regression equation, which was statistically significant (Fig. 6). Cross-validation showed that the constructed model could be used with care to predict the value of

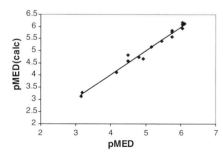

pMED = -0.3506×SHsOH - 19.19×Qv - 1.25×x2 + 3.277×xvp3 + 22.5546

$R^2 = 0.98$; $F=138$; P value = 2.512E-009
Multiple $Q^2 = 0.8025$
Cross validation RSS = 2.83
16 compounds vs. *P. acne* 6922 MICs

Molecular descriptors
SHsOH Sum of the hydrogen estate values for all [– OH] groups
Qv Molecular and group polarity index
x2 Simple second order χ index
xvp3 Valence third order path χ index

FIGURE 4   Statistical correlation for NA structures versus *P. acnes* strain 6922, MIC values.

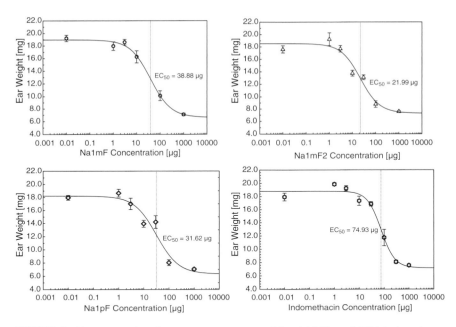

FIGURE 5 Representative dose-response curves of the inhibition of TPA-induced mouse ear edema by three 5-naphthoylsalicylanilides and indomethacin.

pEC_{50}. Indomethacin was the second least potent agent (pEC_{50} = 6.68), yet fitted well within this correlation, which raised the question regarding a common mechanism of action despite the salicylanilides being ca. 10,000-fold more lipophilic. Lipophilicity descriptors were inferior correlates of pEC_{50}. This correlation model offers no interpretation regarding the mechanism of action nor does it directly suggest which molecular modifications may increase inhibitory potency. However, the model may be used to screen hypothetical compounds for anti-inflammatory potential. One mechanism we suspect that the naphthoylsalicylanilides exert their anti-inflammatory activity is via inhibition of enzymes involved in prostaglandin synthesis. This hypothesis is strengthened by the observation that these compounds inhibit both cyclooxygenase 1 and 2, and inhibit PGE_2 production in TPA-treated keratinocytes. Recently, we found that naphthafluor also had very good inhibitory activity against

TABLE 3 EC_{50} Values of Several Salicylanilides and the Anti-inflammatory Drug Indomethacin to Inhibit TPA-Induced Edema in Mouse Ears

Drug	Formula	Formula weight	Hill slope	r2	EC_{50} (µg)	EC_{50} (nm)
Na1	$C_{24}H_{17}NO_3$	367.40	2.7225	0.9898	49.15	133.78
Na1mF	$C_{25}H_{16}F_3NO_3$	435.39	0.9844	0.9050	38.88	89.30
Na1pF	$C_{25}H_{16}F_3NO_3$	435.39	0.9878	0.8546	31.62	72.62
Na1mF2	$C_{26}H_{15}F_6NO_3$	503.39	1.0364	0.8723	21.99	43.68
4MeNa1mF	$C_{26}H_{18}F_3NO_3$	449.42	1.2145	0.9262	28.55	63.54
Indomethacin	$C_{19}H_{16}ClNO_4$	357.81	1.5752	0.9912	74.93	209.42
Salifluor	$C_{22}H_{24}F_3NO_3$	407.40	2.7959	0.9936	127.80	313.71

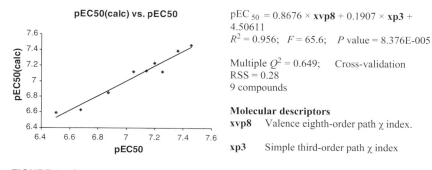

pEC50(calc) vs. pEC50

$pEC_{50} = 0.8676 \times \textbf{xvp8} + 0.1907 \times \textbf{xp3} + 4.50611$

$R^2 = 0.956;\quad F = 65.6;\quad P\ value = 8.376E\text{-}005$

Multiple $Q^2 = 0.649;$ Cross-validation
RSS = 0.28
9 compounds

Molecular descriptors
xvp8   Valence eighth-order path χ index.

xp3   Simple third-order path χ index

FIGURE 6   Statistical correlation for the mouse ear anti-inflammatory data.

several proteases responsible for tissue destruction and/or propagation of the immune response to infection. Therefore, we suspect that part of the anti-inflammatory effect of the naphthoylsalicylanilides, especially against chronic disease, may also arise from their inhibition of pathways yet to be fully elucidated.

CONCLUSIONS

When acne is severe enough to warrant therapy, current treatments often fall short of their curative goal because they do not adequately address the underlying metabolic or pathophysiologic conditions that give rise to the disease, or they are too toxic for effective use. Recent advances in the study of acne firmly implicate that acne's initiation rests with abnormal follicular keratinization and sebum production in the pilosebaceous unit of the skin. This produces an environment for the overgrowth of normal skin flora, such as the bacterium *P. acnes*, leading to acute and progressing to chronic infectious inflammation. These latter events eventually result in tissue destruction and conversion of tissue in the area of the affected pustule.

The rational design of new drugs that have a combination of pharmacologic properties that could address the initiation, progression, or conversion components of this disorder should result in an improved therapy. The LAAD-type salicylanilides, which were originally designed to be topically active antibiotics, were serendipitously discovered to have inherent anti-inflammatory activity. Recent synthetic optimization of this class of novel compounds for both antibacterial and anti-inflammatory active has produced naphthafluor, which is currently in development as both a treatment for acne and another topical infectious multifactorial disorder, gingivitis. Current studies indicate that naphthafluor may have additional properties that would be uniquely beneficial for the treatment of both conditions. Future studies are expected to determine if LAAD-type salicylanilides are, in fact, a major class of pharmacologically active compounds that can be designed to address the many topical inflammatory diseases that are caused or exacerbated by bacterial infection.

REFERENCES

1. Webster GF. Acne vulgaris. Br Med J 2002; 325:475–479.
2. Gollnick H. Current concepts of the pathogenesis of acne: implications for drug treatment. Drugs 2003; 63:1579–1596.

3. Perry AL, Lambert PA. *Propionibacterium acnes*. Lett Appl Microbiol 2006; 43:185–188.
4. Abd El All HS, Shoukry NS, El Maged RA, et al. Immunohistochemical expression of interleukin 8 in skin biopsies from patients with inflammatory acne vulgaris. Diagn Pathol 2007; 2:4.
5. Trivedi NR, Gilliland KL, Zhao W, et al. Gene array expression profiling in acne lesions reveals marked upregulation of genes involved in inflammation and matrix remodeling. J Invest Dermatol 2006; 126:1071–1079.
6. Johnson BM, Nunley JR. Use of systemic agents in the treatment of acne vulgaris. Am Fam Phys 2000; 61:1823–1830.
7. Liao DC. Management of acne. Fam Pract 2003; 52:43–51.
8. Toyodo M, Morohashi M. An overview of topical antibiotics for the treatment of acne. Dermatology 1998; 196:130–134.
9. Gollnick H, Schremm M. Topical drug treatment in acne. Dermatology 1998; 196:119–125.
10. Nishijima A, Kurokawa I, Katoh N, et al. The bacteriology of acne vulgaris and antimicrobial susceptibility of *Propionibacterium acnes* and *Staphylococcus epidermidis* isolate from acne lesions. J Dermatol 2000; 27:318–323.
11. Eady EA, Bacterial resistance in acne. Dermatology 1998; 196:58–66.
12. Eady EA, Jones C, Gardner D. Tetracycline-resistant *Propionibacteria* from acne patients are cross-resistant to doxycycline, but sensitive to minocycline. Br J Dermatol 1993; 128:556–560.
13. Tsuruta D, Someda Y, Sowa J, et al. Drug hypersensitivity syndrome caused by minocycline. J Cutan Med Surg 2006; 10:131–135.
14. Zouboulis CC, Piquero-Martin J. Update and future of systemic acne treatment. Dermatology 2003; 206:37–53.
15. Diamanti-Kandarakis E. Current aspects of anti-androgen therapy in women. Curr Pharm Dis 1999; 5:707–723.
16. Dickerson V. Quality of life issues. Potential role for an oral contraceptive containing ethinyl estradiol and drospirenone. J Reprod Med 2002; 47(Suppl.):985–993.
17. Furuichi Y, Ramberg P, Lindhe J, et al. Some effects of mouthrinses containing salifluor on de novo plaque formation and developing gingivitis. J Clin Periodontol 1996; 23:795–802.
18. Nabi N, Kashuba B, Zucchesi S, et al. In-vitro and in-vivo on Salifluor/PVA/MA copolymer/NaF combination as an antiplaque agent. J Clin Periodont 1996; 23:795–802.
19. Evans RT, Coburn RA, Genco RA, et al. Method of relieving inflammation by using 5-alkylsulfonylsalicylanilides. U.S. Patent 5958911, 1999.
20. Evans RT, Coburn RA, Genco RA, et al. Method of relieving chronic inflammation by using 5-alkylsulfonylsalicylanilides. U.S. Patent 6117859, 2000.
21. Stanley PL, Steiner S, Havens M, et al. Mouse skin inflammation induced by multiple applications of 12-O-tetradecanoyl phorbol-13-acetate. Skin Pharmacol 1991; 4:262–271.
22. Ueno A, Oh-ishi S. Critical roles for bradykinin and prostanoids in acute inflammatory reactions: a search using experimental animal models. Curr Drug Targets Inflamm Allergy 2002; 1(4):363–376.
23. Wilgus TA, Vodovotz Y, Vittadini E, et al. Reduction of scar formation in full-thickness wounds with topical celecoxib treatment. Wound Repair Regen 2003; 11(1):25–34.
24. Lennette A, Balows W, Hausler J, et al., eds. Manual of Clinical Microbiology. 4th ed. Washington, D.C.: American Society for Microbiology, 1997:978–987.

15 Codrugs: Potential Therapies for Dermatological Diseases

Tadeusz Cynkowski and Grazyna Cynkowska
Psivida Inc., Watertown, Massachusetts, U.S.A.

Kenneth A. Walters
An-eX Analytical Services Ltd., Cardiff, U.K.

INTRODUCTION

Implantable drug compositions have been developed that deliver two or more compounds in a single dose and provide controlled delivery of such compounds. In particular, in U.S. Patent 6,051,576, we have described pharmaceutical compounds covalently linking two or more drug compounds (parent drugs) to form a single compound that has relatively low solubility in biological fluids, and that is quickly hydrolyzed to form the parent compounds when dissolved at or near pH 7.4 (1). The potential use of codrugs, or mutual prodrugs, for synergistic biological effect has been described in several therapeutic categories including antimicrobials (2,3), analgesia (4,5), inflammation (6,7), HIV infection (8), oncology (9), alcoholism (10), and ophthalmology (11–14).

There is also a good physicochemical rationale underlying the potential use of codrugs for dermal and transdermal delivery (15). It is well known that permeation across the skin is strongly dependent on the ability of the permeant to partition into and diffuse across serial barriers that are lipophilic and hydrophilic. Initial partition into the stratum corneum (the lipophilic barrier) is related to the oil/water partition coefficient of the permeant, such that the higher this value, the more readily will the compound enter the stratum corneum. The underlying viable epidermis is, however, more hydrophilic, and therefore, partition from the stratum corneum into this layer is easier for compounds with a lower oil/water partition coefficient. There are many examples that illustrate that compounds with a medium octanol/water partition coefficient ($\log P$, between 1 and 3) are the most rapid skin permeants. By using the prodrug approach (16), it is possible to increase P for a hydrophilic compound and thereby increase penetration into the stratum corneum. Subsequent epidermal metabolism (16) will break down the prodrug to release the parent hydrophilic compound and permeation across the viable epidermis will be facilitated.

CODRUG POTENTIAL IN TRANSDERMAL THERAPY

Topical administration of biologically active moieties for systemic effect is becoming increasingly popular. The transdermal mode of drug administration is, however, limited by the ability of potential drug candidates to be absorbed by, or cross, the dermal barrier. As discussed elsewhere in this book, several strategies have been used to decrease the skin barrier to permeation. These include chemical and physical permeation enhancement techniques, microneedles, pressure waves, and high-pressure powder impaction. Because early theoretical analyses indicated the potential of successful transdermal codrug technology (17), attempts have been made to experimentally confirm this optimism. Hammell et al (18) evaluated the transdermal delivery of a dimer (termed "gemini prodrug") of naltrexone by using human skin in vitro. Naltrexone is a drug used in the treatment of narcotic dependence and alcoholism. Skin permeation rates of naltrexone, as a single entity, and the dimer were determined using flow-through diffusion cells. Drug concentrations in the skin were measured at the termination of the diffusion experiment. During the permeation process, the prodrug was hydrolyzed and appeared mainly as naltrexone in the receptor solution. The dimer provided a significantly higher naltrexone equivalent flux across human skin than naltrexone alone (3.0 nmol/cm^2/hr for naltrexone, 6.2 nmol/cm^2/hr for the dimer). Although naltrexone permeability from the dimer exceeded the permeability of naltrexone base by twofold, there was no significant increase in drug concentration in the skin after dimer treatment compared to application of naltrexone alone.

The same group went on to evaluate the enhancement of transdermal delivery of the naltrexone active metabolite 6-β-naltrexol when carbonate linked to hydroxybupropion (10,19). This is an interesting dual therapy concept allowing the treatment of alcohol abuse to be combined with an aid to smoking cessation. In vitro human skin permeation rates and disposition were determined using flow-through diffusion cells. The codrug was partially hydrolyzed on passing through skin, and a combination of intact codrug and parent drugs was found in the receptor medium. Flux of 6-β-naltrexol was significantly higher than the parent drug when applied as the codrug. The extent of parent drug regeneration in the skin ranged from 56% to 86%.

There are a variety of potential dimers or combination codrugs that may find application in the transdermal field. Examples of such codrugs synthesized in our laboratories include:

- Angiotensin-converting enzyme (ACE) inhibitor (benazeprilat) with calcium channel blocker (amlodipine)
- ACE inhibitor (fosinopril) with 3-hydroxy-3-methyl-glutaryd coenzyme A (HMGCoA) reductase inhibitor (lovastatin, simvastatin)
- ACE inhibitor dimers (enalapril, captopril, fosinopril)
- ACE inhibitor (enalapril) with angiotensin II antagonist (telmisartan)

ACE inhibitor (enalapril) with nonsteroidal anti-inflammatory drugs (NSAIDs) (aspirin, diclofenac, naproxen)

- HMGCoA reductase inhibitor (atorvastatin, simvastatin) with antilipemic (ezetimibe)
- HMGCoA reductase inhibitor dimers
- Analgesic (morphine, hydromorphone) with NSAIDs (naproxen, diclofenac, indomethacin, aspirin)
- Antineoplastic (tegafur) with NSAIDs (naproxen)
- Antineoplastic (camptothecin) with NSAIDs (naproxen, flurbiprofen)
- Antineoplastic (combretastatin A4) with antineoplastic (chlorambucil)
- Antineoplastic (combretastatin A4) with corticosteroids
- Various dimers and cross codrugs of NSAIDs (diclofenac, naproxen, flurbiprofen, indomethacin, sulindac, aspirin
- Dimers of antidepressants (paroxetine, fluoxetine)
- Dimers of antiasthmatics (montelucast)

- Dimers of antivirals (ganciclovir, acyclovir)
- Various codrugs and dimers of anti-HIV drugs (AZT, ddC, ddI, indinavir, saquinavir, ritonavir)

CODRUG POTENTIAL IN DERMAL THERAPY

There is tremendous potential for codrug therapy in dermatological diseases. There are several conditions that would benefit from dual therapy including the most prevalent, such as oxidative stress, acne, and psoriasis, and the less common, such as actinic keratosis. However, a review of the available literature indicates that investigation of the codrug concept is limited and evaluation in the clinic rare. Nonetheless, the available reports suggest that the use of codrugs in dermatology could provide a considerable and beneficial therapeutic advancement.

OXIDATIVE STRESS

Oxidative stress and its associated damage to skin is a consequence of environmental factors such as UV light and is a problem of mounting concern. Many cosmetic formulations contain retinoid-based compounds, such as retinyl palmitate, either to protect the skin or to stimulate skin responses that will correct skin damaged by sunlight (20). Another long-chain ester compound, ascorbyl palmitate is also used in cosmetic products as an effective antioxidant that protects tissue integrity. Abdulmajed and Heard (21) synthesized the ester-linked codrug retinyl ascorbate from all-*trans*-retinyl chloride and L-ascorbic acid. The flux across human epidermal membranes was measured and skin penetration was determined by stratum corneum tape stripping of full-thickness human skin. Similar determinations were made for retinyl palmitate and ascorbyl palmitate. Although the codrug had a favourable log P of 2.2, its transdermal flux was, as expected, lower than that obtained for retinyl palmitate and ascorbyl palmitate. Retinyl ascorbate demonstrated higher skin retention than the other two esters and delivered more retinoic acid and ascorbic acid to the viable epidermis than retinol from retinyl palmitate and ascorbic acid from ascorbyl palmitate. The data suggested the potential value of the codrug in treating damage to skin caused by UV-induced production of free radicals. Clearly, prolonged efficacy of agents designed to act in the epidermis is influenced by retention time in the target tissue, and this can be increased by interaction with skin components. Abdulmajed et al. (22) continued their studies on retinyl ascorbate to determine the skin binding properties of the codrug. In their studies they determined the binding of the codrug and its parent compounds, retinoic acid and ascorbic acid, together with retinol, ascorbyl palmitate, and retinyl palmitate to the keratinous tissues, human callus, pig ear skin, and bovine horn. Binding to keratin was assessed using both native tissue and delipidized tissue. Not surprisingly, in delipidized tissue, binding was higher for the polar compounds and dipolar/H bonding to keratin was proposed. The binding characteristic of native tissues was complicated by lipid, creating a dual effect comprising keratin binding and partitioning. Therefore, for highly polar compounds, such as ascorbic acid, lipid content decreased binding, whereas for the more lipophilic retinyl ascorbate binding increased with lipid content, suggesting that a substantial amount is dissolved in the lipid matrix. The authors concluded that this ability to bind with skin components enhanced the suitability of the codrug for topical application.

Further studies by this group suggested that the codrug, retinyl ascorbate, exhibited antioxidant properties that were 30% to 40% more potent than the ascorbates and 70% more potent than the retinoids in the test tube (23), and the greater potency for the codrug was confirmed in cultured human keratinocytes (24).

PSORIASIS

Psoriasis, a T cell–mediated inflammatory skin disease characterized by hyperproliferation and poor differentiation of epidermal keratinocytes, is an example of a skin disease that may benefit from combination therapy. There is considerable evidence to suggest that the hyperproliferation and inflammatory components of the disease can be more rapidly controlled using mixtures of drugs such as the vitamin D3 analog calcipotriol and the steroid betamethasone dipropionate (25,26). Similarly, Clark et al. (27) had found that a combination of methotrexate and cyclosporin was a more effective treatment for severe recalcitrant psoriasis than was either agent alone. There are several drug combinations that may be beneficial in the treatment of psoriasis. These include acitretin, tazarotene, calcipotriene, anthralin, and many steroids, all of which possess one or more functional groups capable of conjugation. More specifically, a codrug comprising a first constituent moiety selected from corticosteroids and NSAIDs, and a second constituent moiety selected from antipsoriatic moieties, such as acitretin, salicylic acid, anthralin, 6-azauridine, calcipotriene, maxacalcitol, pyrogallol, and tacalcitol.

Recently, Ben-Shabat et al. (28) examined the potential use of vitamin D3–based conjugates with polyunsaturated fatty acids (PUFA) as a treatment for psoriasis. Although these conjugates may be considered as prodrugs, the evidence that PUFA may be beneficial in psoriasis (29) implies that they can be considered as codrugs. Using codrugs of linolenic acid or γ-linolenic acid and calcipotriol, prepared by coupling the fatty acid with calcipotriol in the presence of dicyclohexyl-carbodiimide and 4-(dimethylamino)-pyridine, the authors explored the skin bioavailability and cell growth inhibitory activity of the complexes. Application of the codrug resulted in a considerable enhancement of the penetration of calcipotriol into pig skin in vitro. The studies showed that the codrugs penetrated into the skin at higher levels than calcipotriol alone. Analyses of skin and receptor fluid samples indicated that a major portion of calcipotriol-PUFA conjugate was converted into another isomer form before hydrolysis to calcipotriol and PUFA. The antiproliferative activity of the codrug, determined using human keratinocytes, was slightly greater with the calcipotriol-linolenic than with either the γ-linolenic-calcipotriol codrug or calcitriol alone. The biotransformation that occurred after penetration into the skin suggested that the codrugs were fully converted to the parent drugs during absorption.

ACTINIC KERATOSIS

Actinic keratoses are premalignant intraepidermal skin lesions that are caused by excessive exposure to sunlight. The lesions are characterized by disordered epidermal differentiation and have the potential to develop into malignant nonmelanoma skin cancers (30). Many early treatment options involved destructive regimens such as liquid nitrogen freezing, curettage, and chemical peels (31). Less destructive but more prolonged treatment involves topical application of creams and lotions containing 5-fluorouracil (5-FU) (32) and diclofenac (33). Smith et al. (34) conducted a bilateral comparison study of the efficacy and tolerability of diclofenac 3% gel used for 90 days and 5% fluorouracil cream used for 28 days. Although both treatment regimens demonstrated efficacy in the number of lesions cleared, diclofenac induced only mild signs of inflammation in most patients compared to 5-FU, despite the longer treatment period. It appears that inflammation is likely to be required to achieve a therapeutic effect from the daily application of 5% 5-FU cream (35).

Levy et al. (32) compared the flux and skin content of 5-FU from three 0.5% 5-FU formulations with those from a commercially available 5% 5-FU formulation using human skin in vitro. Although the flux from the 5% 5-FU formulation was 20 to 40 times greater than that of the 0.5% 5-FU formulations, a higher percentage of absorbed 5-FU was retained in the skin after 24 hours with the 0.5% formulations. Because the site of action of the 5-FU is within the skin, these data suggest that the lower concentration formulation may be therapeutically equivalent to the high-dose formulation. In a further study, it was found that 0.5% 5-FU cream was at least as effective as 5% 5-FU cream in terms of the percent reduction in actinic keratosis lesions (36). In this and other clinical studies with 5-FU, skin irritation and inflammation is an associated side effect of treatment.

This disease is, therefore, an ideal candidate for codrug therapy. The physicochemical characteristics of 5-FU indicate that it will not penetrate the skin to any great extent, and the issue of skin irritation during therapy can be addressed using anti-inflammatory agents. To this end, we synthesized and evaluated a codrug comprising 5-FU covalently linked to triamcinolone acetonide (CDS-TC-32, FUTA, Fig. 1).

Synthesis of CDS-TC-32

The codrug of triamcinolone acetonide with 5-FU (CDS-TC-32, FUTA) was prepared as shown in Figure 1. Triamcinolone acetonide was selectively chloroformylated in position 21 by using diphosgene (trichloromethyl chloroformate) in the presence of charcoal. The resulting chloroformate was condensed with bis(hydroxymethyl)-

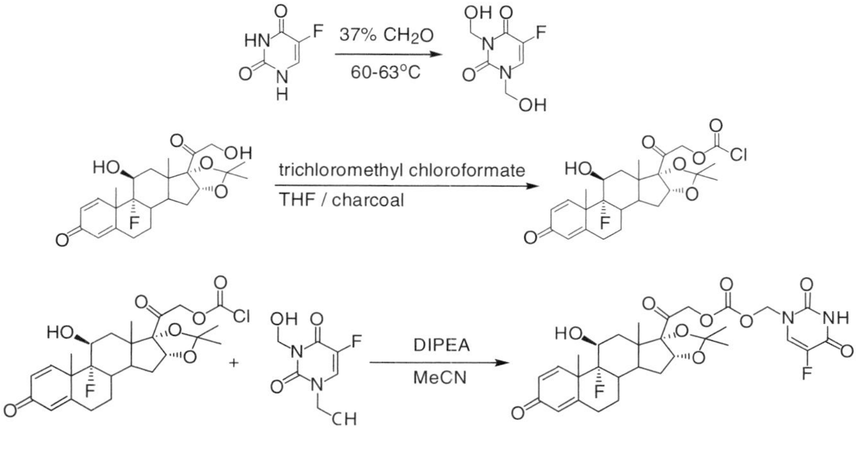

FIGURE 1 Preparation of triamcinolone acetonide–5-fluorouracil (5-FU) codrug CDS-TC-32.

5-fluorouracil prepared separately from 5-FU and formaldehyde. The reaction was performed in acetonitrile in the presence of diisopropylethylamine.

In Vitro Evaluation of CDS-TC-32

In vitro transport of CDS-TC-32 and its parent drugs was evaluated by using both synthetic lipophilic membranes and human skin. In both cases, the relative amount of triamcinolone acetonide and 5-FU that had crossed the membrane was greater after application of the codrug when compared to application of the parent compounds either alone or in combination (Fig. 2). In the case of the human skin membranes, no intact CDS-TC-32 was found in the receptor phase, suggesting that complete hydrolysis had occurred during the permeation process. A further experiment using human skin was designed to determine the amount of intact CDS-TC-32 and parent compounds distributed in various layers through the skin. Twelve replicates were prepared with fresh skin from three donors, which was mounted in diffusion cells within three hours of excision. The integrity of each skin membrane was confirmed by measuring the permeation rate of tritiated water. A target dose of 5 mg/cm^2 of formulation was applied to each cell and receptor phase samples removed, and immediately frozen, at 2, 4, 8, 12, and 24 hours. At 24 hours, the residual formulation was removed with surface wipes, and the skin tape stripped to remove the stratum corneum. The tape strips were grouped (strips 1–2, 3–5, and 6–10). The remaining tissue was dry heat–separated to yield epidermis and dermis samples. Skin samples were extracted and analyzed using two sensitive high-performance liquid chromatography (HPLC) assays, one allowing simultaneous analysis for triamcinolone acetonide and CDS-TC-32. Receptor phase samples were analyzed without modification. Twenty-four hours after application, the majority of the applied CDS-TC-32 was recovered unchanged from the skin surface (77%). However, significant skin penetration and hydrolysis of CDS-TC-32 was observed. Hydrolysis increased with skin depth (Fig. 3), although the available CDS-TC-32 was not completely hydrolyzed in any of the skin strata. No CDS-TC-32 was found in the diffusion cell receptor phases.

The tape strips contained a total of 8.96 ± 0.57% applied CDS-TC-32 (unchanged), with 0.724 ± 0.127% and 0.784 ± 0.095% applied CDS-TC-32 dose recov-

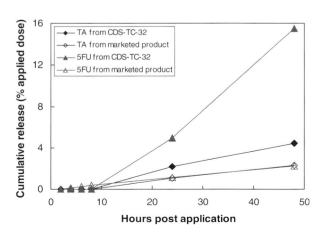

FIGURE 2 In vitro human skin permeation of triamcinolone acetonide and 5-FU when applied as individual marketed products or as CDS-TC-32. Note that the triamcinolone acetonide was present in the application vehicles at equivalent concentrations (0.5% w/w). The marketed 5-FU formulation contained 5% w/w drug, whereas the CDS-TC-32 application vehicle contained 0.21% w/w 5-FU. Values given are expressed in % applied dose permeated.

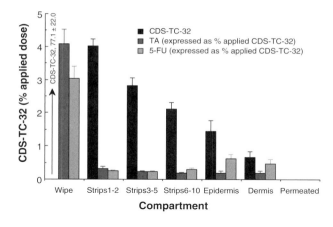

FIGURE 3 In vitro human skin distribution of CDS-TC-32, triamcinolone acetonide, and 5-FU after application of a CDS-TC-32 cream formulation. Values given represent % applied CDS-TC-32 (mean ± SE).

ered as TA and 5-FU, respectively. Epidermis samples contained $1.46 \pm 0.32\%$, $0.194 \pm 0.065\%$, and $0.614 \pm 0.131\%$ applied CDS-TC-32 dose recovered as CDS-TC-32 (unchanged), TA, and 5-FU, respectively. The corresponding values for dermis samples were $0.622 \pm 0.173\%$, $0.202 \pm 0.051\%$, and $0.461 \pm 0.142\%$ applied CDS-TC-32 dose. The total recovery of unchanged CDS-TC-32 was 88.2 ± 1.2 % applied dose. After inclusion of the average recovery of hydrolyzed CDS-TC-32 (5.1%), total recovery was 93.3% of the applied dose.

In Vivo Evaluation of CDS-TC-32

A vasoconstriction (skin blanching assay) and skin surface biopsy (SSB) study was conducted in healthy volunteers and results were compared after application of 0.75% CDS-TC-32 cream (equivalent to 0.5% triamcinolone acetonide) and a marketed 0.5% triamcinolone acetonide cream. Steroids cause local vasoconstriction when applied and the degree of skin blanching is a function of steroid potency and concentration at the active site. The SSB technique removes surface layers of the stratum corneum using cyanoacrylate adhesive and glass slides. Formulations were applied to discrete

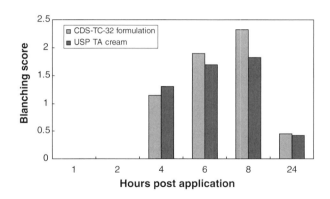

FIGURE 4 In vivo vasoconstriction scores in human volunteers after application of triamcinolone acetonide cream (0.5% w/w) and CDS-TC-32 cream containing the equivalent of 0.5% w/w triamcinolone acetonide. Skin blanching was assessed by trained personnel on a scale of 0 to 3, where 0 = no blanching and 3 = profound blanching. Scores were verified by using a chromameter. Note that for the 24-hour blanching score, the residual formulation had been removed at eight hours.

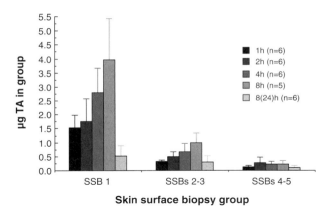

FIGURE 5   In vivo human skin distribution of triamcinolone acetonide in skin surface biopsies after application of 0.5% w/w triamcinolone acetonide formulation. Values are in µg (mean ± SE).

and randomized sites on the backs of 20 volunteers and skin blanching assessed at set time intervals up to 24 hours. Each patient was dosed with three formulations, on separate sites for each formulation and time point. Formulation A was a placebo cream, B a 0.75% CDS-TC-32 cream, and C a marketed 0.5% triamcinolone acetonide cream. SSBs were taken from six patients over the 24-hour period. Five SSBs were

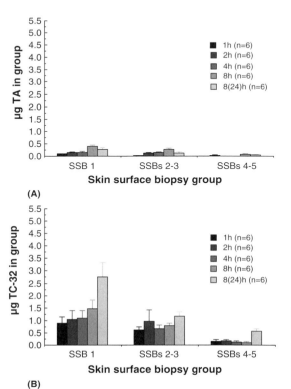

FIGURE 6   In vivo human skin distribution of (A) triamcinolone acetonide and (B) CDS-TC-32 in skin surface biopsies after application of the equivalent of 0.5% w/w triamcinolone acetonide in a CDS-TC-32 formulation. Values are in µg (mean ± SE).

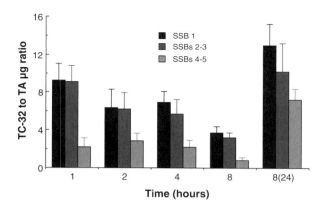

FIGURE 7 The ratio of CDS-TC-32 to triamcinolone acetonide in skin surface biopsies after application of the equivalent of 0.5% w/w triamcinolone acetonide in a CDS-TC-32 formulation. Note that there is more triamcinolone acetonide to CDS-TC-32 in the deeper biopsies, indicating that more CDS-TC-32 is being hydrolyzed in the deeper stratum corneum.

taken from each site, after assay for skin blanching and removal of remaining surface formulation, at 1, 2, 4, 6, and 8 hours. At 8 hours, the formulation was removed from remaining sites, and further SSBs were taken at 24 hours.

No skin blanching was observed at the placebo-treated site. Sites treated with 0.75% CDS-TC-32 cream and the marketed 0.5% triamcinolone acetonide cream showed equivalent blanching (Fig. 4), suggesting that similar amounts of triamcinolone acetonide had reached the dermis from the two formulations.

The TA recovery from the SSB groups for formulation C (0.5% triamcinolone acetonide) is shown in Figure 5. Up to the 8-hour time point, levels of TA in the SSBs increased with time. The subsequent clearance of TA from the skin, after removal of the excess surface formulation at 8 hours, is clearly seen in the reduced 24-hour levels. For formulation B, TA and CDS-TC-32 recoveries from the SSB groups are shown in Figure 6. TA levels were lower than for formulation C, but CDS-TC-32 levels were similar to TA levels from formulation C. The clearance of CDS-TC-32 appeared to be a more gradual process than for TA (from formulation C), with 24-hour SSBs containing much higher levels of CDS-TC-32. The ratio of CDS-TC-32 to TA HPLC peak areas was calculated for formulation B to provide information about how the conversion of CDS-TC-32 varied with skin depth. More conversion was apparent in the deeper SSBs (Fig. 7), suggesting a greater enzymatic activity as the viable epidermis is approached. It was concluded that some conversion of CDS-TC-32 to triamcinolone acetonide and 5-FU occurs, with conversion increasing with skin depth. Overall skin delivery of triamcinolone acetonide was not altered by application as a codrug except that there appeared to be a greater substantivity of the codrug, which indicated the possibility of a cutaneous reservoir of the codrug. The cutaneous reservoir would provide a more sustained release of both triamcinolone acetonide and 5-FU, a factor that may be important in the therapy of actinic keratosis.

FUTURE PERSPECTIVES

There are many skin disorders that may benefit from codrug therapy. The "proliferative skin disorders" mentioned earlier are prime candidates, but dual therapy could be useful in any disease of the skin marked by unwanted or aberrant proliferation of cutaneous tissue. These conditions are typically characterized by epidermal cell proliferation or incomplete cell differentiation and include, for example, X-linked ichthyosis, atopic dermatitis, allergic contact dermatitis, epidermolytic hyperkeratosis, and seborrheic dermatitis.

Acne is another example of a dermatologic condition that may be treated with a combined antiproliferative, antibiotic, and/or keratolytic agent. Acne vulgaris is a multifactorial disease most commonly occurring in teenagers and young adults, and is characterized by the appearance of inflammatory and noninflammatory lesions on the face and upper trunk. The basic defect that gives rise to acne vulgaris is hypercornification of the duct of a hyperactive sebaceous gland. Hypercornification blocks the normal mobility of skin and follicle microorganisms, and in so doing, stimulates the release of lipases by *Propionibacterium acnes* and *Staphylococcus epidermidis* bacteria, and *Pitrosporum ovale*, a yeast. Treatment with an antiproliferative codrug may be useful for preventing the transitional features of the ducts (e.g., hypercornification) that lead to lesion formation. Keratolytic compounds that could be suitable as one or more constituent compounds in a codrug include retinoic acid (vitamin A), resorcinol, salicylic acid, and tetroquinone. Each of these keratolytic compounds possesses one or more functional groups and is thus capable of being linked to one or more of the same keratolytic compound, a different keratolytic compound, or a different pharmaceutically active moiety.

Dermatitis refers to poorly demarcated lesions that are either pruritic, erythematous, scaly, blistered, weeping, fissured, or crusted. These lesions arise from any of a wide variety of causes. The most common types of dermatitis are atopic, contact, and diaper dermatitis. For instance, seborrheic dermatitis is a chronic, usually pruritic, dermatitis with erythema, dry, moist, or greasy scaling, and yellow crusted patches on various areas, especially the scalp, with exfoliation of an excessive amount of dry scales stasis dermatitis, an often chronic, usually eczematous dermatitis. Actinic dermatitis is dermatitis due to exposure to actinic radiation such as that from the sun, ultraviolet waves, or X or gamma radiation. Codrug preparations could be useful in the treatment and/or prevention of certain symptoms of dermatitis caused by unwanted proliferation of epithelial cells. Such therapies for these various forms of dermatitis can also include topical and systemic corticosteroids, antipruritics, and antibiotics.

Skin protection may also benefit from codrug application. For example, sunscreens suitable as one or more constituents of a codrug include *p*-aminobenzoic acid and 4-dimethylaminobenzoic acid.

Thus there are a variety of potential dimers or combination codrugs that may find application in the dermal field. Examples of such codrugs synthesized in our laboratories include the following:

- Analgesic (morphine) with corticosteroids [TA, fluocinolone acetonide (FA), hydrocortisone]
- Analgesic (morphine) with vitamin E
- Topical analgesic (capsaicin) with NSAIDs (diclofenac)
- Antineoplastic (5-FU) with retinoic acid
- Corticosteroids (FA, TA) with selenomethionine
- Retinoids (retinoic acid, tazarotene) with corticosteroids (TA, FA)

CONCLUSIONS

It is possible to make codrugs from many different therapeutic agents. The limited data available indicate that the concept will provide a good therapeutic alternative for many disease states either systemically via the transdermal route or for local dermatological therapy. Many dermatological conditions would benefit from a dual therapeutic approach and the physicochemical rationale for codrug delivery to the skin has obvious advantages.

REFERENCES

1. Ashton P, Crooks PA, Cynkowski T, et al. Means to achieve sustained release of synergistic drugs by conjugation. U.S. Patent 6,051,576, January 1997.
2. Jones RN, Barry AL, Thornsberry C. Antimicrobial activity of Ro 23-9424, a novel ester-linked codrug of fleroxacin and desacetylcefotaxime. Antimicrob Agents Chemother 1989; 33:944–950.
3. Jones RN. Antimicrobial activity of Ro 24-6778, a covalent bonding of desmethylfleroxacin and desacetylcefotaxime. Diag Microbiol Infect Dis 1990; 13:253–259.
4. Chen J, Cynkowski T, Guo H, et al. Morphine pharmacokinetics following intra-articular administration of a novel sustained release opioid (CDS-PM-101) for the relief of post-operative orthopaedic pain. J Control Rel 2005; 101:359–360.
5. Shi W, Liu H, Zhang Y, et al. Design, synthesis, and preliminary evaluation of gabapentin-pregabalin mutual prodrugs in relieving neuropathic pain. Arch Pharm Chem Life Sci 2005; 338:358–364.
6. Sheha M, Khedr A, Elsheriet H. Biological and metabolic study of naproxen-propyphenazone mutual prodrug. Eur J Pharm Sci 2002; 17:121–130.
7. Otagiri M, Imai T, Fukuhara A. Improving the pharmacokinetic and pharmacodynamic properties of a drug by chemical conversion to a chimera drug. J Control Rel 1999; 62:223–229.
8. Sun X-F, Wu Q, Wang N, et al. Novel mutual pro-drugs of 2',3'-dideoxyinosine with 3-octadecyloxy-propane-1,2-diol by straightforward enzymatic regioselective synthesis in acetone. Biotechnol Lett 2005; 27:113–117.
9. Nudelman A, Rephaeli A. Novel mutual prodrug of retinoic and butyric acids with enhanced anticancer activity. J Med Chem 2000; 43:2962–2966.
10. Hamad MO, Kiptoo PK, Stinchcomb AL, et al. Synthesis and hydrolytic behavior of two novel tripartite codrugs of naltrexone and 6β-naltrexol with hydroxybupropion as potential alcohol abuse and smoking cessation agents. Bioorg Med Chem 2006; 14: 7051–7061.
11. Berger AS, Cheng CK, Pearson PA, et al. Intravitreal sustained release corticosteroid-5-fluorouracil conjugate in the treatment of experimental proliferative vitreoretinopathy. Invest Ophthalmol Vis Sci 1996; 37:2318–2325.
12. Yang C-S, Khawly JA, Hainsworth DP, et al. An intravitreal sustained-release triamcinolone and 5-fluorouracil codrug in the treatment of experimental proliferative vitreoretinopathy. Arch Ophthalmol 1998; 116:69–77.
13. Cardillo JA, Farah ME, Mitre J, et al. An intravitreal biodegradable sustained release naproxen and 5-fluorouracil system for the treatment of experimental post-traumatic proliferative vitreoretinopathy. Br J Ophthalmol 2004; 88:1201–1205.
14. Cynkowska G, Cynkowski T, Al-Ghananeem AA, et al. Novel antiglaucoma prodrugs and codrugs of ethacrynic acid. Bioorg Med Chem Lett 2005; 15:3524–3527.
15. Walters K, Shimizu R, Ashton P, et al. Topical delivery of codrugs. U.S. Patent Application: 20030118528, filed November 19, 2002.
16. Stinchcomb AL, Swaan PW, Ekabo O et al. Straight-chain naltrexone ester prodrugs: diffusion and concurrent esterase biotransformation in human skin. J Pharm Sci 2002; 91:2571–2578.
17. Nazemi MH, Brain KR, Heard CM. Design of bifunctional moieties with improved skin delivery potential. Combining dexamethasone and NSAIDs. In: Brain KR, Walters KA, eds. Perspectives in Percutaneous Penetration. Vol. 7a. Cardiff, U.K.: STS Publishing, 2000:67.
18. Hammell DC, Hamad M, Vaddi HK, et al. Duplex "gemini" prodrug of naltrexone for transdermal delivery. J Control Rel 2004; 97:283–290.
19. Kiptoo PK, Hamad MO, Crooks PA, et al. Enhancement of transdermal delivery of 6-β-naltrexol via a codrug linked to hydroxybupropion. J Control Rel 2006; 113:137–145.

20. Tolleson WH, Cherng SH, Xia Q, et al. Photodecomposition and phototoxicity of natural retinoids. Int J Environ Res Public Health 2005; 2:147–155.
21. Abdulmajed K, Heard CM. Topical delivery of retinyl ascorbate co-drug. 1. Synthesis, penetration into and permeation across human skin. Int J Pharmaceut 2004; 280:113–124.
22. Abdulmajed K, Heard CM, McGuigan C, et al. Topical delivery of retinyl ascorbate co-drug. 2. Comparative skin tissue and keratin binding studies. Skin Pharmacol Physiol 2004; 17:274–282.
23. Abdulmajed K, McGuigan C, Heard CM. Topical delivery of retinyl ascorbate co-drug. 4. Comparative anti-oxidant activity towards DPPH. Free Radic Res 2005; 39:491–498.
24. Abdulmajed K, McGuigan C, Heard CM. Topical delivery of retinyl ascorbate co-drug: 6. Determination of toxic dose and antioxidant activity in cultured human epidermal keratinocytes. Pharmazie 2005; 60:794–795.
25. Douglas WS, Poulin Y, Decroix J, et al. A new calcipotriol/betamethasone formulation with rapid onset of action was superior to monotherapy with betamethasone dipropionate or calcipotriol in psoriasis vulgaris. Acta Derm Venereol 2002; 82:131–135.
26. Kragballe K, Noerrelund KL, Lui H, et al. Efficacy of once-daily treatment regimens with calcipotriol/betamethasone dipropionate ointment and calcipotriol ointment in psoriasis vulgaris. Br J Dermatol 2004; 150:1167–1173.
27. Clark CM, Kirby B, Morris AD, et al. Combination treatment with methotrexate and cyclosporin for severe recalcitrant psoriasis. Br J Dermatol 1999; 141:279–282.
28. Ben-Shabat S, Benisty R, Wormser U, et al. Vitamin D3-based conjugates for topical treatment of psoriasis: synthesis, antiproliferative activity, and cutaneous penetration studies. Pharm Res 2005; 22:50–57.
29. Wolters M. Diet and psoriasis: experimental data and clinical evidence. Br J Dermatol 2005; 153:706–714.
30. Callen JP, Bickers DR, Moy RL. Actinic keratoses. J Am Acad Dermatol 1997; 36:650–653.
31. Dinehart SM. The treatment of actinic keratoses. J Am Acad Dermatol 2000; 42:S25–S28.
32. Levy S, Furst K, Chern W. A comparison of the skin permeation of three topical 0.5% fluorouracil formulations with that of a 5% formulation. Clin Ther 2001; 23:901–907.
33. Rivers JK, Arlette J, Shear N, et al. Topical treatment of actinic keratoses with 3.0% diclofenac in 2.5% hyaluronan gel. Br J Dermatol 2002; 146:94–100.
34. Smith SR, Morhenn VB, Piacquadio DJ. Bilateral comparison of the efficacy and tolerability of 3% diclofenac sodium gel and 5% 5-fluorouracil cream in the treatment of actinic keratoses of the face and scalp. J Drugs Dermatol 2006; 5:156–159.
35. Jury CS, Ramraka-Jones VS, Gudi RM, et al. A randomised trial of topical 5% 5-fluorouracil (Efudix cream) in the treatment of actinic keratoses comparing daily with weekly treatment. Br J Dermatol 2005; 153:808–810.
36. Loven K, Stein L, Furst K, et al. Evaluation of the efficacy and tolerability of 0.5% fluorouracil cream and 5% fluorouracil cream applied to each side of the face in patients with actinic keratosis. Clin Ther 2002; 24:990–1000.

16

Topical Therapeutic Agents Used in Wound Care

Sheree E. Cross

Therapeutics Research Unit, School of Medicine, University of Queensland, Princess Alexandra Hospital, Woolloongabba, Queensland, Australia

INTRODUCTION

The administration of topical medications to wound sites in the course of wound care is one of the most documented areas of medical history. This chapter, now updated with advancements achieved in the past 10 years, examines many of the popular wound treatments, most of which stem from folk law rather than true science, and provides a summary of the more recently popular growth factors that are emerging for topical use in chronic or difficult wounds. Beyond the topical agents examined in this chapter, there is also a huge range of agents such as phenytoin, botanical extracts, raw honey, enzymes, minerals, and animal proteins that have been investigated for their effects on wound healing that may warrant more attention in further updates.

TOPICAL WOUND THERAPY

The development of topical medications for wound care is one of the oldest medical dilemmas. In modern pharmacognosy, it is appreciated that plants are the source of some of the most useful medicines in use today. However, without the advantage of sophisticated screening techniques and chemical knowledge, many ancient civilizations were using plants that had powerful properties in wound therapy.

Among the writings of great medical minds such as Hippocrates (460–377 B.C.), Celsus (ca. 20 A.D.), Claudius Galen (129–200 A.D.), and, in the seventh century, Paulus Aegineta, we can find recommendations for the topical application to wounds of a diverse range of solutes, compounds, and mixtures including wine or vinegar for washing, honey, oil and wine for ointments, cobwebs, writing ink, Lemnian clay, wool boiled in water or wine as a useful dressing, copper ore, Cimolian chalk, cold water; myrrh, frankincense, egg white, snails powdered in their shells, verdigris, pine resin, turpentine, radish, lizard dung, and pigeon blood. For the skeptics among us, wine has actually been shown to have profound antibacterial properties, out of proportion with its alcohol content, which have been attributed to the presence of oenosides (polyphenolic compounds) which are more than 30 times more potent than phenol in their antibacterial effects (1,2). In more recent times, substantial in vitro, animal, and human scientific research has led to the discovery and testing of a wide range of topical wound agents, although successful commercialization of many of these products remains to be effectively realized. It should be remembered that the wound bed contains populations of keratinocytes, fibroblasts, melanocytes, lymphocytes, and other cell populations that are very sensitive to the effects of topically applied exogenous compounds, many of which can have deleterious effects on wound healing far outweighing their intended therapeutic action. The remainder of this chapter considers in more detail the range of antiseptics, anti-infective agents, hemostatic agents, antifibrotic agents, and anti-inflammatory agents, and growth factors applied topically to wound sites today.

It should be remembered that wound sites, by definition, do not possess the permeability barrier properties of an intact stratum corneum and are therefore much more susceptible to the application of agents that would be considered fairly innocuous to normal skin. On the other hand, this property also allows the penetration of many agents into granulating eschar and the wound bed that would not be able to gain effective entry through normal skin, thus broadening our palate of potential beneficial agents for use in wound care.

TOPICAL WOUND CARE AGENTS
Antiseptics

It is a widespread misconception that antiseptics can be used to cleanse and protect wound tissue against bacterial infection. Antiseptic solutions (mercurials, quaternary ammonia compounds, iodine and iodophores, alcohol, chlorhexidine, and hydrogen peroxide) are chemical substances designed for application to intact skin, and the merits of antiseptic irrigation of traumatic wounds has received little scientific study (3). Studies have shown that antiseptics have a number of deleterious effects on leukocytes, fibroblasts, epithelialization, and collagen deposition, and consequently, wound healing (4,5) (Table 1). A recent comparison of the toxicity of skin and wound cleansers against fibroblasts and keratinocytes in vitro (Table 2) can be used as a guideline for the use of these supposedly innocuous agents in a clinical setting (6). It should be noted that controversy continues to surround the use of many antiseptic agents because of the lack of sufficient human studies to be accepted as clinically based evidence (3).

Povidone-Iodine

Povidone-iodine (PVD-I) solutions contain polyvinylpyrrolidone iodine, a water-soluble complex containing elemental iodine bound to a synthetic polymer. The complex is designed to provide gradual liberation of bactericidal free iodine, with dilutions of PVD-I solutions increasing the liberation of free iodine. Studies on free iodine have shown that concentrations as low as 1 ppm kill most bacteria in 60 seconds; however, the free iodine is inactivated relatively quickly in the presence of protein, pus, and necrotic tissue (7,8). The use of iodine in wound healing remains controversial as both wound healing stimulation and impairment have both been reported.

The cytotoxicity of PVD-I solutions may be variable dependent on concentration. Conflicting reports have been published regarding the toxicity of PVD-I using cell culture, with 1% PVD-I solutions toxic to fibroblasts, whereas 0.001% solutions were not (9–11). However, Cooper et al. (12) found that the toxicity of a 0.5% solution to keratinocytes and fibroblasts persisted through further dilutions. In vivo studies using animal models have also generated conflicting results. A review by Mayer (13) showed that five of seven reports suggested no beneficial or deleterious effect of PVD-I over saline-treated wounds. Delays in epithelialization and collagen maturation by 0.8% PVD-I used on full-thickness wounds in pigs have been reported (14), whereas more recent studies suggested that a combination of iodine and cadexomer (a modified starch) in an ointment base actually had positive effects on epidermal regeneration in pigs (15) and mice (16).

TABLE 1 Summary of the Actions and Toxicity of Commonly Used Topical Antiseptics

Antiseptic	Product formulation	Action	Local toxicity	Systemic toxicity
PVD-I	Scrub, 10% solution, 1–0.001% cream, 5% polyethylene glycol-based ointment, 10%	Detergent, cleansing agent, bactericidal	Leukocytes, fibroblasts, keratinocytes, epithelialization, collagen maturation, granulation formation	Potential for free iodine absorption and thyroid disease with continued or large-scale use
Sodium hypochlorite (Dakin's solution)	Solution, 0.025% solution, 0.005%	Bactericidal	Leukocytes, fibroblasts, endothelial cells, keratinocytes	None reported
Acetic acid	solution, 0.25%	Limited bactericidal	Fibroblasts, keratinocytes, Cytotoxicity surpasses bactericidal effects	None reported
Hydrogen peroxide	Solution, 3%	Effervescent cleanser, limited bactericidal	Fibroblasts, red blood cells, cytotoxicity surpasses bactericidal effects	None reported
Chlorhexidine	Scrub, 0.1% solution, 4–0.05% cream, 0.15–0.3% dressing, 0.5%	Detergent, cleansing agent, bactericidal	Fibroblasts, keratinocytes, prolonged use may cause contact dermatitis	None reported

Abbreviation: PVD-I, povidone-iodine.

Human in vivo data on local PVD-I effects is limited. Mayer (13) examined the use of 1% and 5% PVD-I solution in the management of surgical wounds and found that a 5% solution caused diminished cell migration and fibroblast activity, with a 1% solution comparable to saline treatment. After 72 hours, little difference was reported between treatments. More recently, PVD-I ointment was shown to have no effect on split-thickness graft-healing times in burn patients (17). However, an increased infection rate of surgical wounds after preclosure treatment with PVD-I has been reported (7). Beyond its local cytotoxic effects, PVD-I has the potential to produce systemic iodine toxicity when used for extended periods or in large open wounds, an effect that is exaggerated in patients showing various degrees of pre-existing thyroid or renal disease (18).

Sodium Hypochlorite (Dakin's Solution)

Sodium hypochlorite is a diluted solution of bleach, usually about 0.25%, although dilutions of 0.005% have been shown to have some bactericidal activity. Similarly to PVD-I, the cytotoxicity data on sodium hypochlorite, although more limited, is conflicting. Kozol et al. (19) found a significant inhibition of neutrophil migration and damage to both fibroblasts and endothelial cells at concentrations of sodium

TABLE 2 Relative Toxicity of Skin and Wound Cleansers Against Fibroblasts and Keratinocytes In Vitro

	Fibroblasts		Keratinocytes	
Cleanser	Nontoxic dilution	Toxicity index[a]	Nontoxic dilution	Toxicity index[a]
Acetic acid (0.25%)	10^{-1}	10	10^{-1}	10
Biolex	10^{-1}	10	No dilution	0
Boric acid (2%)	10^{-1}	10	10^{-1}	10
Cara-Klenz	10^{-1}	10	10^{-1}	10
Dermal wound cleanser	10^{-3}	1000	10^{-2}	100
Dial antibacterial soap	10^{-5}	100,000	10^{-3}	1000
Dove moisturizing body wash	10^{-4}	10,000	10^{-3}	1000
Hibiclens	10^{-4}	10,000	10^{-4}	10,000
Hollister skin cleanser	10^{-4}	10,000	10^{-4}	10,000
Hydrogen peroxide	10^{-3}	1000	10^{-5}	100,000
Ivory liquid gel	10^{-5}	100,000	10^{-3}	1000
Modified Dakin's solution	10^{-1}	10	10^{-5}	100,000
Puriclens	10^{-1}	10	10^{-2}	100
Povidone (10%)	10^{-3}	1000	10^{-5}	100,000
PVD-I (betadine surgical scrub)	10^{-3}	1000	10^{-5}	100,000
Restore wound cleanser	10^{-2}	100	10^{-2}	100
SAF-Clens	No dilution	0	10^{-1}	10
Saline	No dilution	0	10^{-1}	10
Shur-Clens	No dilution	0	No dilution	0
Techni-Care surgical scrub	10^{-3}	1000	No dilution	0

[a]Toxicity index is defined as the dilution required to give experimental cell viability of 85% of control cultures.
Source: Adapted from Ref. 6.

hypochlorite ranging from 0.025% to 0.00025%. In contrast, Heggers et al. (20) reported that solutions of 0.125% had no effect on fibroblasts, whereas 0.125% and 0.5% solutions have been found as toxic and concentrations lower than 0.01% nontoxic to cultured human fibroblasts and keratinocytes (9,12).

In vivo studies have shown that 1% hypochlorite solution caused complete capillary shut down in the rabbit ear chamber granulation model (21), whereas 0.25% solutions increased neodermal thickness in a porcine model (22). However, to date, no human studies appear to have examined local systemic effects after application to wound sites, although adverse effects and tissue damage in dental practice use have been reported (23,24).

Acetic Acid

There are a few studies on the wound toxicity of acetic acid, all of which indicate that its cytotoxicity is far greater than any of its bactericidal effects. Solutions of 0.25% were toxic to fibroblasts and keratinocytes, with dilutions to 0.025% required to eliminate most of this effect (9,12).

Hydrogen Peroxide

Hydrogen peroxide is commonly used as a 3% solution to cleanse wounds by its effervescent action while releasing oxygen in contact with the tissue. Studies suggest that below this concentration its limited bactericidal effects are rapidly diminished (9,11). Solutions of 3% and 0.3% have been shown to be toxic to human fibroblasts, with dilutions of 0.03% still having moderate toxicity (9). Inhibition of neodermal formation was also reported in an in vivo porcine wound healing model after topical application of a 3% hydrogen peroxide solution (22), and application to human appendectomy wounds showed no significant improvement of infection rates (25).

Chlorhexidine
The bactericidal effects of chlorhexidine are utilized as a preoperative disinfectant for the skin, in a 0.5% to 1% solution in aqueous alcohol (70%). Detergent solutions of chlorhexidine, such as scrubs, are soapless because the effects of the compound are easily inactivated by soap. Chlorhexidine is toxic to fibroblasts at concentrations exceeding 0.013%; in fact, all bactericidal concentrations of chlorhexidine are lethal to cultured fibroblasts (26). Adams and Priestly (27) showed that 1% solutions of chlorhexidine arrest the contraction of collagen lattices by human skin fibroblasts. In contrast, in animal in vivo models, Platt and Bucknall (28) found no difference in the healing of infected chlorhexidine-treated sites and control noninfected wounds, and Brennan et al. (29) showed similar healing rates of chlorhexidine- and saline-treated wounds. There do not appear to be any reports on human systemic chlorhexidine toxicity reactions after application to wound sites, although a recent study found that inclusion of chlorhexidine in wound dressings did have a beneficial effect against bacterial growth, although no assessment of changes in healing rates were reported (30).

Antibiotics and Antifungal Agents
Topical antibiotics are most commonly encountered in the treatment of burn wounds, although their use on other wound types is not contraindicated. In burn patients, wound infections are the leading cause of morbidity and mortality (31) and aggressive antibiotic therapy becomes a necessity. The topical route of application of antibiotics can be advantageous in its minimization of systemic absorption and associated side effects, the achievement of high local concentrations of drug, and supposedly decreased induction of antibacterial resistance (32). A summary of many of the topically applied anti-infective agents used on wound sites, along with a number of their potentially deleterious properties that should be considered when applying these agents to open wounds, is shown in Table 3. A few of the more commonly used substances are discussed in more detail below; however, reviews such as those of Lio and Kaye (32) and Howell-Jones et al. (33) are a good source of further information.

Silver Nitrate
Silver nitrate first gained popularity as a topical antiseptic agent and, although extremely toxic to tissues in concentrated forms, a 0.5% solution has been suggested to retain significant antimicrobial activity without significant tissue toxicity (34). However, more recently, it has been established that all silver-based dressings are cytotoxic and should never be used on wounds in the absence of infection (35). In its liquid application form, the insolubility of the silver salts necessitates preparation of the agent in distilled water which leads to the application of extremely hypotonic solutions to wound (36) and potential patient electrolyte imbalance because of the leaching of sodium, potassium, and other solutes into dressings from large surface area wounds.

Methemoglobinaememia, although rare, is another potential complication of silver nitrate therapy due to the production of absorbable nitrite from the nitrate moiety. When the skin or blood of patients show any sign of being cyanotic or gray in the presence of a normal pO_2, therapy should be discontinued. Traditional silver

TABLE 3 Properties of Commonly Used Anti-infective Agents That Affect Local Tolerability and Efficacy After Topical Application

Anti-infective agent	Property						
	Sensitivity reactions	Painful upon application	Inactivated by local substances	Possible side effects	Toxic to local cell populations	Resistance possible	Poorly absorbed
Bacitracin[a]	×	×	×	−	−	×	√
Gentamicin[b]	√	×	−	√	×	√	×
Mafenide solution[c]	√	√	×	√	√	−	×
Mupirocin[d]	×	×	×	−	×	√	√
Nystatin[e]	×	−	−	−	−	√	−
Neomycin[f]	√	−	−	√	√	√	×
Nitrofurazone[g]	−	√	−	−	√	√	−
Neosporin[h]	See individual components						
Polymyxin B sulfate[i]	×	−	−	−	√	×	√
Polysporin[j]	See individual components						
Silver nitrate[k]	×	×	−	√	−	×	√
Silver sulfadiazine[l]	√	×	×	√	√	×	√

[a]Polypeptide, 400–500 U/g white petrolatum–based ointment.
[b]Aminoglycoside, 0.1% in water-miscible base.
[c]Methylated sulfonamide, 10% in water-miscible base.
[d]Pseudomonic acid A, 2% ointment.
[e]Fungacide vs. *Candida*, 5 million U/L solution, cream, or ointment.
[f]Aminoglycoside, 20% neomycin sulfate in petrolatum.
[g]0.2% cream or solution.
[h]Neomycin + polymyxin B sulfate + bacitracin in ointment.
[i]Polypeptide, 5000 or 10,000U/g white petrolatum–based ointment.
[j]Polymyxin B sulfate + bacitracin in ointment.
[k]0.5% solution in distilled water.
[l]Sulfonamide, 1% in water-miscible base.
×, does not possess property; √, does possess property; −, data not reported.

nitrate solution needs to be applied every two to three hours soaked into bulky cotton bandages, making therapy very labor-intensive. Frequent replacement of bandages is also necessary to avoid the buildup of toxic concentrations of silver nitrate at the wound surface due to evaporation of water from the solution (36). A further disadvantage of silver nitrate therapy is that it stains everything (skin, wounds, bandages, clothing). However, impregnation and coating of silver into modern dressings should help reduce excessive deposition and staining of treated sites (37). The timing of application of silver dressings to wounds is also significant, because they appear to have little effect after bacteria have invaded unburned blood vessels and viable tissue adjacent to burn sites (38).

Mafenide
Mafenide cream was the most common topical prophylactic antibiotic for use on burns of all degrees before the introduction of silver sulfadiazine. Mafenide is formulated as a 5% to 10% suspension in a water miscible cream base. It has a fairly wide spectrum of bacteriostatic activity at these concentrations, although little antifungal activity (39,40). A 5% solution, as opposed to the cream, is also used for the irrigation of postoperative graft sites in burn patients (41).

The major advantage of mafenide is that it rapidly penetrates burn eschar and is a useful treatment for invasive wound infections. Mafenide entering the blood stream is deaminated, inhibiting any systemic antimicrobial effects, and excreted in the urine (42). Topical application of mafenide is repeated every 8 to 10 hours to maintain effective concentrations in the wound because of its systemic absorption and breakdown. However, reports recommend not to repeat application <12 hours because of the side effects induced by its absorption.

Hypersensitivity rashes occur in about 50% of patients because of the presence of the sulfa moiety, although these can be controlled to some extent with the use of antihistamines. Pulmonary complications, tachypnea, and hyperventilation, are commonly seen after prolonged use as a consequence of drug-induced acidosis. Additionally, the application of mafenide is painful (43), particularly in the early post-burn period, possibly because of its high osmolarity. Mafenide has been shown to inhibit fibroblasts and keratinocytes in vitro (12,44,45) and suppress neutrophil and lymphocyte activity (46,47), and therefore its use would be expected to delay overall wound healing.

Mupirocin
Mupirocin is more commonly used in the treatment of primary skin infections, such as affected lesions of impetigo and nasal carriage of bacteria, than wounds (32). Despite the fact that it rarely causes local adverse effects and its low absorption, reports of emergence of mupirocin-resistant, methicillin-resistant *Staphylococcus aureus* organisms (48) is likely to restrict the use of this antibiotic topically.

Silver Sulfadiazine
Silver sulfadiazine, available as a 1% preparation in a water-miscible cream, is a highly insoluble compound synthesized from silver nitrate and sodium sulfadiazine (49). Its major advantages include its wide antibacterial spectrum, reasonably low systemic toxicity, minimal pain, and ease of application. The penetration of silver sulfadiazine through eschar is low, although better than silver nitrate. The cream is usually only applied once a daily and is readily removed by washing; although the silver may oxidize to give a gray color, it does not stain skin or cloth (50).

The most common adverse effect of silver sulfadiazine, affecting 5% to 15% of patients, is transient leukopenia, typically within two to three days of treatment, which seems to reverse whether or not the agent is withdrawn (51). Allergies to the sulfa in the cream are unusual and often mild, not requiring the cessation of therapy. There is evidence that silver sulfadiazine is toxic to fibroblasts and keratinocytes in vitro (12,44,45) and tests have also shown some inhibition of neutrophil killing activity and local lymphocyte function (46,47). In addition, studies have suggested that coadministration of epidermal growth factor (EGF) may be useful in reversing the delays in wound healing seen after application of this agent (52); however, rates of epithelialization in a porcine wound model have been shown to be enhanced by treatment (53,54). Interestingly, a faster rate of epithelialization of second-degree burn wounds in adult patients has been found with the use of a combination of silver sulfadiazine with hyaluronic acid, compared to silver sulfadiazine alone, and supports the potential wound healing activity of hyaluronic acid (55).

Gentamicin
Gentamicin has been used as a 0.1% cream or ointment in the control of gram-negative infections in burn wounds. This agent is generally only used topically when

treatment with other agents has failed and its use is discontinued as soon as bacterial colonization is controlled (50). Resistant organisms are always expected with the use of gentamicin. The topical penetration of gentamicin, applied directly to wounds, is rapid, reaching a peak at about 10 days post burn and then diminishing as the water content of the wound decreases (56). Absorption from water-miscible bases is greater and faster than from ointment bases, with gentamicin being identified in the urine within 1 and >2 hours, respectively, from the two formulations (56). A recent study examining the topical application of gentamicin ointment to patients after auricular surgery for the removal of cutaneous malignancies, reported no statistical difference in the control of suppurative and inflammatory chondritis (57). Although absorption into the wound is rapid, concomitant urinary excretion prevents systemic toxicity developing in most cases. Ototoxicity and nephrotoxicity can develop when gentamicin is used on large surface area wounds and systemic absorption is particularly high.

Neomycin
Neomycin is available in cream and ointment bases and is used primarily for its broad spectrum activity. It is most commonly formulated as 20% neomycin sulfate in petrolatum, and often combined with other antibiotics such as bacitracin and polymyxin B. Its effects appear limited to the control of bacterial proliferation on the wound surface. Neomycin does not appear to be toxic to keratinocytes in vitro (58) but it is reported to inhibit the activity of neutrophils (46). Hypersensitivity skin rashes or allergic dermatitis have been reported to occur in about 5% to 8% of patients and could be higher in those with a compromised skin barrier (59,60).

Bacitracin
When bacitracin is applied topically to wounds, its absorption is minimal, thus limiting its usefulness to the treatment of surface infected wounds. Bacitracin has been shown to have little or no effect on keratinocytes in vitro and to augment to antimicrobial action of neutrophils (58). In vivo, bacitracin has been suggested to enhance wound reepithelialization (53,61). Its use in children and infants appears safe, and hypersensitivity or contact dermatitis is rare; however in 2003 it was awarded "Allergen of the Year" by the North American Contact Dermatology Group as its incidence jumped to 9.2% (1998–2000) from 1.5% (1989–1990) (32). Its use in burn and wound care seems to be primarily with superficial partial thickness wounds and burns to the face (50).

Polymyxin B Sulfate
Similarly to bacitracin, polymyxin B sulfate is used as an ointment in the control of surface bacteria in superficial partial thickness wounds and face burns. The phospholipid content of certain bacterial cell walls has been reported to preclude entry of the drug, although formation of polymyxin B sulfate–resistant organisms is rare (62). The topical absorption of polymyxin B sulfate is negligible and systemic toxicity is rare, and related to use over large areas for extended periods of time.

Nystatin
Nystatin is primarily a fungicide used against superficial invasions of *Candida*, but some strains have been shown to develop resistance (63). Dermal hypersensitivity reactions appear to be rare with this agent and no deleterious effects on fibroblasts

or keratinocytes in vitro have been reported (50). Nystatin cream is usually applied one to three times a day to most wounds with signs of fungal invasion. Little is known about the ability of this agent to penetrate wounds and skin.

Nitrofurazone

Nitrofurazone has a fairly wide spectrum of antibacterial activity, although it is less effective than silver sulfadiazine or mafenide against some strains, and without significant fungicidal activity (50). Wound healing is likely to be augmented by use of this agent in the control of surface bacteria as it has been shown to be detrimental to the growth and migration of keratinocytes in vitro (44). The cream is painless to apply and signs of hypersensitivity and dermatitis are rare, although its use on damaged skin has been reported to predispose users to contact allergy (64). Nitrofurazone is usually only applied once daily but is used more frequently on full-thickness wounds (50).

Polysporin® or Neosporin®

Polysporin and Neosporin are simply mixtures containing combinations of bacitracin and polymyxin B sulfate with or without neomycin (Table 3). This combination of agents appears not to cause any further side effects or sensitivities above those of the individual agents, with superiority of the mixtures established over control treatment (65,66) but no significant differences attributable to the presence or absence of neomycin (65).

      Other anti-infective agents under investigation include dressings with potential to release ciprofloxacin into wound sites (67) and investigations into the possibility of inducing the release of natural antibacterial peptides in wound sites through a cutaneous gene therapy approach

Hemostatic Agents

Despite their potential complications, the more common hemostatic chemicals used in surgery do not appear to have changed in over 50 years (68). One of the most commonly used traditional hemostatic agents is Monsel's solution (20% ferric subsulfate). Monsel's solution achieves its hemostatic effect by causing local protein denaturization followed by vascular thrombosis. Other hemostatic agents, such as aluminum chloride solution, produce their effects in a similar manner (69). Monsel's solution has been shown to have lasting cytotoxic effects, causes delays in wound healing, and leads to the production of noticeably larger scars in wounds treated with the solution compared to those treated with pressure or gel foams (70,71). Hemostatic agents also available include products containing gelatin, collagen, fibrin, and thrombin, all associated with a range of dressing materials that can be applied directly to wound sites (72). The effects of these agents on healing has generated conflicting results with granulatomous inflammation observed after implantation of collagen hemostats in rabbits (73) but accelerated healing of punch biopsies in humans treated with bovine collagen matrix (74). One of the most recent reviews in this area recommends use of only minimal required amounts of agent and removal of excess hemostat after achievement of hemostasis to reduce the risk of complications (72). Hydrogen peroxide, 3%, irrigated in wound beds as a dermal hemostatic before graft placement in burn patients, has been associated with promising results (75).

Anti-fibrotic and Anti-inflammatory Agents

The results of aberrant wound healing, manifest as overgranulation, inappropriate fibrosis, or excessive scar formation and contracture, include cosmetic deformity, patient psychological stress and dissatisfaction, and often permanent scarring. Keloids and hypertrophic scars represent two degrees of overhealing, and fibrosis after wound healing, and seem to be related to abnormal persistence of inflammation at the wound site. As our knowledge of the biochemistry of the healing process has grown, the cytokines responsible for each phase of the process and its malfunction are being identified as specific pharmacological targets, such as transforming growth factor beta (76). Despite the research in this area, intralesional steroids and their multiple cytokine effects still appear to be the major weapon in the regression of keloids and hypertrophic scars (77).

Reports on the use of topical vitamin E, the major lipid soluble antioxidant, to minimize scarring and fibrosis, or to improve skin tone and appearance have been appearing in the literature for over 50 years. However, there is little scientific evidence-based medicine suggesting that vitamin E is beneficial in treating the appearance of scars (78).

The topical application of antifibrotics to healing tissue is most well studied in patients after glaucoma filtration surgery. Healing of ocular surgical wounds with minimal scarring and maintenance of the open channel for outflow of fluid from the eye are key outcomes in this procedure. The antiproliferative effect of agents such as 5-fluorouracil and mitomycin C have been investigated and shown to have significant benefit in increasing the success of glaucoma surgery (79); however, these agents are normally administered by injection or in an implantable sponge applied at the time of surgery and have been associated with significant cytotoxicity. Animal studies have demonstrated that mitomycin C applied topically to incisional wounds in rats and laser wounds in rabbits resulted in decreased wound strength and delayed healing, which could be an issue in scar prevention in sites where wound strength is critical (80,81). Recent studies on keloid scar excision sites, in 15 patients, failed to show any benefit of topical mitomycin C, applied before to wound closure, on scar recurrence (82).

Newer agents in this class include the immune modulator, Toll-like receptor agonist thought to induce interferon-alpha production, imiquod, which has been applied as a 5% cream in the successful treatment of keloid scarring. The agent, applied daily for six weeks, was able to prevent occurrence of lesions and provide excellent cosmetic results in eight treatments, five of which had been sites of recurrent lesions after previous keloid removal procedures (83). However, a further study examining its effectiveness in improving scar cosmesis after the surgical removal of melanocytic nevi showed no difference to placebo treatment (84). Other treatments such as steroids and interferon alpha-2b, an antiproliferative cytokine, still require injection to achieve acceptable results in patients (85). However, studies with novel liposome-encapsulated interferon formulations showed that early topical use in skin wounds could reduce scar formation in a guinea pig model (86) warranting further investigation for human application.

The anti-inflammatory effects of corticosteroids and their subsequent ability to retard healing have been documented since the 1950s (87–89). For this reason, topical steroid formulations, common in dermatological practice for the treatment of skin reactions, are not generally recommended for use on open wounds. The ability of steroids to reduce scar formation and contraction has, however, been harnessed for the treatment of scar formation and contraction over the glans of circumcised infants where a combination of topical betamethasone and manual retraction proved to be an effective management of the condition (90). In addition, topical clobetasol (0.05%) has been suggested to be effective in the reduction of facial scar formation in acne keloidalis in African patients (91).

Growth Factors

Topical application of growth factors to stimulate cells involved in wound healing, particularly in patients with a suppressed healing response, has long been an attractive therapeutic approach. Platelet-derived growth factor (PDGF) is released by activated platelets to stimulate recruitment of inflammatory cells into the wound bed, and promote angiogenesis and granulation tissue formation. Treatment of wounds with PDGF has been shown, in the presence of an intact dermis, to limit the role of contracture in wound closure and affect healing through the promotion of granulation and epithelialization (92). Healing of diabetic foot ulcers is improved by the topical application of PDGF and good wound management technique (93), whereas patient autologous platelet lysate did not show any improvement when applied to venous leg ulcers (94). Despite their potential clinical advantages, the price paid for topical growth factor treatment is a growing concern for health service providers, although general opinion appears to be that further studies are needed to more accurately determine their cost effectiveness (95).

EGF stimulates the proliferation and migration of epithelial cells and may accelerate wound contraction through effects on myofibroblast proliferation and collagen deposition (96). These properties would obviously be advantageous in poorly healing wounds and interest in topical EGF has now advanced from animal studies to clinical trials. Application of recombinant (rh) EGF to chronic ulcers in 26 patients significantly reduced healing time compared to saline-treated controls (97) and had positive effects on diabetic foot ulcers in combination with advanced dressing use (98), and application to partial-thickness burn wounds in Chinese patients was shown to result in reduced scar severity and shorter healing times (99,100).

Basic fibroblast growth factor (bFGF) has been associated with beneficial effects such as increased angiogenesis, enhanced epithelialization, reduced contraction rates, and increased granulation tissue formation in animal models (101,102). In the clinical setting, topical bFGF has also been tested for its ability to accelerate wound healing. In a prospective, multicenter clinical trial of 1024 patients with burns, graft donor site wounds, or chronic dermal ulcers and 641 controls, rhFGF was proven to be effective in shortening wound healing time and generally improving wound healing quality (103). Furthermore, a bFGF spray was shown to be useful in the treatment of ischemic ulcer in patients with arteriosclerosis (104). Other growth factors investigated for topical application include transforming growth factor beta (105,106), nerve growth factor (107), human growth hormone (108), hepatocyte growth factor (109,110), insulin-like growth factor (111), and keratinocyte growth factor (112).

The doses of growth factors applied to wounds are still somewhat empirical and achieving the correct concentration around target cells could be vital for clinical success. Obstacles in achieving the optimal dosage and potential biological benefits of topically applied growth factors include their stability within the wound environment together with their ability to penetrate through the eschar to the wound bed and sites of action among living cell populations. Our own work has shown that large-molecular-weight solutes such as bFGF and EGF are only capable of penetrating into the upper layers of granulation tissue at wound sites (113). These findings indicate that calculation of therapeutic doses for topical application must take into consideration levels of drug capable of diffusing to sites of action in the wound bed and not simply match those concentrations shown to have beneficial effects in culture models, which may explain the less-than-satisfactory results observed in a number of clinical trials.

FUTURE PERSPECTIVES

Despite the growing number of agents applied to wounds, their absorption, distribution, and elimination kinetics within wound sites still appear to be relatively poorly defined. Research has tended to focus on clinical efficacy end points rather than understanding in more detail the kinetic processes that contribute to the attainment of these effects. Application of the science of formulation design and dose optimization should now make significant differences in our approach to accepting or rejecting potential clinical advantages of topical agents used in wound care. There may be no bad agent, just a lack of appropriate application vehicle (dressing matrix, liposomal suspension, or complex slow release encapsulation design). The need for development of a rigorous scientific, evidence-based approach to the assessment of topical wound therapies is clear to all, already in practice by some, and will significantly facilitate decision on appropriate therapies for a multitude of wound types.

REFERENCES

1. Majno G. The Healing Hand. Cambridge, Massachusetts: Harvard University Press, 1982.
2. Ribereau-Gayon J, Peynaud E. Traite d'Oenlolgie. Paris: Libr Polytechn, 1961:124.
3. Smith RG. A critical discussion of the use of antiseptics in acute traumatic wounds. J Am Podiatr Med Assoc 2005; 95(2):148–153.
4. Tatnall FM, Leigh IM, Gibson JR. Comparative study of antiseptic cytotoxicity on basal keratinocytes. transformed human keratinocytes and fibroblasts. Skin Pharmacol 1990; 3(3):157–163.
5. Brown CD, Zitelli JA. A review of topical agents for wounds and methods of wounding. Guidelines for wound management. J Dermatol Surg Oncol 1993; 19(8):732–737.
6. Wilson JR, Mills JG, Prather ID, et al. A toxicity index of skin and wound cleansers used on in vitro fibroblasts and keratinocytes. Adv Skin Wound Care 2005; 18(7):373–378.
7. Rodeheaver G, Turnbull V, Edgerton MT, et al. Pharmacokinetics of a new skin cleanser. Am J Surg 1976; 132(1):67–74.
8. LeVeen H, LeVeen R, LeVeen E. The mythology of povidone-iodine and the development of self steralizing plastics. Surg Gynecol Obstet 1993; 176(2):183–190.
9. Lineaweaver W, McMorris S, Soucy D, et al. Cellular and bacterial toxicities of topical antimicrobials. Plast Reconstr Surg 1985; 75(3):94–96.
10. Lineaweaver W, Howard R, Soucy D, et al. Topical antimicrobial toxicity. Arch Surg 1985; 120(3):267–270.
11. McKenna P, Lehr G, Leist P, et al. Antiseptic effectiveness with fibroblast preservation. Ann Plast Surg 1991; 27(3):265–268.
12. Cooper M, Laxer J, Hansbrough J. The cytotoxic effects of commonly used topical antimicrobial agents in human fibroblasts and keratinocytes. J Trauma 1991; 31(6):775–781.
13. Mayer DA. The perils of povidone-iodine use. Ostomy Wound Manage 1994; 40(8):6–8.
14. Welch J. Efficacy and safety of povidone-iodine underscored (letter). J Emerg Nurs 1992; 18(3):191.

15. Lamme EN, Gustafsson TO, Middelkoop E. Cadexomer-iodine ointment shows stimulation of epidermal regeneration in experimental full-thickness wounds. Arch Dermatol Res 1998; 290(1–2):18–24.
16. Langer S, Botteck NM, Bosse B, et al. Effect of polyvinylpyrrolidone-iodine liposomal hydrogel on wound microcirculation in SKH1-hr hairless mice. Eur Surg Res 2006; 38(1):27–34.
17. Vehmeyer-Heeman M, Van den Kerckhove E, Gorissen K, et al. Povidone-iodine ointment: no effect on split skin graft healing time. Burns 2005; 31(4):489–494.
18. Shetty KR, Duthie EH. Thyrotoxicosis induced by topical iodine application. Arch Intern Med 1990; 150(11):2400–2401.
19. Kozol R, Gillies C, Eigebaly S. Effects of sodium hypochlorite (Dakin's solution) on cells of the wound module. Arch Surg 1988; 123(4):420–423.
20. Heggers J, Sazy J, Stenberg B, et al. Bactericidal and wound healing properties of sodium hypochlorite solutions: the 1991 Lindberg award. J Burn Care Rehab 1991; 12(5): 420–424.
21. Brennan SS, Leaper DJ. The effect of antiseptics on the healing wound: a study using the rabbit ear chamber. Br J Surg 1985; 72(10):780–782.
22. Bennett LL, Rosenblum RS, Perlov C, et al. An in vivo comparison of topical agents on wound repair. Plast Reconstr Surg 2001; 108(3):675–685.
23. Witton R, Brennan PA. Severe tissue damage and neurological deficit following extravasation of sodium hypochlorite solution during routine endodontic treatment. Br Dent J 2005; 198(12):749–750.
24. Gernhardt CR, Eppendorf K, Kozlowski A, et al. Toxicity of concentrated sodium hypochlorite used as an endodontic irrigant. Int Endod J 2004; 37(4):272–280.
25. Lau WY, Wong SH. Randomized, prospective trial of topical hydrogen peroxide in appendectomy wound infection. High risk factors. Am J Surg 1981; 142(3):393–397.
26. Sanchez IR, Nusbaum KE, Swaim SF, et al. Chlorhexidine diacetate and povidone-iodine cytotoxicity to canine embryonic fibroblasts and *Staphyococcus aureus*. Vet Surg 1988; 17(4):182–185.
27. Adams LW, Priestly GC. Contraction of collagen lattices by skin fibroblasts: drug-induced changes. Arch Dermatol Res 1988; 280(2):114–118.
28. Platt J, Bucknall RA. An experimental evaluation of antiseptic wound irrigation. J Hosp Infect 1984; 5(2):181–188.
29. Brennan SS, Foster ME, Leaper DJ. Antiseptic toxicity in wounds healing by secondary intention. J Hosp Infect 1986; 8(3):263–267.
30. Martineau L, Shek PN. Evaluation of a bi-layer wound dressing for burn care. II. In vitro and in vivo bactericidal properties. Burns 2006; 32(2):172–179.
31. Yurt RW, McManus AT, Manson AD, et al. Increased susceptibility to infection related to extent of burn injury. Arch. Surg 1984; 119(2):183–188.
32. Lio PA, Kaye ET. Topical antibacterial agents. Infect Dis Clin N Am 2004; 18(3):717–733.
33. Howell-Jones RS, Wilson MJ, Hill KE, et al. A review of the microbiology, antibiotic usage and resistance in chronic skin wounds. J Antimicrob Chemother 2005; 55(2):143–149.
34. Monafo WW, Moyer CA. Effectiveness of dilute aqueous silver nitrate in the treatment of major burns. Arch. Surg 1965; 91:200–202.
35. Paddle-Ledinek JE, Nasa Z, Cleland HJ. Effect of different wound dressings on cell viability and proliferation. Plast Reconstr Surg 2006; 117(7 Suppl.):110S–118S.
36. Moyer CA, Bretano L, Gravens DL. Treatment of large human burns with 0.5 percent silver nitrate solution. Arch Surg 1965; 90:812–867.
37. Walker M, Cochrane CA, Bowler PG, et al. Silver deposition and tissue staining associated with wound dressings containing silver. Ostomy Wound Manage 2006; 52(1):42–44.
38. Chu CS, McManus AT, Mason AD, et al. Topical silver treatment after escharectomy of infected full thickness burn wounds in rats. J Trauma 2005; 58(5):1040–1046.
39. Shuck JM, Thorne LW, Cooper GC. Mafenide acetate solution dressings: an adjunct in burn wound care. J Trauma 1975; 15(7):595–599.
40. Pruitt BA, Goodwin CW. Thermal injuries. In: Davis JH, ed. Clinical Surgery. St Louis: Mosby, 1987:2823–2843.

41. Palmieri TL, Greenhalgh DG. Topical treatment of pediatric patients with burns: a practical guide. Am J Clin Dermatol 2002; 3(8):529–534.
42. Harrison NH, Bales H, Jacoby F. The behaviour of mafenide acetate as the basis for its clinical use. Arch Surg 1971; 103(4):449–453.
43. Montcreif JA, Lindbergh RB, Switzer WE, et al. Use of topical antibacterial therapy in the treatment of the burn wound. Arch Surg 1966; 92:558–562.
44. Smoot EC, Kucan JO, Roth A, et al. In vitro toxicity testing for antibacterials against human keratinocytes. Plast Reconstr Surg 1991; 87(5):917–924.
45. McCauley RL, Linares HA, Pelligrini V, et al. In vitro toxicity of topical antimicrobial agents to human fibroblasts. J Surg Res 1989; 46(3):267–274.
46. Hansbrough JF, Zapata-Sirvent RL, Cooper ML. Effects of topical antimicrobial agents on the human neutrophil respiratory burst. Arch Surg 1991; 126(5):603–608.
47. Zapata-Sirvent RL, Hansbrough JF. Cytotoxicity to human leukocytes by topical antimicrobial agents used for burn care. J Burn Care Rehab 1993; 14(2 pt 1):132–140.
48. Walker ES, Vasquez JE, Dula R, et al. Mupirocin-resistant, methicillin-resistant *Staphylococcus aureus*: does mupirocin remain effective? Infect Control Hosp Epidemiol 2003; 24(5):342–346.
49. Fox CL. Silver sulfadiazine: a new topical therapy for *Pseudomonas* in burns. Therapy of *Pseudomonas* infection in burns. Arch Surg 1968; 96(2):184–188.
50. Ward RS, Saffle JR. Topical agents in burn and wound care. Phys Ther 1995; 75(6):526–538.
51. Choban PS, Marshall WJ. Leukopinea secondary to silver sulfadiazine: frequency, characteristics and clinical consequences. Am Surg 1987; 53(9):515–517.
52. Cho Lee AR, Leem H, Lee J, et al. Reversal of solver sulfadiazine-impaired wound healing by epidermal growth factor. Biomaterials 2005; 26(22):4670–4676.
53. Watcher M Wheeland R. Role of topical antibiotics in the healing of full thickness wounds. J Dermatol Surg Oncol 1989; 15(11):1188–1195.
54. Geronemus RG, Mertz PM, Eaglstein WH. Wound healing. The effects of topical antimicrobial agents. Arch Dermatol 1979; 115(11):1311–1314.
55. Castagliola M, Agrosi M. Second-degree burns: a comparative, multicentre, randomized trial of hyaluronic acid plus silver sulfadiazine vs. silver sulfadiazine alone. Curr Med Res Opin 2005; 21(8):1235–1240.
56. Stone HH, Kolb LD, Pettit J, et al. The systemic absorption of antibiotic from the burned wound surface. Am Surg 1968; 34(9):639–643.
57. Campbell RM, Perlis CS, Fisher E, et al. Gentamicin ointment versus petrolatum for management of auricular wounds. Dermatol Surg 2005; 31(6):664–669.
58. Cooper ML, Boyce ST, Hansbrough JF, et al. Cytotoxicity to cultured human keratinocytes of topical antimicrobial agents. J Surg Res 1990; 48(3):190–195.
59. Sande MA, Mandell GL. Antimicrobial agents: tetracyclines, chloramphenicol, erythromycin and miscellaneous antibacterial agents. In: Gillman AG, Goodman LS, Rall TW, Murad F, eds. The Pharmacological Basis of Therapeutics. New York: Macmillan, 1985:1191–1213.
60. Gette MT, Marks JG, Maloney ME. Frequency of postoperative allergic contact dermatitis to topical antibiotics. Arch Surg 1992; 128(3):365–367.
61. Eaglstein WH, Mertz PM, Alvarez OM. Effect of topically applied agents on healing wound. Clin Dermatol 1984; 2(3):112–115.
62. Brown MRW, Wood SM. Relation between cation and lipid content of cell walls of *Pseudomonas aeruginosa, Proteus vulgaris* and *Klebsiella aerogenes* and their sensitivity to polymyxin B and other antibacterial agents. J Pharm Pharmacol 1972; 24(3):215–218.
63. Dube MP, Heseltine PN, Rinaldi MG, et al. Fungemia and colonisation with nystatin-resistant *Candida rugosa* in a burn unit. Clin Infect Dis 1994; 18(1):77–82.
64. Gujarro SC, Sanchez-Perez J, Garcia-Diez A. Allergic contact dermatitis to ployethylene glycol and nitrofurazone. Am J Contact Dermat 1999; 10(4):226–227.
65. Berger RS, Pappert AS, Van Zile PA, et al. A newly formed topical triple-antibiotic ointment minimizes scarring. Cutis 2000; 65(6):401–404.
66. Lok CE, Stanley KE, Hux JE, et al. Hemodialysis infection prevention with polysporin ointment. J Am Soc Nephrol 2003; 14(1):169–179.

67. Tsou TL, Tang ST, Huang YC, et al. Poly(2-hydroxyethyl methacrylate) wound dressing containing ciprofloxacin and its drug release studies. J Mater Sci Mater Med 2005; 16(2):95–100.
68. Schonauer C, Tessitore E, Barbagallo G, et al. The use of local agents: bone, wax, collagen, oxidized cellulose. Eur Spine J 2004; 13(Suppl. 1):S89–S96.
69. Larson P. Topical hemostatic agents for dermatologic surgery. J Dermatol Surg Oncol 1988; 14(6):623–632.
70. Amazon K, Robinson MJ, Rywlin A. Ferragination caused by Monsel's solution, Am. J. Dermatopath 1980; 2(3):197–205.
71. Epstein E. Effects of tissue destructive techniques on wound healing. J Am Acad Dermatol 1986; 14(6):1098–1099.
72. Tomizawa Y. Clinical benefits and risk analysis of topical hemostats: a review. J Artif Organs 2005; 8(3):137–142.
73. Barbolt TA, Odin M, Leger M, et al. Pre-clinical subdural tissue reaction and absorption study of absorbable hemostatic devices. Neurol Res 2001; 23(5):537–542.
74. Smith KJ, Skelton HG, Barrett TL, et al. Histologic and immunohistochemical features in biopsy sites in which bovine collagen matrix was used for hemostasis. J Am Acad Dermatol 1996; 34(3):434–438.
75. Potyondy L, Lottenberg L, Anderson J, et al. The use of hydrogen peroxide for achieving dermal hemostasis after burn excision in a patient with platelet dysfunction. J Burn Care Res 2006; 27(1):99–101.
76. Leask A, Abraham DJ. TGF-beta signalling and the fibrotic response. FASEB 2004; 18(7): 816–827.
77. Chen MA, Davidson TM. Scar management: prevention and treatment strategies. Curr Opin Otolaryngol Head Neck Surg 2005; 13(4):242–247.
78. Curran JN, Crealey M, Sadadcharam G, et al. Vitamin E: patterns of understanding, use and precscription by health professionals and students at a university teaching hospital. Plast Reconstr Surg 2006; 118(1):248–252.
79. Chang MR, Cheng Q, Lee DA. Basic science and clinical aspects of wound healing in glaucoma filtration surgery. J Ocul Pharmacol Ther 1988; 14(1):75–95.
80. Porter GT, Gadre SA, Calhoun KH. The effects of intradermal and topical mitomycin C on wound healing. Otolaryngol Head Neck Surg 2006; 135(1):56–60.
81. Rho JL, Koo BS, Yoon YH. Effect of topical mitomycin C on the healing of surgical and laser wounds: a hint on clinical application. Otolaryngol Head Neck Surg 2005; 133(6):851–856.
82. Sanders KW, Gage-White L, Stucker FJ. Topical mitomycin C in the prevention of keloid scar recurrence. Arch Facial Plast Surg 2005; 7(3):172–175.
83. Stashower ME. Successful treatment of earlobe keloids with Imiquimod after tangential shave excision. Dermatol Surg 2006; 32(3):380–386
84. Berman B, Frankel S, Villa Am, et al. Double-blind, randomized, placebo-controlled, prospective study evaluating the tolerability and effectiveness of imiquimod applied to postsurgical excisions on scar cosmesis. Dermatol Surg 2005; 31(11 Pt 1):1399–1403.
85. Davison SP, Mess S, Kauffman LC, et al. Ineffective treatment of keloids with interferon alpha-2b. Plast Reconstr Surg 2006; 117(1):247–252.
86. Takeuchi M, Tredget EE, Scott PG, et al. The antifibrogenic effects of liposome-encapsulated IFN-alpha2b cream on skin wounds. J Interferon Cytokine Res 1999; 19(12):1413–1319.
87. Pezzulich RA, Mannix H. Immediate complications of adrenal surgery. Ann Surg 1970; 172(1):109–130.
88. Enquist A, Backer AG, Jarnum S. Incidence of post operative complications in patients subjected to surgery under steroid cover. Acta Chir Scand 1974; 140(3):343–347.
89. Loeb JN. Corticosteroids and growth. N Eng J Med 1976; 295(10):547–552.
90. Palmer JS, Elder JS, Palmer LS. The use of betamethasone to manage trapped penis following neonatal circumcision. J Urol 2005; 174(4pt2):1577–1578.
91. Callender VD, Young CM, Haverstock CL, et al. An open label study of clobetasol propionate 0.05% and betamethasone valerate 0.12% foams in the treatment of mild to moderate acne keloidalis. Cutis 2005; 75(6):317–321.

92. Ehrlich HP, Freedman BM. Topical platelet-derived growth factor in patients enhances wound closure in the absence of wound contraction. Cytokines Cell mol Ther 2002; 7(3):85–90.
93. Steed DL. Clinical evaluation of recombinant human platelet-derived growth factor for the treatment of lower extremity ulcers. Plast Reconstr Surg 2006; 117(7 Suppl):143S–149S.
94. Stacey MC, Mata SD, Trengove NJ, et al. Randomised double-blind placebo controlled trial of topical autologous platelet lysate in venous ulcer healing. Eur J Endovasc Surg 2000; 20(3):296–301.
95. Sibbald RG, Torrance G, Hux M, et al. Cost-effectiveness of becaplermin for nonhealing neuropathic diabetic foot ulcers. Ostomy Wound Manage 2003; 49(11):76–84.
96. Kwon YB, Kim HW, Roh DH, et al. Topical application of epidermal growth factor accelerates wound healing by myofibroblast proliferation and collagen synthesis in rat. J Vet Sci 2006; 7(2):105–109.
97. Zhu JX, Zhang YM. Application of recombinant human epidermal growth factor on chronic ulcer wound. Zhongguo Xiu Fu Chong Jian Wai Ke Za Zhi 2002; 16(1):42–43.
98. Hong JP, Jung HD, Kim YW. Recombinant human epidermal growth factor (EGF) to enhance healing for diabetic foot ulcers. Ann Plast Surg 2006; 56(4):394–398.
99. Wang GY, Xia ZF, Zhu SH, et al. Clinical observation of the long-term effects of rhEGF on deep partial-thickness burn wounds. Zhonghua Shao Shang Za Zhi 2003; 10(3):167–168.
100. Wang SL, Ma JL, Chai JK. Acceleration of burn wound healing with topical application of recombinant human epidermal growth factor ointments. Zhongguo Xiu Fu Chong Jian Wai Ke Za Zhi 2002; 16(3):173–176.
101. Pandit A, Ashar R, Feldman D, et al. Investigation of acidic fibroblast growth factor delivered through a collagen scaffold for the treatment of full-thickness skin defects in a rabbit model. Plast Reconstr Surg 1998; 101(3):766–775.
102. Oda Y, Kagami H, Ueda M. Accelerating effects of basic fibroblast growth factor on wound healing of rat palatal mucosa. J Oral Maxillofac Surg 2004; 62(1):73–80.
103. Fu X, Shen Z, Chen Y, et al. Recombinant bovine basic fibroblast growth factor accelerates wound healing in patients with burns, donor sites and chronic dermal ulcers. Chin Med J (Engl) 2000; 113(4):367–371.
104. Noguchi K, Eishi M, Yamachika S, et al. Three cases of ischaemic ulcer due to arteriosclerosis obliterans responding to basic fibroblast growth factor spray. Heart Vessels 2004; 19(5):252–256.
105. Tyrone JW, Marcus JR, Bonomo SR, et al. Transforming growth factor beta3 promotes fascial wound healing in a new animal model. Arch Surg 2000; 135(10):1154–1159.
106. Sumiyoshi K, Nakao A, Setoguchi, et al. Exogenous Smad3 accelerates wound healing in a rabbit dermal ulcer model. J Invest Dermatol 2004; 123(1):229–236.
107. Generini S, Tuveri MA, Matucci Cerinic M, et al. Topical application of nerve growth factor in human diabetic foot ulcers. A study of three cases. Exp Clin Endocrinol Diabetes 2004; 112(9):542–544.
108. Herndon DN, Hawkins HK, Nguyen TT, et al. Characterization of growth hormone enhanced donor site healing in patients with large cutaneous burns. Ann Surg 1995; 221(6):649–656.
109. Nakanishi K, Uenoyama M, Tomita N, et al. Gene transfer of human hepatocyte growth factor into rat skin wounds mediated by liposomes coated with the sendai virus (hemagglutinating virus of Japan). Am J Pathol 2002; 161(5):1761–1772.
110. Yoshida S, Matsumoto K, Tomioka D, et al. Recombinant hepatocyte growth factor accelerates cutaneous wound healing in a diabetic mouse model. Growth Factors 2004; 22(2):111–119.
111. Rajapaksa S, McIntosh D, Cowin A, et al. The effect of insulin-like growth factor 1 incorporated into a hyaluronic acid-based nasal pack on nasal mucosal healing in a healthy sheep model and a sheep model of chronic sinusitis. Am J Rhino 2005; 10(3):251–256.
112. Rajan MS, Shafiei S, Mohrenfels CV, et al. Effect of exogenous keratinocyte growth factor on corneal epithelial migration after photorefractive keratectomy. J Cataract Refract Surg 2004; 30(10):2200–2206.
113. Cross SE, Roberts MS. Defining a model to predict the distribution of topically applied growth factors and other solutes in excisional full-thickness wounds. J Invest Dermatol 1999; 112(1):36–41.

17

Established and Emerging Oral Antifungals in Dermatology

Gérald E. Piérard and Claudine Piérard-Franchimont
Department of Dermatopathology, University Hospital of Liège, Liège, Belgium

Valérie Vroome
Barrier Therapeutics NV, Geel, Belgium

Jorge Arrese and Pascale Quatresooz
Department of Dermatopathology, University Hospital of Liège, Liège, Belgium

Marcel Borgers
Barrier Therapeutics NV, Geel, Belgium and Department of Molecular Cell Biology, Maastricht University, Maastricht, Netherlands

Geert Cauwenbergh
Barrier Therapeutics Inc., Princeton, New Jersey, U.S.A.

INTRODUCTION

The cutaneous manifestations of fungal diseases are frequently seen in clinical practice. Indeed, they represent the most common forms of fungal disease. They develop in compromised patients and in healthy individuals as well. Humans and animals contract most fungal, actinomycetal, and algal infections by exposure to infectious cells (propagules) usually originating from saprophytes growing in nature. More than 100,000 different species of these microorganisms are ubiquitous in the environment but before the HIV pandemic, only about 150 were recognized to cause disease. Some of these are familiar pathogens, but many more are opportunists and of such low virulence that they seldom cause invasive infection in the healthy, immunocompetent host. A few, such as the agents of actinomycosis and candidiasis, are endogenous and constitute part of the normal body biocenosis.

The course of a particular infection usually depends on several variables, such as the virulence and amount of the etiologic agent, the resistance and immune status of the host, the route of invasion, the anatomic sites affected, the presence of underlying disease or other predisposing factors, and the effectiveness of antifungal therapy or restoration of immunocompetency. With the exception of dermatophytosis, tinea (pityriasis) versicolor, and candidiasis of the newborn, no evidence is available that fungal infections are contagious. However, systemic infections can be transmitted by accidental percutaneous inoculation or contamination of open wounds with infectious material.

In dermatology, it is usual to distinguish the superficial dermatomycoses from the semi-invasive and invasive deep mycoses. Oral antifungal therapy is indicated in extensive superficial dermatomycoses and in those that prove to be difficult-to-treat conditions by topical compounds alone (1). In particular, tinea capitis and onychomycosis, both of which have varied etiology, are usually treated by oral antifungals. These drugs are mandatory for the semi-invasive and disseminated mycoses. When considering oral antifungal therapy, it is important to distinguish the mycoses restricted to the cornified structures (stratum corneum, nail, hair) from those localized in living tissues. This distinction is attributable to the fact that drug pharmacokinetics and pharmacodynamics are influenced by these localizations of the pathogen fungus (2). To eradicate fungal disease, adequate concentrations of an antimycotic must remain in the affected tissues. Because the physicochemical properties of each antifungal agent are different, variations in drug delivery and excretion exist, leading to potentially different levels of efficacy.

The efficacy of antifungal drugs in onychomycoses and tinea capitis is difficult to predict from conventional in vitro testing (3–5). Indeed, the response of fungi to antifungals is largely influenced by the presence of cornified cells (5). Hence, the in vitro evaluations of antifungal activity in culture media should not be taken at face value in the dermatological field. For instance, the extrapolation of in vitro fungicidy to the in vivo situation proves to be irrelevant and probably misleading in some instances (4). Any antifungal drug may be selected on the basis of the specific clinical presentation (what part of the body is infected?), the specific infected site (does it penetrate into and bind inside the affected tissue?), the organism involved and its biologic status (does it kill spores?), and the status of the patient's defence against fungi. Of course, other considerations remain important. These include ease of drug administration, the low and acceptable adverse effect profile, the cost of the drug, as well as consideration of the nutritional status, hygiene, concurrent medications, and the general health status of the affected individual (6).

In most onychomycoses, tinea capitis, semi-invasive mycoses, and invasive mycoses, prolonged therapy is needed to achieve resolution. Complete cure cannot be guaranteed with confidence because the potential for treatment failures exists with each of the current antifungals. These considerations are in contrast with the expectations based on some in vitro antifungal susceptibility testing. Treatment failures, recurrences, and relapses are not exceptional (1,4). Notwithstanding the fact that the need to combat life-threatening deep fungal infections is of great importance, there remains an unmet need for compounds to treat superficial infections, especially chronic ones such as onychomycosis and tinea capitis.

To be effective, an antifungal drug must successfully penetrate the affected body tissues and the cell membranes of the causative organism. Therefore, the use of oral drugs assumes that the drugs reach the given tissue(s) after absorption, resulting in the desired antifungal tissue concentration and optimal therapeutic effect. It remains that antifungal drug efficacy in onychomycoses is impeded by slow nail growth and by specific conditions that retard the rate of nail growth, such as advanced age. In addition, if a systemic drug is only taken up in the newly formed nail during treatment, it will take a long time for the nail to become fully impregnated with the drug (2).

MAIN ANTIMYCOTIC DRUG CLASSES IN DERMATOLOGY

The mechanistic and structural correlates of antifungal action explain the mode of action of the principal antimycotic drug categories (7,8). The main classes of oral antifungals comprise the polyene antimicrobials, griseofulvin, flucytosine, the azole derivatives, the allylamines, the echinocandins, and the sordarins. These compounds vary greatly from each other as far as their spectrum of activity, potency, and safety are concerned. These properties are largely determined by their particular mode of action and pharmacokinetics. Antimycotic drugs interfere with the normal life cycle of fungi by inhibiting normal functioning of one or several vital cellular structures such as plasma membranes and cell wall components (8). The effects of these agents are reflected in altered patterns of growth, differentiation, transformation, ultrastructure, and viability of the fungi. The molecular target sites and subcellular targets for antimycotic action have been identified for most antifungal drug classes (8). Not only their mode of action, but also the pharmacokinetics, the fungicidal or fungistatic effects, spectrum of activity, potency, and safety vary greatly. This chapter is a selected review of oral antifungals of interest in dermatology. They are presented in alphabetical order.

Amphotericin B

Amphotericin B belongs to the polyene antimicrobials. The drug binds to the fungal ergosterol mainly, and forms cylindrical channels in the fungal cell membrane, altering its permeability and leading to cell death. For decades, amphotericin B was the only treatment option for systemic fungal infections. However, although amphotericin B has a higher affinity for ergosterol, it also binds to cholesterol, a component of mammalian cell membranes, causing cytotoxicity in human tissues. Thus, despite the fact that almost all fungi are susceptible to amphotericin B, its clinical use is limited by toxicity expressed as chills, nausea, and vomiting, as well as liver, renal, and cardiovascular complications. Developing lipidic versions of the drug with reduced toxicity was one of the first biotechnology efforts in the antifungal arena (8). This compound has no indication in common dermatomycoses.

Caspofungin

Caspofungin is a member of the echinocandin class. The drug inhibits β-1,3-D-glucan, a component of the fungal cell wall, resulting in osmotic fragility and lysis of the susceptible fungi. It has shown efficacy in the treatment of aspergillosis, candidemia, and esophageal candidiasis. So far, caspofungin has not been used in any of the dermatomycoses.

Fluconazole

Fluconazole is an orally active synthetic bis-triazole antifungal agent. It is active against dermatophytes and *Candida* species with the exception of *Candida krusei* (9). Fluconazole is primarily fungistatic by inhibiting the fungal enzyme lanosterol 14-demethylase. This prevents the conversion of lanosterol to the fungal membrane lipid ergosterol. As a result, fungal cell membrane permeability increases causing loss of intracytoplasmic components, thus inhibiting fungal cell growth and replication. When administered as a single oral 150 mg dose, fluconazole is more selective for fungal CYP 450 enzymes than for CYP 450 enzymes in mammalian organs. Compared with other azoles, fluconazole appears to be a weak inhibitor of CYP 450–mediated drug oxidative pathways tested on human hepatic microsomes in vitro. Fluconazole administered as a single oral 150 mg dose does not adversely affect the steroid biosyntheses in humans.

Pharmacokinetics

After oral administration, fluconazole is well absorbed, metabolically stable, and widely distributed as free drug in body fluids and tissues. The peak plasma concentrations of fluconazole range between 2.4 and 3.6 mg/L after a single 150 mg dose. Continued administration leads to a 2.5-fold increase in peak plasma concentrations (10). Steady-state plasma concentrations are achieved within four to seven days when no loading dose is given. The half-life of fluconazole in plasma is about 31 to 37 hours. The long half-life results in drug accumulation with multiple dosing.

The apparent distribution of fluconazole, which is not extensively bound to tissue, protein, or fat, is approximately that of total body water (10). The effect of the patient status may influence the pharmacokinetic properties of fluconazole. Its plasma concentrations may become elevated in elderly patients. Fluconazole half-life is prolonged in patients with renal dysfunction; therefore, dosage adjustment is recommended. The drug is excreted in large part unchanged in urine (11).

Fluconazole penetrates well into body fluids and tissues, including skin and nails. The concentrations of fluconazole in skin blister fluid and nails were found to be similar. The drug was reported to be still present inside nails 6 months after termination of therapy (12). However, drug concentration in the nail may remain lower than the minimum inhibitory concentration (MIC) values for the fungal pathogens. Indeed, tissue affinity of fluconazole appears limited and keratin adherence was reported to be weak (2).

Adverse Events and Drug Interactions
Much attention has been paid to potential adverse events and drug interactions related to the intake of antifungals (13–16). Before initiating therapy with fluconazole, a detailed drug history should be obtained. The more common adverse events are headache, gastrointestinal troubles, and skin rash. In humans, fluconazole inhibits both CYP3A4 and CYP2C9 in a dose-dependent manner, and may consequently increase plasma concentrations of drugs metabolized by these pathways. Therefore, a number of drugs that are metabolized by these enzymes are contraindicated or require close monitoring (6,14,15).

Griseofulvin
Griseofulvin is a traditional oral antifungal agent derived from *Penicillium griseofulvium*. It is fungistatic and its spectrum of antifungal activity is restricted to dermatophytes. It was the first drug available to manage onychomycosis, but it is no longer in common use in dermatology except for the treatment of tinea capitis (17). Griseofulvin inhibits the formation of the cell wall and intracellular microtubules, disrupts the nucleic acid synthesis and the mitotic process, and thus prevents cell division of dermatophytes (17,18).

Pharmacokinetics
Griseofulvin is poorly soluble in water and poorly absorbed after oral administration. Its bioavailability is improved when taken with a fatty meal. Absorption is also increased by reducing the size of the drug particles (ultramicrosize griseofulvin) (19). The peak plasma level is achieved two to four hours after drug administration. The average half-life of griseofulvin is 11 to 14 hours, and the drug is completely excreted in the urine within 72 hours as its metabolite 6-demethylgriseofulvin (20). Griseofulvin apparently reaches the upper part of the stratum corneum from the sweat. The nail does not benefit from this mechanism. Griseofulvin is progressively incorporated in the nail from the matrix. The drug persists in the nail for only one to two weeks after discontinuation of treatment (2).

Adverse Events and Drug Interactions
Adverse events of griseofulvin intake are generally caused by hypersensitivity (skin rash, urticaria). Headache (15% in adults), oral thrush, nausea, vomiting, diarrhea, fatigue, and insomnia may be observed (17). The occurrence of severe reactions is rare and results from high doses and/or long duration therapy (6). Griseofulvin should not be administered during pregnancy because of the risk of developing conjoint twins. It is contraindicated in individuals with porphyria and hepatocellular failure. Griseofulvin induces CYP3A4, leading to lower plasma levels of drugs metabolized by this pathway. Resistance development of dermatophytes against griseofulvin has become an issue in the past decade or so.

Itraconazole
Itraconazole is a lipophilic and keratophilic bis-triazole exhibiting fungistatic activity (2,3,8,21,22). It inhibits the CYP 450 enzyme lanosterol 14-demethylase, which prevents its conversion to ergosterol. Hence, methylated sterols accumulate in fungal cells. This action reduces membrane-bound enzyme activity and interrupts chitin synthesis resulting in abnormal permeability and function of the cell membrane (23). The spectrum of antifungal activity is wide and includes dermatophytes, yeasts, and selected moulds (3,8,21,22,24–26).

Pharmacokinetics
Itraconazole is metabolized in the liver by oxidative mechanisms involving the CYP 3A4 isoenzyme system. More than 30 metabolites have been identified. Hydroxy-itraconazole is a major metabolite also showing antifungal activity. Itraconazole and its major metabolites are excreted in the urine and feces. The elimination of itraconazole from plasma follows a biexponential pattern with a dose- and time-dependent elimination half-life in the range of 25 to 40 hours. Hydroxyitraconazole is eliminated more rapidly, but its plasma concentrations at steady state is 1.5- to 2-fold higher than that of itraconazole. Thus, plasma concentrations of itraconazole measured by bioassay are approximately 3.5 times higher than those determined by high-performance liquid chromatography (27).

Although itraconazole is widely distributed in lipophilic tissues, it also exhibits a high affinity for cornified cells (28) and is incorporated into the nail plate. When the drug reaches the nail unit, a fast diffusion occurs and during treatment the levels of itraconazole in the nail increase with time. In nails, the MIC for dermatophytes is approximately 100 ng/g and better therapeutic results are achieved with itraconazole levels in nails exceeding 400 ng/g. Continuous therapy with itraconazole consists of a regimen of 200 mg/day for 6 to 12 weeks for onychomycoses. The drug is also effective in the treatment of dermatophyte and *Candida* onychomycoses as well as in those due to some nondermatophyte moulds (29–36). Itraconazole also show efficacy in treating tinea capitis (37).

Pharmacokinetic studies (28) provide a good rationale for the development of improved dosing strategies. For example, doubling the dose of itraconazole from 100 to 200 mg/day results in a 10-fold increase in nail drug levels. Itraconazole is present in the distal end of the fingernail after one week and in the toenail two weeks after beginning therapy because of diffusion via the nail bed. The concentration of orally administrated antifungal agent in the lateral portion of the nail plate may be less compared to the central part of the nail (2). Continuous treatment is not necessary to maintain therapeutic levels of itraconazole in the nail. Its ability to reach the nail quickly (within seven days of starting treatment) and to remain there up to nine months after therapy while being quickly eliminated from the plasma, make it an ideal drug to use in a intermittent therapy regimen (30). This regimen consists of twice-daily 200 mg dosing for one week per month for two months for fingernails and three or four months for toenails (28). As a result, higher maximum itraconazole plasma concentrations are achieved, but the total systemic exposure is lower compared with the continuous regimen (38). No significant difference was found in the clinical response on mycologic cure rates between continuous and pulse treatment regimens (38). There were no significant efficacy differences between three and four pulses (28). A treatment regimen for onychomycosis consisting of one week of treatment per month for three months reduces the total drug dose, cost of treatment, and most likely increases patient compliance, safety, and guarantees optimal tolerance. There may be other ways to use intermittent antifungal treatment. For instance, onychomycosis may be treated with intermittent low-dose itraconazole 200 mg/day for one week every four weeks, a regimen repeated six times (39).

Itraconazole Capsules
The oral bioavailability of itraconazole capsules is maximized when taken with a meal or an acidic beverage. Steady-state concentration is achieved in 15 days with oral doses of 50 to 400 mg/day. Itraconazole is distributed in lipid-enriched tissues with about 95% of the blood value bound to plasma proteins, and 0.2% available as circulating free drug. Plasma half-life varies between 15 and 25 hours after a single dose, and between 30 and 40 hours during multiple dosing when steady state is reached. In comparison with itraconazole, peak plasma levels of hydroxyitraconazole are on average 70%, and area under the curve values 130% higher, but with a shorter half-life of about 14 hours.

Itraconazole Solution
Itraconazole exists in an oral solution using hydroxypropyl-β cyclodextrin (HP-β-CD) as vehicle. The oral delivery of HP-β-CD itraconazole suspension enhances the drug bioavailability of itraconazole by molecular dispersion, protection from degradation, and delivery to the surfaces of the intestinal wall (25,40,41). Compared to the capsule presentation, the oral HP-β-CD itraconazole suspension confers enhanced oral bioavailability by about 30% (40). An additional 25% to 30% increase in oral bioavailability and increased peak plasma concentrations can be achieved when the drug in HP-β-CD suspension is taken on an empty stomach (41,42). HP-β-CD exhibits minimal to undetectable systemic effects because of the absence of absorption. However, this carrier exerts osmotic activity in the intestinal tract, which may lead to gastrointestinal intolerance, in particular at dosages exceeding 400 mg (43,44).

Adverse Events and Drug Interactions
Although with much less avidity than on fungal cells, itraconazole also binds to the mammalian CYP 450 3A4 system in the liver where the drug is metabolized (15,16,45). This mechanism is responsible for most aspects of potential itraconazole toxicity and clinically relevant drug-drug interactions (46,47). The most common adverse reactions after itraconazole intake are headache and gastrointestinal tract upset. Dermatologic disorders including Stevens-Johnson syndrome have been reported. Asymptomatic abnormalities of hepatic function occur in less than 3% of patients (47). Reversible hepatobiliary effects are estimated at 1:500,000. Hepatitis occurs most often with continuous therapy and usually after four or more weeks of therapy (47).

Monitoring hepatic enzyme test values is recommended in patients with preexisting hepatic function abnormalities, those who have experienced liver toxicity with other medications, and those receiving continuous itraconazole for more than one month or at any time a patient develops symptom suggestive of liver dysfunction.

Congestive heart failure and pulmonary oedema have been reported and itraconazole should not be administered at high dosage in patients with systemic mycoses and evidence of ventricular dysfunction or a history of congestive heart failure (48). The relative risk for any pregnancy loss is 1.75. Itraconazole inhibits 14-α-demethylase, a fungal CP450 enzyme, and a member of the same group of enzymes that is present in the human liver is responsible for the metabolism of many drugs. Itraconazole specifically inhibits the CP 450 3A4 isoenzyme system (CYP3A4), and, consequently, may increase plasma concentrations of drugs metabolized by this pathway. Itraconazole is also known to increase the levels of a series of drugs (6). Because itraconazole is itself metabolized by CYP3A4, any inducers or inhibitors may decrease or elevate itraconazole levels, respectively. Absorption of itraconazole may be decreased by the concomitant administration of antacids, H_2 blockers, and proton pump inhibitors.

Ketoconazole
Ketoconazole was the first oral imidazole available for the treatment of fungal infections with a broad spectrum of action, including dermatophytes and yeasts (9,17,49). It represented a major therapeutic breakthrough at the time it was introduced on the market. The drug is poorly soluble in water at pH above three. Because of the risk of adverse reactions, the drug is not currently used as a first-line antifungal drug in dermatomycoses.

Posaconazole
Posaconazole is a triazole structurally related to itraconazole. This drug shows potent broad-spectrum activity against opportunistic fungal pathogens such as *Candida* spp., *Cryptococcus neoformans*, *Aspergillus* spp., *Fusarium* spp., dermatophytes, and zygomycetes (50,51). Posaconazole works principally by inhibition of CP 450 14-α-demethylase and is a more potent inhibitor of sterol C14 demethylation than itraconazole (51). Posaconazole is presently formulated in oral tablet and suspension preparations. No data are available about the efficacy of posaconazole in the treatment of onychomycosis and other cutaneous mycoses.

Pramiconazole
Pramiconazole is a novel triazole that exhibits low solubility in water and acids. Its solubility in aqueous solvents is increased by HP-β-CD. The drug is very potent against dermatophytes (*Trichophyton* spp., *Microsporum canis*, *Epidermophyton floccosum*), yeasts (*Candida* spp. and *Malassezia* spp.), and many other fungi and actinomycetes (8,52–57). Pramiconazole has the highest in vitro activity against *Malassezia* spp. (56). The high activity of pramiconazole is ascribed to its prominent affinity to fungal CYP 450.

Pharmacokinetics
After a single oral dose of pramiconazole in solution with 40% HP-β-CD, peak plasma levels are reached between one and three hours in animals. The absolute

oral bioavailability of pramiconazole in HP-β-CD solution ranges between 65% and 85% in animals. The compound is eliminated from the plasma with a terminal half-life of 23 hours in laboratory animals (52). The metabolism of pramiconazole was studied in vitro using isolated hepatocytes and subcellular liver fractions of different species. The compound is extensively metabolized by liver enzymes by two metabolic pathways, namely, hydroxylation at the 2,4-difluorophenyl or *N*-oxidation at the 1,2,4-triazole-1-ylmethyl ring and oxidative dioxolane scission.

Animal models have demonstrated the in vivo efficacy of pramiconazole in dermatophyte infections. The results indicated a 4- to 8-fold superiority of potency of this compound over itraconazole, especially in superficial fungal infections (52). In humans, the drug efficacy in onychomycosis is not yet established (6). However, the corneofungimetry bioassay has revealed the antifungal activity of the drug in human stratum corneum after oral intake (55). Human corneofungimetry was performed with *Candida albicans*, *Malassezia globosa*, *M. canis*, *Trichophyton rubrum*, and *T. mentagrophytes* at different time intervals during and after one week of oral dosing with 100 or 200 mg pramiconazole. The drug clearly reduced the fungal growth of all strains at day 7, thereby reaching statistical significance for four of five strains. The clinical efficacy of pramiconazole with one single intake was also proven in seborrhoeic dermatitis (57), as well as in pityriasis versicolor and various dermatophytoses after one to five days of treatment (8).

Adverse Events and Drug Interactions
Inhibition experiments with pramiconazole in human liver microsomes revealed that CYP 3A4 was the CYP 450 form that was the most sensitive to inhibition. Pramiconazole showed a much lower interaction potential with CYP 450 3A4 compared to ketoconazole and itraconazole. Pramiconazole did not significantly inhibit the human CYP 450 1A2, 2D6, 2C9, 2A6, and 2E1 (8). Studies in healthy volunteers have demonstrated that a single dose of pramiconazole up to 1200 mg was safe and well tolerated. Neither cardiovascular adverse effects nor changes in clinical laboratory parameters were noticed. Limited adverse events have been reported, including gastrointestinal pain and diarrhea, effects known to be induced by HP-β-CD. The incidence of headache or diarrhea was similar in the placebo and the active treatment groups, and were therefore probably not drug- and dose-related. The proposed single dose of 200 mg is therefore expected to be safe and well tolerated. This was verified in a clinical study (57).

Ravuconazole
Ravuconazole is a triazole derivative with antifungal capabilities against a broad spectrum of fungi (7,51,58,59) including *Aspergillus* spp., *C. neoformans*, *Candida* spp., and dermatophytes. Its activity against the latter is greater than that of fluconazole and itraconazole (51). Its structure is related to that of voriconazole.

Pharmacokinetics and Efficacy
Ravuconazole has a long half-life of approximately 100 hours. A dosage of 200 mg/day for 12 weeks appears to be effective for treating moderate to severe dermatophyte toenail onychomycosis (6,51,59). However, the cure rate was not higher than that obtained with terbinafine and itraconazole, and therefore ravuconazole at 200 mg/day does not appear to be a better option for onychomycosis treatment than the available antifungals. As with all azole antifungal agents, ravuconazole works

principally by inhibition of CP 450 14-α-demethylase (CP450 14DM). Its potency and binding affinity for CP450 14DM is similar to that of itraconazole. The metabolism is similar to that of voriconazole.

Adverse Events and Drug Interactions

Adverse events associated with ravuconazole treatment include abdominal problems, headache, dizziness, pruritus, and rash (59). Ravuconazole is not a potent inhibitor of the CYP 3A4 metabolic pathway as other azoles, and may therefore have fewer drug interactions. However, this is not firmly established.

Terbinafine

Terbinafine is a lipophilic and keratinophilic allylamine indicated for the treatment of dermatophyte onychomycosis. The drug inhibits fungal ergosterol biosynthesis at the point of squalene epoxidation. Its in vitro fungicidal activity on fungi growing in culture media might be caused by the accumulation of high levels of intracellular squalene. However, when fungi are cultured in contact with cornified cells, they modify their metabolism and they become considerably less sensitive to terbinafine (5,24). This is probably relevant to the in vivo situation where terbinafine does not readily kill all fungi responsible for onychomycoses (4). Thus, the concept of fungicidy cannot be extrapolated at face value to the in vivo conditions, particularly onychomycosis and tinea capitis.

Pharmacokinetics

Terbinafine is absorbed within two hours after oral administration (60), and is not affected by food intake. Peak plasma concentrations ranging between 0.8 and 1.5 μg/mL appear within about two hours after administration of single 250- to 500-mg dosages. Terbinafine is distributed in skin, adipose tissue, and nails (61,62) after one week of treatment. Plasma half-life is triphasic, with half-lives of 1.1, 16 to 26, and about 100 hours, respectively. Low plasma concentrations can be measured up to six weeks after therapy is discontinued (63). Approximately 70% of the administered dose is slowly eliminated in the urine.

Patient status may influence the pharmacokinetic properties of terbinafine. A decreased plasma clearance of terbinafine is observed in cases of liver failure, and adjustment to the dose is recommended when liver alteration is severe. An impaired elimination of the drug is also observed in cases of renal disease (60) and dosage should be reduced when creatinine clearance is less than 50 mL/min.

Orally administered terbinafine reaches the distal part of the nail between one and 18 weeks (62,63). When the drug reaches the nail, a rapid diffusion takes place, resulting in a steady state with drug levels varying between 250 and 550 ng/g (64). During treatment, the levels of terbinafine in the nail do not increase with time. They persist for about nine months after discontinuation of therapy (62). This pharmacokinetic aspect suggests that terbinafine most likely penetrates into the nail, not only by diffusion, but also by incorporation into the matrix. Continuous terbinafine is an effective treatment of dermatophyte onychomycosis (65,66). Intermittent therapy can also be used successfully for treating onychomycosis (65–68).

Adverse Events and Drug Interactions

The more common adverse events while patients are on terbinafine treatment involve the gastrointestinal system (diarrhea, dyspepsia, abdominal pain, nausea, flatulence), dermatological signs (rash, pruritus, urticaria), and headache. Asymptomatic liver enzyme abnormalities occur in about 3.3% of patients (13–16). Signs of hepatobiliary dysfunction reach 1:45,000 to 1:120,000. Hepatitis may appear without preexisting liver disease. Taste disturbance was reported in 2.8% of patients. Neutropenia was observed in 1:400,000 patients. Terbinafine is metabolized by CP 450 enzymes and plasma clearance of terbinafine is increased by the P450-inducer rifampicin and decreased by the P 450-inhibitor cimetidine. Terbinafine is also reported to decrease cyclosporine levels by increasing cyclosporine clearance. It was also shown that terbinafine inhibits CYP2D6, a CP 450 isoenzyme that metabolizes a few other drugs.

Voriconazole

Voriconazole is a triazole antifungal agent, structurally related to fluconazole. It is indicated for the primary treatment of acute invasive aspergillosis, as salvage therapy for severe systemic infections by *Scedosporium apiospermum* and *Fusarium* spp., and for refractory *Candida* infections (69,70). Similar to other azole antifungals, voriconazole inhibits the fungal CP 450–mediated 14-α-lanosterol demethylation. The inhibition of CP 450 14-α-demethylase is dose-dependent and, compared to fluconazole, provided with an increased potency. The accumulation of 14-α-methyl sterols is added to the loss of ergosterol in the fungal cell wall and may account for the strong antifungal activity of the compound.

Pharmacokinetics

Voriconazole is metabolized by the human hepatic CP 450 enzymes, CYP2C19, CYP2C9, and CYP3A4, with less than 2% of the dose excreted unchanged in the urine. The major metabolite of voriconazole is the *N*-oxide, which exhibits minimal antifungal activity and consequently does not contribute to the overall efficacy of voriconazole. This antifungal is active both in oral and intravenous administrations. It is available as a lyophilized powder for solution for intravenous infusion, film-coated tablets for oral administration, and as a powder for oral suspension. Dosages are 200 mg twice daily orally and 3 to 6 mg/kg every 12 hours intravenously.

Adverse Events and Drug Interactions

Levels of voriconazole are significantly reduced by the concomitant administration of a series of drugs (6). It is, therefore, necessary to monitor or adjust the dose of other drugs. The most common adverse effects of voriconazole are visual disturbances that affect 40% of patients and include abnormal vision, color vision change and photophobia, elevations of liver enzymes (20%), and skin rashes (6%). Adverse effects often lead to discontinuation of voriconazole therapy. Liver function tests should be evaluated at the start of and during the course of the treatment. Acute renal failure has been observed in severely ill patients. The mechanisms underlying the dermatologic adverse effects of voriconazole are unknown. A photosensitivity reaction may occur with long-term treatment. A case of photoaging caused by voriconazole therapy has been reported in a 15-year-old patient (71). Voriconazole has never been evaluated for the treatment of onychomycosis.

COMBINATION THERAPIES

Combination and sequential antifungal therapies are not indicated in dermatomycoses, except in rare cases (72). In systemic mycoses, these procedures are sometimes used. Potentialization can be achieved by some specific combinations, but inhibition is observed with other antifungal combinations (6,72–80).

ANTIFUNGALS IN ATOPIC DERMATITIS

The head-and-neck type of atopic dermatitis has been shown to respond to itraconazole (81,82). This effect is presumably due to the intervention of *Malassezia* spp.*** in the pathogenesis of this disorder.

CONCLUSION

Besides the five main considerations for choosing a drug (efficacy, safety, cost, compliance, and availability), choice of treatment depends on many factors including patient's age and preference, etiologic agent, number of nails affected, degree of nail involvement, whether toenails or fingernails are infected, and whether other drugs are taken.

A better knowledge of pharmacokinetics of the antifungals has influenced the manner in which oral antifungal agents are dosed. In addition, the claim for the fungicidal effect of terbinafine had led some clinicians to mistakenly extrapolate this characteristic to the in vivo situation, thus prescribing this drug as if it guaranteed cure in a short-term treatment. The era of griseofulvin or ketoconazole where the patient had to be treated daily as long as the nail was abnormal is over but the quest to discover the ideal treatment continues today.

REFERENCES

1. Arrese JE, Piérard GE. Treatment failures and relapses in onychomycosis: a stubborn clinical problem. Dermatology 2003; 207:255–260.
2. De Doncker P. Pharmacokinetics of orally administered antifungals in onychomycosis. Int J Dermatol 1999; 38:S10–S27.
3. Arrese JE, De Doncker P, Odds F, Piérard GE. Reduction in the growth of non-dermatophyte moulds by itraconazole: evaluation by corneofungimetry bioassay. Mycoses 1998; 41:461–465.
4. Arrese JE, Pierard-Franchimont C, Piérard GE. A plea to bridge the gap between antifungals and onychomycosis management. Am J Clin Dermatol 2001; 2:281–284.
5. Osborne CS, Leitner I, Favre B, Ryder NS. Antifungal drug response in an in vitro model of dermatophyte nail infection. Med Mycol 2004; 42:159–163.
6. Baran R, Gupta AK, Piérard GE. Pharmacotherapy of onychomycosis. Expert Opin Pharmacother 2005; 6:609–624.
7. Gupta AK, Tomas E. New antifungal agents. Dermatol Clin 2003; 21:565–576.
8. Borgers M, Degreef H, Cauwenbergh G. Fungal infections of the skin: infection process and antimycotic therapy. Curr Drug Targets 2005; 6:849–862.
9. Piérard GE, Rurangirwa A, Piérard-Franchimont C. Bioavailability of fluconazole and ketoconazole in human stratum corneum and oral mucosa. Clin Exp Dermatol 1991; 16:168–171.
10. Humphrey MJ, Jevons S, Tarbit MH. Pharmacokinetic evaluation of UK-49,858, a metabolically stable triazole antifungal drug, in animals and man. Antimicrob Agents Chemother 1985; 28:648–653.
11. Debruyne D, Ryckelynck JP: Clinical pharmacokinetics of fluconazole. Clin Pharmacokinet 1993; 24:10–27.
12. Faergemann J, Laufen H. Levels of fluconazole in normal and diseased nails during and after treatment of onychomycosis in toenails with fluconazole 150 mg once weekly. Acta Derm Venereol 1996; 76:219–221.

13. Katz HI. Drug interactions of the newer oral antifungal agents. Br J Dermatol 1999; 141: S26–S32.
14. Gupta AK, Katz HI, Shear NH. Drug interactions with itraconazole, fluconazole and terbinafine and their management. J Am Acad Dermatol 1999; 41:237–249.
15. Shear N, Drake L, Gupta A, et al. The implications and management of drug interactions with itraconazole, fluconazole and terbinafine. Dermatology 2000; 201:196–203.
16. Shapiro LE, Shear NH. Drug interactions: proteins, pumps, and P-450s. J Am Acad Dermatol 2002; 47:467–484.
17. Pierard GE, Arrese JE, Pierard-Franchimont C. Treatment of onychomycosis. Traditional approaches. J Am Acad Dermatol 1993; 29:S41–S45.
18. Sloboda RD, Van Blaricom G, Creasey WA, et al. Griseofulvin: association with tubulin and inhibition of in vitro microtubule assembly. Biochem Biophys Res Commun 1982; 105:882–888.
19. Schäfer-Korting M, Korting HC, Mutschler E. Human plasma and skin blister fluid levels of griseofulvin following a single oral dose. Eur J Clin Pharmacol 1985; 29:109–113.
20. Bates TR, Sequeira JAL. Use of 24 hr urinary excretion to assess the bioavailability of griseofulvin in humans. J Pharm Sci 1975; 64:709.
21. Van Cutsem J, Van Gerven F, Janssen PAJ. Activity of orally, topically, and parenterally administered itraconazole in the treatment of superficial and deep mycoses: animal models. Rev Infect Dis 1987; 9:S15–S32.
22. Pierard GE, Arrese JE, Pierard-Franchimont C. Itraconazole. Exp Opin Pharmacother 2000; 1:287–304.
23. Groll AH, Piscitelli SC, Walsh TJ. Clinical pharmacology of systemic antifungal agents: a comprehensive review of agents in clinical use, current investigational compounds, and putative targets for antifungal drug development. Adv Pharmacol 1998; 44:343–500.
24. Piérard GE, Arrese JE, De Doncker P. Antifungal activity of itraconazole and terbinafine in human stratum corneum: a comparative study. J Am Acad Dermatol 1995; 32:429–435.
25. Piérard GE, Kharfi M, Salomon-Neira MD, et al. Itraconazole in human aspergillosis revisited. J Mycol Med 2004; 14:192–200.
26. Piérard GE, Arrese JE, Pierard-Franchimont C. Itraconazole corneofungimetry bioassay on Malassezia species. Mycoses 2004; 47:418–421.
27. Warnock DW, Turner A, Burke J. Comparison of high performance liquid chromatographic and microbiological methods for determination of itraconazole. J Antimicrob Chemother 1988; 21:93–100.
28. Cauwenbergh G, Degreef H, Heykants J, et al. Pharmacokinetic profile of orally administered itraconazole in human skin. J Am Acad Dermatol 1988; 18:263–268.
29. De Doncker PD, Decroix J, Pierard GE, et al. Antifungal pulse therapy for onychomycosis. A pharmacokinetic and pharmacodynamic investigation of monthly cycles of 1-week pulse therapy with itraconazole. Arch Dermatol 1996; 132:34–41.
30. De Doncker P, Scher R, Baran R, et al. Itraconazole therapy is effective for pedal onychomycosis caused by some nondermatophyte molds and in mixed infection with dermatophytes and molds: a multicenter study with 36 patients. J Am Acad Dermatol 1997; 36: 73–177.
31. Havu V, Brandt H, Heikkila H, et al. Continuous and intermittent itraconazole dosing schedules for the treatment of onychomycosis: a pharmacokinetic comparison. Br J Dermatol 1999; 140:96–101.
32. De Doncker P, Gupta AK, Marynissen G, et al. Itraconazole pulse therapy for onychomycosis and dermatomycoses: an overview. J Am Acad Dermatol 1998; 37: 969–974.
33. Haneke E, Abeck D, Ring J. Safety and efficacy of intermittent therapy with itraconazole in finger- and toenail-onychomycosis: a multicentre trial. Mycoses 1998; 41:521–527.
34. Wang DL, Wang AP, Li RY, Wang R. Therapeutic efficacy and safety of one-week intermittent therapy with itraconazole for onychomycosis in a Chinese patient population. Dermatology 1999; 199:47–19.
35. Gupta AK, De Doncker P, Haneke E. Itraconazole pulse therapy for the treatment of Candida onychomycosis. J Eur Acad Dermatol Venereol 2000; 15(5):112–115.

36. Gupta AK, Maddin S, Arlette J, et al. Itraconazole pulse therapy is effective in dermatophyte onychomycosis of the toenail: a double-blind placebo-controlled study. J Dermatol Treat 2000; 11:33–37.
37. Ginter-Hanselmeyer G, Smolle J, Gupta A. Itraconazole in the treatment of tinea capitis caused by *Microsporum canis*: experience in a large cohort. Pediatr Dermatol 2005;22: 499–502.
38. Havu V, Brandt H, Heikkila H, et al. A double-blind, randomized study comparing itraconazole pulse therapy with continuous dosing for the treatment of toe-nail onychomycosis. Br J Dermatol 1997; 136:230–234.
39. Ingber A. Intermittent low dose itraconazole treatment for onychomycosis—long term follow-up. Med Mycol 2001; 39:471–473.
40. Barone JA, Moskovitch BL, Guarnieri J, et al. Enhanced bioavailability of itraconazole in hydroxypropyl-β-cyclodextrin solution versus capsules in healthy volunteers. Antimicrob Agents Chemother 1998; 42:1862–1865.
41. Van De Velde VJS, Van Peer AP, Heykants JJP, et al. Effects of food on the pharmacokinetics of a new hydroxypropyl-beta-cyclodextrin formulation of itraconazole. Pharmacotherapy 1996; 16:424–428.
42. Menichetti F, Del Favero A, Martino P, et al. Itraconazole oral solution as prophylaxis for fungal infections in neutropenic patients with hematologic malignancies: a randomized, placebo-controlled, double-blind, multicenter trial. Clin Infect Dis 1998; 28:250–255.
43. Glasmacher A, Haln C, Molitor E, et al. Itraconazole trough concentrations in antifungal prophylaxis with six different dosing regiments using hydroxypropyl-beta-cyclodextrin oral solution or coated-pellet capsules. Mycoses 1999; 42:591–600.
44. Stevens DA. Itraconazole in cyclodextrin solution. Pharmacotherapy 1999; 19:603–611.
45. Groll AH, Piscitelli SC, Walsh TJ. Clinical pharmacology of systemic antifungal agents: a comprehensive review of agents in clinical use, current investigational compounds, and putative targets for antifungal drug development. Adv Pharmacol 1998; 44:343–500.
46. Venkatakrishnan K, Von Moltke LL, Greenblatt DJ. Effects of the antifungal agents on oxidative drug metabolism: clinical relevance. Clin Pharmacokinet 2000; 38:111–180.
47. Gupta AK, Chwetzoff E, Del Rosso J, Baran R. Hepatic safety of itraconazole. J Cutan Med Surg 2002; 6:210–213.
48. Ahmad SR, Singer SJ, Leissa BG. Congestive heart failure associated with itraconazole. Lancet 2001; 357:1716–1717.
49. Arrese JE, Fogouang L, Piérard-Franchimont C, Pierard GE. Euclidean and fractal computer-assisted corneofungimetry. A comparison of 2% ketoconazole and 1% terbinafine topical formulations. Dermatology 2002; 204:222–227.
50. Barchiesi F, Arzeni D, Camiletti V, et al. In vitro activity of posaconazole against clinical isolates of dermatophytes. J Clin Microb 2001; 39:4208–4209.
51. Gupta AK, Kohli Y, Batra R. In vitro activities of posaconazole, ravuconazole, terbinafine, itraconazole and fluconazole against dermatophyte, yeast and non-dermatophyte species. Med Mycol 2005; 43:179–185.
52. Odds F, Ausma J, Van Gerven F, et al. Activity in vitro and in vivo activities of the novel azole antifungal agent R126638. Antimicrob Agents Chemother 2004; 48:388–391.
53. Vanden Bossche H, Ausma J, Bohets H, et al. The novel azole R126638 is a selective inhibitor of ergosterol synthesis in *Candida albicans, Trichophyton* spp. and *Microsporum canis*. Antimicrob Agents Chemother 2004; 48:3272–3278.
54. Meerpoel L, Backx LJJ, van der Veken LJE, et al. Synthesis and in vitro and in vivo structure-activity relationships of novel antifungal triazoles for dermatology. J Med Chem 2005; 48:2184–2193.
55. Piérard-Franchimont C, Ausma J, Wouters L, et al. Activity of the triazole antifungal R126638 as assessed by corneofungimetry. Skin Pharmacol Physiol 2006; 19:49–56.
56. Faergemann J, Ausma J, Borgers M. The in vitro activity of R126638 and ketoconazole against *Malassezia* species. Acta Dermatol Venereol 2006; 86:312–315.
57. Piérard GE, Ausma J, Henry F, et al. A pilot study on seborrheic dermatitis using pramiconazole as a potent oral anti-*Malassezia* agent. Dermatology 2007; 214:162–169.
58. Fung-Tome JC, Huezko E, Minassian B, Bonner DP: In vitro activity of a new oral triazole, BMS-207147 (ER-30346). Antimicrob Agents Chemother 1998; 42:313–318.

59. Gupta AK, Leonardi C, Stoltz RR, et al. A phase I/II randomized, placebo-controlled, dose-ranging study evaluating the efficacy, safety and pharmacokinetics of ravuconazole in the treatment of onychomycosis. J Eur Acad Dermatol 2005; 19:437–443.
60. Jenssen JC: Pharmacokinetics of terbinafine in humans. J Dermatol Treat 1990; 1:S15–S18.
61. Faergemann J, Zehender H, Boukhabza A et al. A double-blind comparison of levels of terbinafine and itraconazole in plasma, skin, sebum, hair and nails during and after oral medication. Acta Derm Venereol 1997; 77:74–76.
62. Schatz F, Brautigam M, Bobrowolski E, et al. Nail incorporation kinetics of terbinafine in onychomycosis patients. Clin Exp Dermatol 1995; 20:377–383.
63. Finlay AY, Lever LR, Thomas R, Dykes PJ. Nail matrix kinetics of oral terbinafine in onychomycosis and normal nails. J Dermatol Treat 1990; 1:S51–S54.
64. Finlay AY. Pharmacokinetics of terbinafine in the nail. Br. J. Dermatol. 1992, 126: S28–S32.
65. Evans G, Sigurgeirsson B. Double blind, randomized, study of continuous terbinafine compared with intermittent itraconazole in treatment of toenail onychomycosis. Br Med J 1999; 318:1031–1035.
66. Tosti A, Piraccini BM, Stinchi C et al. Treatment of dermatophyte nail infections: an open randomized study comparing intermittent terbinafine therapy with continuous terbinafine treatment and intermittent itraconazole therapy: J Am Acad Dermatol 1996; 34(4):595–600.
67. Zaias N, Rebell G. The successful treatment of *Trichophyton rubrum* nail bed (distal subungal) onychomycosis with intermittent pulse-dosed terbinafine. Arch Dermatol 2004; 140:691–695.
68. Gupta AK, Del Rosso JQ. An evaluation of intermittent therapies used to treat onychomycosis and other dermatomycoses with the oral antifungal agents. Int J Dermatol 2000; 39:401–411.
69. Piérard GE, Arrese JE, Quatresooz P, Pierard-Franchimont C: Voriconazole (Vfen®). Rev Med Liège 2003; 58:351–355.
70. Van Loo D: Voriconazole: an evaluation of activity and use. J Infect Dis Pharmacother 2003; 6:15–37.
71. Racette AJ, Roenigk HH, Hansen R, et al. Photoaging and phototoxicity from long-term voriconazole treatment in a 15-year-old girl. J Am Acad Dermatol 2005; 52:82–85.
72. Gupta AK, Lynde CW, Konnikov N. Single-blind, randomized, prospective study of sequential itraconazole and terbinafine pulse for the treatment of toenail onychomycosis. J Am Acad Dermatol 2001; 44:485–491.
73. Medoff G, Kobayashi GS, Kwang CN, et al. Potentialisation of rifampicin and flucocytosine as antifungal antibiotics by amphotericin B. Proc Soc Exp Biol Med 1971; 138:571–574.
74. Polack A. The past, present and future of antimycotic combination therapy. Mycoses 1999; 42:355–370.
75. Rubin MA, Carroll KC, Cahill BC: Caspofungin in combination with itraconazole for the treatment of invasive aspergillosis in humans. Clin Infect Dis 2002; 34:1160–1161.
76. Steinbach WJ, Stevens DA, Denning DW. Combination and sequential antifungal therapy for invasive aspergillosis: review of published in vitro and in vivo interactions and 6281 clinical cases from 1966 to 2001. Clin Infect Dis 2003, 37:S188–S224.
77. Kontoyiannis DP, Hachem R, Lewis RE, et al. Efficacy and toxicity of caspofungin in combination with liposomal amphotericin B as primary or salvage treatment of invasive aspergillosis in patients with hematologic malignancies. Cancer 2003, 98:292–299.
78. Sugar AM: Use of amphotericin B with azole antifungal drugs: what are we doing? Antimicrob Agents Chemother 1995; 39:1907–1912.
79. Bohme A, Just-Nubling G, Bergmann L, et al. Itraconazole for prophylaxis of systemic mycoses in neutropenic patients with haematological malignancies. J Antimicrob Chemother 1999; 42:443–451.
80. Santos DA, Hamdan JS. In vitro antifungal oral drug and drug-combination activity against onychomycosis causative dermatophytes. Med Mycol 2006; 44:357–362.
81. Faergemann J. Atopic dermatitis and fungi. Clin Microbiol Rev 2002; 15:545–563.
82. Nikkels AF, Pierard GE: Framing the future of antifungals in atopic dermatitis. Dermatology 2003; 206:398–400.

18

Hydroxy Acids and Retinoids in Cosmetic Products

Robert L. Bronaugh

Office of Cosmetics and Colors, Food and Drug Administration, College Park, Maryland, U.S.A.

INTRODUCTION

Alpha hydroxy acids (AHAs) and retinol (free or palmitate ester) are frequently used ingredients in cosmetic products. These products are often advertised to reduce fine lines and wrinkles and to improve skin condition in general. Chemically, the two classes of ingredients are quite different. AHAs are generally smaller, more hydrophilic molecules, whereas retinol and its esters, such as retinyl palmitate, are much more lipophilic. Skin absorption studies of these chemicals have increased our understanding of the potential local and systemic exposure from topical use of products containing these ingredients. In addition, studies have been conducted to evaluate the effect of hydroxy acids on skin sensitivity to UV light.

HYDROXY ACIDS

It is generally believed that hydroxy acids exert their effect of enhancing desquamation of skin by reducing cohesion between corneocytes in the lower, newly formed levels of the stratum corneum (1,2). The activity of hydroxy acids on skin is likely influenced by the ability of these chemicals to be absorbed into the stratum corneum and possibly deeper into the skin. Absorption into the various layers of skin and through the skin was markedly affected by the pH of the formulation (3). Stratum corneum levels of glycolic acid and lactic acid were greater at the lower pH by 4.8- and 2.0-fold, respectively, when absorption values from oil-in-water (O/W) emulsions at pH 3 and pH 7 were compared (Table 1). At pH 3.0, the AHAs were unionized and therefore much more readily absorbed into skin because of their increased lipophilicity. Activity of AHAs in eliciting desquamation is greatly increased by reducing the pH of the formulation to the pK_a (or lower) of the AHA, which for glycolic acid is 3.8.

Because of the effects of AHAs on the desquamation of the stratum corneum, studies have been conducted to assess the barrier integrity of skin after treatment with

TABLE 1 Percent Applied Dose Absorbed of 5% AHA

Location	5% Glycolic acid		5% Lactic acid	
	pH 3	pH 7	pH 3	pH 7
Receptor fluid	2.6 ± 0.7	0.8 ± 0.3	3.6 ± 1.2	0.4 ± 0.1
Stratum corneum	5.8 ± 2.8	1.2 ± 0.4	6.3 ± 1.4	3.2 ± 0.8
Viable epidermis	6.6 ± 2.5	0.8 ± 0.3	6.6 ± 0.9	3.2 ± 0.8
Dermis	12.2 ± 1.4	0.6 ± 0.2	13.9 ± 2.3	2.9 ± 1.3
Total in skin	24.6 ± 4.0	2.6 ± 0.6	26.8 ± 4.5	9.4 ± 2.1
Total absorption	27.2 ± 3.3	3.5 ± 0.9	30.4 ± 3.3	9.7 ± 2.0

Values are the mean ± SE of two to five determinations in each of three donors.

TABLE 2 In Vitro Skin Absorption of Two Cosmetic Ingredients After Pretreatment of Hairless Guinea Pig Skin

	Pretreatment formulations			
	Untreated	VIC	5% GA	10% GA
HQ				
Receptor fluid	4.3 ± 0.6	5.9 ± 0.3	6.4 ± 0.9	4.4 ± 0.5
Skin	15.0 ± 0.7	13.2 ± 1.0	15.4 ± 1.0	16.1 ± 1.8
Total	19.3 ± 0.4	19.0 ± 1.0	21.8 ± 1.9	20.5 ± 2.1
Musk xylol				
Receptor fluid	30.3 ± 2.5	23.6 ± 0.2	20.7 ± 4.2	21.6 ± 3.6
Skin	18.0 ± 2.6	18.8 ± 1.2	16.1 ± 3.2	18.8 ± 2.1
Total	48.3 ± 1.7	42.4 ± 1.1	36.7 ± 1.3	40.4 ± 1.7

Note: Values are percent of applied dose absorbed in 24 hours and are the mean ± SE of determinations in three animals (usually three replicates per animal). One-way ANOVA ($p < 0.05$) found no significant differences between treatment groups except for total absorption of musk xylol. VIC and 5% GA were not different from each other but each was significantly different from untreated skin.
Abbreviations: ANOVA, analysis of variance; GA, glycolic acid; HQ, hydroquinone; VIC, Vaseline Intensive Care.

AHAs. Hairless guinea pigs were treated daily for three weeks with glycolic acid in a 5% or 10% O/W emulsion at pH 3.0 (4). The decrease in turnover of hairless guinea pig stratum corneum with the 5% and 10% glycolic acid formulations (compared to control emulsion) was 29% and 36%, respectively. This decreased turnover time compared favorably to the 29% decrease reported for human skin treated with 3% glycolic acid, pH 3.0 (5). After the in vivo treatment of hairless guinea pig skin with glycolic acid, the animals were sacrificed and the skin was removed and dermatomed (250–300 μm thick) for in vitro diffusion cell measurement of the percutaneous absorption of the model compounds [^{14}C]hydroquinone and [^{14}C]musk xylol. No significant difference in the 24-hour absorption of either test compound was observed for skin treated with the control lotion or the glycolic acid formulations (Table 2).

An investigation of the effects of the AHAs glycolic acid and lactic acid on the skin barrier was recently conducted using hairless mice (6). The mice were treated daily for 14 days with 5% solutions of the two AHAs in a vehicle composed of distilled water, ethanol, and propylene glycol (2:2:1) at pH 3.8. Mice were treated on the opposite side of the back with a control vehicle (without AHA). Transepidermal water loss (TEWL) measurements on treated skin at the end of 14 days showed no increase over the normal TEWL range and no significant difference from TEWL values measured on control skin. The hydration of the stratum corneum measured by its capacitance was similar in treated and control skin at the end of the study. Epidermal thickness was histologically measured with a light microscope and resulted in values of 24.4, 24.2, 24.8, and 24.4 μm for skin treated with lactic acid, glycolic acid, control vehicle, and no treatment, respectively. The number of stratum corneum layers was reduced with AHA treatment but the stratum corneum lipid layers in the intercellular space appeared normal with the electron microscope. Therefore, it could be concluded that the barrier properties of hairless mice skin appeared to be undamaged by AHA treatment.

Effects of UV Light and AHAs on Skin
Several clinical studies have examined the effects of UV light irradiation on skin pretreated with glycolic acid. One study selected 15 volunteers with skin types sug-

gesting increased sensitivity to sun (Fitzgerald skin types I and II) and applied a formulation containing 10% glycolic acid at pH 3.5 once daily for four days (7). Other test sites on the volunteers were treated daily with either 8% glycerin or by rubbing with a moistened mechanical sponge for 15 seconds. At the end of the daily treatments, the test sites were irradiated with one minimum erythema dose (MED) of primarily UVB light 15 minutes after the last dosing. The formation of sunburn cells was evaluated in biopsies taken from the test sites. The glycolic acid formulation did not statistically increase sunburn cell formation when compared to the 8% glycerin, mechanical exfoliating sponge, or untreated skin.

A second study was conducted using similar procedures except that the treatment of skin test sites continued for 12 weeks. This study examined two groups (16 subjects each) with different glycolic acid formulations. Group A used 10% glycolic acid in a thickened aqueous vehicle at pH 4.0. Group B used a 10% formulation of glycolic acid at pH 3.5. In both groups, treatment with glycolic acid for 12 weeks and subsequent UV irradiation resulted in a significant increase in sunburn cells compared to control vehicles and untreated skin.

Other investigators conducted a clinical study that examined the effects of daily glycolic acid treatment (6 days per week) on the MED, sunburn cells, and cyclobutyl pyrimidine dimers after 4 weeks of treatment followed by exposure to UV light (8). The backs of 29 White volunteers were treated with either a 10% glycolic acid formulation (pH 3.5) or a placebo (formulation without glycolic acid). Subjects were primarily Fitzgerald skin type III and were assigned to group 1 or group 2.

Subjects in group 1 were irradiated with a solar simulator after 4 weeks of treatment and again at five weeks to determine recovery. Both the MED and sunburn cell formation were determined in biopsies removed from the test sites. After four weeks of treatment with the glycolic acid formulation, there was a statistically significant decrease in the MED of the treated skin as compared to the placebo or to untreated skin. After glycolic acid treatment was discontinued for one week, the MED on the treated site returned to normal. The number of sunburn cells induced by UV light after four weeks of glycolic acid treatment increased 1.9-fold compared to sunburn cells formed in the sites treated with the placebo. However, after one week of discontinued treatment, the number of sunburn cells at the glycolic acid–treated sites and the placebo sites were not significantly different.

The 12 subjects in group 2 received four weeks of treatment with glycolic acid and placebo followed by 1.5 MED irradiation with UV light. There was no significant difference in cyclobutyl pyrimidine dimers measured in the glycolic acid–treated sites compared to placebo.

In January 2005, the U.S. Food and Drug Administration (FDA) issued a Guidance for Industry entitled, "Labeling for Topically Applied Cosmetic Products Containing Alpha Hydroxy Acids as Ingredients." Because of evidence suggesting that topically applied cosmetic products containing AHAs might increase the sensitivity of skin to sunlight, the FDA recommends that the following statement appear on the labels of these products:

> "Sunburn Alert: This product contains an alpha hydroxy acid (AHA) that may increase your skin's sensitivity to the sun and particularly the possibility of sunburn. Use a sunscreen, wear protective clothing, and limit sun exposure while using this product and for a week afterwards."

The Scientific Committee on Cosmetic Products and Non-Food Products Intended for Consumers (SCCNFP) issued an opinion on the safety of AHAs in 2000 (10). The committee suggested that glycolic acid could be used safely at a level up to 4% and a pH of 3.8 or higher. It also recommended that lactic acid be used up to a maximum level of 2.5% and a pH of 5.0 or higher. Warning statements were recommended for consumers to avoid eye contact with AHAs and to avoid UV light or use protection from UV light because of possible increased susceptibility to damage from UV light while using cosmetic products with AHAs. An updated position paper was prepared in 2004 after receipt of new data from the cosmetic industry (11). However, because of the inadequate nature of the data submitted, the SCCNFP maintained its previous opinion on the safety of AHAs.

RETINOIDS

Retinoic acid (tretinoin) shows some effectiveness in treating the appearance of photoaging (12). The mechanisms responsible for this action may include the proliferation of keratinocytes resulting in increased shedding of corneocytes (13) and may also be associated with the formation of new collagen in the upper dermis (14). The activity of retinoic acid in skin may be ultimately associated with stimulation of retinoid receptors (15). Retinol application to skin has been reported to induce expression of cellular binding proteins and result in other molecular changes that are similar to those seen after treatment with retinoic acid (16).

Retinol and its ester retinyl palmitate are widely used in cosmetic products. Retinyl palmitate was found to be absorbed into human and hairless guinea pig skin using in vitro techniques that maintain the viability of skin (17). With human skin, 18% of the applied dose was found in skin at the end of a 24-hour study, with only 0.2% of the dose absorbed through the skin (Table 3). Almost half of the retinyl palmitate found in skin had been metabolized to retinol. If further metabolism of retinol to retinoic acid occurred, it was in small amounts and lower than the level of detection in this in vitro system.

Retinol absorption from cosmetic formulations has been measured through excised human skin in diffusion cell studies (18). Absorption through skin into the receptor fluid was 0.3% of the applied dose from a gel vehicle and 1.3% from an emulsion vehicle in 24-hour studies. Retinol and retinoic acid absorption was observed in vivo in human subjects with induction of retinoic acid 4-hydroxylase activity used as an endpoint for comparison (19). Retinoic acid treatment (under occlusion) resulted in significant induction in enzyme activity at concentrations as

TABLE 3 Percutaneous Absorption and Metabolism of Retinyl Palmitate

Skin type	Skin		Receptor fluid	
	Radioactivity absorbed (%)[a]	Metabolized (%)[b]	Radioactivity absorbed (%)[a,c]	Metabolized (%)[b]
Guinea pig				
Male	30 ± 4	38 ± 13	0.5 ± 0.2	100
Female	33 ± 2	30 ± 16	0.6 ± 0.3	100
Human				
Female	18 ± 1	44 ± 5	0.2 ± 0.01	100

Note: Values are the mean ± SE of determinations from two human donors (three to four repetitions per donor) and three animals (three repetitions per animal).
[a]Absorption is expressed as % of the applied dose in skin and receptor fluid.
[b]Metabolism is expressed as % of the absorbed retinyl palmitate hydrolyzed to retinol.
[c]0- to 24-hour fractions combined.

low as 0.001%. Retinol (also under occlusion) required a concentration of 0.025% to have significant effects on 4-hydroxylase activity.

Liposomes have been reported to enhance the penetration of retinol through human skin assembled in diffusion cells (20). The skin absorption rates after infinite dosing of retinol were compared after application of retinol in either deformable (flexible) liposomes made with polysorbate 20, or in a control vehicle without liposomes. At the end of 24 hours, approximately 30 $\mu g/cm^2$ skin of retinol had been absorbed through skin from the flexible liposomes, whereas control retinol absorption was found to be about 1 $\mu g/cm^2$.

Enhanced absorption of retinol was found from solid lipid nanoparticles incorporated into an O/W cream compared to a conventional formulation (21). Highest retinol concentrations were found in the stratum corneum and the upper viable epidermal layer. The penetration of retinyl palmitate was influenced even more by incorporation into the solid lipid nanoparticles.

CONCLUSIONS

In conclusion, hydroxy acids and certain retinoids (retinol, retinyl palmitate) are commonly found in cosmetic products formulated to improve the appearance of skin. More studies are required to completely understand the mechanisms of action of these ingredients. Skin irritation can result at higher dosage levels for both classes of ingredients, especially with sun exposure; therefore, care must be taken when using cosmetic products containing hydroxy acids and retinoids.

REFERENCES

1. Van Scott EJ, Yu RJ. Alpha hydroxy acids: procedures for use in clinical practice. Cutis 1989; 43:222–228.
2. Van Scott EJ, Yu RJ. Actions of alpha hydroxy acids on skin compartments. J Geriatric Dermatol 1995; 3(Suppl. A):19A–24A.
3. Kraeling MEK, Bronaugh RL. In vitro percutaneous absorption of alpha hydroxy acids in human skin. J Soc Cosmet Chem 1997; 48:187–197.
4. Hood HL, Kraeling MEK, Robl MG, et al. The effects of an alpha hydroxy acid (glycolic acid) on hairless guinea pig skin. Food Chem Toxicol 1999; 37:1105–1111.
5. Smith WP. Hydroxy acids and skin aging. Cosmet Toiletr 1994; 109(9):41–48.
6. Kim T-H, Choi EH, Yang YC, et al. The effects of topical α-hydroxyacids on the normal skin barrier of hairless mice. Br J Dermatol 2001; 144:267–273.
7. Anderson FA, ed. Final report on the safety assessment of glycolic acid, ammonium, calcium, potassium, and sodium glycolates, methyl, ethyl, propyl, and butyl glycolates, and lactic acid, ammonium, calcium, potassium, sodium, and tea-lactates, methyl, ethyl, isopropyl, and butyl lactates, and lauryl, myristyl, and cetyl lactates. Int J Toxicol 1998; 17(Suppl. 1):1–241.
8. Kaidbey KK, Sutherland B, Bennett P, et al. Topical glycolic acid enhances photodamage by ultraviolet light. Photodermatol Photoimmunol Photomed 2003; 19:21–27.
9. Anonymous. Labeling for Topically Applied Cosmetic Products Containing Alpha Hydroxy Acids as Ingredients, 2006. (Accessed September 19, 2007, at www.cfsan.fda .gov~dms/ahaguid2.html.)
10. Anonymous. Position Paper on the Safety of Alpha-Hydroxy Acids. SCCNFP/030/00, 2000.
11. Anonymous. Consumer Safety of Alpha Hydroxy Acids, SCCNFP/0799/04, 2004.
12. Kang S, Leyden JJ, Lowe NJ, et al. Tazarotene cream for the treatment of facial photodamage: A multicenter, investigator-masked, randomized, vehicle-controlled, parallel comparison of 0.01%, 0.025%, 0.05% and 0.1% tazarotene creams with 0.05% tretinoin emollient cream applied once daily for 24 weeks. Arch Dermatol 2001; 137:1597–1604.

13. Baumann L, Vujevich J, Halern M, et al. Open-label pilot study of alitretinoin gel 0.1% in the treatment of photoaging. Cutis 2005; 76:69–73.
14. Gilchrest BA. Treatment of photodamage with topical tretinoin: an overview. J Am Acad Dermatol 1997; 36:S27-S36.
15. Elder JT, Astrom A, Pettersson U, et al. Differential regulation of retinoic acid receptors and binding proteins in human skin. J Invest Dermatol 1992; 98:673–679.
16. Kang S, Duell EA, Fisher GJ, et al. Application of retinol to human skin in vivo induces epidermal hyperplasia and cellular retinoid binding proteins characteristic of retinoic acid but without measurable retinoic acid levels or irritation. J Invest Dermatol 1995; 105:549–556.
17. Boehnlein J, Sakr A, Lichtin JL, et al. Characterization of esterase and alcohol dehydrogenase activity in skin metabolism of retinyl palmitate to retinol (vitamin A) during percutaneous absorption. Pharm Res 1994; 11:1155–1159.
18. Yourick JJ, Jung CT, Bronaugh RL. Percutaneous absorption of retinol in fuzzy rat (in vivo and in vitro) and human skin (in vitro) from cosmetic vehicles. The Toxicologist 2006; 90(S1), Abstract no. 810, 164.
19. Duell EA, Kang S, Voorhees JJ. Unoccluded retinol penetrates more effectively than unoccluded retinyl palmitate or retinoic acid. J Invest Dermatol 1997; 109:301–305.
20. Oh Y-K, Kim MY, Shin J-Y, et al. Skin penetration of retinol in Tween 20-based deformable liposomes: in vitro evaluation in human skin and keratinocyte models. J Pharm Pharmacol 2006; 58:161–166.
21. Jenning V, Gysler A, Schafer-Korting M, et al. Vitamin A loaded solid lipid nanoparticles for topical use: occlusive properties and drug targeting to the upper skin. Eur J Pharm Biopharm 2000; 49:211–218.

| 19 | Natural Ingredients Used in Cosmeceuticals |

Anthony C. Dweck
Dweck Data, Salisbury, Wiltshire, U.K.

INTRODUCTION

The term "cosmeceuticals" should be used with caution, because there are separate pieces of legislation that apply to pharmaceutical and cosmetics in the United Kingdom that have corresponding legislation that applies to the European Union (see Chapter 1). The manufacture of cosmetics and toiletries is more regulated than the food industry but not to the extent of the pharmaceutical industry. The comparison between the production of pharmaceuticals in terms of Good Manufacturing Practice (GMP) and the cosmetics and toiletries industry is not that dissimilar. In European countries, United States, and Japan, the laws are quite specific, and although these countries strive to achieve parity, there are still many differences between the various legislative documents, particularly in the area of sun care, antiperspirants, and toothpaste.

The European Economic Community (EEC) have Council Directive 76/768/ EEC up to the 27th Amending Directive 2003/15/EC and including the previous 26 amendments and this has to be translated into the language of each member state. In the United Kingdom, the law is Statutory Instrument 2004 No. 2152, The Cosmetic Products (Safety) Regulations 2004. In addition, products must not infringe the Medicines for Human Use (Marketing Authorizations, etc.) Regulations 1994, a very common infringement with today's eagerness to have "alluring" pack copy. The regulations provide that, unless exempt, any "medicinal product" to which Chapters II to V of Directive 2001/83/EEC apply must not be placed on the U.K. market unless it has a marketing authorization (product license) granted by the European Commission or by the U.K. Licensing Authority. The Act similarly provides that, unless exempt, any other "medicinal product" must not be sold or supplied without a marketing authority. A marketing authorization or product license is only granted for a product that meets statutory standards of safety, quality, and efficacy.

The status of many products that are on the "borderline" between medicinal products and food supplements, cosmetic, or medical devices can be difficult to determine. The MHRA have produced a Guidance Note 8 document to explain how and on what basis the MCA decides whether products are medicines or not. It includes guidance on the statutory procedures in Regulation 3A of the Regulations introduced by the Medicines for Human Use (Marketing Authorizations, etc.) Amendment Regulations 2000 (S.I. 2000/292). There is also the requirement to ensure that claims made on the packaging comply with the Trade Descriptions Act 1968, Control of Misleading Advertising Regulations 1988 (as amended). Products must also comply with the Weights and Measures Act 1985. Certain categories (e.g., insect repellants and products that contain this property) may also be subject to the Statutory Instrument 2003 No. 429, The Biocidal Products (Amendment) Regulations 2003.

Compliance with these laws is mandatory in Europe and many countries have adopted them with little alteration. It will be the way of things to come and most countries are in the process of harmonizing and adopting these legal safeguards. Any company that does not react ahead of the inevitable is going to find it an arduous and almost impossible task to implement in the time frames that are normally allowed for full compliance.

DEFINITION OF NATURAL

A natural is any material that is harvested, mined, or collected, and which may have subsequently been washed, decolorized, distilled, fractionated, ground, milled, separated, or concentrated, leaving a chemical or chemicals that would be available and detectable in the original source material. It is also the modification of natural material by the action of microorganisms, enzymes, or yeasts to modify or increase the yield of material by this process. Naturally derived materials are defined by the use of a natural raw material as the starting point in a chemical process that produces a new chemical or chemicals that in themselves may not be available in nature or in the starting material. Nature-identical materials are substances that have been synthetically produced, not usually from a natural starting material, in order to produce a material that is identical to that naturally occurring in nature.

SOURCES OF DATA FOR PRODUCTS THAT MAY HAVE TOPICAL COSMECEUTICAL BENEFIT

Many ethnopharmaceutical applications for topical application that have been used for countless generations have been tried and tested in those countries where their use is prevalent. In many cases, these are well described in the literature and have been identified from their phytochemical composition, preparation, part used, and dosage. This search is no longer restricted to the European systems of herbal medicine but now extends to Russian, Chinese, Indian systems of Ayurvedic medicine and Unani, African, and more recently, Aboriginal traditional medicine. Less reliable sources are "grandmother's recipes" or folklore, which pass from generation to generation without any real scientific basis. The works of the old herbalists such as Galen, Dioscorides, Culpeper, Hildegarde von Bingen, and Paracelsus (Theophrastus Bombastus von Hohenheim) may give some insights to future investigation. In some cases, these remedies may be discounted after serious evaluation, but there are still many occasions when science substantiates their beneficial use.

PLANTS ARE COMPLEX CHEMICAL FACTORIES

A plant is a complex and ever-active chemical factory that produces a wide range of chemical moieties that it requires for protection against yeast and moulds, resistance to insect attack, even protection against UV and drought conditions in some specialist plants. Other coastal region plants require very specific protection against salts and excess minerals. It is this complex environment that produces many dozens of chemical entities that may have benefit in human treatments for various skin conditions. The composition may vary according to the area of growth (country), the soil, the weather conditions, the time of harvest, the processing, and, of course, the part of the plant that is being extracted. The storage conditions of the plant, the time of extraction, and the solvents used in that extraction will all have a significant implication on the final chemical composition, for example, the content of natural preservatives produced by plants to protect the fruit and the leaves will fall dramatically once they have been separated from the main plant. This can be easily demonstrated by smelling a fresh bloom on a living rose and then cutting off that flower. In a matter of minutes, the rose note will alter drastically as the chemical composition alters.

The pharmaceutical industry and the purists would always prefer to work with single chemical entities derived from a single plant. Although this sounds a perfect solution for reproducibility, the truth is very different. Plants tend to have a full orchestra of individual phytochemically active materials that work synergistically. The overall result is that the effect of the individual components is far outweighed by the blend. In traditional Chinese medicine (TCM), the normal herbal treatment is tailored for an individual and targets both underlying causes and their effects. In the Far East, it is recognized that in some seasons a particular plant may lack potency but that another plant attributed with having the same effect is substantially rich and effective, that is, one plant thrives in a rainy season but suffers in a hot dry season and vice versa. Blends that involve eight or more herbal materials is not uncommon with each pair acting on different indications, such as pruritis, erythema, edema, circulation, granulation, reepithelialization, and cicatrization. Although the terminology used in TCM may seem strange to Westerners, the correlation to terms we do understand and theirs is an almost perfect match.

Fatty Acids

The simplest treatment of dry skin conditions is with fixed vegetable oils. Many of these vegetable, nut, seed, and kernel oils are simple blends of fatty acids with varying carbon chain lengths. Coconut, sunflower, safflower, rapeseed, corn, or sesame seed oil will give perfectly acceptable skin coverage and are most often used as carrier oils for essential oils. These oils will coat the skin to occlude and protect it by slowing down transepidermal water loss and so increasing hydration within the stratum corneum and top layers of the dermis. They will also "glue down" dry and desquamatous skin cells to make the skin look less rough and scaly. Some oils such as castor seed oil (*Ricinus communis*) are renowned not only for their very high gloss (and so a frequent component in lipsticks and lip salves), but also for their high degree of occlusiveness which makes them ideal for skin protection, for example, diaper or nappy rash creams, where the most traditional and best-known example would be zinc and castor oil cream.

Other oils such as evening primrose oil (*Oenothera biennis*), borage (starflower) seed oil (*Borago officinalis*), and blackcurrant seed oil (*Ribes nigrum*) are particularly useful because of their high γ-linolenic acid content (Fig. 1). Evening primrose used to hold a pharmaceutical license for use on atopic dermatitis, but subsequently lost this status on the publication of further clinical trial data. It is still widely taken orally for mastitis (breast pain).

A new oil, made commercially available in 2006, is inchi oil (*Plukentia volubilis*), which also has the name Aztec peanut—although it is totally unrelated to the peanut (*Arachis hypogaea*). This oil is abundant in omega-3, omega-6, and omega-12 fatty acids, and could well show huge promise in skin care. Another plant that is rich in γ-linolenic acid is a particular species of rose hip seed oil (*Rosa* aff. *rubiginosa*) that is collected in the foothills of the Chilean Andes and often called *Rosa moschata*. This

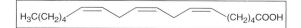

$H_3C(CH_2)_4$ ... $(CH_2)_4COOH$

FIGURE 1 γ-Linolenic acid.

oil is reputed to contain vitamin A according to some references. A large body of evidence (mainly anecdotal clinical) suggests that this oil has exceptional cicatrizing properties and is an excellent oil for restoring skin elasticity especially for postsurgical conditions where tightness has become a problem for the patient. It was also shown to be effective for treating the hyperpigmentation of certain scar tissues.

Flavonoids

"Flava" means yellow in Greek and the collective name of flavonoids for this group of compounds was proposed by Geissman in 1952. This is a very large group of compounds showing extraordinary diversity and variation and as the Greek root for the word suggests, many of these compounds are yellow in color. They consist of a number of structurally related groups of products, which are often identified as polyphenols. Many have a basic skeleton (Fig. 2) that contains 15 carbon atoms, which are usually subdivided into one part made up from a phenolic (6C) moiety and another which has a cinnamic acid molecule (C13) as a building block. The group called the chalcones may be considered as the Friedel-Crafts reaction product of a (substituted) cinnamic acid and a phenol.

The flavonoids in red wine (*Vitis vinifera*) such as quercetin, kaempferol, and anthocyanidins account for the free radical–scavenging activity. In green tea (*Camellia sinensis* or *Thea viridis*), it is the catechins and catechin gallate esters that are shown to be effective antioxidants against free radicals. The dietary effectiveness of these materials has been known for generations and similar antioxidant effectiveness has been shown to occur when these materials are topically applied to protect skin cells.

Flavonoids also are a source of natural color, with yellows from the chalcones and flavonols, and reds, blues, and violets from the anthocyanidins. The flavones are colorless, but are still able to absorb UV strongly and so act as a beacon to pollinating insects. The exploitation of these molecules as a source of natural color in cosmetics and toiletries is just beginning, but their poor light stability is often a stumbling block. Flavonoids may be found as their glycosides. These are molecules that are substituted on one or more of the hydroxyl groups with a sugar such as galactose, glucose, mannose, or rhamnose, etc. The aglycons do not carry a sugar moiety.

Chalcones

Chalcones act as precursors for an enormous range of flavonoid derivatives. Reductive ring closure of chalcones results in the formation of a flavone. Naringenin chalcone (Fig. 3A) is converted to a flavanone, naringenin (Fig. 3B), from which apigenin (Fig. 3C) (4′,5,7-trihydroxyflavone) is formed. Flavones are generally found in herbaceous families such as Labiatae, Umbelliferae, and Compositae. Flavones have the skeleton 2-phenylchromen-4-one and include apigenin, baicalein, chrysin, diosmetin, diosmin, flavone, luteolin, tangeretin, techtochrysin, rhamnazin, nobiletin,

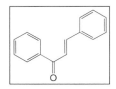

FIGURE 2   Chalcone skeleton.

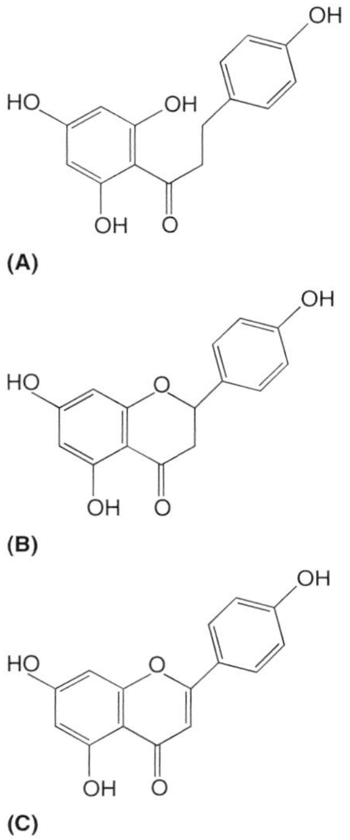

FIGURE 3 Chalcone conversions: (**A**) naringenin chalcone, (**B**) naringenin, and (**C**) apigenin.

and natsudaidain. The most common flavones are apigenin found in celery (*Apium graveolens*) and parsley (*Carum petroselinum*); luteolin found in German chamomile (*Matricaria recutita*) and horsetail (*Equisetum arvense*), and diosmetin found in rosemary (*Rosmarinus officinallis*). All these materials are known for their soothing, calming, and cicatrizing effects, although each has additional properties that are a result of other chemical moieties within their constituents, for example, the silicate content in horsetail gives it nail strengthening properties. The flavones often occur as glycosides. Flavones also occur in nature in association with tannins (polyesters of gallic acid; 3,4,5-trihydroxybenzoic acid). Gallic acid and its esters (e.g., propyl gallate, dodecyl gallate) are well-known powerful antioxidants, and it is probable that these products fulfill a similar role in higher plants.

Flavones
The simplest representative of the group of flavones is "flavone" (Fig. 4), which does not carry any hydroxy, methoxy, or glycosidic groups.

Flavanone Glycosides
The flavanone glycosides are very important, because they include naringin (Fig. 5A), which has been found specifically in grapefruit peel and seeds, and hesperidin (Fig. 5B) found in citrus peels and seeds. These materials have been shown to exhibit antimicrobial activity and have been used as preservatives (even though they are not listed in Annex VI of permitted preservatives).

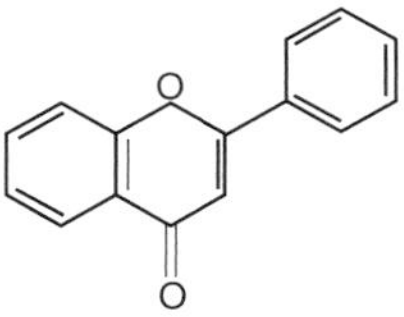

FIGURE 4   Flavone.

Aurones

Some aurones occur naturally. In this group, the six-membered heterocyclic ring is replaced by a five-membered ring. An example of an aurone is sulfuretin, 6,3',4'-trihydroxyaurone (Fig. 6) found in *Rhus verniciflua* and *Dalbergia odorifera*, which are being studied for their anti-inflammatory properties.

Flavonols

The most common flavonols (3-hydroxyflavones) are kaempferol, quercetin (Fig. 7), and rhamnetin. The name for quercetin comes from the genus in which the chemical was first identified, namely, *Quercus* spp., or oak, but the highest levels have been seen in evening primrose leaf (*O. biennis*) and the sap of mayapple (*Podophyllum peltatum*). Kaempferol (Fig. 7B) is found in neem or Nimba flowers (*Azadirachta indica*) and pea (*Pisum sativa*). It is also widely found throughout the *Brassica* spp., such as cabbage, kohlrabi cauliflower, and kale. Interestingly, these plants have not been exploited for their anti-inflammatory activity. The flavonols also exist as flavonol glycosides such as rutin (Fig. 8), found in buckwheat (*Fagopyrum esculentum*) and rue (*Ruta graveolens*).

Isoflavones

The isoflavones (Fig. 9A) are mainly found within the Leguminosae (specifically in the sub-family Papilionoideae), although many other species (e.g., Compositae, Iridaceae, Myristicaceae, and Rosaceae) contain these chemical moieties (1). These

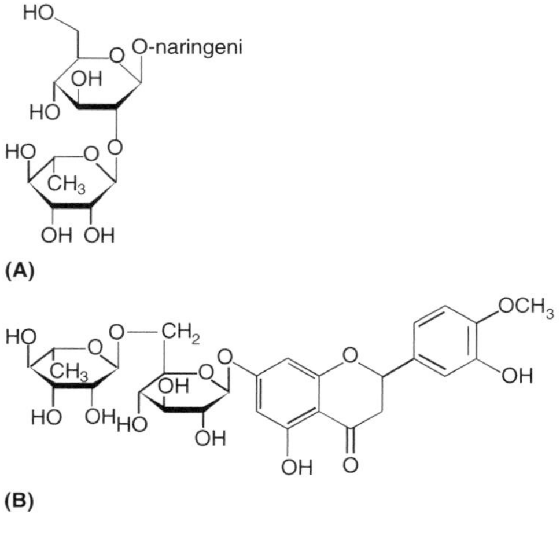

FIGURE 5   Flavone glycosides: (**A**) naringin and (**B**) hesperidin.

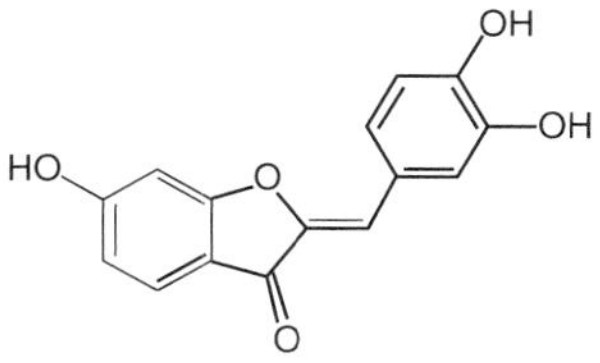

FIGURE 6   Sulfuretin.

isoflavones can act as steroidal mimics by filling the stereochemical space that could be occupied by estrogenic compounds. This spatial chemistry helps explain the effects of many nutritional herbal supplements and topical preparations (Fig. 9B,C).

Daidzein is a phytoestrogen (also called a phenolic estrogen, to distinguish it from a steroidal estrogen such as 17β-estradiol). The activity of phytoestrogen is much weaker than steroidal estrogens, varying from 0.005% to 2% (2). The estrogenic properties are insufficient in strength to replace steroidal estrogens, but they do have significant value in reducing the effects of aging and improving the quality of the skin. Phytoestrogens may also be viewed in relation to the phytochemical division of terpenoids, which comprise the largest group of natural plant products. All terpenoids are biogenetically derived from isoprene. The largest group of terpenoids are the triterpenoids, which include, among other divisions, the triterpenoid and steroid saponins and the phytosterols.

Nature has a rich portfolio of phytosterols, and it is easy to understand why compounds such as stigmasterol and β-sitosterol (Fig. 10A,B) have anti-inflammatory effects and are capable of reducing swelling and erythema when their structure is compared to corticosterone (Fig. 10C) and hydrocortisone (Fig. 10D).

The most commonly occurring isoflavones are:

- Biochanin A   5,7-Dihydroxy-4′-methoxyisoflavone
- Daidzein   4′,7-Dihydroxyisoflavone
- (±)-Equol   4′,7-Isoflavandiol
- Formonometin   7-Hydroxy-4′-methoxyisoflavone
- Glycitein   4′,7-Dihydroxy-6-methoxyisoflavone
- Genistein   4′,5,7-Trihydroxyisoflavone
- Genistein-4′,7-dimethylether   5-Hydroxy-4′,7-dimethoxyisoflavone
- Prunetin   4′,5-Dihydroxy-7-methoxyisoflavone

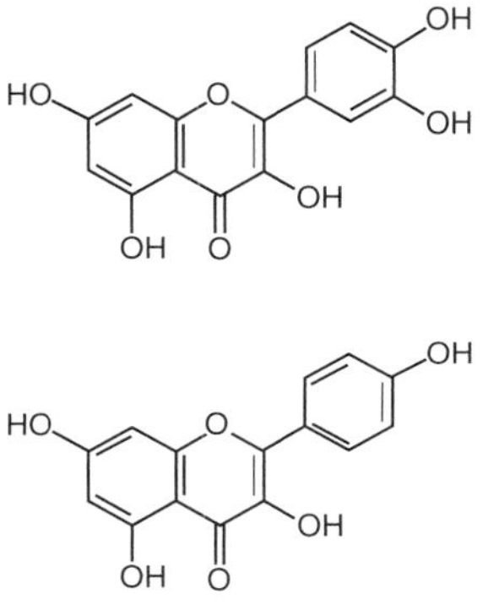

FIGURE 7   Flavonols: (**A**) quercetin and (**B**) kaempferol.

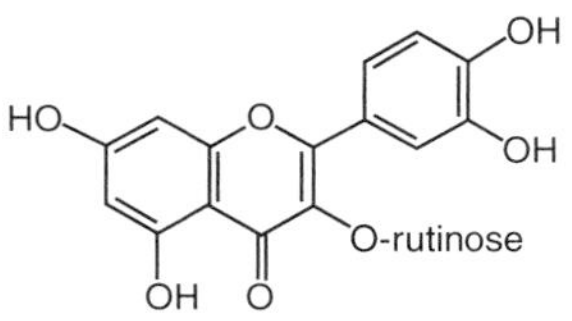

FIGURE 8   Rutin.

With the associated glucosides:

- Genistin   Glucosyl-7-genistein
- Glycitin   4',7-Dihydroxy-6-methoxyisoflavone-7-D-glucoside
- Ononin   Formononetin-7-O-glucoside
- Sissotrin   Biochanin A-7-glucoside

Daidzein

Daidzein (7-hydroxy-3-(4-hydroxyphenyl)-4*H*-1-benzopyran-4-one,4',7-dihydroxyiso-flavone) is a solid substance that is virtually insoluble in water. Daidzin, which has greater water solubility than daidzein, is 7-β glucoside of daidzein. Daidzein, the aglycone of daidzin, is an isoflavone and a phytoestrogen. The isoflavone is found naturally as the glycoside daidzin and as the glycosides 6"-O-malonyldaidzin and 6"-O-acetyldaidzin (Fig. 11A,B). Daidzein and its glycosides are mainly found in the Leguminosae family that includes soybeans and chickpeas. Daidzein glycosides are the second most abundant isoflavones in soybeans and soy foods; genistein glyco-sides are the most abundant. Nonfermented soy foods, such as tofu, contain daidzein,

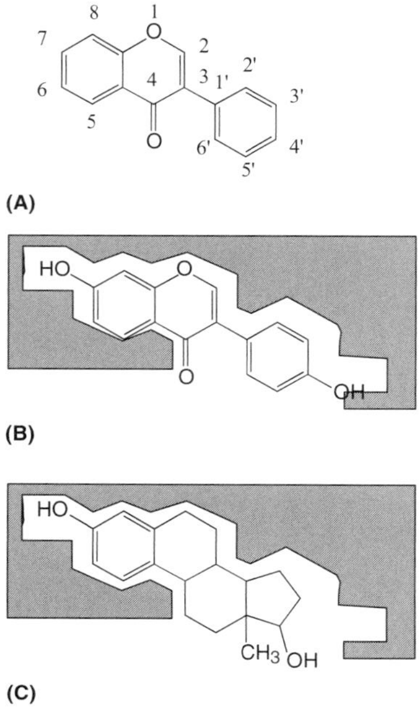

(A)

(B)

(C)

FIGURE 9   Isoflavones: (**A**) isoflavone skeleton struc-ture, (**B**) estrogen receptor with daidzen, and (**C**) estro-gen receptor with 17β-estradiol.

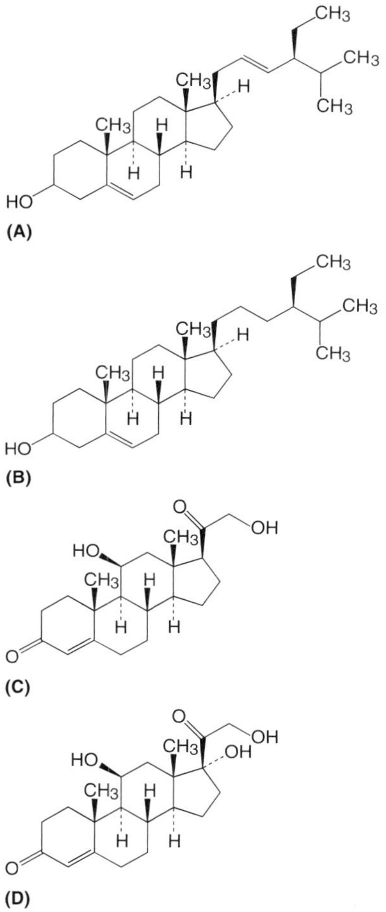

FIGURE 10   (**A**) Stigmasterol, (**B**) β-sitosterol, (**C**) corticosterone, and (**D**) hydrocortisone.

principally in its glycoside forms. Fermented soy foods, such as tempeh and miso, contain significant levels of the aglycone.

Kudzu Vine (Pueraria labata)
The root of *P. labata* is an herbal medicine commonly known as the kudzu vine. It has been used for the treatment of alcohol abuse for centuries in TCM and thought to be effective because of the daidzein and daidzin found in the herb (3).

White Kwao Krua (Pueraria mirifica)
In addition to genistein, daidzein, daidzin, and genistin, the plant contains some unique isoflavones such as kwakhurin, kwakhurin hydrate (Fig. 12A), and puerarin (Fig. 12B) (4). The roots also contain mirificoumestan (Fig. 12C), deoxymiroestrol (Fig. 12D), and coumestrol (Fig. 12E). The traditional use of the plant is clearly for the hormonal properties, because in Thailand, it is used for breast development. When *P. mirifica* is taken as a dietary supplement, its phytoestrogen constituents

(A)

(B)   FIGURE 11   (A) Malonyldaidzin and (B) acetyldaidzin.

will naturally alleviate symptoms occurring as a result of the aging process and a deficiency in estrogen levels. Aging signs and symptoms will, to a certain extent, be reversed. The rich source of sterols and phytohormones also indicates the plant for the topical treatment of wrinkles and aging skin conditions.

Red Clover (Trifolium pratense L.) (Leguminosae)
Red clover flower heads contain the following isoflavones: biochanin A, daidzein, formononetin, genistein, pratensein, and trifoside. The plant has alterative, antispasmodic, expectorant properties and is a sedative dermatological agent. Its main use is for skin complaints such as psoriasis and eczema, as well as an expectorant in coughs and bronchial conditions (5). Biochanin A (Fig. 13A) and formononetin (Fig. 13B) are two isoflavones from red clover. They are very similar to genistein and daidzein, except that the hydroxyl groups have been methylated. These two isoflavones are considerably less estrogenic in their original forms; the stereochemistry of the methoxy groups means they are not able to efficiently bind to estrogen receptors. However, once ingested, they are demethylated by bacteria in the colon; biochanin A becomes genistein (Fig. 13C) and formononetin becomes daidzein. Daidzein can be further metabolized to equol (Fig. 13D). Internally, therefore, biochanin A and formononetin are a source of considerable estrogenic activity. It may well be that these mechanisms give red clover its reputation as an alterative remedy, cleansing the system yet mild enough for many children's skin problems, even eczema. A lotion of red clover can be used externally to give relief from itching and other skin disorders (6). Red clover is recommended for athlete's foot, sores, burns, and ulcers (7), and has been used in the herbal treatment of cancer, especially of the breast or ovaries (8). It is also a very popular alternative remedy for hormone replacement therapy.

Sweet Yellow Melilot (Melilotus officinalis)
Melilot is soothing, astringent, and anti-irritant possessing similar properties to red clover. It may also be anti-inflammatory, antiedema, and anesthetic (9). However, it is perhaps not the isoflavones at force here, but possibly the β-sitosterol or coumarin contained in the roots. *M. officinalis* L. extract, containing 0.25% coumarin (Fig. 14),

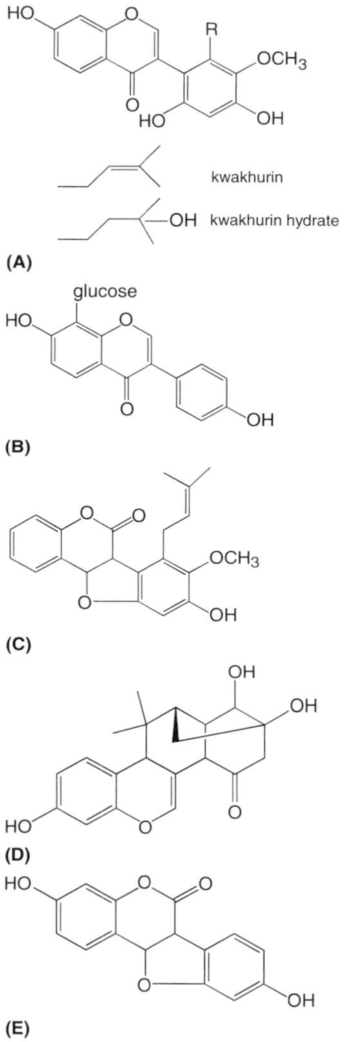

FIGURE 12 Chemicals contained in white kwao krua: (**A**) kwakhurin, kwakhurin hydrate; (**B**) puerarin; (**C**) mirificoumestan; (**D**) deoxymiroestrol; and (**E**) coumestrol.

was studied on acute inflammation induced with oil of turpentine in rabbits. The extract demonstrated anti-inflammatory effects similar to those of hydrocortisone sodium hemisuccinate (10).

Phytosterols and Related Compounds

The benefits of phytosterols may be seen in herbal materials indicated for arthritis, such as frankincense (*Boswellia serrata*). The boswellic acid (Fig. 15) present inhibits two inflammatory enzymes, 5-lipoxygenase (which produces leukotrienes) and human leukocyte elastase (which degrades elastase). The Department of Biochemical Pharmacology of the Imperial College School of Medicine has prepared a paper

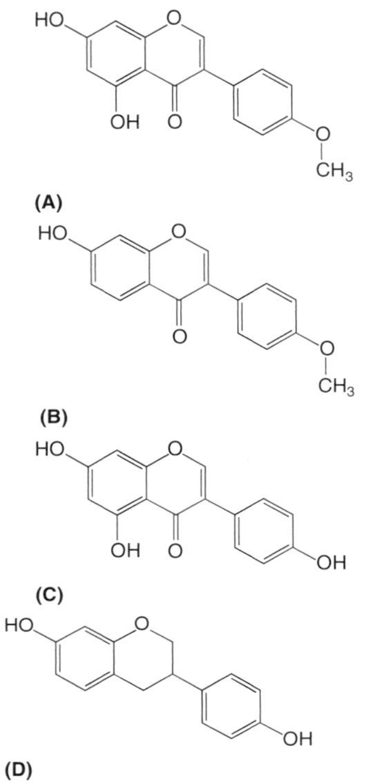

(A)

(B)

(C)

(D)

FIGURE 13 Isoflavones from red clover and their metabolites: (**A**) biochanin A, (**B**) formononetin, (**C**) genistein, and (**D**) equol.

for discussion: "Assessment of the estrogenic potency of phyto-compounds." This reviewed the available information on cellular and molecular mechanisms and phytoestrogen potencies. Taking all estrogen receptor binding assays into account, the review proposed the following rank order of phytoestrogen potency: estradiol >> coumestrol > 8-prenylnaringenin > equol ≥ genistein > biochanin A > daidzein > genistein glucuronide* > daidzein glucuronide* > formononetin (the activity of those compounds marked * may be attributable to the presence of activating enzymes present in the receptor preparation). Phytoestrogens stimulated in vitro cell proliferation at concentrations of 0.1 to 10 mM (3- to 4-fold less than estradiol). They did not induce the maximal proliferative effect of estradiol because higher concentrations inhibited proliferation. Most endogenous estrogens (>90%) were not freely available but bound to plasma proteins. Phytoestrogens bound at 1/100th to 1/1000th of the affinity of estradiol. The availability of phytoestrogens in plasma relative to estradiol will be greater. Coumestrol, 8-prenylnaringenin, and equol were more than 1000-fold less potent than estradiol and the isoflavones more than 10,000-fold less potent.

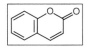

FIGURE 14 Coumarin.

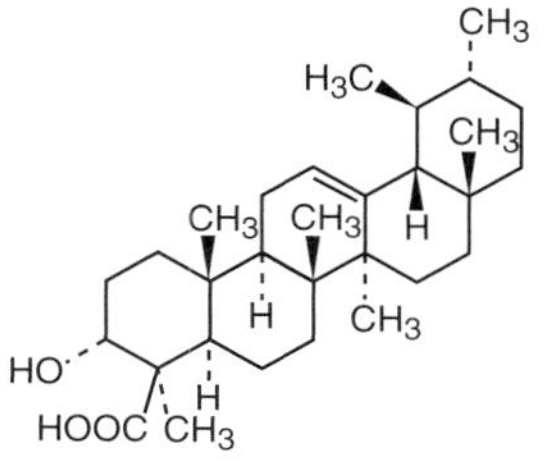

FIGURE 15   Boswellic acid

Wild Yam (Dioscorea villosa)

The wild yam (*D. villosa*) was the source of diosgenin (Fig. 16A), a steroidal saponin used as the starting point for the commercial source of pregnanolone (Fig. 16B) and progesterone (Fig. 16C), which were used in the first birth control pills. The root of *Dioscorea* is used for numerous purposes, but its major use is for the suppression of menopausal symptoms such as hot flashes (11). During pregnancy, small frequent doses of wild yam will help allay nausea (12). As an antispasmodic, it is valuable in neuralgic affections such as spasmodic hiccup and spasmodic asthma (13). It has

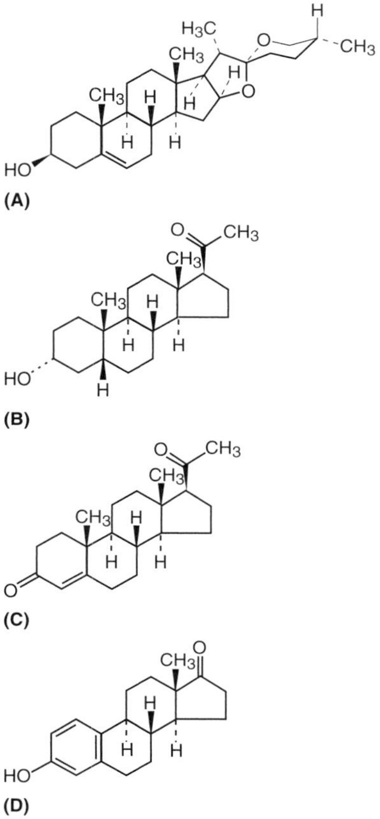

(A)

(B)

(C)

(D)

FIGURE 16   (**A**) Diosgenin, (**B**) pregnanolone, (**C**) progesterone, and (**D**) estrone.

potential in skin care and body care, being anti-inflammatory and anti-rheumatic. It is also cited for dysmenorrhea, and ovarian and uterine pain (14,15).

It is interesting to note that *Vitex agnus-castus* is a source of natural progesterone, and many documented studies have investigated the use of these products to treat various gynecological disorders (16). The fruit of *Vitex* contains essential oils (including limonene, 1,8-cineole, and sabinene), iridoid glycosides (agnuside and aucubin), and flavonoids (including castican, orientin, and isovitexin). The active constituents have been determined as 17-α-hydroxyprogesterone (leaf), 17-hydroxyprogesterone (leaf), androstenedione (leaf), δ-3-ketosteroids (leaf), epitestosterone (flower), progesterone (leaf), testosterone (flower and leaf) (17,18).

It is highly unlikely that diosgenin in the plant could ever be metabolized to a corticosteroid or hormonal derivative on application to the skin. However, it does seem likely that this material (being the precursor to these estrogenic molecules) will, to some extent, mimic the function of those pharmaceutical active materials and benefit the skin (19). However, the production of wild yam was unable to sustain the demand for diosgenin as the starting precursor, for the production of birth control materials, which was dominated by estrone (Fig. 16D).

Fenugreek (Trigonella foenum graecum)

The world turned its attention to fenugreek (*T. foenum graecum*) for its source of diosgenin. Fenugreek seeds are emollient and accelerate the healing of suppuration and inflammation. Seeds are cooked with water into a porridge and used as hot compresses on boils and abscesses in a similar manner to the usage of linseed (20). A cataplasm obtained by boiling the flour of the seeds with vinegar and saltpeter is used for swelling of the spleen (21). Extracts of the seeds are incorporated into several cosmetics claimed to have effect on premature hair loss and as a skin cleanser (22), and it is also present in hair tonics and claimed to cure baldness (23). Many of the herbal materials found to have an effect on hair growth have a hormonal or hormonal-mimetic basis. Likewise, there are a number of references to fenugreek having galactagogue (increase milk in nursing mothers) activity (8,24,25), which again is indicative of an estrogen-like activity. Fenugreek is reputed to be oxytocic and uterine stimulant activity has been documented in vitro (16), so its use during pregnancy and lactation is not advisable.

Pomegranate (Punica granatum)

The seeds of pomegranate, an ancient symbol of fertility, contain an estrone identical to the genuine hormone, and they are the best source of plant estrone (26). Pomegranate fermented juice and seed oil showed strong antioxidant activity (determined by measuring the coupled oxidation of carotene and linoleic acid), close to that of butylated hydroxyanisole (Fig. 17) and green tea, and significantly greater than that of red wine (27). This is clearly a fruit worthy of further exploration. The rind is used as an astringent (28) and the leaf has antibacterial properties (29).

Date Palm (Phoenix dactylifera)

A decrease of normal body hormones plays a role in skin aging, reduced skin thickness, and the disturbance of normal collagen turnover, which in turn results in a decrease in collagen I and III synthesis. Date palm kernel has seven compounds with regenerative, anti-oxidizing, firming, and soothing properties, extracted: phytosterols, phytosteroids, ursolic acid, isoflavones, policosanols, provitamin A, and vitamin E. Some studies suggest that dehydroepiandrosterone (DHEA) (Fig. 18), known for its

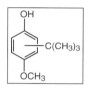

FIGURE 17 Butylated hydroxyanisole.

capacity to promote keratinization of the epidermis, would have a beneficial effect against signs of aging. The effects of date palm kernel extract were compared with those of DHEA using ex vivo skin. There was a decrease of wrinkles within five weeks of date palm kernel extract application and the skin structure was also improved in a way superior to that of DHEA (30). The seed and the pollen have both been shown to contain estrone and this may further explain the reasons for this activity (31,32).

Hops (Humulus lupulus)
The hop contains β-sitosterol, estradiol, stigmasterol, and estrone, together with many other materials that are known for their sedative attributes. Regular doses of the herb can help regulate the menstrual cycle (33). It had long been known that menstrual periods came early in young girls hop picking. Considerable amounts of estrogen (30,000–300,000 IU per 100 g) have been found in hops. The presence of antiandrogens may explain why hops will suppress sexual excitement in men (26). Hop extract recovered the proliferation of hair follicle derived keratinocyte suppressed by androgen, stimulated the proliferation of hair follicle keratonicytes and demonstrated a potent acceleration of hair growth (34).

Sarsaparilla (Smilax ornate)
Sarsaparilla is used in concoctions with other plants as a tonic or aphrodisiac (35). It was formerly used in the treatment of syphilis (36), gonorrhea (37), rheumatism, and certain skin diseases. Used in soft drinks, the genins are also used in the partial synthesis of cortisone and other steroids (6). It is especially useful as part of a wider treatment for chronic rheumatism. It has also been shown that sarsaparilla contains chemicals with properties that aid testosterone activity in the body (15). Sarsaparilla contains saponins, sarsaponin, and parallin, which yield isomeric sapogenins, sarsapogenin, and smilogenin. It also contains sitosterol and stigmasterol in the free form and as glucosides. It is antirheumatic, antiseptic, antipruritic, and indicated for psoriasis and other cutaneous conditions. It is specifically used in cases of psoriasis especially where there is desquamation (14).

Sugars, Polysaccharides, and Mucopolysaccharides
The skin appears to have an affinity for sugars, and there are many examples where they have been shown to have a significant cutaneous effect. In Third World countries

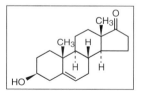

FIGURE 18 Prasterone or dehydroepiandrosterone.

and poorer communities, honey, the first choice as a natural source of these sugars, has been shown to be of great benefit in the treatment of burns, scalds, and wounds, especially because it has antibacterial properties when used undiluted. Reepithelialization is accelerated, granulation is even, and there is less necrotic tissue formed. Honey absorbs exudates and makes noninvasive cleaning simple and painless.

Mucopolysaccharides are present in numerous plant materials, including the ribwort and greater plantains (*Plantago lanceolata* and *Plantago ovata*). Mucilages are found in numerous species of seaweeds, for example, bladderwrack (*Fucus vesiculosus*), sea lettuce (*Ulva lactuca*), and oarweed, tangleweed, or kombu (*Laminaria digitata*). These plants have similar effects and they are used for dry, desquamatous, pruritic skin conditions.

SPECIALIST PLANTS

There are a number of plants that have unique chemical entities and are specific for treating skin diseases and damage.

Gotu Kola (*Centella asiatica*)

C. asiatica (Indian pennywort or cotyle) is an important medicinal herb in India. Its Sanskrit name is Brahmi and in Tamil it is known as *Mandukaparni*. An infusion of the leaves and stems has long been used in India for leprosy and other skin diseases. Asiaticoside (Fig. 19) was found to be active against leprosy (by dissolving the waxy coating of *Mycobacterium leprae*) and an oxidized form, oxyasiaticoside, inhibited growth of tubercle bacillus in vitro and in vivo (38,39).

C. asiatica extracts are used for the treatment of skin ailments, particularly ulcers, wounds, and for prevention of keloid and hypertrophic scars. *Centella* extracts have been found to accelerate wound healing, particularly in cases of chronic, postsurgical, and posttraumatic wounds. Extracts have also been successfully used as a therapy in the treatment of second- and third-degree burns. The pharmacological activity of *C. asiatica* is thought to be attributable to several saponin constituents, including the asiatic acid and madecassic acid, and both compounds stimulate the production of human collagen I, a protein involved in wound healing. Asiaticoside

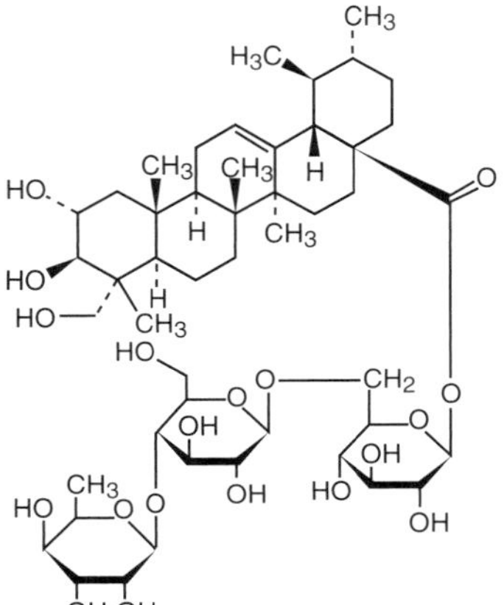

FIGURE 19   Asiaticoside.

is effective in accelerating the healing of superficial postsurgical wounds and ulcers by an acceleration of cicatricial action.

Topical application of asiaticoside has been shown to promote wound healing in rats and significantly increased the tensile strength of the newly formed skin. Extracts of *C. asiatica*, and in particular asiaticoside, have also been shown to be valuable in the treatment of hypertropic scars and keloids. The mechanism is because of the effect of the plant on the synthesis of collagen and acidic mucopolysaccharides, and by the inhibition of the inflammatory phase of hypertropic scars and keloids. Asiaticoside is likely to interfere with scar formation by acting on myofibroblasts and immature collagen (40).

Licorice (*Glycyrrhiza glabra*)

Theophrastus recommended licorice for quenching thirst, to combat cramps caused by stomach ulcers and asthma. Napoleon chewed licorice root regularly and eventually blackened his teeth (41). Licorice is one of the most commonly used plant materials in TCM, and various species, including *Glycyrrhiza glabra*, *Glycyrrhiza uralensis*, and *Glycyrrhiza inflata*, are used. The roots are most often used with other herbs to mediate their effects (41). It was introduced into Britain by the Black Friars in the 16th century and was later cultivated extensively in the Pontefract district of Yorkshire (43). Glycyrrhizin, a triterpenoid saponin found in the roots, has anti-inflammatory and antiallergic activity, the former attributed to the corticosteroid-like activity of glycyrrhetinic acid or enoxolone (Fig. 20A) and glycyrrhizin (Fig. 20B) (40).

Comfrey (*Symphitum officinale*)

Comfrey's medieval reputation for knitting broken bones is reflected in its name of knitbone, which comes from the Latin *conferre*, meaning to bring together (45). The plant contains allantoin (Fig. 21), which acts as a vulnerary because of its cell proliferant effect. The demulcent action is because of the high mucilage content. Significant anti-inflammatory activity has been demonstrated in vivo (46). The plant also contains

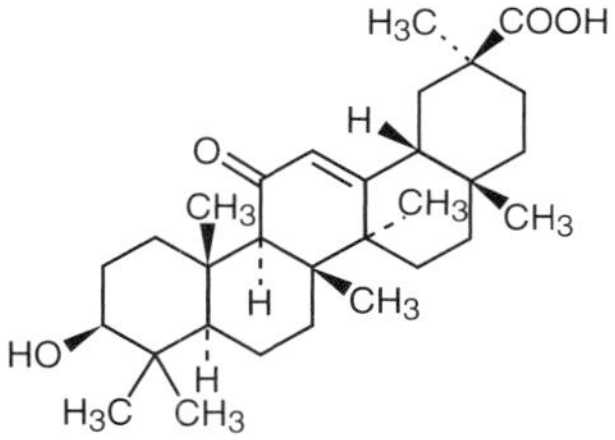

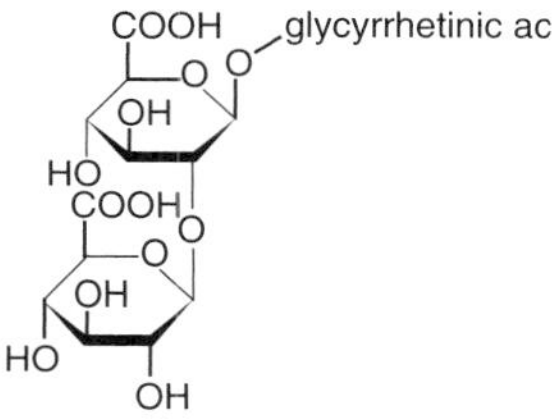

FIGURE 20 (**A**) Glycyrrhetinic acid (enoxolone) and (**B**) glycyrrhizic acid.

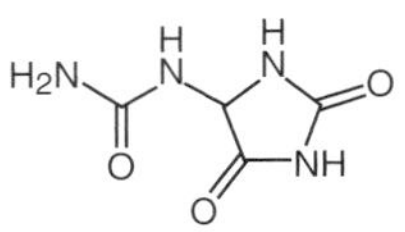

FIGURE 21   Allantoin.

mucilage, tannins, starch, and two alkaloids, consolidine and symphytocynglossine. Large amounts of potassium, phosphorus, and vitamins A and C are also present (47).

Aloe Vera (*Aloe barbadensis*)

There are many studies on the healing power of aloe vera. Aloe-treated wounds in dogs had smaller unhealed areas than untreated controls and wounds treated with antibiotics (48). Mannose-6-phosphate is the major sugar in aloe, and mice receiving 300 mg/kg of mannose-6-phosphate had improved wound healing over saline controls (49).

After full-face dermabrasion, the abraded face was divided in half. One side was treated with a standard polyethylene oxide gel wound dressing, and the other was treated with a similar gel dressing saturated with stabilized aloe vera. By 24 to 48 hours, there was dramatic vasoconstriction and accompanying reduction in edema on the aloe-treated side. By the third to fourth day, there was less exudate and crusting at the aloe site, and by the fifth to sixth day the reepithelialization at the aloe site was complete. Overall, wound healing was approximately 72 hours faster at the aloe site. This acceleration in wound healing was important to reduce bacterial contamination, subsequent keloid formation, and pigmentary changes (50).

The influence of oral and topical aloe vera on wound healing (induced using a biopsy punch) in mice was studied. In the oral study, test animals received aloe vera (100 mg/kg/day) in drinking water for 2 months, and the controls received water only. In the topical study, test animals were given 25% aloe vera cream and the controls received cream only. There was a 62.5% reduction in wound diameter (oral aloe vera group) and a 50.8% reduction (topical aloe vera group). These data suggest that aloe vera is effective by both oral and topical routes of administration (51).

Eight topical agents in current use were studied for their effects on wound contraction and rate of reepithelialization of full-thickness skin excisions in pigs. The following were applied daily for 27 days: scarlet red ointment, benzoyl peroxide lotion, bacitracin ointment, silver sulfadiazine cream, aloe vera gel, tretinoin cream, capsaicin cream, and mupirocin ointment. Reepithelialization was significantly enhanced by capsaicin, bacitracin, silver sulfadiazine, and scarlet red, and was markedly retarded by tretinoin. Wound contraction was significantly retarded by mupirocin, bacitracin, and silver sulfadizine. Knowledge of the effects of topical agents on various aspects of healing allows the clinician to choose the most appropriate material to use in a given clinical situation to optimize the healing process (52).

Aloe vera (100 and 300 mg/kg daily for 4 days) blocked the wound healing suppression of hydrocortisone acetate by up to 100% using the wound tensile strength assay. The growth factors present in aloe vera mask wound healing inhibitors such as sterols and certain amino acids. The sterols showed good anti-inflammatory activity in reducing the croton oil-induced ear swelling (53,54). The use of aloe in treating leg ulcers has been described (55). Kligman writes in his conclusions, "It is our opinion that the Aloe vera materials tested did not interfere with the normal rate of superficial dermal wound reepithelialization nor did they enhance the process any faster than the covered nontreated control wounds at the end of three

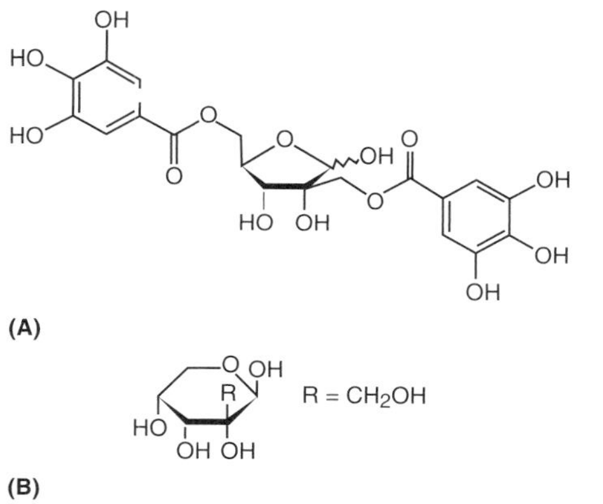

(A)

(B)

FIGURE 22 (**A**) Hamamelitannin and (**B**) hamamelose.

weeks. It can be stated that the wounds treated with Aloe vera healed better than uncovered wounds and were more cosmetically gratifying" (56). A review of the literature showed that the healing, soothing, and cooling claims routinely made for aloe are justified (57). Aloe vera also has a prophylactic effect in the protection of the skin against UV radiation (58) and also protects the skin against the radiation produced in radiotherapy treatment (59–61).

Witch Hazel (*Hamamelis virginiana*)

Known as hamamelis, snapping hazel, winter bloom, spotted alder, tobacco wood, and hamamelis water, witch hazel is a well-known plant with a long history of use in the Americas. Uses include the treatment of hemorrhoids, burns, and eye irritation. Preparations have been used topically for symptomatic treatment of itching and other skin inflammation, and its drying and astringent effects help treat skin inflammation (62) and also protects against infection. The astringent action is because of the hamamelitannin (Fig. 22A) and hamamelose (Fig. 22B). Inflammation of mucous membranes including mouth, throat, and gums may also be treated with a witch hazel gargle. It is also used for swollen or tired eyes, to relieve the pain of sunburn, as a face splash for oily skin, and to control minor pimple formation. It reduces the pain of insect bites and can be used cold or with ice to reduce the pain of sprains or athletic injuries including bruises. It is used in some hospital recovery rooms to reduce the swelling from intravenous feeding (63).

CONCLUSIONS

A plant is a complex chemical factory, where each chemical component delivers specific properties that in concert are often synergistic in their performance. In addition to some of the simple categories discussed herein, there are numerous plant species that have chemicals that are unique to them.

REFERENCES

1. Boland GM, Donnelly DMX. Isoflavonoids and related compounds. Nat Prod Rep 1998:241–260.

2. Brand-Garnys E, van Dansic P, Brand HM. Flavonoids: looking in the face of cosmeceuticals. SÖFW 2001; 127(1/2):8.
3. Keung W-M, Vallee BL. Daidzin and daidzein suppress free-choice ethanol intake by Syrian Golden hamsters. Proc Natl Acad Sci USA 1993; 90:10008–10012.
4. Dweck AC. The Pueraria family with special interest in *Pueraria mirifica*. Pers Care Mag 2003; 4(1):7–8.
5. Wren RC. Rewritten by EM Williamson and FJ Evans: Potter's New Cyclopaedia of Botanical Drugs and Preparations, C.W. Daniels, 1994.
6. Evans WC. Trease and Evans Textbook of Pharmacognosy. 13th ed. Balliere Tindall, 1989.
7. Leung AY. Encyclopedia of Common Natural Ingredients Used in Food, Drugs and Cosmetics. 1st ed. John Wiley, 1980.
8. Mills SY. The A-Z of modern herbalism. A Comprehensive Guide to Practical Herbal Therapy. Thorsons, 1989 (retitled).
9. Council of Europe. Plant Preparations used as Ingredients of Cosmetic Products. 1st ed. Strasbourg: HMSO, 1989.
10. Plesca-Manea L, Parvu AE, Parvu M, et al. Effects of *Melilotus officinalis* on acute inflammation. Phytother Res 2002; 16(4):316–319.
11. Watson C. Love Potions—A guide to aphrodisiacs. Optima Books, 1993.
12. Lust J. The Herb Book—The Most Complete Herb Book Ever Published. 1st ed. Benedict Lust Publications, 1974.
13. Grieve M. A Modern Herbal—The Medicinal, Culinary, Cosmetic and Economic Properties, Cultivation and Folklore of Herbs, Grasses, Fungi, Shrubs and Trees With All Their Modern Scientific Uses. London, U.K.: Tiger Books International, 1998.
14. The British Herbal Pharmacopoeia. British Herbal Manufacturers Association (B.H.M.A), 1983.
15. Hoffmann D. The New Holistic Herbal. Element. 2nd impression, 1991.
16. Newall CA, Anderson LA, Phillipson, JD. Herbal Medicines—A Guide for Health-Care Professionals. London, U.K.: The Pharmaceutical Press, 1996.
17. Brown DJ. Herbal Research review: *Vitex agnus castus*—clinical monograph. Q Rev Nat Med, Summer 1994.
18. Phytochemical and Ethnobotanical Databases (www.ars-grin.gov/duke/.)
19. Dweck AC. The wild yam—a review. Pers Care Mag 2002; 3(3):7–9.
20. Fluck H. Medicinal Plants. W. Foulsham & Co. Ltd., 1988.
21. Boulos L. Medicinal Plants of North Africa. Algonac, Mich: Reference Publications, 1983.
22. Iwu MM. Handbook of African Medicinal Plants. CRC Press, 1993.
23. Leung AY, Foster S. Encyclopedia of Common Natural Ingredients Used in Food, Drugs and Cosmetics. 2nd ed. John Wiley, 1996.
24. Bunney S. The Illustrated Book of Herbs. Octopus, 1984.
25. Burkill HM. The Useful Plants of West Topical Africa. 2nd ed, Vol. 3. Families J-L. Royal Botanic Gardens Kew, 1985.
26. Weiss RF. Herbal Medicine (Translated from the 6th. German edition of Lehrbuch der Phytotherapie by A.R. Meuss). The Bath Press, 1986.
27. Schubert SY, Lansky EP, Neeman I. Antioxidant and eicosanoid enzyme inhibition properties of pomegranate seed oil and fermented juice flavonoids. J Ethnopharmacol 1999; 66(1):11–17.
28. Lust J. The Herb Book. 16th impression. Bantam Publishing, 1986.
29. Stuart M. Illustrated Guide to Herbs. CPG (Cambridge Physic Garden) Edgerton International Ltd., 1994.
30. Dal Farra C. Date palm kernel extract exhibits anti-aging properties and significantly reduces skin wrinkles. Proceeding of the Active Ingredients Conference, Paris, June 17–19, 2003.
31. Morton, J. Date. p. 5–11. In: Fruits of Warm Climates. Miami, Fla: Julia F. Morton, 1987: 5–11 (www.hort.purdue.edu/newcrop/morton/Date.html.).
32. Duke JA. 1983. Handbook of Energy Crops (www.hort.purdue.edu/newcrop/duke_energy/Phoenix_dactylifera.html.)
33. Keville K. The Illustrated Herb Encyclopaedia—A Complete Culinary, Cosmetic, Medicinal and Ornamental Guide to Herbs. Grange Books, 1991.

34. Okano Y, Rin K, Okamoto N, et al. Hop extract as a new potent ingredient for hair growth. Preprint, Vol. 3. 18th International IFSCC Congress, Venice, 1994.
35. Seaforth CE. Natural Products in Caribbean Folk Medicine. University of the West Indies, 1988.
36. Carrington S. Wild Plants of the Eastern Caribbean. London, U.K.: Macmillan Education, 1998.
37. Honychurch PN. Caribbean Wild Plants and Their Uses. Macmillan, 1994.
38. Bep O. Medicinal Plants in Nigeria. Published as a private edition 1960 by the Nigerian College of Arts, Science and Technology.
39. Lewis WH, Elvin-Lewis MPF. Medical Botany—Plants Affecting Man's Health. John Wiley & Sons, 1977.
40. World Health Organisation: WHO Monograph on Selected Medicinal Plants, Vol. 1. Geneva, Switzerland: World Health Organisation, 1999.
41. Schauenberg P, Paris F. Guide to Medicinal Plants. Lutterworth Press, 1990.
42. Tang S, Palmer M. Chinese Herbal Prescriptions—A Practical and Authoritative Self-Help Guide. Rider & Company, an imprint of Century Hutchinson Ltd., 1986.
43. Gordon L. A Country Herbal. Webb and Bower Ltd., 1980.
44. Sela MN, Steinberg D. Glycyrrhizin: the basic facts plus medical and dental benefits. In: Grenby TH, ed. Progress in Sweeteners. London, U.K.: Elsevier, 1989, 7:1–96.
45. Back P. The Illustrated Herbal. Hamlyn Publishers, 1987.
46. Bradley PR. British Herbal Compendium. Vol. 1. 1992.
47. Spoerke DG. Herbal Medications. Santa Barbara: Woodbridge Press, 1990.
48. Swaim SF. Riddell KP, McGuire JA. Effects of topical medications on the healing of open pad wounds in dogs. J Am Anim Hosp Assoc 1992; 28(6):499–502.
49. Davis RH, Donato JJ, Hartman GM, Haas RC. Anti-inflammatory and wound healing activity of a growth substance in Aloe vera. J Am Podiatr Med Assoc 1994; 84(2):77–81.
50. Fulton JE. The stimulation of postdermabrasion wound healing with stabilized aloe vera gel-polyethylene oxide dressing. J Dermatol Surg Oncol 1990; 16(5):460–467.
51. Davis RH, Leitner MG, Russo JM, Byrne ME. Wound healing. Oral and topical activity of Aloe vera. J Am Podiatr Med Assoc 1989; 79(11):559–562.
52. Watcher MA, Wheeland RG. The role of topical agents in the healing of full-thickness wounds. J Dermatol Surg Oncol 1989; 15(11):1188–1195.
53. Davis RH, DiDonato JJ, Johnson RW, Stewart CB. Aloe vera, hydrocortisone, and sterol influence on wound tensile strength and anti-inflammation. J Am Podiatr Med Assoc 1994; 84(12):614–621.
54. Davis RH, Kabbani JM, Maro NP. Aloe vera and wound healing. J Am Podiatr Med Assoc 1987; 77(4):165–169.
55. Zawahry ME, Hegazy MR, Helal M. Use of aloe in treating leg ulcers and dermatoses. Int J Dermatol 1973; 12(1):68–73.
56. Kligmann AM. Wound healing assay. Test report 3791 Ivy Research Laboratories Inc., 1979.
57. Reynolds T, Dweck AC. Aloe vera leaf gel—a review update. J Ethnopharmacol 1999; 68:3–37.
58. Strickland FM, Pelley RP, Kripke ML. Prevention of ultraviolet radiation-induced suppression of contact and delayed hypersensitivity by *Aloe barbadensis* gel extract. J Invest Dermatol 1994; 102(2):197–204
59. Sato Y, Ohta S, Shinoda M. Studies on chemical protectors against radiation: XXXI. Protection effects of *Aloe arborescens* on skin injury induced by X-irradiation. J Pharm Soc Japan 1990; 110(11):876–884.
60. Iena IM. [The therapeutic properties of aloe]. Vrach-Delo 1993; (2–3):142–145.
61. Lushbaugh CC, Hale DB. Experimental acute radiodermatitis following beta irradiation. Cancer 1958; 6:690–698.
62. Swoboda M, Meurer J. The treatment of atopic dermatitis with an ointment containing *Hamamelis virginiana* extract: a double-blind study. Br J Phytother 1992; 2(3).
63. Buchman DD. Herbal Medicine: The Natural Way to Get Well and Stay Well. Century Hutchinson, 1987.

20

Influence of Formulation Design on the Clinical Performance of Topically Applied Formulations

Johann W. Wiechers

JW Solutions, Gouda, Netherlands

SUMMARY

Although enormous amounts of time and money are spent on identifying the right drug or active ingredient to overcome skin ailments, relatively little effort is given to the design of the topical formulation in which that drug or active ingredient is ultimately applied on the skin. As a consequence, some or, in the worst case, all of the intrinsic activity of the active ingredient may be lost. Of course, this is not deliberate, but topical product developers are also people with certain habits, and it is only logical to use the same formulation base that was previously successful for that new drug, active ingredient, or cosmeceutical.

This chapter proposes a rather radical approach, called "formulating for efficacy," which is based on the optimization of two opposing effects: (1) to increase the absolute solubility of the drug or active ingredient in the formulation to ensure that there is sufficient material that can reach minimal effective concentrations (MECs) at the target site in the skin; (2) to reduce the relative solubility of the drug or active ingredient in the formulation to ensure an optimal driving force away from the formulation and into the skin. Examples will be shown illustrating that this approach leads to significantly higher skin penetration that subsequently results in significantly better clinical efficacy.

In addition, it will be shown that the application of this concept can also help to lower the dose of active ingredients without a loss of clinical efficacy, making the benefits of formulating for efficacy very visible: (1) to create an efficacious product; (2) to enhance the efficacy of an already efficacious formulation; (3) to reduce the amount of active ingredient used in a cosmeceutical product without the loss of clinical efficacy.

INTRODUCTION

The first half of the 1990s was characterized by the advent of active ingredients. Every cosmetic product needed to contain a chemical entity with some biological activity to allow it to be successful in the market place. In vitro evidence for this biological activity was often sufficient to convince both the cosmetic product formulator as well as the consumer that there were clear benefits to be obtained from using this product. Cosmetic advertisements such as "Product X contains ingredient Y that is known to do Z" were both common and attractive. So-called cosmetic ingredient claims emerged on every product label and in advertisements in glossy magazines.

But time changes everything and consumers of cosmetic products started to realize that the antiaging creams that they bought did not necessarily prevent wrinkles forming. The efficacy of these cosmeceutical products was simply not enough. Cosmetic marketers became unhappy and started asking for more efficacious products while at the same time, regulators of cosmetic products started to ask for clinical evidence for the claims that were made. Cosmetic claim substantiation became a cosmetic discipline. Customers of cosmetic products wanted to see a real consumer-perceivable benefit, cosmetic marketers wanted to deliver this benefit, and cosmetic regulators wanted to see the evidence. In the meantime, cosmetic formulators were the ones who had to deliver the clinical effect via the delivery of the active ingredient to the site of action in the skin at sufficiently high concentrations for a sufficiently long period of time. They tried new active ingredients with promising intrinsic activity profiles but were often not able to create efficacious products when using their standard cosmetic formulations. Suppliers of the new active ingredients were blamed. Some suppliers were smart and realized that the lack of skin delivery was the root cause of this and started to provide cosmetic delivery systems to the cosmetic industry: liposomes, nanosomes, microcapsules, and the like emerged into the market, and these were popular for some time and continue to be so in selected applications where they have demonstrated their benefit. But skin delivery systems cannot be used generically. Something that is good for one active ingredient, drug, or cosmeceutical, is not necessarily good for another. Moreover, not everyone wanted to include costly gadgets into their topical preparations that would hopefully give them enhanced delivery. There was need for a more generic approach that would work with every active ingredient, under every condition (concentration) at no extra cost.

In 2003, I presented, together with my colleagues, a paper at the International Federation of Societies of Cosmetic Chemists Conference in Seoul, South Korea, that went a long way in providing exactly that. It was not set up to meet this objective, but started as a means to explain some seemingly contradictory requirements for skin delivery to my colleagues. When I was finally able to explain this to my colleagues, the formulating for efficacy concept was born. Although very simple in principle, its consequences are far-reaching from both a marketing perspective as well as a consumer perspective. The use of this concept allows the formulator to create a more efficacious product at lower concentrations of active ingredient, a target that would delight people both within as well as outside the cosmetic or pharmaceutical industry.

In this chapter, I will first discuss the various factors influencing skin delivery from topical formulations, such as formulation type, structure, and composition. I will explain the theoretical background of the formulating for efficacy concept, show how this has been used to enhance the skin penetration of active ingredients into the skin, and show clinical results from formulations that were and that were not optimized via this concept. This will be followed by new clinical results indicating that the dose of active ingredient can be lowered without a loss of efficacy. The chapter will end with some further perspectives of possible improvements that could be made to the formulating for efficacy concept.

FACTORS INFLUENCING SKIN DELIVERY FROM TOPICAL FORMULATIONS

Various factors influence skin penetration. In short, they are the condition of the skin (whether it is healthy or diseased), the physicochemical properties of the penetrating molecule, the formulation in which the penetrating molecule is applied, and finally, the dosing conditions (1). The condition of skin, which includes such aspects as skin lipid structure and organization, and how this may be influenced by various disease states, is discussed elsewhere in this book. It has been shown in patients suffering from atopic dermatitis, for instance, that the barrier function of the skin is reduced because of changes in the packing rigidity of skin lipids (2). The physicochemical properties that favor skin penetration in short are the following: (1) a [10]log octanol/water partition coefficient of 1 to 2, that is, the molecule should be 10- to 100-fold more soluble in octanol than in water; (2) a low molecular weight (ideally, lower than 500, but when higher, generally the lower the better); (3) uncharged over the physiological pH range encountered during skin penetration; (4) a high dipole moment (1). A molecule such as dimethyl sulfoxide fulfills all these requirements and it penetrates human skin within seconds. The influence of formulation design on skin penetration is the subject of this chapter. The dosing conditions are generally of relatively minor importance, although in individual cases, they may have a big impact. This encompasses issues such as application under occlusion, which was shown to be very relevant for the topical application of corticosteroids, the number of daily applications, and the skin temperature. In the following, it is assumed that a formulation is applied onto healthy skin and contains a drug, an active ingredient, or a cosmeceutical, which has the right chemical characteristics to penetrate the skin.

Formulation Type

There are three fundamental levels on which a formulation can influence topical delivery. On the first level, there is the influence of formulation type, that is, whether the drug or active ingredient is dosed in a gel, an oil-in-water (O/W) emulsion or a water-in-oil (W/O) emulsion, a microemulsion, or an oil. In a systematic study, four model drugs of differing polarities (the polar 5-fluorouracil, the intermediate polarity hydrocortisone, the lipophilic testosterone, and the very lipophilic ketoconazole) were dosed at 1% w/w from the five formulation types mentioned earlier. Both transdermal and dermal delivery were measured and results are discussed accordingly.

For transdermal delivery, the microemulsions were almost always superior to the other formulations tested (Fig. 1). In the table attached to Figure 1, a score of 1 means that that particular formulation type delivered the greatest amount of drug and a score of 5 means that it delivered the least amount. Please note that this is not an equidistant scale; 2 and 3 may be close together, whereas 1 and 2 may be numerically far apart. The graph in Figure 1 clearly indicates that 5-fluorouracil penetration from a microemulsion is significantly higher than from any of the other formulation types tested. It must be said that considerably higher levels of surfactants were used to create this microemulsion and the microemulsions containing the other polarity drugs. It is therefore assumed that the higher transdermal penetration can be explained from the high levels of surfactant in the formulation because these are known to act as skin penetration enhancers. Transdermal delivery from these microemulsions was consistently high but the dermal delivery was variable (results not shown).

Although this was not very surprising, the next finding was. When comparing the transdermal delivery from O/W and W/O emulsions, it was noted that this was always roughly the same with average scores ranging from 2 to 4. This suggested that transdermal delivery from an O/W emulsion is roughly the same as that from a W/O emulsion. However, when comparing the dermal delivery,

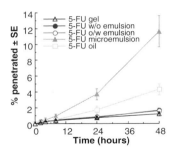

Formulation	hydrophilic 5-fluoro-uracil	medium polarity hydro-cortisone	lipophilic testos-terone	very lipophilic keto-conazole
gel	5	3	5	5
w/o	3	4	2	4
o/w	3	5	3	2
micro	1	1	1	3
oil	2	2	4	1

FIGURE 1 Transdermal delivery of 5-fluorouracil, a model polar penetrant, from five different formulation types: gel, W/O emulsion, O/W emulsion, microemulsion, and oil. Penetration after 48 hours was ranked from 1 (highest) to 5 (lowest). When results were statistically insignificant, the same higher score (higher number) was given. The table on the right gives the transdermal skin penetration results of all four model penetrants from all five formulations. Note that the microemulsions delivered in three out of four cases the highest amount, most likely due to the high levels of surfactants used to create these microemulsions. *Abbreviations*: W/O, water-in-oil; O/W, oil-in-water.

a completely different picture was obtained. Here, we saw that dermal delivery from W/O emulsions was poor for the lipophilic model penetrants, whereas the dermal delivery from O/W emulsions was poor for the more hydrophilic penetrants! This was remarkable because generally accepted knowledge dictates that delivery is better from the external phase because the drug has immediate access to the skin. Therefore, if this generally accepted wisdom is indeed correct, the delivery of the lipophilic model penetrants ketoconazole and testosterone should have been higher from W/O emulsions, but there is no evidence for this in the transdermal results. In the dermal results, it is exactly the opposite. Also, dermal delivery of the hydrophilic 5-fluorouracil and intermediate polarity hydrocortisone is higher when it is incorporated in the internal phase, that is, in a W/O emulsion. An easy explanation for this would be that the internal phase has a smaller volume than the external phase. At constant loading levels of 1%, the local concentration in the internal phase would therefore be higher, hence the thermodynamic activity would be higher, but that is incorrect because all formulations (apart from ketoconazole in oil) were formulated at maximum thermodynamic activity! This is shown in Figure 2, where the transdermal delivery differences ranked as in Figure 1 are shown on the left and dermal delivery differences on the right.

Although this study yielded some very interesting observations, care should be taken not to extrapolate these findings to general guidelines. The chemicals used to make these formulations were the same within the same formulation (i.e., all gels had the same composition apart from the drug), but there were differences between the chemicals used for the different formulation types. This study did confirm, however, that the most prominent characteristic determining skin penetration is the physicochemical nature of the penetrating molecule. In other words, when dealing with a molecule that does not have the intrinsic capability to penetrate the skin (because it is too big, of the wrong polarity, or ionized), then clever topical formulation design is not going to make it happen. Other means of skin penetration enhancement such as iontophoresis or encapsulation might still work. But for the

Formulation	hydrophilic 5-fluoro-uracil	medium polarity hydro-cortisone	lipophilic testos-terone	very lipophilic keto-conazole	Formulation	hydrophilic 5-fluoro-uracil	medium polarity hydro-cortisone	lipophilic testos-terone	very lipophilic keto-conazole
gel	5	3	5	5	gel	3	2	3	3
w/o	3	4	2	4	w/o	2	1	5	5
o/w	3	5	3	2	o/w	5	5	1	3
micro	1	1	1	3	micro	4	4	2	1
oil	2	2	4	1	oil	1	3	3	1

FIGURE 2 Comparison of the transdermal (*left*) and dermal delivery (*right*) of four model penetrants from five different formulations, with particular emphasis on the W/O and O/W emulsions. Although transdermal delivery is on average the same for the various penetrants from O/W and W/O emulsions, their dermal delivery is distinctly different, favoring the penetration from the actives that are present in the internal phase.

classical topical formulations, it can be concluded that when the physical chemistry is not right, the drug or active ingredient will not penetrate skin.

Formulation Structure

A second level of influence is the physical formulation structure and in particular the influence of droplet size on skin penetration. Here, again, some rather interesting observations were made, which are contradictory to what most cosmetic and pharmaceutical formulators believe to be true. In a series of skin penetration experiments using tetracaine as the model penetrant in a series of formulations, all containing exactly the same ingredients but processed in different ways to give a range of different droplet sizes, no influence of droplet size on either transdermal or dermal delivery could be seen. In a first "Total Surfactant" experiment, the overall level of surfactant in the formulation was kept constant. Smaller droplets, however, need more surfactant to stabilize the emulsion because of the larger total interfacial surface of the smaller droplets. As a consequence, less free surfactant was present in the formulations with smaller droplet sizes, and one could explain that the observed lack of influence of droplet size was the net result of two opposing effects. If, on the one hand, skin penetration was enhanced from the smaller droplet size emulsions, but, on the other hand, also enhanced at higher free surfactant concentrations (present in larger droplet size emulsions), then the net result of droplet size could be zero. We therefore repeated the experiment, adapting the amount of surfactant used to the droplet surface area keeping the concentration of free surfactant constant, the "Free Surfactant" experiment. Again, no influence of droplet size on transdermal and dermal delivery of tetracaine was noted. Although this initially surprised us, because we were expecting an increased penetration with reducing droplet size, our finding can in hindsight be easily rationalized from the fact that in skin penetration, each molecule is assumed to penetrate individually and in accordance with its physicochemical characteristics as expressed in the Potts-Guy equation (3). Therefore, it should not make any difference whether an active ingredient, drug, or cosmeceutical is incorporated in a small or large droplet; the skin delivery should be the same. The reason why it is generally assumed that smaller droplet size emulsions enhance skin penetration is most likely because a large excess of surfactant is used to create the smaller droplet size emulsions (similar to the microemulsions in the formulation type study described earlier). This droplet size study was the first systematic investigation that used exactly the same formulation components and only differed in the way the formulations were manufactured (4).

Results from the Total Surfactant and the Free Surfactant experiments are shown in Figure 3. Dermal delivery, expressed as microgram of tetracaine per milligram of skin, is plotted on the left-hand Y axis (open symbols), whereas transdermal delivery, expressed as the percentage of the dose that penetrated skin within 24 hours, is plotted on the right-hand Y axis (closed symbols). Droplet size is plotted logarithmically on the X axis. Although the lines are not perfectly straight, the observed differences are far from statistically significant and it can therefore be concluded that there is no influence of emulsion droplet size on both transdermal and dermal delivery.

Again, as described earlier for the influence of formulation type on skin penetration, care should be taken not to generalize this finding. After all, we evaluated only one active ingredient (tetracaine) and one surfactant system (C_{12-15} Pareth-7, commercial name Synperonic A7). However, feedback has been received from other cosmetic scientists who claim to have found the same results using another emollient as the active ingredient and another surfactant system, but they never published their findings because they go very much against normally accepted rules.

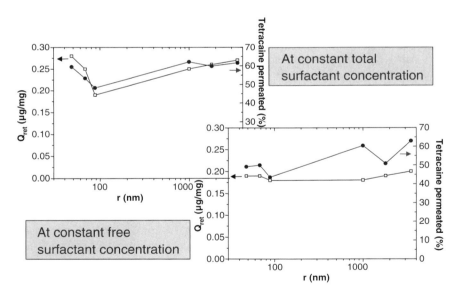

FIGURE 3 Dermal (*open squares*) and transdermal (*filled in circles*) delivery of tetracaine from macroemulsion and nanoemulsion either at a constant total free surfactant concentration or a constant free surfactant concentration. Both experiments show that there is no influence of droplet size on either dermal or transdermal delivery because observed differences are not statistically significant ($P > 0.05$). These findings contradict the general belief that skin penetration from smaller droplet sizes is enhanced, a finding that is based on studies in which the formulations vary not only in droplet size but also in surfactant concentrations required to stabilize emulsions with smaller droplet sizes, which is probably the reason for this enhancement. The formulations used in this study only differed in the way they were mechanically processed and not in chemical composition.

The conclusion of all these studies is that there is some influence of formulation type but not of formulation structure on dermal and transdermal delivery. Most of the claimed differences of droplet size seem to be due to the presence of (excess) surfactant in the formulation, that is, the composition of the formulation seems to be influencing skin delivery of a given active ingredient more than anything else. As a consequence, formulation design could very well become a trial-and-error process before one will find the best composition to optimize the skin delivery of a particular active. Therefore, a more systematic approach, based on understanding rather than on a trial-and-error method, is needed. Formulating for efficacy is such a systematic approach that was developed on a fundamental understanding of skin delivery processes. In the following, the theoretical background of formulating for efficacy will be explained as well as the use of this concept in formulation design. Clinical results will be shown for formulations that were and were not optimized by this concept to show the validity of this concept.

THEORETICAL BACKGROUND OF FORMULATING FOR EFFICACY

Both dermal and transdermal delivery aim to achieve one goal summarized in the four R's of delivery: to deliver the right chemical at the right concentration to the right site in (dermal delivery) or beyond (transdermal delivery) the skin for the correct period of time. If one of these four R's is not achieved, there is no delivery and as a result no clinical efficacy can be obtained. The active ingredient or drug needs to be stable in the formulation as well as during its passage through the stratum corneum and viable epidermis and dermis, although in certain cases, prodrugs that penetrate the skin better and rely on skin metabolism to transform the prodrug to the parent drug that subsequently has the right intrinsic activity, are used. The right site is often achieved in topical delivery by applying the drug to the relevant surface area of the body but this site definition goes much further. One may want to target a specific cell type within the viable epidermis and the common way to achieve this is to simply dose enough on the skin surface in an attempt to deliver sufficient quantities of active ingredient to the site of action. The correct length of time is seldom an issue in topical delivery; topical formulations are applied indefinitely and the only issue could be a too-short application time because of accidental removal of the formulation by the mechanical movement of clothes or our body movements. This leaves only the right concentration. Efficacy is only obtained if we deliver more than the MEC and less than the toxic concentration, two concentrations that can be obtained from in vitro experiments using the drug, cosmeceutical, or active ingredient.

Two separate issues need to be ensured if you want to deliver enough material to reach levels beyond the MEC. On the one hand, one needs to ensure that there is enough active ingredient in the formulation that the MEC can be reached. This requires a high absolute solubility of the cosmeceutical in the formulation. This can be achieved by matching the polarity of the formulation to the polarity of the drug or active ingredient. If the two are similar, the solubility of the active ingredient in the formulation will be high but its driving force for delivery will be low. One therefore also needs to optimize the driving force to ensure that the cosmeceutical will leave the formulation and penetrate into the skin in order to reach its site of action. For this, it needs to have a low solubility in the formulation relative to its solubility in the stratum corneum. The two requirements seem contradictory, but what one is really looking for is for the active ingredient to be very soluble in the formulation but even more soluble in the stratum corneum. Our work revealed that it is possible to calculate the optimal polarity of the phase in which the active ingredient is incorporated that will give you the maximally achievable skin delivery possible for that specific molecule (5). The formula for the polarity of the formulation from which you will achieve 50% skin penetration is:

polarity of formulation = polarity of penetrant ± penetrant polarity gap

The penetrant polarity gap is the polarity difference between the active ingredient and the stratum corneum. Polarity of penetrants, stratum corneum, and formulations can be calculated via polarity index (PI) values, which are a mixture of many different molecular physicochemical characteristics that influence solubility and skin penetration. The polarity of the stratum corneum was assumed to be slightly more polar than n-butanol based on literature reports (6). In formulating for efficacy terminology, the relative polarity index (RPI) is the difference between the PI values of active ingredient and the formulation component under study, whereas the penetrant polarity gap is the difference between the PI values of active ingredient and the stratum corneum (5). The optimal polarity of a formulation can now be realized by mixing a primary emollient with a low RPI (hence a high solubility of the active ingredient in that emollient) with a secondary emollient with a high RPI (hence a low solubility of the active ingredient in that emollient but therefore with high driving force to leave the emollient) in the right proportions to achieve the best of both worlds, that is, a high solubility and a high driving force. This is schematically illustrated in Figure 4.

Experimentally, one uses a primary emollient with a small RPI (i.e., with a polarity that is very similar to the active ingredient that one wants to formulate) to dissolve the desired amount of active ingredient (green arrow in Fig. 4) and then adds a secondary emollient with a large RPI (i.e., with a polarity that is very different from the active ingredient that one wants to formulate) to maximize the driving force for diffusion (red arrow). The resulting mixture, indicated by the blue arrow, has the optimal polarity to ensure a maximum driving force for the amount of active ingredient incorporated into the formulation.

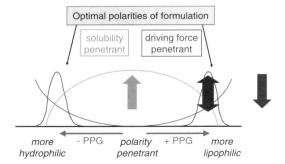

FIGURE 4   A schematic overview of formulating for efficacy. The active ingredient is dissolved in the primary emollient with a low relative polarity index (RPI) in which it is very soluble (*light grey arrow*). Subsequently, a secondary emollient with a high RPI ensuring a high driving force for diffusion (*medium grey arrow*) is added. The proportions of primary and secondary emollient relative to the concentration of the active ingredient will ensure that the optimal polarity for the formulation is achieved (*dark grey arrow*) where skin delivery is maximal.

SKIN DELIVERY AND CLINICAL EVIDENCE VALIDATING THE FORMULATING FOR EFFICACY CONCEPT

We have used the formulating for efficacy concept to make skin delivery–optimized formulations containing octadecenedioic acid, a novel skin whitener. Formulation A was made without using the Formulation for Efficacy concept and contained 2% active ingredient. Formulation B was made using the formulating for efficacy concept and also contained 2% octadecenedioic acid. The exact composition of the formulations is provided in Table 1. The only difference between the formulations is the choice of the emollients. Propylene glycol isostearate is used as the primary emollient in formulation B, whereas triethylhexanoin was used as the secondary emollient. Skin delivery experiments using the two formulations on full-thickness pig skin were performed and showed a statistically significant, 3.5-fold increase in dermal delivery (Fig. 5) (5).

The delivery result (Fig. 5) illustrates that the formulating for efficacy concept delivers significantly more octadecenedioic acid into the skin. The fact that this increase was 3.5-fold is accidental because this depends on the extent of skin delivery from the formulation that was not optimized for skin delivery. Therefore, it cannot in general be stated by what factor skin delivery will increase using the formulating for efficacy concept. But both formulations contained 2% active, yet the delivery was much more effective from the second optimized formulation.

This enhanced skin delivery suggests that the clinical efficacy should also increase. Octadecenedioic acid is a new skin-whitening molecule that interacts with the γ isoform of the peroxisome proliferator–activated receptor, PPARγ. This interaction results in reduced tyrosinase mRNA production, which subsequently results in reduced tyrosinase production (7). As tyrosinase is the rate-limiting enzyme in skin melanogenesis, its reduced production means that skin should become whiter. Clinical studies in which skin color was measured using a chromameter were carried out. In both studies, 20 subjects applied either formulation A or B for a period of eight weeks twice a day. The chromameter measures the L, a, and b values that characterize the color of any object. The L scale is the luminosity

TABLE 1 Composition of the Nonoptimized (A) and Two Skin Delivery Optimized Formulations (B and C)

INCI name	Function	Concentration (% w/w)		
		Formulation A	Formulation B	Formulation C
Octadecenedioic acid	Active ingredient	2.0	2.0	1.0
Propylene glycol isostearate	Primary emollient	–	15.0	7.5
Triethylhexanoin	Secondary emollient	–	3.0	1.5
Caprylic/capric Triglyceride	Emollient	10.0	–	–
Cetyl alcohol	Emollient	2.0	–	–
Glyceryl stearate SE	Self-emulsifying emollient	2.0	–	–
Steareth-21	Emulsifier	5.0	5.0	5.0
Steareth-2	Coemulsifier	1.0	1.0	1.0
Glycerin	Moisturizer	4.0	4.0	4.0
Xanthan gum	Thickener	–	0.2	0.2
Preservative	Preservative	0.2	0.7	0.7
2-Amino-2-methyl-1-propanol	pH modifier	qs	–	–
Water		qs 100	qs 100	qs 100

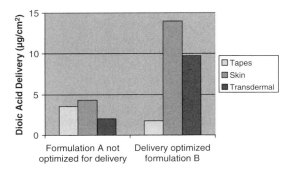

FIGURE 5 Skin delivery of octadecene-dioic acid from formulations not optimized (A) and optimized (B) for skin delivery (for composition, see also Table 1). Note that the latter delivers significantly more dioic acid to the skin.

scale and its extreme colors are black and white; the ΔL value represents the color difference on the L scale relative to the start of the study. The results of these two studies are compared in Figure 6.

The skin delivery–optimized formulation B showed not only an increased skin delivery but also an increased skin efficacy. Theoretically, there should be a direct correlation between skin delivery and clinical efficacy, and this was confirmed in the enhancement factors, 3.5-fold for skin delivery and 3.2-fold for clinical efficacy.

However, there is more that the formulating for efficacy concept can achieve. In a delivery-optimized formulation, it is the ratio between the primary emollient, the secondary emollient, and the drug, active ingredient, or cosmeceutical that optimizes the flux of the penetrant relative to its concentration. What will happen to the skin delivery of the active ingredient if the percentage of the oil phase is reduced and in doing so the amount of a lipophilic active in the formulation is also reduced? Because the ratio between the three constituents of the oil phase is not changed by this reduction, delivery expressed as $\mu g/cm^2/hr$ should remain the same, although delivery expressed as a percentage would increase.

To prove this point, a third formulation was prepared, formulation C, in which the oil phase was halved relative to formulation B (see Table 1 for composition), and this formulation was also clinically tested for its skin whitening efficacy. The clinical results of formulations A, B, and C are shown in Figure 7. Relative to formulation A (which contained 2% octadecenedioic acid and was not optimized for skin delivery), the clinical effect of formulation C (which contained 1% octadecenedioic acid but was optimized for skin delivery) was enhanced by a factor of 3.9. There was no statistically significant difference in clinical efficacy between formulations B and C,

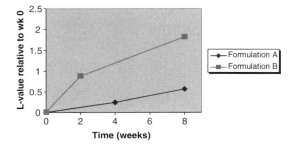

FIGURE 6 Clinical efficacy of two formulations both containing 2% octadecenedioic acid. Formulation A was not optimized for skin delivery, whereas formulation B was. The clinical efficacy of formulation B at week 8 is 3.2-fold enhanced relative to formulation A ($P < 0.05$).

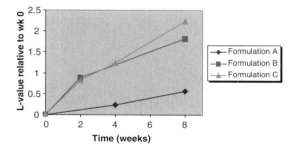

FIGURE 7 Clinical efficacy of three formulations containing octadecenedioic acid, the same formulations A and B that were shown in Figure 6 containing 2% of the active ingredient but also formulation C containing 1% octadecenedioic acid and optimized for skin delivery. Relative to formulation A, the clinical efficacy of formulation C is enhanced by a factor of 3.9 ($P < 0.002$), whereas there is no statistically significant difference between formulations B and C as was expected on theoretical grounds. This graph shows that it is not the concentration of the active that determines the extent of clinical efficacy but the ratio between drug, primary emollient, and secondary emollient, which can be found via the formulating for efficacy concept.

whereas there was between formulations A and B ($P < 0.05$) and formulations A and C ($P < 0.002$). This proves that it is the ratio between drug, primary emollient, and secondary emollient that is of importance, and not the absolute concentration of the drug in a formulation, that determines the clinical efficacy. However, this does not mean that one can infinitely reduce the concentration of the cosmeceutical in the formulation because there will be point that there is simply not enough drug left in the vehicle to obtain the minimum effective concentration at the target site. Studies in which the concentration is continuously reduced, that is, from 1.0% down to 0.05% octadecenedioic acid, are underway to determine the optimal concentration in the formulation. The optimal concentration (or OC_{100}) in the formulation is defined here as the minimum concentration of the active ingredient at which maximal efficacy can be obtained and should not be confused with the minimum effective concentration (or MEC) at the target site.

The discussion above illustrates that formulating for efficacy has three potential applications as shown in Figure 8. In a formulation that is not optimized for skin delivery, there is a constant increase in the amount delivered to the target site in the skin when the concentration of the active ingredient in the formulation is increased. At the point of saturation of the active ingredient in the formulation, maximal thermodynamic activity is reached and a further increase in the concentration of the active ingredient does not bring any additional cosmeceutical to the target site. If you have a situation where there is insufficient delivery to exceed the MEC, use of the formulating for efficacy concept may create an effective product because levels above the MEC are reached and clinical effect can be obtained. This is indicated as situation A in Figure 8. If you are already exceeding the MEC, your formulation, which is not optimized for delivery, will have a suboptimal efficacy. Use of the formulating for efficacy concept will maximize the clinical effect at the same level of active ingredient loading (situation B in Fig. 8). The comparison between formulations A and B in Figure 6 is an example of this situation in which we have enhanced or maximized clinical effect. Finally, you may already have obtained maximum clinical efficacy but at a high concentration of active ingredient. Situation C in Figure 8

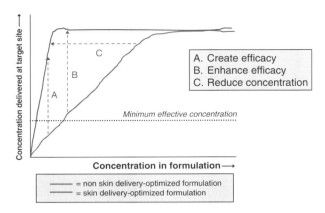

FIGURE 8 The three possible benefits of formulating for efficacy. When one does not have sufficient delivery to reach the minimum effective concentration, use of the formulating for efficacy
concept can make your formulation clinically effective (situation A). When one has insufficient skin
delivery to have maximal clinical efficacy, use of the formulating for efficacy concept can enhance
the clinical efficacy of your formulation (situation B). Finally, when you have a formulation with maximal clinical efficacy, use of the formulating for efficacy concept will allow you to reduce the concentration of your active in your formulation without losing clinical efficacy (situation C). Mixed forms of
benefit where you reduce the concentration yet achieve more clinical efficacy are also possible.

illustrates that you can reduce the concentration without losing clinical efficacy. This
was shown in the comparison between formulations B and C in Figure 7.

CONCLUDING REMARKS

In order for cosmetic products to exert clinical efficacy, the active ingredient or cosmeceutical will need to penetrate the skin to reach the site of action at a sufficiently
high concentration for a sufficiently long period of time. The most important determinant for skin penetration is the physicochemical nature of the molecule, in
particular its octanol-water partition coefficient and molecular weight and volume.
If a molecule does not have the right physicochemical properties to penetrate, nothing can be done via formulation design to enable the chemical to penetrate the skin
apart from special delivery systems such as transfersomes, etc.

Assuming the chemical of interest does have the right physicochemical properties, the formulation type in which the active ingredient is incorporated does have
an influence on skin delivery, but the influence depends on the polarity of the cosmeceutical. Information as provided in Figure 2 may give some guidance towards
the influence of formulation type although it should be realized that more than
20 formulations are needed to conclusively state the influence of formulation type
on skin delivery.

Reducing the droplet size in emulsions is often claimed to enhance the skin
delivery of cosmeceuticals but we were not able to confirm this when we kept the
composition of the formulations exactly the same and only changed the way in
which the emulsions were mechanically processed: neither dermal nor transdermal
delivery showed a dependence on droplet size. Formulation composition, on the
other hand, had a pronounced influence on skin delivery.

Our research indicated that the emollients determine how much active ingredient penetrates into the skin, whereas the emulsifiers determine where it penetrates into the skin. The formulating for efficacy concept allows calculation of the required polarity of the formulation that will maximize the skin delivery. This should not only result in more skin delivery but also in increased efficacy of the topically applied formulation as was shown for formulations containing octadecenedioic acid. In essence, use of formulating for efficacy should allow three different scenarios: (1) to create a clinically effective formulation from a previously noneffective formulation at the same dosage of active ingredient; (2) to enhance the clinical efficacy of a suboptimal delivering formulation, again at the same dosage of active ingredient; and (3) to reduce the level of the active ingredient of an already optimized formulation without losing any clinical efficacy. Of course, mixed possibilities such as obtaining greater efficacy at a lower dose level of active ingredient are also possible.

Cosmetic and pharmaceutical product developers should realize that topical formulation design is no longer a matter of trial and error but that it can be optimized by concepts such as formulating for efficacy. This, in turn, should result in more efficacious products so that there is no longer an excuse for lack of clinical efficacy from a formulation that contains sufficient active material.

REFERENCES

1. Wiechers JW. The barrier function of the skin in relation to percutaneous absorption of drugs. Pharm Weekbl Sci Ed 1989; 11:185–198.
2. Pilgram GSK, Vissers DCJ, van der Meulen H, et al. Aberrant lipid organization in stratum corneum of patients with atopic dermatitis and lamellar ichthyosis. J Invest Dermatol 2001; 117:710–717.
3. Potts RO, Guy RH. Predicting skin permeability. Pharm Res 1992; 9:663–669.
4. Izquierdo P, Wiechers JW, Escribano E, et al. A study on the influence of emulsion droplet size on the skin penetration of tetracaine. Skin Pharmacol Physiol, accepted for publication, 2007; 20:263–270.
5. Wiechers JW, Kelly CL, Blease TG, et al. Formulating for efficacy. Int J Cosmet Sci 2004; 26:173–182.
6. Scheuplein RJ, Blank IH. Mechanism of percutaneous absorption: IV. Penetration of non-electrolytes (alcohols) from aqueous solutions and from pure liquids. J Invest Dermatol 1973; 60:286–296.
7. Wiechers JW, Rawlings AV, Garcia C, et al. A new mechanism of action for skin whitening agents: binding to the peroxisome proliferator-activated receptor. Int J Cosmet Sci 2005; 27:123–132.

21

Dry Skin and Moisturizers

Anthony Vincent Rawlings
AVR Consulting Ltd., Northwich, Cheshire, U.K.

Paul John Matts
Procter & Gamble Beauty, Egham, Surrey, U.K.

INTRODUCTION

Over a decade ago, Rawlings et al. (1) summarized the knowledge on the state of the art of stratum corneum (SC) biology and dry skin, and this was recently elaborated by Rawlings and Matts (2). This chapter builds on these publications and Chapter 7 to discuss the latest understanding of dry skin (Fig. 1) and the effect of moisturizers on this most common dermatological problem. First, however, we need to consider the role of water loss through the SC. We are all losing water through our skin unless we live in 100% relative humidity (RH) climates. Under normal circumstances, the SC must be as impermeable as possible, except for a small amount of water loss, to (1) hydrate the outer layers of the SC to maintain flexibility and (2) provide enough water to allow enzyme reactions that facilitate SC maturation events, together with corneodesmolysis and, ultimately, desquamation (Fig. 2) (3–6). This inbuilt mechanism of transepidermal water loss (TEWL) is vital for the normal functioning of the SC. Naturally, in this process, water gradients are generated within the tissue. However, a key to precipitating the condition we call "dry skin" is a perturbation of these water gradients within the SC, and Warner and his team at Procter & Gamble were the first to demonstrate the changes in SC water gradients in dry skin (7) where about one-third of the outer layers of the SC are reported to contain less than 10% water content (Fig. 3). At this level of water, the SC will be dysfunctional and brittle (8).

The SC uses the following three main mechanisms to hold onto water:

1. The presence of intercellular lamellar lipids, whose physical conformation, predominantly an orthorhombic laterally-packed gel and a 13-nm-long periodicity lamellar phase induced by linoleate-containing, long-chain ceramides, provide a tight and semi-permeable barrier to the passage of water through the tissue
2. The presence of fully matured, resilient, corneodesmosome-bound and ceramide-hydrophobed corneocytes, which influence the tortuosity of the SC and thereby the diffusion path length of water
3. The presence of both intracellular and extracellular hygroscopic materials called natural moisturizing factors (NMFs)

STRATUM CORNEUM AND EPIDERMAL STRUCTURE

The original picture of the SC with a basket-weave appearance at the histological level and a stratum compactum–stratum disjunctum at the electron microscope level has come under scrutiny over the last decade. For instance, Pfeiffer et al. (10) developed new, high-pressure freezing followed by freeze substitution techniques

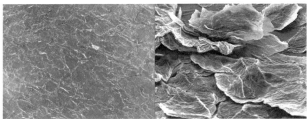

Visible light macrograph of dry skin on the outer lower leg (approx 50x), showing lifting squame

SEM micrograph of carbon tape applied to dry outer lower leg skin (500x); note compacted corneocytes in disarray

FIGURE 1 Typical photographs of cosmetic dry skin. *Source*: From Ref. 2.

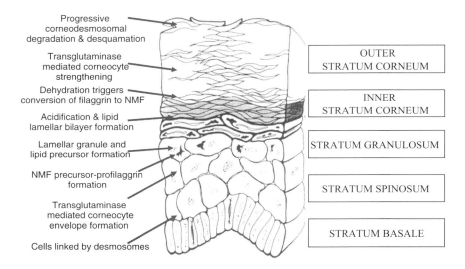

Progressive corneodesmosomal degradation & desquamation

Transglutaminase mediated corneocyte strengthening

Dehydration triggers conversion of filaggrin to NMF

Acidification & lipid lamellar bilayer formation

Lamellar granule and lipid precursor formation

NMF precursor-profilaggrin formation

Transglutaminase mediated corneocyte envelope formation

Cells linked by desmosomes

OUTER STRATUM CORNEUM

INNER STRATUM CORNEUM

STRATUM GRANULOSUM

STRATUM SPINOSUM

STRATUM BASALE

FIGURE 2 Typical structure of the epidermis and critical steps in formation of the SC. *Source*: From Ref. 1 and 9.

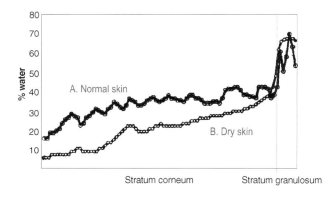

A. Normal skin

B. Dry skin

Stratum corneum   Stratum granulosum

FIGURE 3 (**A**) Water profile averaged over a single rectangular region of a cryosection contained from an individual with good skin, grade 0.5. The horizontal axis is distance across the SC with the SC/granulosum junction indicated by a vertical line. (**B**) Water profile averaged over a single rectangular region of a cryosection obtained from an individual with dry skin, grade 4. *Source*: From Ref. 7.

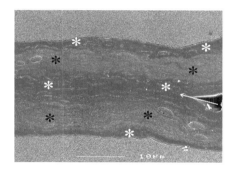

FIGURE 4 High-magnification cryoscanning electron microscopy images of two sheets of stratum corneum (SC) hydrated to 90% w/w. Both sheets show an increased hydration level in their central regions and a low hydration in the superficial and lowest part of the SC. *Source*: From Ref. 13.

for electron microscopy methods and visualized an SC that appeared more compact with smaller intercellular spaces and, hence, tighter cell-cell interactions. More controversial, however, was the lack of keratohyalin granules in the epidermis. Norlen (11) has also developed novel cryotransmission electron microscopy techniques to image vitreous sections of skin without the use of cryoprotectants and, again, a more densely packed SC was apparent compared with conventional images and new organelles or tubular structures were observed in the epidermis. Norlen (12) has further proposed a cubic rod-packing model for SC keratin structures. However, even with a more compacted SC, several swelling regions have been established by Bouwstra et al. (13) and Richter et al. (14) upon skin hydration that appear to be related to loss of barrier function and loss of NMF in the outer layers of the SC, hydrolysis of filaggrin to NMF and lysis of nonperipheral corneodesmosomes, allowing greater intercorneocyte freedom and transglutaminase-mediated maturation of corneocytes toward the surface layers of the SC (Fig. 4). All these events become aberrant in dry skin.

STRATUM CORNEUM LIPID CHEMISTRY AND BIOPHYSICS

All SC lipids are important for barrier function of the skin, but because of their unique properties and structure, the ceramides have been of most interest in recent years. Ceramides constitute (on a weight basis) approximately 47% of the SC lipids (15). A new nomenclature based on structure, rather than the original chromatographic migration characteristics, was proposed by Motta et al. (16). In this system, ceramides are classified in general as CER FB, where F is the type of fatty acid and B indicates the type of base. When an ester-linked fatty acid is present, a prefix E is used. Normal fatty acids (saturated or unsaturated), α-hydroxy fatty acids, and ω-hydroxy fatty acids are N, A, and O, respectively, whereas sphingosines, phytosphingosines, and 6-hydroxysphingosine are indicated by S, P, and H, respectively. Sphinganine (not previously classified) is proposed to be SP in this nomenclature system. A novel long-chain ceramide containing branched-chain fatty acids is also found in vernix caseosa (17). Typical structures of human ceramides are given in Figure 5. Newly identified ceramides have also been found attached to the corneocyte envelope. In addition to ceramide A (sphingosine) and ceramide B (6-hydroxysphingosine), Chopart et al. (18) recently identified covalently bound ω-hydroxyl fatty acid containing sphinganine and phytosphingosine ceramides. These covalently bound ceramides should now be named CER OS, CER OH, CER OSP, and CER OP.

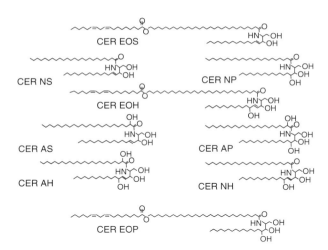

FIGURE 5 Structures of human SC ceramides.

Ceramides are produced as precursors in the form of glucosylceramides, epidermosides, or sphingomyelin. Epidermosides are glycated precursors of ω-hydroxyl–containing ceramides. Hamanaka et al. (19) have demonstrated that sphingomyelin provides a proportion of CER NS and CER AS, whereas the glucosylceramides are precursors to ceramides and epidermosides are precursors to the covalently bound ceramides, together with CER EOS, CER EOH, and CER EOP.

It is the lipid packing states, however, and not only the chemical structures of the SC lipids that are important for barrier function. Lipids in vivo appear to exist as a balance between a solid crystalline state (orthorhombic packing) and gel (hexagonal packing) or liquid crystalline states. The former lipids are the most tightly packed conformation and have optimal barrier properties but a greater proportion of hexagonally packed lipid conformations are known to occur in the outer layers of the SC (20). This is consistent with a weakening of the barrier toward the outer layers of the SC. It is possible that short-chain fatty acids derived from sebum contribute to the crystalline to gel transition in the upper SC layers (21).

Bouwstra et al. (22) recently proposed a sandwich model for the lamellar lipids consisting of two broad lipid layers with a crystalline structure separated by a narrow central lipid layer with fluid domains (Fig. 6). It seems that cholesterol and ceramides are important for the formation of the lamellar phase, whereas fatty acids play a greater role in the lateral packing of the lipids. Cholesterol may be located with the fatty acid tail of CER EOS in the fluid phase. CER EOS, EOH, and EOP play essential roles in formation of the additional lamellar arrangements. The repeat distances were found to be 13 nm in dimension, composed of two units measuring approximately 5 nm each and one unit measuring approximately 3 nm in thickness. These repeat lamellar patterns were also observed by X-ray diffraction studies and were named the long- and short-periodicity phases (LPP and SPP, respectively).

For total lipid mixtures in the absence of CER EOS, mostly hexagonal phases are observed, and no LPP phase is formed. Moreover, the importance of ceramide 1 or CER EOS–linoleate in facilitating the formation of the LPP has been further elaborated by understanding the influence of the type of fatty acid esterified to the ω-hydroxyl fatty acid (Fig. 7) (23). As a consequence, greater amounts of the LPP is observed mainly with linoleate-containing CER EOS, less with oleate-containing CER EOS and

SANDWICH MODEL

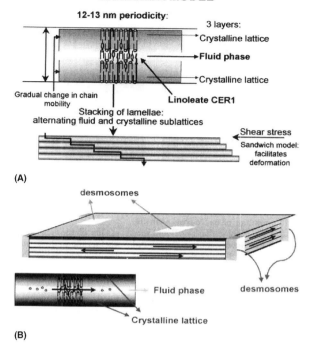

(A)

(B)

FIGURE 6 (**A**) "Sandwich model," the characteristics of which are the following: (1) the liquid sublattice is located in the central lipid layer of this phase; in this layer mainly unsaturated linoleic acid and cholesterol are present. (2) in the sublattice adjacent to the central layer, a gradual change in lipid mobility occurs due to the presence of less mobile long saturated hydrocarbon chains. (3) only a small fraction of lipids forms a fluid phase in the SC; therefore, one can assume that this central lipid layer is not a continuous phase. (**B**) The liquid phase parallel to the basal layers of the lamellae facilitates transport and therefore communication between the desmosomes. *Source*: From Ref. 22.

is absent if only stearate-containing CER EOS is present in the lipid mixtures. These studies indicate that for formation of the LPP, a certain fraction of the lipids has to form a liquid phase. If the liquid phase is too high (as with the oleate-containing CER EOS) or too low (as with stearate-containing CER EOS), the levels of the SPP increase at the expense of the LPP. It is important to remember that the fatty acid composition of CER EOS is highly complex but contains a large proportion of linoleic acid.

Compositional changes in SC lipids could, therefore, dramatically influence the condition of the skin. In this respect, using electron microscopy of tape strippings from the outer layers of normal healthy SC, Rawlings et al. (24) reported complete loss of lamellar ordering in the outer layers of the SC (Fig. 8). These results have been confirmed by Warner et al. (25) and more recently by Berry et al. (26).

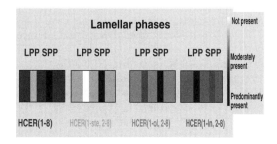

FIGURE 7 A summary of the lamellar phases and CER EOS in various lipid mixtures. HCER(1–8) mixtures in which HCER (EOS) is replaced with synthetic stearate–containing CER EOS, oleate-containing CER EOS, or linoleate-containing CER EOS. *Source*: From Ref. 23.

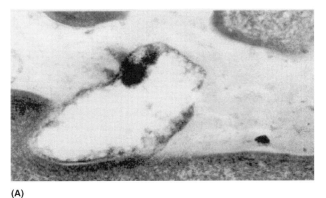

(A)

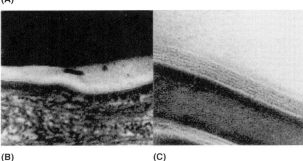

(B)   (C)

FIGURE 8 Organization of SC lipids in tape strippings of individuals with clinically normal skin. Transmission electron micrographs of tape strippings. Ultrastructural changes in lipid organization toward the surface of the SC: (**A**) first strip, absence of bilayers and presence of amorphous lipidic material; (**B**) second strip, disruption of lipid lamellae; (**C**) third strip, normal lipid lamellae (×200,000). *Source*: From Ref. 24.

CORNEODESMOSOMES AND CORNEODESMOLYSIS

Corneodesmosomes (27) are macromolecular glycoprotein complexes incorporated into the corneocyte envelope (CE) that consist of the cadherin family of transmembrane glycoproteins, desmoglein 1 (Dsg 1), and desmocollin 1 (Dsc 1). These glycoproteins span the cornified envelope into the lipid enriched intercellular spaces between the corneocytes and provide cohesion by binding homeophilically with proteins on adjacent cells. Within the corneocytes, Dsg 1 and Dsc 1 are linked to keratin filaments via corneodesmosomal plaque proteins such as plakoglobin, desmoplakins and plakophilins. The corneodesmosomal protein, corneodesmosin (Cdsn), after secretion by the lamellar bodies together with the intercellular lipids and certain proteases, becomes associated with the desmosomal proteins just before transformation of desmosomes into corneodesmosomes. - these proteins are cross-linked into the complex by transglutaminase, their controlled disruption must occur by proteolysis to allow desquamation to proceed. Indeed, Rawlings et al. (24) and Fig. 9 demonstrated degradation of the corneodesmosomes toward the surface of the SC in humans.

   Corneodesmolysis, and ultimately desquamation, is facilitated by the action of specific hydrolytic enzymes in the SC that degrade the corneodesmosomal linkages. Currently, several serine, cysteine, and aspartic enzymes are believed to be involved in this process, namely, SC chymotryptic enzyme (SCCE), SC tryptic enzymes (SCTE), SC thiol protease (SCTP now known as cathepsin L-2), cathepsin E, and the aspartic protease cathepsin D. SCCE and SCTE are alkaline-optimal en-

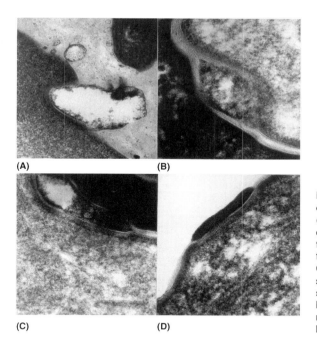

(A)   (B)

(C)   (D)

FIGURE 9 Electron micrographs of tape strippings of normal skin (grade 1). Degradation of corneodesmosomes (CD) toward the surface of the SC: (**A**) First strip, CD fully degraded; (**B**) second strip; CD partially degraded and encapsulated by lipid lamellae; (**C**) third strip; CD partially degraded, vaculation of structure. (**D**) Third strip, normal CD in contact with lamellar lipids. *Source*: From Ref. 24.

zymes, whereas the latter ones are acidic-optimum enzymes (28–32). Cathepsin L has also recently been implicated in Cdsn hydrolysis (33). Only SCTE and not SCCE, however, was capable of degrading Dsg 1 (34). This enzyme was also reported to be involved in the processing of pro-SCCE. Bernard et al. (35) have also identified an endoglycosidase, heparanase 1, within the SC, thought to play a role in the pre-proteolytic processing of the protecting sugar moieties on corneodesmosomal proteins. Cdsn undergoes several proteolytic steps. Cleavage of the N-terminal glycine loop domain occurs first at the compactum-disjunctum interface (48–46- to 36–30-kDa transition), followed by cleavage of the C-terminal glycine loop domain in exfoliated corneocytes (36–30- to 15-kDa transition) (36). The last step appears to be inhibited by calcium resulting in residual intercorneocyte cohesion. Nevertheless, the presence of oligosaccharides did not protect Cdsn against proteolysis by SCCE (34). A complete list of the putative desquamatory enzymes is given in Table 1.

These enzymes are secreted with the lamellar bodies and have been immunolocalized to the intercorneocyte lipid lamellae. Sondell et al. (37) used antibodies that immunoreact precisely with pro-SCCE to confirm that this enzyme was transported to the SC extracellular space via lamellar bodies. In later studies, using antibodies to both pro-SCCE and SCCE, Watkinson et al. (38) demonstrated that the processed enzyme was more associated with the corneodesmosomal plaque. More recently, Igarashi et al. (39) have immunolocalized cathepsin D to the intercellular space, whereas cathepsin E was localized within the corneocytes. Finally, KLK8 has also been reported to be localized to the intercellular spaces of the SC (40).

Naturally, as the desquamatory enzymes are present in the intercellular space, the physical properties of the SC lipids, together with the water activity in this microenvironment, will influence their activity. However, SCCE appears to have a

TABLE 1 Desquamatory Enzymes

Sphingoid hydrolases	Ceramidase	
	Glucocerebrosidase	
	Sphingomylinase	
	Sphingomyelin deacylase	
	Glucosylceramide deacylase	
Sulfatases	Steroid sulfatase	
Glycosidases	Heparanase 1	
Serine proteases	SC chymotryptic-like enzyme	(SCCE/KLK7)
	SC tryptic-like enzyme	(SCTE/KLK5)
Cysteine proteases	SC thiol protease	(SCTP/L2)
	SC cathepsin L-like enzyme	(SCCL)
Aspartic proteases	SC cathepsin D-like enzyme	(SCCDE)
	SC cathepsin E-like enzyme	(SCCEE)
	Skin aspartic protease	(SASPase)
	Caspase 14	

Abbreviation: SC, stratum corneum.

greater tolerance to water deprivation than other proteolytic enzymes and this may be an adaptation to maintain enzyme activity even within the water-depleted SC intercellular space (41). However, a variety of inhibitors are also present to attenuate their activities, cholesterol sulfate being one. Other protein and peptide inhibitors are present such as elfin, covalently bound to the corneocyte envelope, antileuko-proteinase, α-1-antitrypsin, α-1-antichymotrypsin, and the SPINK5-derived pep-tides (42). Antileukoprotease is believed to be the major physiological inhibitor of SCCE; the serpins are too low in concentration to be physiologically relevant (43). Caubet et al. (34) recently speculated in a new model of desquamation that SPINK5 may also inhibit SCTE.

Currently, little is understood of the molecular activation mechanisms of SCCE or other enzymes within the SC, but Brattsand et al. (44) have proposed a model for the activation of the kallikreins (Fig. 10). Clearly, SC pH and water content will in-fluence enzymic activity. As the SC pH declines toward the surface of the skin, the

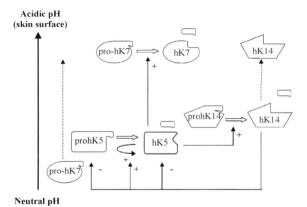

FIGURE 10 Proposed kallikrein activation cascade in human SC. *Source*: From Ref. 44.

activity of SCTE and SCCE may be reduced and perhaps the acid-optimal cathepsin enzymes mediate the final desquamatory steps. The role of the newly identified skin aspartic protease and caspase 14 is still awaiting clarification.

CORNEOCYTE ENVELOPE MATURATION AND THE ROLE OF TRANSGLUTAMINASES

The corneocyte envelope is an extremely insoluble proteinaceous layered structure whose stability is attributed to the degree of cross-linking of envelope proteins by either disulfide, glutamyl-lysine isodipeptide bonds or glutamyl polyamine cross-linking of glutamine residues of several corneocyte envelope proteins (45). The enzymes, responsible for catalysing the γ-glutamyl-ε-lysine isodipeptide bond formation, are the calcium-dependent transglutaminases (TGase; glutamyl-amine aminotransferases EC 2.3.2.13), of which four are expressed in the epidermis: TGase 1, 2, 3, and 5. However, only TGase 1, 3, and 5 are thought to be involved in keratinocyte differentiation.

During the formation of the corneocyte envelope at early time points in the keratinocyte differentiation process, envoplakin and periplakin are expressed and become associated with desmosomes in the viable epidermis. Subsequently, involucrin (the glutamyl-rich protein that covalently binds to lipids) is expressed at the same time as TGase 1 (46–48). TGase 1 then cross-links involucrin to the other early expressed proteins, such as members of the small proline rich (SPRR) family, and subsequently, other plasma membrane proteins become cross-linked and these form a scaffold for further reinforcement and maturation events (49).

When viewed by Normarski microscopy, corneocyte envelopes (CEs) were shown to have a crumpled surface when isolated from the lower layers of the SC and a smoother, more flattened surface when isolated from the upper SC (Fig. 11). These two populations of corneocyte envelopes were named fragile (CEf) and rigid (CEr). Mils et al. (50) reported that about 80% of corneocytes from volar forearm skin were smooth and rigid, whereas 90% from foot sole were rough or fragile cells. They can also be further differentiated by their binding of tetra methyl rhodamine isothiocyanate (TRITC), with the rigid envelopes staining to a greater extent (51), however, Hirao et al. (52) used a more elegant method to identify corneocyte envelopes based on their hydrophobicity (staining with Nile red) and antigenicity (to anti-involucrin). It is clear from these studies that immature envelopes (CEf) occur in the deeper layers of the SC (involucrin-positive and weak staining to Nile red or TRITC) and that mature envelopes occur in the surface layers of healthy skin (apparent

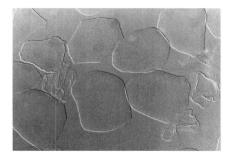

FIGURE 11 Normaski phase contrast microscopy of TRIC stained cornified envelopes demonstrating increased fluorescence labeling of Cer compared with CEf. *Source*: From Ref. 51.

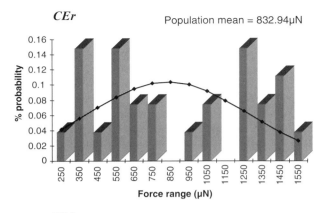

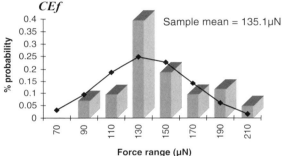

FIGURE 12 Distribution profile of the maximal compressional forces (μN) of individual CEs. Top panel shows the force range for Cer and the bottom for CEf. The maximal compression force was significantly different between the corneocytes. *Source*: From Ref. 51.

involucrin staining lessened and increased staining with Nile red or TRITC). More recent work from Kashibuchi et al. (53) using atomic force microscopy confirmed these structural changes in corneocytes from the deeper layers of the SC.

The classification of fragile and rigid envelopes has subsequently been found to be a pertinent classification system as, mechanically, they have fragile and rigid characteristics under compressional force (Fig. 12) (51). Supporting this concept of increasing CE strength, γ-glutamyl-lysine cross-links also increase in the subsequent layers of the SC, due to enhanced TGase activity. Three pools of TGase activity have been identified in the SC, which have been classified based upon their solubility characteristics: a water-soluble TGase (mainly TGase 1 and 3), a detergent-soluble TGase (TGase 1) and a particulate form that cannot be liberated from the corneocyte. Whether all enzyme fractions are active in this maturation process of CEf to CEr is currently unknown.

STRATUM CORNEUM NATURAL MOISTURIZING FACTORS

Readers should refer to older reviews for a historical perspective on filaggrin biology (1) where it is described that NMF allows the outermost layers of the SC to retain moisture against the desiccating action of the environment. Traditionally, it was believed that this water plasticized the SC, keeping it resilient by preventing cracking and flaking that might occur through mechanical stress. The general mechanisms by which these NMF components influence SC functionality have been studied extensively. The specific ionic interaction between keratin and NMF, accompanied by a decreased mobility of water, leads to a reduction of intermolecular forces between the keratin fibers and an increased elastic behavior. Recent studies have emphasized that it is the neutral and basic free amino acids (54), in particular, that are important for the plasticization properties of the SC. The generation of NMF is summarized by Mechin et al. (Fig. 13) (55) who highlight the importance of peptidylarginine deminases involved in the processing of filaggrin allowing its hydrolysis to NMF.

Hyaluronic acid and glycerol have recently been shown to be present naturally in the SC (56). Glycerol can also be derived from sebaceous triglyceride breakdown and again, to emphasize the importance of this molecule, studies by Fluhr et al. (57) have indicated that topically applied glycerol can restore to normal the quality of SC observed in asebic mice (lacking sebaceous secretions). The importance of glycerol as a natural skin moisturizng molecule has also been shown by Elias et al. (58). These two molecules have been largely ignored in descriptions of NMF composition (1). A further understanding of the effect of lactate on SC properties was recently described. Lactate and potassium were found to be the only components of NMF that correlated significantly with the state of hydration, stiffness, and pH, in the SC (59).

An acid pH within the SC, or the so-called acid mantle, is critical to the correct functioning of this tissue. Studies point to the role of free fatty acids, generated through phospholipase activity, as being vital for SC acidification (60), whereas Krein and Kermici (61) have recently proposed that urocanic acid (UCA) plays a vital role in the regulation of SC pH. Although this is in dispute, it is likely that all NMF components contribute significantly to the overall maintenance of pH.

Other components of NMF, not derived from filaggrin and urea, like lactate may also be derived in part from sweat. However, the presence of sugars in the SC represents primarily the activity of the enzyme β-D-glucocerebrosidase, as it catalyses the removal of glucose from glucosylceramides to initiate lipid lamellae organization in the deep SC (1).

In the last decade new tools have been developed for the measurement of such compounds in vivo. Caspers et al. (62) have pioneered the use of confocal Raman

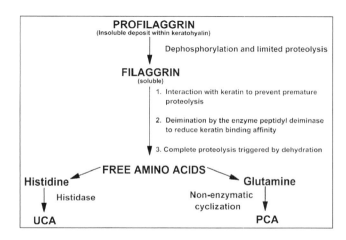

FIGURE 13 Schematic representation of profilaggrin catabolism and filaggrin hydrolysis to NMF and activation of peptidylarginine deiminase. *Source*: From Ref. 4.

microspectroscopy to determine the concentration of defined NMF components, non-invasively, in vivo within the SC.

THE EFFECT OF HUMIDITY ON EPIDERMAL DIFFERENTIATION AND SC QUALITY

Before considering the biology of dry skin, it is important to review the effect of environmental conditions on the SC and the epidermis, as these are the primary initiating events for the precipitation of the condition. Rogers et al. (63) demonstrated that there was a significant reduction in the levels of SC ceramides and fatty acids, together with linoleate-containing CER EOS in subjects in winter compared with summer. Similar differences in scalp lipid levels have been observed between the wet and dry seasons in Thailand (64). More importantly, Declercq et al. (65) have reported an adaptive response in human barrier function, where subjects living in a dry climate such as in Arizona (compared with a humid climate in New York) had much stronger barrier function and less dry skin due to increased ceramide levels and increased desquamatory enzyme levels (SCCE and SCTE).

Elias et al. have conducted several studies that support these findings. TEWL was reduced by approximately 30% in animals exposed to a dry (<10% RH) environment due to increased lipid biosynthesis, increased lamellar body extrusion and a slightly thicker SC layer, whereas in animals exposed to a high humidity environment (80% RH), this induction of lipid biosynthesis was reduced (66). However, abrupt changes in environmental humidity can also influence SC moisturization (67). After transferring animals from a humid (80% RH) to dry (<10% RH) environment, a sixfold increase in TEWL occurred. Barrier function returned to normal within seven days due to normal lipid repair processes. These changes did not occur in animals transferred from a normal to dry humidity environment. Changes in barrier function have also been reported in a group of Chinese workers who were exposed to very low humidity conditions. However, the changes in barrier function take longer to reach equilibrium than anticipated from the animal studies (68). Similar findings were reported for the water-holding capacity and free amino acid content of the SC. Katagiri et al. (69) demonstrated that exposure of mice to a humid environment, and subsequent transfer to a dry one, reduced skin conductance and amino acid levels, even at seven days following transfer; after transfer from a normal environment, however, decreased amino acid levels recovered within three days.

Exposure to low humidity conditions also increases epidermal DNA synthesis and amplifies the DNA synthetic response to barrier disruption (70). Equally, when in a dry environment epidermal interleukin 1 levels increased and levels of this cytokine were greater when the barrier was experimentally challenged (71). More recently, the same group also reported increased numbers of mast cells and increased dermal histamine levels (but unchanged epidermal histamine levels) (72).

These changes in barrier properties of the SC are attributable to changes in SC moisture content and provide evidence that changes in environmental humidity contribute to the seasonal exacerbation or amelioration of xerotic skin conditions, which are characterized by a defective barrier, epidermal hyperplasia, and inflammation.

WINTER- AND SOAP-INDUCED DRY SKIN

In dry, flaky skin conditions, corneodesmosomes are not degraded efficiently and corneocytes accumulate on the skin's surface layer leading to scaling and flaking.

Increased levels of corneodesmosomes in soap-induced dry skin were first reported by Rawlings et al. (24) but have been confirmed more recently by Simon et al. (73). Many corneodesmosomal proteins are increased in the SC and surface layers of xerotic skin (24, 72–74). Interestingly, however, in winter xerosis, the accumulation of the corneodemosomal proteins, Dsg1, and plakoglobin, correlated with each other. Cdsn protein levels, which were also increased, do not, however, have such an association suggesting that different proteolytic mechanisms occur for the different corneodesmosomal components during desquamation. As suggested by Simon et al. (73), as plakoglobin is a cytoplasmic protein, this would indicate that at least the cytoplasmic domain of Dsg1 may be cleaved. In fact, immunoreactivity to the carboxy-terminal tail of the cytoplasmic portion of Dsg1 was observed. Perhaps the intracellular portions of Dsg1 are also degraded within the corneocyte (for example, plakoglobin by the trypsin-like activity or cathepsin E activity reported within the corneocyte matrix). Conversely, Cdsn might be degraded by SCCE, SCTE or cathepsin D in the lamellar matrix. This is consistent with early electron microscope images (24) showing that corneodesmosomes become internally vacuolated, followed by complete detachment of the protein structures from the corneocyte envelope (Fig. 9).

The lamellar lipid matrix is also perturbed dramatically in dry skin (Fig. 14) (24). As the main desquamatory enzymes are found within this lipid matrix, the physical properties of the lamellar lipids will, therefore, influence enzyme activity.

Reduced levels of SCCE were originally reported by Rawlings et al. (5) in the outer layers of xerotic SC compared with normal skin. This was confirmed recently in more extensive studies by Van Overloop et al. (75) who found that the equally important SCTE activity was also reduced. Conversely, in sodium lauryl sulfate

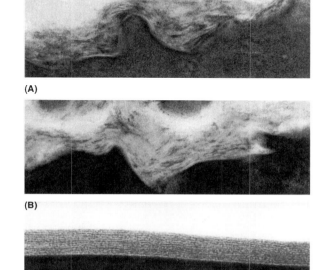

(A)

(B)

(C)

FIGURE 14 Organization of SC lipids in tape stripping of subjects with winter xerosis. Transmission electron micrographs of tape strippings of individuals with severe xerosis. Perturbation in lipid organization toward the surface of the SC. (**A**) First strip, disorganized lipid lamellae; (**B**) second strip, disorganized lipid lamellae; (**C**) third strip, normal lipid lamellae (×200,000). *Source*: From Ref. 24.

(SLS)–induced dry skin, increased activities of these enzymes were reported (29). More recently, the overactivation of the plasminogen cascade has been associated with dry skin. Normally, only observed in the epidermal basal layers, skin plasmin is widely distributed through the epidermis in dry skin. A urokinase-type plasminogen activator also exists in the SC (76). Clearly, these and other enzymes are potentially involved in the inflammatory and hyperproliferative aspects of dry skin.

It is now well established that in hyperproliferative disorders such as dry skin there is a change in SC lipid composition. In particular, the composition of the ceramide subtypes change and a predominance of sphingosine-containing ceramides (at the expense of the phytosphingosine-containing ceramides) have been observed in the SC of subjects with dry skin. Fulmer and Kramer (77) first identified these changes in SDS induced dry skin (increased levels of ceramide 2 and 4, and reduced levels of ceramide 3). However, Saint-Leger et al. (78) could not find any changes in ceramide levels in dry skin, but found increased fatty acid levels. Rawlings et al. demonstrated reduced levels of ceramides at the surface of the SC in winter xerosis (24). At this time, the full complexity of the different ceramide structure was not known but Chopart et al. (79) observed dramatic reductions in the levels of phytosphingosine-containing ceramides in dry skin (approximately 50%), together with a shortening and lengthening of the acyl-sphingoid bases sphingosine and 6-hydroxysphingosine. Van Overloop et al. (75) also demonstrated that the phytosphingosine-containing ceramides were reduced to a greater extent than other ceramides, with increasing dryness levels. Fulmer and Kramer (77) also observed dramatic reductions in the levels of long-chain fatty acids in dry skin. Imokawa et al. (80) did not find reduced ceramide levels in xerotic skin (but only average levels, rather than superficial levels, were measured).

These changes in lipid composition will, of course, influence the lamellar packing of the lipids. In fact, Schreiner et al. (81) established a reduction of CER EOS and EOH with increased concentrations of sphingosine-containing ceramides (CER NS and CER AS) and crystalline cholesterol in association with a loss of the LPP. However, although the lipid ultrastructure is clearly aberrant in the outer layers of dry skin (24), more work is needed to ascribe a particular lipid phase.

The proportions the different corneocyte envelope phenotypes also change in subjects with dry skin (44,51). Soap washing leads to a dramatic increase in the levels of the fragile envelope phenotype at the expense of the rigid phenotype. It is known that SC transglutaminase activities increase toward the surface of the SC, particularly the detergent-soluble and particulate fractions. Although the same trend of the relative increase in TGase between the inner and outer corneum is true of dry skin, TGase activities are dramatically lowered in dry skin compared with healthy skin, particularly the detergent-soluble fraction, which contains mainly TGase 1.

Reduced NMF levels are also implicated in dry skin conditions. The loss of NMF generally reported with increased ageing, however, is not consistent with the recent observations (82) of increased NMF in subjects with senile xerosis, and suggests that our understanding of this process is far from complete.

THE DRY SKIN CYCLE MODEL

Recently, it has been proposed that the induction and propagation of dry skin conditions may be best and most intuitively expressed as a cyclical model, dependent on SC integrity and particularly upon barrier function and homeostasis (2). In this model, it is emphasized that a spiralling deterioration in skin condition occurs that, without intervention, would lead to a progressive worsening in model endpoints. Additionally, it is implicit that intervention at one, or preferably multiple, points within this cycle is necessary to arrest the progression of this continuing downward spiral. The model describes several phases within this cycle and, therefore, possible targets against which treatments could be directed. Reference to the graphical depiction of the model (Fig. 15) may facilitate complete understanding of the relationship of these phases.

The induction phase can be mediated by a variety of different factors:

- Low environmental temperature and humidity
- Abrupt changes in environmental conditions that includes the effect of modern indoor climate-controlled environments
- Surfactant dissolution of SC lipid and NMF
- Chronological ageing and genetics

Once the skin is provoked by one or more of these factors, there is an inevitable sequence of events that may be described conveniently as a cycle.

Blank (8) estimated that the SC loses its flexibility once its water content falls below approximately 10%, the provocation for which may constitute one or a combination of the factors noted above. Without intervention, this quickly leads to a steeper SC hydration gradient, a decrease in net recondensation on the SC surface, a corresponding increase in evaporative water loss from the SC surface, a consequent further drop in SC water concentration, and so on. The inevitable rapid consequence of this series of events is a decrease in the plastic or viscous properties of the SC (commonly interpreted as skin softness or suppleness), an increase in SC fragility/brittleness and an impairment of SC barrier function (83–86). This surface dehydration is the first step in the development of the dry skin cycle and is further exacerbated by destruction of the normal barrier lipid lamellae in the outer layers of the SC during bathing (24). The impaired barrier in the superficial layers of the SC allows leaching of NMF from the outermost skin cells, thereby reducing SC water activity. Whiteness between the dermatoglyphics (caused by backscatter from multiple tissue–air interfaces) and minor scaling due to the dehydration of individual

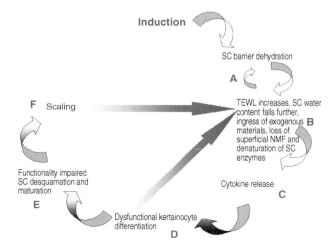

FIGURE 15 Schematic diagram showing pivotal events within the dry skin cycle. *Abbreviations:* NMF, natural moisturizing factor; SC, stratum corneum; TEWL, transepidermal water loss. *Source*: From Ref. 2.

corneocytes are the first visible steps in the cycle. Perturbation to the barrier then leads to further development of dry skin.

Enhanced keratinocyte proliferation, consequent hyperkeratosis, and mild inflammatory changes, one of the hallmarks of dry skin conditions, occur as the skin attempts to repair itself. This response is mediated via production and secretion of cytokines and growth factors, with many researchers citing the ratio between interleukin-1 receptor antagonist protein and interleukin 1α as a key marker of this process (87–90). The degree of hyperproliferation is dependent upon the corresponding degree of barrier perturbation (91), probably reflecting both the ingress of exogenous irritants through the impaired barrier and the growing realization that the SC barrier is itself a biosensor and that corneocytes and keratinocytes are participating in the release of these messengers. The hyperproliferation of the epidermis probably occurs as a result of the double paracrine signalling events between the epidermis and dermis. Interleukin 1 acts on fibroblasts that, in turn, secrete KGF and GMCSF inducing hyperproliferation and dysfunctional differentiation of keratinocytes (92).

The induction of this inflammatory hyperproliferative state is absolutely a key in the cycle of dry skin as it fundamentally leads to aberrant differentiation and the overhasty production of a variety of poor quality materials and structures vital to the proper functioning of the SC barrier and normal healthy skin. These include

1. the production of smaller and immature corneocyte envelopes;
2. changes in epidermal lipid and particular ceramide biology;
3. reduced protease and transglutaminase activity;
4. reduced filaggrin synthesis and NMF levels.

Finally, a loss in efficiency of desquamation, due to reduced activity of desquamatory enzymes at the surface of the dry SC, and ensuing scaling, thickening and loss of hygroscopicity of the SC occurs. Marked scaling is one of the obvious consumer-noticeable expressions of dry skin. The formation of a thicker SC with impaired desquamation has, again, immense biophysical importance. The water gradient across the thicker SC becomes steeper, leading to further increases in evaporative water loss, reducing further water concentration in the outer SC and propagating directly another round of the dry skin cycle.

Corneocytes that should be in a mature fully hydrophobed format are now replaced by fragile corneocytes. The resulting barrier protecting these corneocytes and their contents is now weaker due to changes in barrier lipid profiles and surface hydrophobicity. Equally, the hygroscopic (though highly water-labile) NMF present within corneocytes of normal SC, are depleted gradually through normal everyday activities such as cleansing and/or occupational duties (1,60). The corneocytes of dry SC are, therefore, subject to exaggerated insult due to their changed biochemical and biophysical properties. The dry skin cycle, thus, is propagated further by an increased loss of NMF relative to normal skin and a corresponding loss in SC hygroscopicity.

Finally and most importantly, the development of an increasingly thick, dry SC results in a layer characterized, from a biomechanical viewpoint, by a dramatic increase in hardness and brittleness. The consumer perceives this as tightness. These properties create an SC barrier inherently susceptible to mechanical stress and fracture, another factor driving the impairment in barrier function cyclical nature of the dry skin cycle.

The clinical endpoint of dry skin cannot be regarded as static but rather is most fully described as a cycle that, without intervention, tends to perpetuate itself. Pivotal to every stage of this cycle and its propagation is a compromised SC barrier. Interventions that truly break the dry skin cycle, therefore, by definition need to repair and augment SC barrier function.

MOISTURIZERS AND THE MANAGEMENT OF DRY SKIN
Humectants and Occlusive Agents
Traditionally, humectants, occlusives, and emollients have been, and will continue to be, the mainstay of cosmetic treatments (93), and arguably, the most widely used and effective humectant used for xerotic skin is glycerol, due to its excellent safety profile, cost, and outstanding water-retaining (humectant) and hygroscopic properties. There is now much evidence, however, that glycerol is not only a mere humectant, but also (*i*) is a lipid fluidizer (94), modulating the temperature-dependent rheology

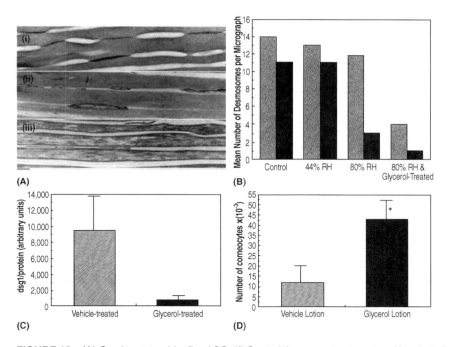

FIGURE 16   (**A**) Osmium tetroxide–fixed SC. (*i*) Control tissue, no treatment and incubated at 44% RH. Note electron dense corneodesmosomes fully intact. (*ii*) Tissue incubated at 80% RH for seven days. Note partial degradation of corneodesmosomes. (*iii*) Tissue incubated at 80% RH following 5% glycerol treatment. Note paucity of corneodesmosomes and virtually complete degradation of their structures. (**B**) Comparison of the number of corneodesmosomes in control SC and SC incubated at 44%, 80%, and 80% RH following 5% glycerol treatment. Note the decrease in intact corneodesmosomes in 80% RH-treated samples and the significantly reduced number of intact (black boxes) and total (gray boxes) corneodesmosomes in glycerol-treated tissue incubated at 80% RH. (**C**) Comparison of the effect of 5% glycerol on Dsg 1 digestion at 80% RH. Note the dramatic decrease in Dsg 1 levels in glycerol-treated samples. (**D**) Comparison of the effect of lotions with and without the addition of 5% glycerol on corneocyte release. *Source*: From Ref. 95.

of SC lipids, thus preventing a loss of fluidity of their lamellar structure at low relative humidities, and (*ii*) has ^{corneodesmolytic} activity, facilitating the proteolytic digestion of superficial corneodesmosomes in dry skin (Fig. 16) (95).

Humectants are also an essential requirement for most of the additional approaches. In O/W creams, occlusives and bilayer-forming lipids (described below) also require glycerol to alleviate dry skin. Moreover, humectants are required for the transglutaminase-mediated corneocyte envelope maturation required for a healthy SC (Fig. 17) (96). In this respect, combinations of humectants including glycerol have been shown to be more effective than using glycerol alone. Glycerol has also been shown to enhance the barrier function of the SC (97).

Like glycerol, urea is a natural component of the SC NMF and has been used as a humectant in creams since 1943 (98). Urea (10%) has been shown to be more efficacious than salicylic acid and petroleum jelly. Urea-containing moisturizers have been reported to improve barrier function, reduce TEWL, increase skin capacitance, and reduce irritation (99–102).

As a principal component of NMF there is considerable interest in the ability of pyrrolidone carboxylic acid (PCA) and its derivatives to moisturize the SC. Creams and lotions containing the sodium salt of PCA are reported to hydrate the SC and improve dry, flaky skin (103–107).

Petroleum jelly acts primarily as an occlusive agent having been shown to reduce TEWL by over 98%, whereas other oils only manage a 20% to 30% reduction. Yet this agent does not simply act as an occlusive film over the surface of the skin. It has been shown to diffuse into the SC intercellular domains, which may add to its efficacy. On penetrating the epidermis, it was also shown to accelerate lipid biosynthesis thereby aiding barrier repair (108).

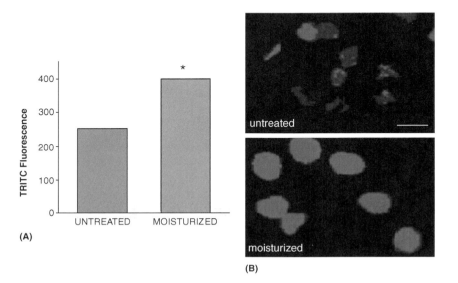

FIGURE 17 Enhanced CE maturation in dry skin following moisturization. (**A**) Evidence of increased TRITC staining (*P* < 0.00001); (**B**) as visualized under a fluorescent microscope. *Source*: From. Ref. 51.

Bilayer-Forming Lipids

From current understanding of the compositional changes in dry skin, five aspects of SC lipid biochemistry need to be corrected:

1. The lowered levels of ceramides generally
2. The phytosphingosine-containing ceramide insufficiency
3. The ceramide 1 linoleate (CEOS) insufficiency
4. The lowered covalently bound ceramides
5. The precise chain length of the ceramide sphingoid bases and free fatty acids

Overall, however, the lipid lamellar architecture in the outer layers of the SC needs to be normalized in dry, flaky skin conditions. Evidence also indicates that a reduction in long-chain fatty acids also occurs in SLS-induced dry skin. As these lipids are important for inducing an orthorhombic lateral packing state they also need to be supplied to the skin to more effectively correct barrier function. Moreover correction of the reduction of SC NMF levels, correction of the aberration of corneocyte envelope maturation and the impaired corneodesmolysis is needed for dry skin treatments.

Several clinical studies evaluating the effects of ceramides have been conducted recently. However, it is important to remember that to derive the full benefits

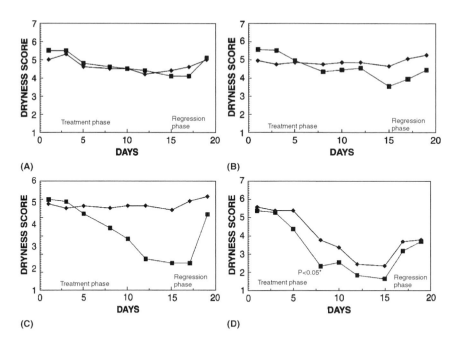

FIGURE 18 Moisturization efficacy tests: (**A**) Comparing the effect of 1% glycerol (square) with a no-treatment control (triangle); (**B**) comparing the effect of a lotion containing 1% phospholipids, 2% cholesterol and 1% stearic acid (square) with a no-treatment control (triangle); (**C**) comparing the effect of a lotion containing 1% phospholipids, 2% cholesterol, and 1% stearic acid plus 1% glycerol (square) with a no-treatment control (triangle); (**D**) comparing the effect of a lotion containing 1% phospholipid, 2% cholesterol, 1% stearic acid plus 5% glycerol (square) with a lotion containing 1% petrolatum, 2% cholesterol, 1% stearic acid plus 5% glycerol (triangle). *Source*: From Ref. 115.

of ceramide technology, formulation into heavy emulsions where other emollients dominate the formulation will be difficult to discern unless the ceramides are at a high enough concentration. Two studies investigated the properties of Locobase Repair cream and found opposite effects on barrier recovery. Barany et al. (109) did not find any improvements over placebo, whereas Kucharekova et al. (110) found that the CER NP containing cream significantly reduced TEWL, erythema, and epidermal proliferation compared with placebo cream. Further improvements in function are observed with complete lipid mixtures. De Paepe et al. (111) demonstrated improvements in barrier functionality and SC hydration from a lipid mixture of CER NP (0.2%), CER AS (0.1%), and CER UP (0.2%) together with cholesterol (0.25%), linoleic acid (0.25%), and phytosphingosine (0.5%) compared with placebo lotions and a lotion containing only CER NP (0.6%) and CER UP (0.4%). The increases in TEWL and SC hydration are shown in Fig. 15. Berardesca et al. (112) have also established that balanced lipid mixtures containing CER NP are effective in improving the barrier properties and clinical condition of skin in subjects with contact dermatitis. Equally convincing are the studies of Chamlin et al. (113) showing that a ceramide dominant barrier repair cream alleviated childhood atopic dermatitis. Over the six-week treatment period, TEWL values decreased by 50% and the number of D-squame tape strippings required to break the barrier increased from approximately 12 to 22 indicating a stronger SC barrier function. In addition to ceramides, which have been introduced to supplement the SC barrier (114), phospholipids are also bilayer-forming lipids and when combined with glycerol have been shown to be clinically superior to petroleum jelly in relieving dry skin (Fig. 18) (115).

Hydroxyacids
Hydroxyacids are used to facilitate desquamation and improve lipid biosynthesis and barrier function. The influence of α- and β-hydroxy acids (116) on desquamation is well established (Fig. 19) but new lipophilic variants of salicylic acid appear to influence corneodesmolysis differently. Whereas lactic and salicylic acid act on all corneodesmosomes, LSA only acted on the stratum disjunctum corneodesmosomes. These lipophilic variants appear to act on the whole structure of the corneodesmosomes, whereas the "ordinary" acids fractionate the corneodesmosomes. Fartarsch et al. (117) also demonstrated that the action of glycolic acid on corneodesmolysis

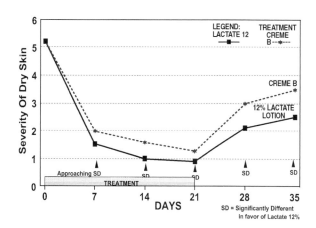

FIGURE 19 Improvement in dry skin condition following twice daily applications of a 12% lactic acid formulation. *Source*: From Ref 121.

was restricted to the stratum disjunctum suggesting a targeted action without compromising barrier function. Medium-chain fatty acids have also been reported to improve SC flexibility and assist in the relief of dry skin in combination with barrier lipids. Further enhanced dry skin relief was observed in the presence of barrier lipids (118), and the L-isomer, in particular, increased SC extensibility and keratinocyte ceramide synthesis (Fig. 20) (119). In SC extensibility studies, using extensions where only lipids are believed to be extended, longer chain α-hydroxyacids also plasticize the corneum (120).

SC turnover time, measured by dansyl chloride (a measure of epidermal proliferation matched by desquamation), increased by 15% after applying a moisturizing cream at pH 3.8. Further increases were obtained by increasing the concentration of the free acid of glycolic acid or by decreasing the pH of the base. At 8% glycolic acid (4% free acid), Johnson (122) reported approximately 30% increase in SC turnover time. The increased turnover time must be matched by increased desquamation otherwise retention hyperkeratosis would occur. Desquamation is enhanced by further activating acidic-optimum enzymes or by chelating calcium, which is known to reduce the final processing steps of Cdsn degradation.

Not all hydroxyacids perform equally and some appear to enhance the skin's sensitivity to UV irradiation (e.g., glycolic acid). However, glucanolactone and tartaric acid have been shown to be superior to glycolic acid and lactic acid in improving barrier function (Fig. 21) and do not increase sunburn cell formation (123).

Moisturization Augmentation by Inducing Epidermal Differentiation and Lipogenesis

Unsaturated fatty acids are ligands for nuclear receptors such as the peroxisomal proliferator–activated receptor, and have been shown to improve epidermal

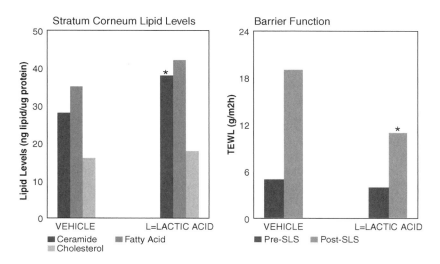

FIGURE 20 Effect of lactic acid on SC lipid levels and barrier function following a one-month topical application of 4% lactic acid in an aqueous vehicle. TEWL evaluated before application of SLS patch and 24 hours after removal (*$P < 0.05$). *Source*: From Ref. 119.

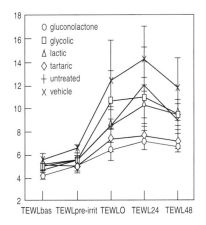

FIGURE 21 TEWL after sodium lauryl sulfate challenge (g/m²/hr). Lower barrier damage was detected in α-hydroxy acid–treated sites compared with vehicle and untreated sites. *Source*: From Ref. 123.

differentiation and increase ceramide and filaggrin levels (124). This superfamily of nuclear transcription receptors includes receptors for retinoic acid, steroids, thyroid, and vitamin D, together with the peroxisome proliferator–activated receptor (PPAR), the farnesol-activated receptor (FXR), and the liver-activated receptor (LXR). These transcription factors bind their respective ligands and regulate many aspects of cellular proliferation and differentiation. Fatty acids are important ligands for the PPAR receptor, farnesol for the FXR, and hydroxylated cholesterol derivatives or cholestenoic acid for the LXR. All of these pathways stimulate epidermal differentiation and increased the synthesis of involucrin, filaggrin, and enzymes of the ceramide synthesis pathway.

The transcription factor most intensively investigated is the PPAR. There are three main PPAR isoforms α, β/δ, and γ. Nevertheless, PPAR-δ was recently observed to be the predominant PPAR subtype in human keratinocytes, whereas PPAR-α and PPAR-γ were only induced during epidermal differentiation suggesting nonredundant functions during differentiation (125). Respective ligands for all of these isoforms increase epidermal differentiation. Pharmaceutical ligands for the PPAR receptors increase ceramide synthesis in vitro by increasing the expression of SPT, glucosyl ceramide synthase and glucocerebrosidase but not sphingomyelinase (126). More recently, PPAR-δ ligands were found to be the most potent in inducing epidermal differentiation (tetrathioacetic acid) by increasing involucrin and transglutaminase while decreasing proliferation.

Petroselenic acid (127) and conjugated linoleic acid (128) have been identified as potent PPAR-α activators, improving epidermal differentiation, reducing inflammation, increasing extracellular matrix components and eliciting skin lightening. Increased levels of transglutaminase, involucrin, filaggrin and corneocyte envelope formation were observed in keratinocytes in vitro after treatment with petroselenic acid. These effects were confirmed in vivo by short-term patch testing over three weeks and increased involucrin and filaggrin were also observed (Fig. 22). Improvements in the signs of photodamage, skin tone, and dry skin were also observed in a 12-week clinical study on forearm skin (129). Octadecenedioic acid has also recently been identified as a pan-PPAR agonist (with a preference for PPAR-γ). It has been shown to reduce skin hyperpigmentation and is also expected to improve epidermal differentiation (130).

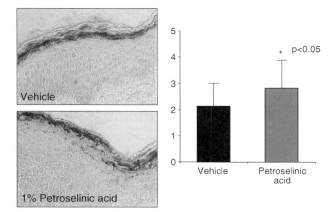

FIGURE 22 Increased synthesis of profilaggrin/filaggrin in human axilla skin detected by immunohistochemistry following a three-week application of a 1% petroselinic acid formulation. *Source*: From Ref. 131.

Changes in lipid levels and types can be corrected by topical application of agents to manipulate lipid synthesis within the epidermis. However, as described above in dry skin conditions, the epidermis produces less phytosphingosine-containing ceramides, changes the carbon chain lengths of other sphingoid bases and produces less long-chain fatty acids. These results suggest that changes in the levels or activities of the different fatty acid synthetases and the enzymes involved in phytosphingosine synthesis occur in dry skin. The biology of these enzymes is yet to be described in these conditions.

Elias et al. (132) used lipid mixtures to aid barrier recovery in acetone damaged barrier studies. Cholesterol was shown to aid barrier recovery in a tape-stripping model in aged skin but not young skin. In fact any incomplete mixture of the three major lipid species slows barrier recovery in this model. An equimolar mixture of the three dominant SC lipids allows normal rates of barrier recovery in normal skin, whereas adjustment to a 3:1:1 (ceramide/cholesterol/fatty acid) molar ratio accelerates barrier recovery. As expected the requirements for optimal barrier recovery in aged skin is different and it has been shown that a cholesterol dominant lipid mixture accelerates barrier recovery in aged skin, whereas a fatty acid dominant mixture delays barrier recovery. In young skin any lipid species can be dominant and the barrier will recover quickly but in atopic dermatitis a ceramide dominant mixture is required (133). Further studies on the use of long-chain fatty acids are recommended. It has been shown that mevalonic acid, the product of the rate limiting enzyme HMGCoA reductase, increases cholesterol biosynthesis (134).

There are several other means to increase ceramide synthesis in vivo and improve barrier function. As described above α-hydroxy acids, well known for their desquamatory properties, stimulate lipid biosynthesis. Lactic acid, especially the L-isomer, increases ceramide biosynthesis in vitro and in vivo. Presumably, lactic acid achieves this by acting as a general lipid precursor by providing acetate and more reducing power in the form of NADH or NADPH (135). Interestingly, lactic acid also increased the levels of linoleate-containing CER EOS, which may contribute to the improvements in skin functionality.

The pleotropic skin benefits of niacinamide have been the subject of intense study and have been excellently reviewed by Matts et al. (136). Niacinamide has been reported to stimulate the synthesis of glucosylceramides, sphingomeylin, cholesterol

TABLE 2 Agents That Increase Ceramide Biosynthesis

Lipids	Optimized mixtures of ceramides, cholesterol, fatty acids
Lipid precursors	Phytosphingosine, tetraacetylphytosphingosine, ω-hydroxy fatty acids, linoleic acid
α-Hydroxy acids	L-Lactic acid
Humectants	Glycerol, urea
Vitamins	Niacinamide, lipoic acid, ascorbic acid
Protease inhibitors	Aminocyclohexanecarboxylic acid, egg white lysozyme
Minerals	Magnesium, calcium
Histamine receptor	H1 receptor antagonist
Antagonists	H2 receptor antagonist
PPAR	PPAR-α agonists
Electrical potential	Negative potential
Triterpenoids	Ursolic acid
GABA agonists	GABA type A agonists (musimol, isoguvacine)
Purinergic receptor	P2Y antagonists
Fragrances	Fragrances
GC receptor	Glucocorticoid receptor antagonists

Abbreviations: PPAR, peroxisome proliferator–activated receptor; GABA, γ-aminobutyric acid.
Source: From Ref. 143.

and fatty acids by keratinocytes in vitro (129). The increases in ceramide synthesis were achieved by enhancing the activity of SPT together with the expression of LCB 1 and 2. In vivo, however, increased levels of SC fatty acid (67%) and ceramide (34%) levels were observed. Similar to studies with lactic acid, increases in the levels of SC cholesterol are refractory to change. Tanno et al. (137) have also been researching the changes in skin functionality in sensitive skin. In their most recent studies topical application of niacinamide improved the barrier of the most severely affected

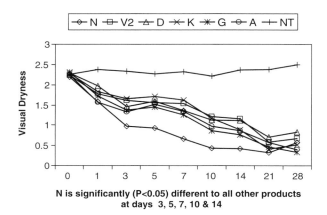

N is significantly (P<0.05) different to all other products
at days 3, 5, 7, 10 & 14

FIGURE 23 Results from the treatment phase of a Kligman-type regression study (products applied twice daily at 2 mg/cm² to randomized sites on the outer, lower leg of female subjects (n = 36) with inclusion of a no-treatment control). Products represented high-efficacy commercial moisturizers with ingredients of differing dry skin relief mechanism. *Abbreviations*: NT, no treatment control; N, niacinamide-containing lotion; A, lactic acid–containing moisturizer; other product codes represent commercial products with high loadings of traditional humectants and emollients (including glycerin and petrolatum). *Source*: From Ref. 2.

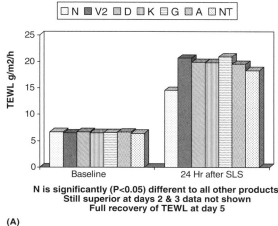

N is significantly (P<0.05) different to all other products
Still superior at days 2 & 3 data not shown
Full recovery of TEWL at day 5

(A)

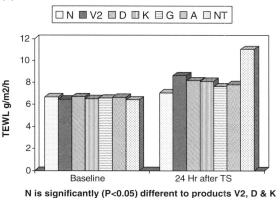

N is significantly (P<0.05) different to products V2, D & K

(B)

FIGURE 24 (**A**) Change in TEWL in posttreatment phase after SLS patch chemical insult expressed as difference from pretreatment baseline. (**B**) Change in TEWL in posttreatment phase after tape-stripping mechanical insult expressed as difference from pre-treatment baseline *Source*: From Ref. 147.

subject with sensitive skin with a concomitant improvement in stinging score. Ertel et al. (138) observed similar improvements in barrier functionality together with an increased SC turnover rate using a 2% niacinamide cream. Others (139) observed significant improvements in SC barrier function and improvement in global skin condition in subjects with stage I/II rosacea.

Topical application of phytosphingosine and its derivatives have also been shown to increase SC ceramide levels and barrier function (140). This is especially important as the phytosphingosine-containing ceramides are deficient in dry skin. Although increases in the total levels of ceramides were observed, greater increases in CER EOS and CER AS were found when combined with juniperic acid and linoleic acid. Linoleic acid on its own is incorporated into CER EOS in vivo (141), which is important for lipid phase behavior and skin properties. Lipid fractions from unsaponifiable fractions of avocado (furanyl-8-11- *cis* heptadecadiene) and sunflower oleodistillates (mainly linoleic and oleic acids) also increase ceramide and cholesterol biosynthesis ex vivo (142).

The effects of increasing SC lipid levels by stimulating ceramide biosynthesis have been investigated extensively by Denda et al. (141). Histamine antagonists and certain fragrances stimulate lipid biosynthesis. Mixtures of magnesium and calcium salts have also been shown to accelerate skin barrier recovery and improve surfactant- or tape-stripping–induced dry skin. Although these studies indicate the importance of these ions for epidermal homeostasis, more work is needed with cosmetic formulations. More recently, it has been demonstrated that γ-aminobutyric acid (GABA) type A receptor agonists, muscimol, and isoguvacine accelerate barrier recovery following disruption. Conversely, ATP (purinergic) receptor (P2X) agonists delay barrier recovery, whereas P2Y antagonists accelerate it. These also reduced the epidermal hyperproliferative response induced by acetone treatment under low environmental humidity (summary on Table 2).

Other agents have been shown to stimulate ceramide synthesis in vitro. Lipoic acid and *N*-acetylcysteine were also reported to increase ceramide synthesis in vitro (144). Recently vitamin C has been shown to activate PKC and increase ceramide synthesis and improve the ceramide subspecies profile in epidermal skin equivalents (145). Others (146) have also demonstrated that ursolic acid increased ceramides in human skin.

Recently, niacinamide has been formulated in lotions, together with glycerol and other NMF components, which effectively alleviate dry skin and provide significant improvement in SC barrier function (147). These lotions are more effective than traditional emollient and lactic acid–containing moisturizers in relieving dry skin in the treatment phase of a typical Kligman-type regression study (Fig. 23), to-

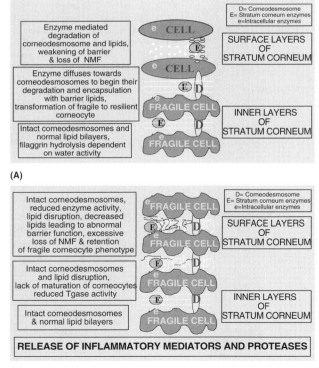

FIGURE 25 Summary of SC maturation and corneodesmolysis in (**A**) normal and (**B**) dry skin. *Source*: From Ref. 2.

gether with the changes in moisturization and barrier function as well as improving resistance to SLS and tape-stripping–induced barrier perturbation (Fig. 24) (100). Increased SC thickness due to increased SC hydration was also proven in vivo using Raman microspectroscopy following topical application of niacinamide lotions (148).

SUMMARY AND CONCLUSIONS

Tremendous advances in our knowledge of SC biology have been made over the last decade but more importantly the understanding of the aberration of the normal functioning of the SC in dry, flaky skin conditions has become clearer and a new model of dry skin has been described (Fig. 25). On perturbation of SC barrier function, superficial dehydration of the SC occurs and release of inflammatory mediators, induction of hyperproliferation, and disruption of epidermal differentiation is induced. As has become apparent, reductions in SC water and NMF levels, changes in lipid ultrastructure and reductions in enzyme activities contribute to the reduced corneodesmolysis that occurs in these conditions (Fig. 24). Although occlusives, emollients, and humectants have been the mainstay of cosmetic treatments, their effects on epidermal and SC biology have only recently been described. New ingredients, such as ceramides and other bilayer forming lipids, hydroxyacids, ligands for nuclear receptors such as PPAR and agents such as niacinamide, have been evaluated. The combination of traditional and new approaches has resulted in new therapies for the treatment of dry skin.

REFERENCES

1. Rawlings AV, Scott IR, Harding CR, et al. Stratum corneum moisturization at the molecular level. J Invest Dermatol 1994; 103:731–740.
2. Rawlings AV, Matts PJ. Stratum corneum moisturization at the molecular level: an update in relation to the dry skin cycle. J Invest Dermatol 2005; 124:1099–1110.
3. Rawlings AV. Skin waxes: their composition, properties, structures and biological significance. In: Hamilton, RJ, ed. Waxes: Chemistry, Molecular Biology and Functions. Dundee, Scotland: The Oily Press, 1994:221–256.
4. Harding CR, Watkinson A, Rawlings AV. Dry skin, moisturization and corneodesmolysis. Int J Cosmet Sci 2000; 22:21–52.
5. Rawlings AV, Harding CR, Watkinson, et al. Dry and xerotic skin conditions. In: Leyden JJ, Rawlings AV, eds. Skin Moisturization. New York: Marcel Dekker, 2002:119–143.
6. Rawlings AV. Trends in stratum corneum research and the treatment of dry skin conditions. Int J Cosmetic Sci 2003; 25:63–95.
7. Warner RR, Lilly NA. Correlation of water content with ultrastructure in the stratum corneum. In: Elsner P, Berardesca E, Maibach HI, eds. Bioengineering of the Skin: Water and the Stratum Corneum. Boca Raton, Fla: CRC Press, 1994:3–12.
8. Blank IH. Factors which influence the water content of the stratum corneum. J Invest Dermatol 1952; 18:433–440.
9. Rawlings AV, Harding CR. Moisturization and skin barrier function. Dermatol Ther 2004; 17: 43–48.
10. Pfeiffer S, Vielhaber G, Vietzke JP, et al. High-pressure freezing provides new information on human epidermis: simultaneous protein antigen and lamellar lipid structure preservation. Study on human epidermis by cryoimmobilization. J Invest Dermatol 2000; 114(5):1030–1038.
11. Norlen L. Skin barrier structure and function: The single gel phase model. J Invest Dermatol 2001; 117:830–836.

12. Norlen L, Al-Amoudi A. Stratum corneum keratin structure, function, and formation: the cubic rod-packing and membrane templating model. J Invest Dermatol 2004; 123(4):715–732.
13. Bouwstra JA, de Graaff A, Gooris GS, et al. Water distribution and related morphology in human stratum corneum at different hydration levels. J Invest Dermatol 2003; 120(5):750–758.
14. Richter T, Peuckert C, Sattler M, et al. Dead but highly dynamic—the stratum corneum is divided into three hydration zones. Skin Pharmacol Physiol 2004; 17(5):246–257.
15. Downing DT, Stewart ME. Epidermal composition. In: Loden M, Maibach HI, eds. Dry Skin and Moisturizers. Boca Raton, Fla: CRC Press, 2000:13–26.
16. Motta SM, Monti M, Sesana S, et al. Ceramide composition of psoriatic scale. Biochim Biophys Acta 1993; 1182: 147–151.
17. Oku H, Mimura K, Tokitsu Y, et al. Biased distribution of the branched-chain fatty acids in ceramides of vernix caseosa. Lipids 2000; 35(4):373–381.
18. Chopart M, Castiel-Higounenc I, Arbey E, et al. A new type of covalently bound ceramide in human epithelium. Stratum Corneum 2001; III (poster).
19. Hamanaka S, Hara M, Nishio H, et al. Human epidermal glucosylceramides are major precursors of stratum corneum ceramides. J Invest Dermatol 2002; 119:416–423.
20. Pilgram GSK, Engelsma-van Pelt AM, Bouwstra JA, et al. Electron diffraction provides new information on human stratum corneum lipid organisation studied in relation to depth and temperature. J Invest Dermatol 1999; 113:403–409.
21. Brancaleon L, Bamberg MP, Sakamaki T, et al. Attenuated total reflection-fourier transform infrared spectroscopy as a possible method to investigate biophysical parameters of stratum corneum in vivo. J Invest Dermatol 2001; 116:380–386.
22. Bouwstra J, Pilgram G, Gooris G, et al. New aspects of the skin barrier organization. Skin Pharmacol Appl Skin Physiol 2001; 14:52–62.
23. Bouwstra J, Gooris GS, Dubbelaar FER, et al. Phase behaviour of stratum corneum lipid mixtures based on human ceramides: The role of natural and synthetic ceramide 1. J Invest Dermatol 2002; 118:606–617.
24. Rawlings AV, Watkinson A, Rogers J, et al. Abnormalities in stratum corneum structure lipid composition and desmosome degradation in soap-induced winter xerosis. J Soc Cosmet Chem 1994; 45:203–220.
25. Warner RR, Boissy YL. Effect of moisturizing products on the structure of lipids in the outer stratum corneum of humans. In: Loden M, Maibach HI, eds. Dry Skin and Moisturisers. Boca Raton, Fla: CRC Press, 2000:349–372.
26. Berry N, Charmeil C, Gouion C, et al. A clinical, biometrological and ultrastructural study of xerotic skin. Int J Cosmet Sci 1999; 21:241–249.
27. Serre G, Mils V, Haftek M, et al. Identification of late differentiation antigens of human cornified epithelia, expressed in re-organized desmosomes and bound to cross-linked envelope. J Invest Dermatol 1991; 97:1061–1072.
28. Lundstorm A, Egelud T. Cell shedding from human plantar skin in vitro: evidence that two different types of protein structures are degraded by a chymotrypsin-like enzyme. Arch Dermatol Res 1990; 282:234–237.
29. Suzuki Y, Nomura J, Koyama J, et al. The role of proteases in stratum corneum: involvement in stratum corneum desquamation. Arch Dermatol Res 1994; 286:249–253.
30. Horikoshi T, Igarashi S, Uchiwa H, et al. Role of endogenous cathepsin D-like and chymotrypsin-like proteolysis in human epidermal desquamation. Br J Dermatol 1999; 141:453–459.
31. Horikoshi T, Arany I, Rajaraman S, et al. Isoforms of cathepsin D human epidermal differentiation. Biochimie 1998; 80:605–612.
32. Watkinson A. Stratum corneum thiol protease (SCTP): a novel cysteine protease of late epidermal differentiation Arch Dermatol Res 1999; 291:260–268.
33. Bernard D, Mehul B, Thomas-Collignon A, et al. Analysis of proteins with caseinolytic activity in a human stratum corneum extract revealed a yet unidentified cysteine protease and identified the so-called 'stratum corneum thiol protease' as cathepsin L2. J Invest Dermatol 2003; 120:592–600.
34. Caubet C, Jonca N, Brattsand M, et al. Degradation of corneodesmosome proteins by two serine proteases of the kallikrein family. J Invest Dermatol 2004; 122:1235–1244.

35. Bernard D, Mehul B, Delattre C, et al. Purification and characterization of the endogly-cosidase heparanase 1 from human plantar stratum corneum: a key enzyme in epidermal physiology. J Invest Dermatol 2001; 117:1266–1273.
36. Simon M, Jonca N, Guerrin M, et al. Refined characterization of corneodesmosin proteolysis during terminal differentiation of human epidermis and its relationship to desquamation. J Biol Chem 2001; 276:20292–20299.
37. Sondell B, Thornell LE, Stigbrand T, et al. Immunolocalization of SCCE in human skin. Histo Cyto 1994; 42:459–465.
38. Watkinson A, Smith C, Coan P, et al. The role of Pro-SCCE and SCCE in desquamation. 21st IFSCC Congress 2000:16–25.
39. Igarashi S, Takizawa T, Yasuda Y, et al. Cathepsin D, and not cathepsin E, degrades des-mosomes during epidermal desquamation. Br J Dermatol 2004; 151(2):355–61.
40. Ishida-Yamamoto A, Simon M, Kishibe M, et al. Epidermal lamellar granules transport different cargoes as distinct aggregates. J Invest Dermatol 2004; 122:1145–1153.
41. Watkinson A, Harding C, Moore A, et al. Water modulation of stratum corneum chymo-tryptic enzyme activity and desquamation. Arch Dermatol Res 2001; 293:470–476.
42. Komatsu N, Takata M, Otsuki N, et al. Elevated stratum corneum hydrolytic activity in Netherton syndrome suggests an inhibitory regulation of desquamation by spink5-derived peptides. J Invest Dermatol 2002; 118:436–443.
43. Franzke CW, Baici A, Bartels J, et al. Antileukoprotease inhibits stratum corneum chymotryptic enzyme. J Biol Chem 1996; 271:21886–21890.
44. Brattsand M, Stefansson K, Lundh C, et al. A proteolytic cascade of kallikreins in the stratum corneum. J Invest Dermatol 2005; 124:198–203.
45. Watkinson A, Harding CR, Rawlings AV. The cornified envelope: its role on stratum corneum structure and maturation. In: Leyden JJ, Rawlings AV, eds. Skin Moisturization. New York: Marcel Dekker, 2002:95–117.
46. Candi E, Tarcsa E, Idler WW, et al. Transglutaminase cross-linking properties of the small proline rich 1 family of cornified envelope proteins. J Biol Chem 1999; 274:7226–7237.
47. Kim IG, Gorman JJ, Park SC, et al. The deduced sequence of the novel protransglutaminase-E (TGase 3) of human and mouse. J Biol Chem 1993; 268:12682–12690.
48. Nemes Z, Marekov LN, Steinert PM. Involucrin cross-linking by transglutaminase 1. J Biol Chem 1999; 274:11013–11021.
49. Cabral A, Voskamp P, Cleton-Jansen M, et al. Structural organisation and regulation of the small proline rich family of cornified envelope precursors suggest a role in adaptive barrier function. J Biol Chem 2001; 276:19231–19237.
50. Mils V, Vincent C, Croute F, et al. The expression of desmosomal and corneodesmosomal antigens shows specific variations during the terminal differentiation of epidermis and hair follicle epithelia. J Histochem Cytochem 1992; 40:1329–1337.
51. Harding CR, Long S, Richardson J, et al. The cornified cell envelope: an important marker of stratum corneum maturation in healthy and dry skin. Int J Cosmet Sci 2003; 25:1–11.
52. Hirao T, Denda M, Takahashi M. Identification of immature cornified envelopes in the barrier-impaired epidermis by characterization of their hydrophobicity and antigenicities of the components. Exp Dermatol 2001; 10:35–44.
53. Kashibuchi N, Hirai Y, O'Goshi K, et al. Three-dimensional analyses of individual corneocytes with atomic force microscope: morphological changes related to age, location and to the pathologic skin conditions. Skin Res Technol 2002; 8:203–211.
54. Jokura Y, Ishikawa S, Tokuda H, et al. Molecular analysis of elastic properties of the stratum corneum by solid-state C13-nuclear magnetic resonance spectroscopy, J Invest Dermatol 1995; 104:806–812.
55. Mechin MC, Enji M, Nachat R, et al. The peptidylarginine deiminases expressed in human epidermis differ in their substrate specificities and subcellular locations. CMLS D01 2005:1–12; 62(17):1984–95.
56. Sakai S, Yasuda R, Sayo T, et al. Hyaluronan exists in the normal stratum corneum. J Invest Dermatol 2000; 114:1184–1187.
57. Fluhr JW, Mao-Qiang M, Brown BE, et al. Glycerol regulates stratum corneum hydration in sebaceous gland deficient (Asebia) mice. J Invest Dermatol 2003; 120:728–737.
58. Choi EH, Man MQ, Wang F, et al. Is endogenous glycerol a determinant of stratum corneum hydration in humans. J Invest Dermatol 2005; 124:1–6.

59. Nakagawa N, Sakai S, Matsumoto M, et al. Relationship between NMF (potassium and lactate) content and the physical properties of the stratum corneum in healthy subjects, J Invest Dermatol 2004; 122:755–763.
60. Fluhr JW, Kao J, Jain M, et al. Generation of free fatty acids from phospholipids regulates stratum corneum acidification and integrity. J Invest Dermatol 2001; 117:44–51.
61. Krien PM, Kermici M. Evidence for the existence of a self-regulated enzymatic process within the human stratum corneum—an unexpected role for urocanic acid. J Invest Dermatol 2000; 115:414–420.
62. Caspers PJ, Lucassen GW, Carter EA, et al. In vivo confocal raman microspectroscopy of the skin: non-invasive determination of molecular concentration profiles. J Invest Dermatol 2001; 116:434–442.
63. Rogers J, Harding CR, Mayo A, et al. Stratum corneum lipids: the effect of ageing and the seasons. Arch Dermatol Res 1996; 288:765–770.
64. Meldrum H, et al. The characteristic decrease in scalp stratum corneum lipids in dandruff is reversed by use of a ZnPTO containing shampoo. IFSCC Mag 2003; 6(1):3–6.
65. Declercq L, Muizzuddin N, Hellemans L, et al. Adaptation response in human skin barrier to a hot and dry environment. J Invest Dermatol 2002; 119:716.
66. Denda M, Sato J, MasudaY, et al. Exposure to a dry environment enhances epidermal permeability barrier function. J Invest Dermatol 1998; 111:858–863.
67. Sato J, Denda M, Chang S, et al. Abrupt decreases in environmental humidity induce abnormalities in permeability barrier homeostasis. J Invest Dermatol 2002; 119:900–904.
68. Chou TC, Lin KH, Wang SM, et al. Transepidermal water loss and skin capacitance alterations among workers in an ultra-low humidity environment. Arch Dermatol Res 2005; 296:489–495.
69. Katagiri C, Sato J, Nomura J, et al. Changes in environmental humidity affect the water-holding capacity of the stratum corneum and its free amino acid content, and the expression of filaggrin in the epidermis of hairless mice. J Dermatol Sci 2003; 31:29–35.
70. Denda M, Sato J, Tsuchiya T, et al. Low humidity stimulates epidermal DNA synthesis and amplifies the hyperproliferative response to barrier disruption: Implication for seasonal exacerbation of inflammatory dermatoses. J. Invest Dermatol 1988; 111:873–878.
71. Ashida Y, Ogo M, Denda M. Epidermal interleukin-1 generation is amplified at low humidity: implications for the pathogenesis of inflammatory dermatoses. Br J Dermatol 2001; 144:238–243.
72. Ashida Y, Denda M. Dry environment increases mast cell number and histamine content in dermis in hairless mice. Br J Dermatol 2003; 149:240–247.
73. Simon M, Bernard D, Minondo AM, et al. Persistence of both peripheral and non-peripheral corneodesmosomes in the upper stratum corneum of winter xerosis skin versus only peripheral in normal skin. J Invest Dermatol 2001; 116:23–30.
74. Long S, Banks J, Watkinson A, et al. Desmocollins: a key marker for desmosome processing in stratum corneum. J Invest Dermatol 1996; 106:872.
75. Van Overloop L, Declercq L, Maes D. Visual scaling of human skin correlates to decreased ceramide levels and decreased stratum corneum protease activity. J Invest Dermatol 2001; 117:811.
76. Kawai E, Kohno Y, Ogawa K, et al. Can inorganic powders provide any biological benefit in stratum corneum while residing on the skin surface. IFSCC Congress, Edinburgh, 2002, 10.
77. Fulmer AW, Kramer GJ. Stratum corneum lipid abnormalities in surfactant-induced scaly skin. J Invest Dermatol 1986; 86:598–602.
78. Saint-Leger D, Francois AM, Leveque JL, et al. Stratum corneum lipids in skin xerosis. Dermatologica 1989; 178:151–155.
79. Chopart M, Castiel-Higounenc C, Arbey E, et al. Quantitative analysis of ceramides in stratum corneum of normal and dry skin. Stratum Corneum 2001; III (poster).
80. Imokawa G. Ceramides as natural moisturizing factors and their efficacy in dry skin. In: Leyden JJ, Rawlings AV, eds. Skin Moisturization. New York: Marcel Dekker, 2002:267–302.
81. Schreiner V, Gooris GS, Pfeiffer S, et al. Barrier characteristics of different human skin types investigated with x-ray diffraction, lipid analysis and electron microscopy imaging. J Invest Dermatol 2000; 114:654–660.
82. Tezuka T. Electron-microscopic changes in xerosis senilis epidermis. Its abnormal membrane-coating granule formation. Dermatologica 1983; 166:57–61.

83. Matts PJ, Goodyer E. A new instrument to measure the mechanical properties of human skin in vivo. J Cosmet Sci 1998; 49:321–333.
84. Matts PJ. Hardware and measurement principles: the gas-bearing electrodynamometer and linear skin rheometer. In: Elsner P, Beradesca E, Wilhem KP, et al, eds. Bioengineering of the Skin: Skin Biomechanics. Boca Raton, Fla: CRC Press, 2002; 335–48.
85. Cooper ER, Missel PJ, Hannon DP, et al. Mechanical properties of dry, normal and glycerol-treated skin as measured by the gas-bearing electrodynamometer. J Cosmet Sci 1985; 36:335–348.
86. Christensen MS, Hargens CW, Nacht S, et al. Viscoelastic properties of intact human skin: instrumentation, hydration effects, and the contribution of the stratum corneum. J Invest Dermatol 1977; 69(3):282–286.
87. Denda M, Wood LC, Emami S, et al. The epidermal hyperplasia associated with repeated barrier disruption by acetone treatment or tape stripping cannot be attributed to increased water loss. Arch Dermatol Res 1996; 288(5–6):230–238.
88. Kikuchi K, Kobayashi H, Hirao T, et al. Improvement of mild inflammatory changes of the facial skin induced by winter environment with daily applications of a moisturizing cream. A half-side test of biophysical skin parameters, cytokine expression pattern and the formation of cornified envelope. Dermatology 2003; 207(3):269–275.
89. Terui T, Hirao T, Sato Y, et al. An increased ratio of interleukin-1 receptor antagonist to interleukin-1 in inflammatory skin diseases, Exp Dermatol 1998; 7:327–334.
90. Proksch E, Jensen J, Elias PM. Skin lipids and epidermal differentiation in atopic dermatitis. Clinics in Dermatology 2003; 21:134–144.
91. Proksch E, Feingold KR, Man MQ, et al. Barrier function regulates epidermal DNA synthesis. J Clin Invest 1991; 87(5):1668–1673.
92. Angel P, Szabowski A. Function of AP-1 target genes in mesenchymal-epithelial cross-talk in skin. Biochem Pharmacol 2002; 64(5–6):949–956.
93. Rawlings AV, Canestrari DA, Dobkowski B. Moisturizer technology versus clinical performance. Dermatol Ther 2004; 17:49–56.
94. Mattai J, Froebe CL, Rhein LD, et al. Prevention of model stratum corneum lipid phase transitions in vitro by cosmetic additives. J Soc Cosmet Chem 1993; 44:89–100.
95. Rawlings AV, Watkinson A, Hope J, et al. The effect of glycerol and humidity on desmosome degradation in stratum corneum. Arch Dermatol Res 1995; 287:457–464.
96. Hirao T, Takahashi M, Kikuchi K, et al. A novel non-invasive evaluation method of cornified envelope maturation in the stratum corneum provides new insight for skincare cosmetics. IFSCC Congress, Edinburgh 2002, 51.
97. Fluhr JW, Gloor M, Lehmann L, et al. Glycerol accelerates recovery of barrier function in vivo. Acta Derm Venereol 1999; 79:418–421.
98. Rattner H. Dermatologic uses of urea. Acta Derm Venereol 1943; 37:155–165.
99. Fredrikkson T, Gip L. Urea creams in the treatment of dry skin and hand dermatitis. Int J Dermatol 1990; 14:442–444.
100. McCallion R, Po AL. Modelling TEWL under steady state conditions and relative humidities. Int J Pharmaceut 1994; 105:103–112.
101. Loden M. Urea containing moisturisers influence barrier properties of normal skin. Arch Dermatol Res 1996; 288:103–107.
102. Pigatto PD, Bigardi AS, Cannistraci C, et al. 10% urea cream for atopic dermatitis J Dermatol Treat. 1996; 7:171–175.
103. Scott IR, Harding CR. A filaggrin analogue to increase natural moisturising factor synthesis in skin. Dermatology 2000, 1993:773.
104. Kwoyo Hakko Kogyo. Pyrrolidone carboxylic acid esters compositions to prevent loss of moisture from the skin. Patent JA 4882046, 1982.
105. Org Santerre. Pyrrolidone carboxylic acid sugar compounds as rehydrating ingredients in cosmetics. Patent FR 2277823, 1977.
106. Clar EJ, Foutanier A. L'acide pyrrolidone carboxylique et la peau. Int J Cosmet Sci 1981; 3:101–113.
107. Middelton JD, Roberts ME. Effects of a skin cream containing the sodium salts of pyrrolidone carboxylic acid on dry and flaky skin. J Soc Cosmet Chem 1978; 29:201–205.
108. Ghadially R, Halkiersorenson L, Elias PM. Effects of petrolatum on stratum corneum structure and function. J Am Acad Dermatol 1992; 26:387–396.

109. Barany E, Lindberg M, Loden M. Unexpected skin barrier influence from non-ionic emulsifiers. Int J Pharmaceut 2000; 195:189–195.
110. Kucharekova M, Schalkwijk J,Van De Kerkhof PC, et al. Effect of a lipid-rich emollient. Contact Dermatitis 2002; 46:331–338.
111. De Paepe K, Roseeuw D, Rogiers V. Repair of acetone- and sodium lauryl sulphate–damaged human skin barrier function using topically applied emulsions containing barrier lipids. JEADV 2002; 16:587–594.
112. Berardesca E, Barbareschi M, Veraldi S, et al. Evaluation of efficacy of a skin lipid mixture in patients with irritant contact dermatitis, allergic contact dermatitis or atopic dermatitis: a multicenter study. Contact Dermatitis 2001; 45:280–285.
113. Chamlin SL, Kao J, Frieden IJ, et al. Ceramide-dominant barrier repair lipids alleviate childhood atopic dermatitis: changes in barrier function provide a sensitive indicator of disease activity. J Am Acad Dermatol 2002; 47:198–4208.
114. Wollenweber U, Korevaar K, Rawlings AV, et al. Application of a skin-identical lipid concentrate for enhanced skin moisturization and protection. SOFW J 2004; 130:9.
115. Summers RS, Summers B, Chandar P, et al. The effect of lipids with and without humectant on skin xerosis. J Soc Cosmet Chem 1996; 47:27–39.
116. Leveque JL, Saint-Leger D. Salicylic acid and derivatives. In: Leyden JJ, Rawlings AV, eds. Skin Moisturization. New York: Marcel Dekker, 2002:353–364.
117. Fartasch M, Teal J, Menon GK. Mode of action of glycolic acid on human stratum corneum: ultrastructural and functional evaluation of the epidermal barrier. Arch Dermatol Res 1997; 289:404–409.
118. Bowser P, Evenson A, Rawlings AV. Cosmetic composition containing a lipid and a hydroxyl or ketocarboxylic acid. EP0587288B1.
119. Rawlings AV, Davies A, Carlomusto M, et al. Effect of lactic acid isomers on keratinocyte ceramide synthesis, stratum corneum lipid levels and stratum corneum barrier function. Arch Dermatol Res 1996; 288:383–390.
120. Rawlings AV, Hope J, Ackerman C, et al. Hydroxycaprylic acid improves stratum corneum extensibility at low relative humidity and protects desmosomes against mechanical damage. IFSCC Congress, Yokohama, 1992:1.
121. Wehr R, Krochmal L, Bagatell F, Ragsdale WA. Controlled two center study of lactate 12% lotion and a petrolatum-based cream in patients with xerosis. Cutis 1986; 23:205.
122. Johnson AW. Hydroxyacids. In: Leyden JJ, Rawlings AV, eds. Skin Moisturization. New York: Marcel Dekker, 2002:323–352.
123. Berardesca E, Distante F, Vignoli GP, et al. Alpha hydroxy acids modulate stratum corneum barrier function. Br J Dermatol 1997; 137:934–938.
124. Hanley K, Jiang Y, He SS, et al. Keratinocyte differentiation is stimulated by activators of the nuclear receptor PPAR alpha. J Invest Dermatol 1998; 110:368–375.
125. Westergaard M, Henningsen J, Svendsen ML, et al. Modulators of keratinocyte gene expression and differentiation by PPAR selective ligand tetradecylthioacetic acid. J Invest Dermatol 2001; 116:702–712.
126. River M, Castiel I, Safonova I, et al. Peroxisome proliferator-activated receptor-alpha enhances lipid metabolism in a skin equivalent model. J Invest Dermatol 2000; 114:691–687.
127. Alaluf S, Barrett KE, Green MR, et al. A cosmetic composition for treating aged wrinkled skin through topical application of a composition containing petroselenic acid. US6042841.
128. Alaluf S, Rawlings AV. A topical composition comprising from petroselenic acid and conjugated linoleic acid. US6423325.
129. Lee R, Paterson S, Marti V, et al. Peroxisome proliferator activated receptor alpha activators: petroselenic acid as a novel skin benefit agent for antiperspirants. IFSCC Congress, Edinburgh, 2002:11.
130. Wiechers JW, Rawlings AV, Garcia C, et al. A new mechanism of action for skin whitening agents: binding to the peroxisome proliferator activated receptor. Int J Cosmet Sci 2005; 27:123–132.
131. Harding CR, Rawlings AV. Effects of NMF and lactic acid isomers on skin function. In: Loden M, Maibach HI, eds. Dry skin and moisturizers, 2006: 187–210.

132. Mao-Qiang M, Feingold KR, Elias PM. Exogenous lipids influence permeability barrier function. Arch Dermatol 1993; 129:729–738.
133. Chamlin SL, Frieden IJ, Fowler A, et al. Optimization of physiological lipid mixtures for barrier repair. J Invest Dermatol 1996; 106:1096–1101.
134. Haratake A, Ikenaga K, Katoh N, et al. Topical mevalonic acid stimulates de novo cholesterol biosynthesis and epidermal permeability barrier homeostasis in aged mice. J Invest Dermatol 2000; 114:247–252.
135. Rawlings AV, Davies A, Carlomusto M, et al. Effect of lactic acid isomers on keratinocyte ceramide synthesis, stratum corneum lipid levels and stratum corneum barrier function. Arch Dermatol Res 1996; 288:383–390.
136. Matts PJ, Oblong JE, Bissett DL. A review of the range of effects of niacinamide in human skin. IFSCC Mag 2002; 5:285–290.
137. Tanno O, Ota Y, Hikima R, et al. An increase in endogenous epidermal lipids improves skin barrier function. IFSCC International Congress 2000, 347–358.
138. Ertel KD, Berge CA, Mercurio MG, et al. New facial moistuizer technology increase exfoliation without compromising barrier function. 58th Annual Meeting of the American Academy of Dermatology, San Francisco 2000.
139. Draelos ZD, Ertel E, Berge C, et al. A facial moisturizing product as an adjunct in the treatment of rosacea. 59th Annual Meeting of the American Academy of Dermatology, San Francisco 2001.
140. Davies A, Verdejo P, Feinberg C, et al. Increased stratum corneum ceramide levels and improved barrier function following treatment with tetraacetylphytosphingosine. J Invest Dermatol 1996; 106:918.
141. Conti A, Rogers P, Verdejo P, et al. Seasonal influences on stratum corneum ceramide 1 fatty acids and the influence of topical essential fatty acids. Int J Cosmet Sci 1996; 18:1–12.
142. Msika P, Piccirilli A, Chesne C. Effects of two specific lipidic ingredients on the synthesis of epidermal lipids in human skin explants in culture. IFSCC Congress, Berlin, 2000:1–5.
143. Denda M. New stategies to improve skin barrier homeostasis. Adv Drug Del Rev 2002; 54:123–130.
144. Zhang K, Kosturko K, Rawlings AV. The effect of thiols on epidermal lipid biosynthesis. J Invest Dermatol 1995; 104:687.
145. Uchida Y, Behne M, Quice D, et al. Vitamin C stimulates sphingolipid production and markers of barrier formation in submerged human keratinocyte cultures. J Invest Dermatol 2001; 117:1307–1313.
146. Yarosh DB, Both D, Brown D. Liposomal ursolic acid (merotaine) increases ceramides and collagen in human skin. Horm Res 2000; 54:318–321.
147. Matts PJ, Gray J, Rawlings AV. The "dry skin cycle"—a new model of dry skin and mechanisms for intervention. The Royal Society of Medicine Press Ltd, International Congress and Symposium Series 2005; 256:1–38.
148. Sieg A, Crowther J, Blenkiron P, et el. Confocal Raman microspectroscopy: measuring the effects of topical moisturizers on stratum corneum water gradients in vivo. Proc SPIE. 2006; 6093:1–7.

22

Antioxidants in the Skin: Dermatological and Cosmeceutical Aspects

Maxim Darvin and Juergen Lademann
Universitätsklinikum Charité, Klinik für Dermatologie,
Venerologie und Allergologie, Berlin, Germany

ANTIOXIDANTS—THE PROTECTION SYSTEM OF HUMAN SKIN AGAINST THE INFLUENCE OF FREE RADICALS

Human skin as a boundary organ between the environment and the organism is constantly in contact with solar radiation and environmental substances, which provoke the production of free radicals in the skin. Free radicals have a powerful oxidative activity, which means that they immediately interact with the surroundings and oxidize DNA, lipids, and proteins of living cells (1–4). As a result of such attacks, the membranes of living cells can be destroyed, which in turn gives rise to cell death and disorganization in the living bio-media (2,5). Additionally, oxygen free radicals are constantly produced in the organism as a result of metabolic processes. It is well known that approximately 2–3% of oxygen on the mitochondrial level is transferred to the oxygen free radicals. Some of these radicals are useful for the living organism, acting as weapons against viruses and bacteria. The remainder are harmful for living cells and should be neutralized before the harmful interaction can take place.

For effective protection against the negative action of these highly reactive substances, human skin has developed a defense system in the form of antioxidant substances, such as vitamins (A, C, D, and E), carotenoids (beta-carotene, lycopene, and lutein/zeaxanthin), enzymes (superoxide dismutase, catalase, and glutathione peroxidase), and others (flavonoids, lipoic acid, uric acid, selenium, coenzyme Q10, etc.). Beta-carotene and lycopene are the main carotenoids present in the human skin. Approximately 70% of the total amount of carotenoids in the skin are beta-carotene and lycopene (6). These substances act effectively against the destructive action of free radicals and other reactive substances, thus neutralizing them. During the processes of neutralization, the energy of the excited radicals is transferred to the carotenoid molecules, which after the interaction with their surroundings, revert to the carotenoid ground state and dissipate excess energy as heat (7). Carotenoid molecules can neutralize several attacks of free radicals before being destroyed (8).

Some antioxidants are synthesized by the organism, but the majority, including carotenoids, cannot be produced and must be taken in via food or supplements that contain these substances (9).

IN VIVO DETERMINATION OF CAROTENOIDS IN THE SKIN

There are three methods for measuring carotenoid antioxidants in the human skin: high-pressure liquid chromatography (HPLC), reflection spectroscopy, and resonance Raman spectroscopy. The HPLC method is widely used for the determination of carotenoids in serum, but it is difficult to perform on skin tissue as it requires large tissue biopsies and special preparation (10). Moreover, HPLC is a highly invasive in vitro method, which is relatively expensive and time consuming.

Reflection spectroscopy is a noninvasive optical method, which is used for measuring carotenoids in the skin (11). This method is based on the absorption properties of the carotenoids, by means of which, in this spectral region, the backscattered light from the skin is reduced. The main disadvantage of reflection spectroscopy is the influence of different substances in the skin, which influence reflection measurements. Moreover, reflection spectroscopy cannot isolate individual carotenoids.

Resonance Raman spectroscopy is a noninvasive and selective optical method, which is based on the differences in the absorption coefficients for the carotenoids beta-carotene and lycopene in the blue and green ranges of spectra. As a result of different absorption values for beta-carotene and lycopene, resonance Raman scattered wavelengths are also different. These clearly detected Raman lines are used for the noninvasive, selective, and in vivo determination of the concentration of carotenoid substances in the human skin (12,13).

Resonance Raman Spectroscopic Determination of Antioxidants in the Human Skin

Carotenoids, alpha-carotene, beta-carotene, lutein, zeaxanthin, lycopene, phytoene, phytofluene, and others are found at different concentrations in the human blood and skin (10,14–17). Food carotenoids are usually C40 tetraterpenoids, which are built from eight C5 isoprenoid units, joined in one sequence. The "skeleton" of these molecules consists of alternating carbon single and double bonds. Namely, the quantity of conjugated carbon double bonds along its backbone provides a rich yellow–orange–red color of carotenoid molecules and defines the absorption properties in the visible blue–green range of spectra. The absorption spectrum of most carotenoids has three characteristic peaks (Fig. 1). The greater number of conjugated carbon double bonds in the structure of carotenoid molecule gives rise to the shift in the absorption spectrum toward the longer wavelengths. For example, beta-carotene has nine conjugated carbon double bonds, is orange, and maximally

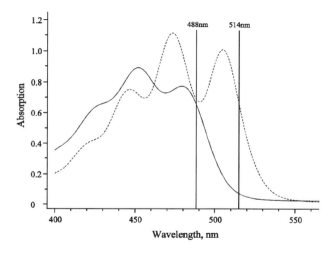

FIGURE 1 Absorption spectra of solutions of beta-carotene (solid line) and lycopene (dotted line) carotenoid antioxidant substances in ethanol.

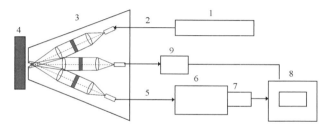

FIGURE 2 Scheme of the experimental setup: (1): Ar+ multiline laser, (2), (5): optical fibers, (3): optical imaging system, (4): measuring object (skin), (6): spectrograph, (7): CCD camera, (8): personal computer, and (9): detector measuring back-reflected light from the skin.

absorbs at 425, 450, and 478 nm, whereas lycopene has 11 conjugated double bonds, is red, and absorbs at 446, 472, and 503 nm (8).

The majority of the detectable carotenoids in the human organism have nine conjugated carbon double bonds in their structure; thus, they have approximately the same absorption values in the blue range of spectra, with the exception of phytoene and phytofluene, which absorb in the UV range of the spectra. Consequently, lycopene is distinguished from other carotenoids in the direction of absorption at the longer wavelengths. Beta-carotene and lycopene represent the largest group, making up approximately 70% of the carotenoids in the human skin (6). Absorption spectra of carotenoid substances beta-carotene and lycopene are presented in Figure 1.

Carotenoids are active Raman molecules, which mean that a small amount of light is scattered with the change of wavelength (Raman shift) induced by a resonance laser excitation wavelength. The utilization of specially developed filters, an optical analysis system as well as a software, allows the measurement of the intensity of the Raman bands which originate from the carotenoids. The experimental arrangement for the Raman measurements of carotenoids is shown in Figure 2.

The irradiation of an Ar^+ multiline laser is transferred, filtered, and focused onto the skin. The Raman signal from the skin is collected by a lens system and transferred into a fiber bundle to a spectrograph. The spectrum is recorded by a CCD camera and visualized on a personal computer. The usage of the specially developed software allows the intensity of the Raman signal to be measured without being influenced by the fluorescence background.

The three Raman bands can be detected on the large fluorescence background, which is caused by collagen, porphyrins, elastin, and other substances of the skin and not by carotenoids (Figs. 3A, B).

The Raman bands at 1523, 1156, and 1005 cm^{-1} originate, respectively, from the carbon–carbon double bond, from carbon–carbon single-bond stretching vibrations of the conjugated backbone, and from the rocking motions of the methyl groups of the carotenoid molecules. The strong 1523 cm^{-1} carbon–carbon double-bond stretching vibration Raman line is used for the determination of the concentration of carotenoids in the human skin.

At present, there are three different methods for the in vivo determination of carotenoids in the skin, based on the resonance Raman spectroscopy:

1. Measurement of a total concentration of carotenoids in the skin without separation. This method is based on the utilization of one excitation wavelength in the blue optical range of spectra (e.g., 488 nm of an Ar^+ laser). This wavelength excites all carotenoids, whose absorption spectrum lies in the blue–green optical

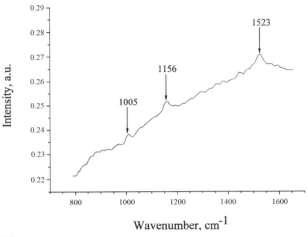

(A)

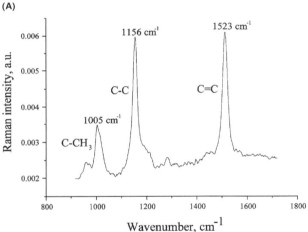

(B)

FIGURE 3 Typical Raman spectrum obtained from human skin under an excitation wavelength at 488 nm (**A**) and the skin Raman spectrum after subtraction of fluorescence background (**B**).

range of spectra (Fig. 1), simultaneously. As a result, the total level of carotenoids may be detected.

2. Separate measurements of beta-carotene and lycopene concentrations in the skin. This method is based on the utilization of two different excitation wavelengths in the blue and in the green optical range of spectra (e.g., 488 and 514.5 nm of an Ar+ laser). As shown in Figure 1, beta-carotene and lycopene have approximately the same absorption values at 488 nm but different absorption values at 514.5 nm. As a result, the scattered resonance Raman lines, originating from beta-carotene and lycopene, will reflect the same tendency. These differences are used for the separate detection of carotenoids beta-carotene and lycopene in the human skin using two different excitation wavelengths (12,16).

3. Measurement of the antioxidant lycopene in the human skin with the use of one excitation wavelength in the green optical range of spectra (preferably

around 514.5 nm). Using the green excitation wavelength at 514.5 nm, strong excitation of lycopene occurs. Other carotenoids are also excited, but they are in the dip of the absorption curve at 514.5 nm (Fig. 1) and, as a result, their contribution is small compared with lycopene. Moreover, the absence of re-absorption at 558 nm (the corresponding wavelength of the 1523 cm^{-1} Raman shift under excitation at 514.5 nm) makes Raman measurements independent from the influence of other carotenoids, which are present in the skin (13).

DISTRIBUTION OF CAROTENOIDS IN THE SKIN AND THEIR KINETICS

Darvin et al. (12) investigated the distribution of the carotenoids at different body sites (inner palm, forehead, flexor forearm, and back) of healthy volunteers by Raman spectroscopy. They found that beta-carotene and lycopene distribution in the human skin strongly depended on the skin region and that there were drastic inter-individual differences, reflecting the lifestyle of the volunteers. The beta-carotene and lycopene concentrations in the skin were lower in smokers than in nonsmokers and higher in vegetarian groups (12).

The highest concentration of carotenoids was found on the forehead and the palm, which corresponded to the body sites with the highest density of sweat glands (18). Therefore, it seems that the lipophilic carotenoids are delivered with the sweat to the skin surface. This hypothesis is supported by the observation of Ekanayake-Mudiyanselage (19) that lipophilic vitamin E is transported by the sweat to the skin surface.

The daily concentration of carotenoids in the skin of volunteers was investigated over several months using Raman spectroscopy (20). The results showed the individual variations in the level of carotenoids in the skin of the volunteers, which strongly correlated with the specific lifestyle conditions such as dietary supplementation rich in carotenoids and the influence of possible stress factors. Carotenoid-rich diets, based on high amounts of fruits and vegetables that have high levels of carotenoids, apparently increase the measured carotenoid antioxidant level of the skin. On the other hand, the carotenoid level in the skin of the volunteers was decreased subsequent to stress factors, such as exhaustion, illness, smoking, and alcohol consumption. This decrease occurred relatively quickly, over 24 hours, whereas the corresponding increase lasted up to three days (20).

During the summer and autumn, an increase in the average level of carotenoids in the skin was measured in all volunteers. The seasonal variation can be explained by an increased consumption of fruits and vegetables, rich in carotenoids, during summer and autumn months. The average seasonal increase of the carotenoid content in the skin was 1.3-fold (20).

Potential Methods of Increasing the Carotenoid Level in the Skin

The human organism can obtain most of the antioxidant substances including carotenoids only through fruits and vegetables, which naturally contain a high amount of different carotenoids. It was shown that a one-time supplementation with a high dosage of foodstuffs containing high amount of carotenoids increased the level of the carotenoids in the skin. The increase in the carotenoid level could usually be observed the next day after the supplementation (21,22). The studies demonstrated that the antioxidants that were taken up from food partly accumulated in the skin and were stored there, thereby increasing the antioxidative potential of the skin.

ANTIOXIDANTS PROTECT THE SKIN AGAINST AGING

During the Raman spectroscopic investigation of carotenoids in the human skin, it was observed that volunteers with a higher concentration of antioxidants had a younger looking skin with regard to furrows and wrinkles (20). To quantify this observation, a study was performed whereby the skin surface structure (depth and density of furrows and wrinkles) was compared with the skin concentration of beta-carotene and lycopene. The investigation was carried out on volunteers aged between 40 and 50 years, who had not significantly changed their lifestyle during the last three decades. No correlation ($R^2 = 0.009$) was found between the skin surface structure (roughness) and the age of the volunteers, whereas a strong correlation ($R^2 = 0.79$) was obtained for the relation between the skin concentration of lycopene and the skin roughness (20). The results demonstrate that a correlation between the appearance of the skin, in particular with regard to furrows and wrinkles, and the level of carotenoids in the skin evidently exists.

Supplementation with fruits and vegetables reduced the formation and development of furrows and wrinkles on the skin with age. In this case, the skin looks younger. The results presented in the study were obtained from healthy volunteers. The lycopene concentration in the skin had originated from their habitual diet and not from special food additives or cosmetic products. It will be a topic of further research to investigate whether similar results can be obtained by food supplements or topically applied antioxidant substances.

INFLUENCE OF IRRADIATION ON CAROTENOID CONCENTRATIONS IN THE SKIN
UV Irradiation

It is well known that high doses of UV irradiation are harmful to living skin (1). Under exposure to UV light, skin sensitizer molecules, such as melanin, flavin, porphyrin, and others, are excited from their singlet ground state to an intermediate singlet excited state. From this state, the excess energy of these molecules is relaxed nonradioactively to an excited triplet state. The excited sensitizer molecule in the triplet state easily interacts with oxygen in the ground triplet state, which is contained in the skin. As a result of this reaction, excited singlet oxygen is produced, and the sensitizer molecule is returned to the ground state. More than 99% of the reaction between the triplet sensitizer and triplet oxygen gives rise to the production of singlet oxygen radicals (23). Singlet oxygen possesses a high oxidative activity and serves as a free radical.

If the number of radicals formed in the tissue is significantly increased, the defense mechanism of the body is not able to neutralize all the reactive molecules (24). In this case, chain reactions are initiated, which again high amounts of free radicals form and oxidative stress occurs. The free radicals that are produced subsequent to UV irradiation give rise to the inflammation processes and the formation of erythema. The systematic irradiation of the skin with UV irradiation can lead to the formation of skin cancer (25).

Free radicals immediately react with the surroundings, oxidizing the DNA, lipids, and proteins of living cells (2,3). This gives rise to irreversible changes and conformations on the cellular level and disorganization between the cells. The accumulation of such harmful changes results in preliminary aging that can be seen by the dryness and deepening and the expansion of furrows and wrinkles of the skin.

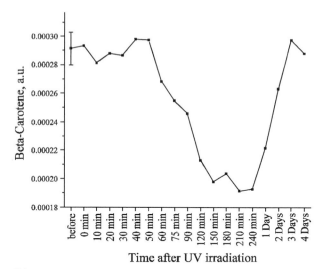

(A)

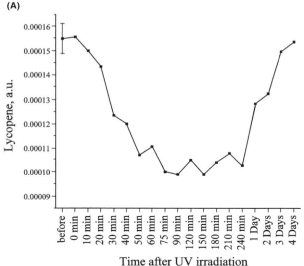

(B)

Time after UV irradiation

FIGURE 4 Kinetics of the skin's beta-carotene (**A**) and lycopene (**B**) concentrations after UV irradiation of the skin.

Using Raman spectroscopy, the kinetics of the concentration of carotenoids in the human skin subsequent to irradiation with UV light was investigated in vivo. The irradiation was carried out using an erythema tester (Dr. Höhle Meßtechnik GmbH, Germany) as a source of UVB irradiation. The skin of the forearm of healthy volunteers was irradiated with a UVB dose of 30 mJ/cm², which was sufficient for the formation of a light erythema. An example of the reaction of the beta-carotene (A) and lycopene (B) concentrations to the UV irradiation dose is shown in Figure 4. Both carotenoids showed different kinetics. Lycopene degraded relatively quickly (<30 minutes) after UV irradiation, whereas the response time of the beta-carotene concentration varied from 30 to 90 minutes. The differences in the response time of beta-carotene and lycopene can be explained by the different quenching rates concerning the neutralization of free radicals. This quenching rate is higher for lycopene than for beta-carotene (26). No differences were found between the response time and the individual level of the carotenoids in the skin. On the other hand, the experiments demonstrated that the magnitude of degradation was dependent on the individual antioxidant level of the volunteers.

The strong correlation can be explained by the production of the same amount of free radicals after UV exposure of the skin because volunteers had received the same dose of irradiation. As a result, the quantity of produced radicals will be approximately the same for all volunteers. It can be expected that the same amount of carotenoids will be destroyed. In this case, the volunteers with low levels of carotenoids showed a higher magnitude of destruction, which was observed in the experiments.

Infrared Irradiation

In an analogy to UV irradiation experiments, the influence of infrared (IR) irradiation on the skin was investigated (27). IR irradiation is widely used in medicine for accelerating wound healing processes (28) and for warming muscles, whereby blood and lymph flow is increased and the rate of metabolism and recovery increased.

IR irradiation of living skin leads to a decrease in the concentration of the carotenoids, beta-carotene and lycopene, in the irradiated area (27). The power density of the IR irradiation on the skin was 190 mW/cm^2. The time of irradiation was 30 minutes. The average magnitude of reduction was 27% for beta-carotene and 38% for lycopene.

The temperature of the skin surface increased to $41 \pm 1°C$ after IR irradiation of the skin. Taking into consideration the relative temperature stability of carotenoids, at least up to 50°C, and the absence of absorption in the IR range of spectra, the most likely outcome of the reduced levels of carotenoids subsequent to IR irradiation is the reduction of neutralization of free radicals, which can be produced in the skin by IR irradiation. There was a strong correlation between the individual level of beta-carotene and lycopene in the skin of volunteers and the magnitude of destruction of carotenoids (27).

Under the IR irradiation of the skin, carotenoids beta-carotene and lycopene start to decrease almost immediately, with a small time delay of about 10 minutes for beta-carotene. The differences in the response time for UV and IR can be explained by the essential differences in the power densities of UV and IR irradiations (0.3 mW/cm^2 for UV irradiation and 190 mW/cm^2 for IR irradiation) as well as exposure times (100 seconds and 30 minutes correspondingly).

The recovery time of carotenoid levels in the skin after the influence of stress from factors such as irradiation depends on the carotenoid stock in the adipose tissue and on nutrition. There are three main pathways for the transport of carotenoids to the skin: by blood flow, from adipose tissue with the aid of diffusion, and via sweat.

APPLICATION STRATEGIES OF ANTIOXIDANT SUBSTANCES

The application of antioxidant substances systemically and topically for medical treatment and the prophylaxis of many diseases and the added protection of skin against the destructive action of free radicals and other reactive species have become very popular over the past few years. The available literature is very extensive, and the results published are often contradictory. Nevertheless, there are some clear tendencies concerning the systemic and topical application of antioxidant substances in medicine and cosmetics (29). Stimulated by the positive results of a fruits and vegetables diet in the support of medical treatment and cosmetology, synthetic and natural antioxidant substances have been broadly applied (15,30–32). Surprisingly, not only positive but also strongly negative results have been obtained by different authors (33–39).

According to study reports, synthetic and natural antioxidant substances support various types of medical therapies if they are applied in mixtures of different compounds at low concentrations (35,36,40–42). In the case of application of a high concentration of some single compounds, side effects were often observed (36,42,43).

Following skin treatment with systemically delivered antioxidants, positive cosmetic effects were observed on photoprotection (44–46), stimulation of the synthesis of collagen, and cell proliferation (47). It has been also shown that supplementation of antioxidants prevents the formation of skin carcinoma (48). Almost no side effects were reported apart from a number of allergic reactions. One reason for this seems to be the lower concentration of systemically applied antioxidant substances when compared with a medical application. The topical application of antioxidants is mainly related to cosmetic treatment for skin protection and anti-aging (49–52) where positive results were obtained.

All antioxidant substances act as a "protection chain," which means that different antioxidants possess a synergic effect and protect each other from direct destruction when neutralizing free radicals and other reactive species (53–55). Therefore, they act effectively only in combination with the other types of antioxidant substances. This relation becomes disturbed if one component is artificially increased by supplementation. It can even happen that the antioxidants act not only as radical quenchers, but also as radical producers (56) if their concentration is higher than the critical level. In this case, antioxidants can manifest pro-oxidant activity on the organism. Furthermore, different antioxidants have different effectiveness on the neutralization of the free radicals that determine the rate and ability of individual antioxidants to interact with free radicals (57). These effects seem to depend on the concentration and on the mixture of the applied antioxidant substances.

CONCLUSIONS

Antioxidant substances protect our body from the action of highly reactive free radicals. Most of the antioxidants cannot be produced in sufficient amounts endogenously. Therefore, they have to be provided by the diet. The content of antioxidants in the human skin can be increased by eating different fruits and vegetables. The use of food supplements also leads to an increase in skin antioxidants.

Noninvasive online Raman spectroscopic measurements of antioxidant concentration in the human skin are an efficient means to analyze the influence of food supplementation and stress factors on the antioxidant potential of the skin. A comparison between electron spin resonance spectroscopy (58,59) and Raman spectroscopy demonstrated that antioxidants can be used as markers for the analysis of the antioxidant defense system within the skin. The antioxidant substances in the organism form protection chains (53–55), in which they protect each other from the damage caused by the action of free radicals. Thus, the systemic application of mixtures of antioxidant substances by foods and vegetables or by mixtures of antioxidant extracts seems to be very efficient in protecting our body in comparison with the application of single compounds. There is a critical concentration where antioxidants can obtain pro-oxidative properties. It seems that this critical value depends on several factors such as the concentration and composition of the antioxidants in the mixture.

Because of the increased application of noninvasive optical and spectroscopic diagnostic methods for the analysis of antioxidants, an increase in knowledge concerning the action and optimal concentration of antioxidants in the skin can be expected.

REFERENCES

1. Biesalski HK, Hemmes C, Hopfenmuller W, et al. Effects of controlled exposure of sunlight on plasma and skin levels of beta-carotene. Free Radic Res 1996; 24: 215–224.
2. Dumay O, Karam A, Vian L, et al. Ultraviolet AI exposure of human skin results in Langerhans cell depletion and reduction of epidermal antigen-presenting cell function: partial protection by a broad-spectrum sunscreen. Br J Dermatol 2001; 144: 1161–1168.
3. Flora SJ. Role of free radicals and antioxidants in health and disease. Cell Mol Biol 2007; 53:1–2.
4. Young AR, Sheehan JM, Chadwick CA, Potten CS. Protection by ultraviolet A and B sunscreens against in situ dipyrimidine photolesions in human epidermis is comparable to protection against sunburn. J Invest Dermatol 2000; 115:37–41.
5. Taylor CR, Sober AJ. Sun exposure and skin disease. Annu Rev Med 1996, 47, 181–191.
6. Hata TR, Scholz TA, Ermakov IV, et al. Non-invasive Raman spectroscopic detection of carotenoids in human skin. J Invest Dermatol 2000; 115:441–448.
7. Darvin ME, Gersonde I, Ey S, et al. Non-invasive detection of beta-carotene and lycopene in human skin using Raman spectroscopy. Laser Phys 2004; 14:231–233.
8. Guggenbuhl N. Les antioxydants a la source. Bull Soc Belge Ophtalmol 2006; 301:41–5.
9. Shao A, Hathcock JN. Risk assessment for the carotenoids lutein and lycopene. Regul Toxicol Pharmacol 2006; 45:289–98.
10. Talwar D, Ha Tom KK, Cooney J, et al. A routine method for the simultaneous measurement of retinal, α-tocopherol and five carotenoids in human plasma by reverse phase HPLC. Clin Chim Acta 1998; 270:85–100.
11. Stahl W, Heinrich U, Jungmann H, et al. Increased dermal carotenoid level assessed by non-invasive reflection spectrophotometry correlate with serum levels in women ingesting betatene. J Nutr 1998; 128:903–907.
12. Darvin ME, Gersonde I, Meinke M, et al. Non-invasive in vivo determination of the carotenoids beta-carotene and lycopene concentrations in the human skin using the Raman spectroscopic method. J Phys D Appl Phys 2005; 38:1–5.
13. Darvin ME, Gersonde I, Meinke M, et al. Non-invasive *in vivo* detection of the carotenoid antioxidant substance lycopene in the human skin using the resonance Raman spectroscopy. Laser Phys Lett 2006; 3:460–463.
14. Walfisch Y, Walfisch S, Agbaria R, et al. Lycopene in serum, skin and adipose tissues after tomato-oleoresin supplementation in patients undergoing haemorrhoidectomy or perianal fistulotomy. Br J Nutr 2003; 90:759–766.
15. Khachik F, Carvalho L, Bernstein PS, et al. Chemistry, distribution, and metabolism of tomato carotenoids and their impact on human health. Exp Biol Med 2002; 227:845–851.
16. Ermakov I, Ermakova M, Gellermann W, et al. Noninvasive selective detection of lycopene and beta-carotene in human skin using Raman spectroscopy. J Biomed Opt 2004; 9:332–338.
17. Stahl W, Sies H. Perspectives in biochemistry and biophysics. Lycopene: a biologically important carotenoid for humans? Arch Biochem Biophys 1996; 336:1–9.
18. Hadgraft J. Penetration routes through human skin. Proc 10-th EADV Congress. Skin and Environment; Perception and Protection, Munich, 2001; 463–468.
19. Ekanayake-Mudiyanselage S, Thiele JJ. Sebaceous glands as transporters of vitamin E. Hautarzt 2006, 57, 291–296.
20. Darvin ME. Non-invasive measurements of the kinetics of the carotenoid antioxidant substances in the skin. PhD thesis, Universitätsmedizin Berlin-Charite, 2007.

21. Darvin ME, Gersonde I, Albrecht H, et al. Non-invasive in-vivo Raman spectroscopic measurement of the dynamics of the antioxidant substance lycopene in the human skin after a dietary supplementation. Proc SPIE (in press).
22. Darvin ME, Gersonde I, Albrecht H, et al. Resonance Raman spectroscopy for the detection of carotenoids in foodstuffs. Influence of the nutrition on the antioxidative potential of the skin. Laser Phys Lett 2007 (in press).
23. Min D, Boff JM. Chemistry and reaction of singlet oxygen in foods. Compr Rev Food Sci Food Safety 2002; 1:58–61.
24. Jackson MJ. An overview of methods for assessment of free radical activity in biology. Proc Nutr Soc 1999; 58:1001–1006.
25. Moon JS, Oh CH. Solar damage in skin tumors: quantification of elastotic material. Dermatology 2001; 202:289–292.
26. Darvin ME, Gersonde I, Albrecht H, et al. In-vivo Raman spectroscopic analysis of the influence of UV radiation on carotenoid antioxidant substance degradation of the human skin. Laser Phys 2006; 16:833–837.
27. Darvin ME, Gersonde I, Albrecht H, et al. In vivo Raman spectroscopic analysis of the influence of IR radiation on the carotenoid antioxidant substances beta-carotene and lycopene in the human skin. Formation of free radicals. Laser Phys Lett (in press).
28. Danno K, Mori N, Toda K, et al. Near-infrared irradiation stimulates cutaneous wound repair: laboratory experiments on possible mechanisms. Photodermatol Photoimmunol Photomed 2001; 17:261–265.
29. Darvin M, Zastrow L, Sterry W, et al. Effect of supplemented and topically applied antioxidant substances on human tissue. Review. Skin Pharmacol Physiol 2006; 19:238–247.
30. Osganian SK, Stampfer MJ, Rimm E, et al. Dietary carotenoids and risk of coronary artery disease in women. Am J Clin Nutr 2003; 77:1390–1399.
31. Montonen J, Knekt P, Jarvinen R, et al. Dietary antioxidant intake and risk of type 2 diabetes. Diabetes Care 2004; 27:362–366.
32. Franceschi S, Bidoli E, La Vecchia C, et al. Tomatoes and risk of digestive-tract cancers. Int J Cancer 1994; 59:181–184.
33. Biesalski HK, Obermueller-Jevic UC. UV light, beta-carotene and human skin—beneficial and potentially harmful effects. Arch Biochem Biophys 2001; 389:1–6.
34. Stahl W, Sies H. Perspectives in biochemistry and biophysics. Lycopene: a biologically important carotenoid for humans? Arch Biochem Biophys 1996; 336:1–9.
35. http://home.howstuffworks.com/ antioxidant4.htm (accessed 2002)
36. Lowe GM, Booth LA, Young AJ, et al. Lycopene and beta-carotene protect against oxidative damage in HT29 cells at low concentrations but rapidly lose this capacity at higher doses. Free Radic Res 1999; 30:141–151.
37. Pryor WA, Stahl W, Rock CL. Beta carotene: from biochemistry to clinical trials. Nutr Rev 2000; 58:39–53.
38. Lee BM, Park KK. Beneficial and adverse effects of chemopreventive agents. Mutat Res 2003; 523–524:265–278.
39. Bjelakovic G, Nikolova D, Simonetti R, et al. Antioxidant supplements for preventing gastrointestinal cancers. Cochrane Database Syst Rev 2004; 18:CD004183.
40. Cesarini JP, Michel L, Maurette JM, et al. Immediate effects of UV radiation on the skin: modification by an antioxidant complex containing carotenoids. Photodermatol Photoimmunol Photomed 2003; 19:182–189.
41. http://www.crnusa.org/benpdfs/CRN007benefits_can.pdf (accessed June 2002).
42. Eichler O, Sies H, Stahl W. Divergent optimum levels of lycopene, beta-carotene and lutein protecting against UVB irradiation in human fibroblastst. Photochem Photobiol 2002; 75:503–506.
43. Jenkins GJ, Stephens LA, Masnavi N, et al. Molecular analysis of the chemoprotective effects of topical sunscreen and vitamin C in preventing UV-induced and reactive oxygen species-induced DNA damage, respectively, using the PCR inhibition methodology. Anticancer Res 2002; 22:3873–3877.
44. Heinrich U, Gärtner Ch, Wiebusch M, et al. Supplementation with β-carotene or a similar amount of mixed carotenoids protects humans from UV-induced erythema. J Nutr 2003; 133:98–101.

45. Greul AK, Grundmann JU, Heinrich F, et al. Photoprotection of UV-irrdiated human skin: an antioxidative combination of vitamins E and C, carotenoids, selenium and proanthocyanidins. Skin Pharmacol Appl Skin Physiol 2002; 15:307–315.

46. Stahl W, Heinrich U, Jungmann H, et al. Carotenoids and carotenoids plus vitamin E protect against ultraviolet light-induced erythema in humans. Am J Clin Nutr 2000; 71: 795–798.

47. Hata R, Senoo H. L-Ascorbic acid 2-phosphate stimulates collagen accumulation, cell proliferation, and formation of a three-dimensional tissue like substance by skin fibroblasts. J Cell Physiol 1989; 138:8–16.

48. Ponnamperuma RM, Shimizu Y, Kirchhof SM, et al. Beta-Carotene fails to act as a tumor promoter, induces RAR expression, and prevents carcinoma formation in a two-stage model of skin carcinogenesis in male Sencar mice. Nutr Cancer 2000; 37:82–88.

49. Mukhtar H, Katiyar SK, Agarwal R. Green tea and skin anticarcinogenic effects. J Invest Dermatol 1994; 102:3–7.

50. Lupo MP. Antioxidants and vitamins in cosmetics. Clin Dermatol 2001, 19:467–476.

51. Kligman AM, Grove GL, Hirose R, et al. Topical tretinoin for photoaged skin. J Am Acad Dermatol 1986; 15:836–859.

52. Darr D, Combs S, Dunston S, et al. Topical vitamin C protects porcine skin from ultraviolet radiation-induced damage. Br J Dermatol 1992; 127:247–253.

53. Katiyar SK, Ahmad N, Mukhtar H. Green tea and skin. Arch Dermatol 2000; 136:989–994.

54. Weiss JS, Ellis CN, Headington JT, et al. Topical tretinoin in the treatment of aging skin. J Am Acad Dermatol 1988; 19:169–175.

55. Evelson P, Ordonez CP, Llesuy S, et al. Oxidative stress and in vivo chemiluminescence in mouse skin exposed to UVA radiation. J Photochem Photobiol B 1997; 38:215–219.

56. Moon TE, Levine N, Cartmel B, et al. Effect of retinol in preventing squamous cell skin cancer in moderate-risk subjects: a randomized, double-blind, controlled trial. Southwest Skin Cancer Prevention Study Group. Cancer Epidemiol Biomarkers Prev 1997; 6:949–956.

57. Rao AV. Lycopene, tomatoes and the prevention of coronary heart disease. Nutr Res 2002; 19:305–323.

58. Fuchs J, Groth N, Herrling T. In vivo measurement of oxidative stress status in human skin. Methods Enzymol 2002; 352:333–339.

59. Herrling T, Fuchs J, Rehberg J, et al. UV-induced free radicals in the skin detected by ESR spectroscopy and imaging using nitroxides. Free Radic Biol Med 2003; 35:59–67.

23 Absorption and Evaporation of Volatile Compounds Applied to Skin

Gerald B. Kasting and Matthew A. Miller
James L. Winkle College of Pharmacy, University of Cincinnati Academic Health Center, Cincinnati, Ohio, U.S.A.

Johannes M. Nitsche
Department of Chemical Engineering, State University of New York at Buffalo, Buffalo, New York, U.S.A.

INTRODUCTION

The disposition of volatile products following application to the skin plays a role in both their safety and efficacy. The absorption rate determines systemic levels and skin concentrations, both of which must be factored into risk assessments. The evaporation rate determines efficacy for certain products, for example, a fine fragrance or an insect repellant. These two factors are interdependent as both depend on and, in turn, affect the residual concentration of the compound in or on the skin.

The problem of predicting skin disposition of volatiles has been of interest in our laboratory for several years. We have investigated two general approaches to this problem: a well-stirred compartment or pharmacokinetic model (1–6) and a diffusion model (7,8). The former is simpler and has merit for interpolation within a closely related set of compounds and exposure conditions. Its application to risk assessment for perfume raw materials (or fragrance ingredients) has been discussed (6). The pharmacokinetic approach will not be further considered here; the focus of this chapter is how to make predictions using the diffusion model.

A suitable starting point for a skin diffusion model for volatile chemicals is shown in Figure 1. This is a one-dimensional model composed of four layers: a vehicle layer or donor solution, stratum corneum, viable epidermis, and dermis. The upper two layers correspond to the diffusion model described in Ref. 7. If only systemic absorption estimates are required and the compound is not highly lipophilic (9), then the solution of the diffusion equation in these two layers with sink conditions at the base of the stratum corneum provides an adequate description of the problem. Analytical solutions to this problem for a number of exposure conditions may be found (7,10,11). If, on the other hand, skin and underlying tissue concentrations are of interest, it is necessary to include an explicit representation of the skin layers and (perhaps) the underlying fat and muscle. We will not consider the subdermal layers here; for a useful discussion, see Ref. 12. A distributed model for partitioning, diffusion, and clearance in the dermis has recently been described by workers from our laboratories (13,14). This model forms the basis for the viable skin model presented here. It is noteworthy that less is known about the transport properties of viable epidermis than dermis. Our working approach, discussed later, is to treat viable epidermis as unperfused dermis. Because the diffusive resistance of viable epidermis appears to be low, this assumption has a minimal impact on systemic absorption estimates. However, it does affect the tissue concentration calculation in that layer. For problems such as allergic contact dermatitis, where the putative site of action is the Langerhans cell surface in the mid-epidermis, a physiologically accurate representation of the epidermis is desirable. The cellular nature of this tissue, in contrast to the largely acellular (but fibrous) dermis, in all probability imparts to it different selectivity for transport of chemical permeants.

A study of the schematic diagram shown in Figure 1 gives rise to three important questions: (1) Is it reasonable that a slab model with no internal microstructure can accurately represent skin transport? (2) How can appropriate transport parameters for the slab model be chosen prospectively? (3) How can the calculation be implemented? Each of these questions is addressed in the following sections. An example calculation for the fragrance ingredient benzyl alcohol is then presented showing the power of the technique but also revealing some of its limitations. Complexity is incurred because many small semipolar molecules like benzyl alcohol affect skin permeability, presumably by interacting with stratum corneum lipids. A general method of predicting these interactions is not yet known.

EFFECTIVE MEDIUM THEORY

Although the stratum corneum, viable epidermis, and dermis slabs each have complex microstructures, they can be described macroscopically as effective homogeneous continua characterized by average diffusion and partition coefficients. A theory for this type of coarse graining has a distinguished history in mathematical physics, going back to the pioneering analyses of macroscopic conduction properties of composite media by Maxwell (15) and Rayleigh (16). The scope of the approach was later extended by Brenner et al., as summarized by Brenner and Edwards (17). An important finding from this research is that such an approach may

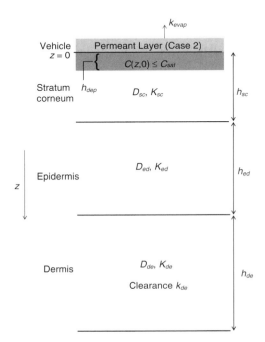

FIGURE 1 Schematic diagram of diffusion/evaporation model for skin disposition of potentially volatile permeants.

TABLE 1 Required Permeant Physical Properties for Skin Transport Calculations

Parameter	Units	Definition
MW	Da	Molecular weight
log K_{oct}	–	Log of octanol/Water partition coefficient
S_w	g/cm³	Water solubility of unionized form
P_{vp}	Torr	Vapor pressure
pK_a	–	Ionization constant(s)[a]
f_u	–	Fraction unbound in a 2% albumin solution[b]
ρ	g/cm³	Density

All properties were determined at skin temperature, normally taken to be 32°C. For a discussion, see Ref. 7.
[a]The fraction nonionized (f_{non}) in the stratum corneum (pH 5) and viable skin tissues (pH 7.4) must be estimated. All pK_a values relevant to this calculation should be included.
[b]In the absence of experimental data, the method of Yamazaki and Kanaoka (28) may be employed to obtain this value (14).

be justified so long as the timescale of the phenomenon of interest is long compared with those of the relevant microscopic transport processes contributing to the observed effect. Long-standing belief that transport through the stratum corneum is describable as Fick's law diffusion through an effective homogeneous membrane (18,19) has been confirmed recently in, for example, an experimental study by Kalia et al. (20) and theoretical studies by Frasch and Barbero (21–23). Using a two-dimensional brick-and-mortar microstructural representation of stratum corneum, the latter investigators derived an effective diffusivity and partition coefficient for the system and showed how to more accurately predict the diffusive lag time from these parameters.

Our combined research groups have further developed the effective medium approach for modeling transport in the stratum corneum (7,8,24–26) and the dermis (13,27). Substantial predictive power is evident in both cases. In the following section, formulas for the transport properties resulting from these investigations are presented. They are all derivable from the simple set of physical properties shown in Table 1.

EFFECTIVE TRANSPORT PARAMETERS FOR SKIN
Stratum Corneum
Model-based calculation

The microstructural model from which the stratum corneum parameters are derived is shown schematically in Figure 2. The model is described in considerable detail in Refs. 24–26. The features that distinguish this model from earlier entries in the field are the following: (1) a more realistic geometry with lipid pathways calibrated from microscopic examination of human stratum corneum (29), (2) anisotropic lamellar lipids (30) with six bilayers separating opposing corneocytes, and (3) permeable corneocytes that swell when the skin is hydrated (31,32) and also bind permeants (26). To describe this system in the slab form shown in Figure 1, three parameters are needed: h_{sc}, D_{sc}, and K_{sc}. Here, K_{sc} is short for $K_{sc/pH}$, where $K_{sc/pH}$ reflects the partition coefficient of the permeant between stratum corneum and buffer at a pH at which it is 100% unionized. Derivations of the formulas reported here may be found in Refs. 25 and 26.

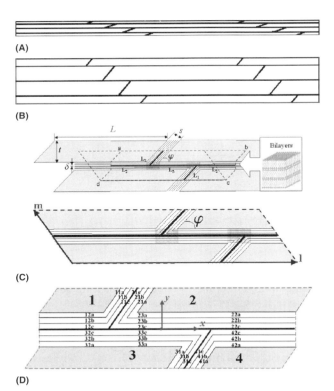

FIGURE 2 Definition sketch showing assumed model microstructure. (**A**) Structure for partially hydrated skin. (**B**) Structure for fully hydrated skin. (**C**) Schematic drawings indicating notation (not to scale). (**D**) Labeling scheme used to identify individual lipid bilayers and corneocytes within a unit cell.

We focus on the solution described as Model 2 for partially hydrated skin (25). Model 2 refers to the postulated lipid bilayer arrangement between corneocytes and is the more likely of the two limiting arrangements described in Ref. 25. "Partially hydrated" means that the stratum corneum containing an average water content of 30% w/w or 0.43 g H_2O/g dry stratum corneum. Stratum corneum properties in the partially hydrated state are quite different from those in the fully hydrated state (73% w/w, 2.75 g H_2O/g dry stratum corneum), which applies to most steady-state permeability measurements in vitro. The calculation of corneocyte phase transport properties D_{cor} and K_{cor} in Ref. 24 has furthermore been simplified to require only the molecular weight (MW) of the permeant. In Ref. 25, these properties are estimated from the molar volume of the permeant (V_A) using hindered diffusion arguments. In the formulas below, D_{cor} and K_{cor} are calculated directly from MW by regressing the more accurately calculated V_A-based values against MW for the 97 permeants analyzed in Ref. 25. A maximum error of 41% in the D_{cor} values and 12% in the K_{cor} values is introduced by this procedure, leading to an rms error of 0.6% and a maximum error of 5% in the macroscopic properties P_{sc} and D_{sc}. The higher accuracy for the latter parameters arises because most of the diffusive resistance of the stratum corneum lies in the lipid phase rather than the corneocytes.

The simplified formulas for partially hydrated stratum corneum transport properties are shown in Table 2. In these equations, MW is the gram molecular weight of the permeant and K_{oct} is its octanol/water partition coefficient. The "reduced" molecular weight $MW_r = MW / 100$ is introduced as a matter of convenience for scaling the coefficients. Values of the partially hydrated stratum corneum permeability P_{sc} calculated from the relationships in Table 2 are lower than hydrated skin permeabilities by approximately a factor of 3, deriving mainly from the lipid disruption factor H_{trans} [Eq. (4)]. However, geometrical swelling and corneocyte permeability factors also play a role. By combining the value of P_{sc} with the partition coefficient for partially hydrated stratum corneum K_{sc} (26) and its thickness h_{sc}, the effective diffusivity D_{sc} is obtained at the end of the process [Eq. (15)].

For finite dose calculations, the concept of a deposition depth h_{dep}, a saturation concentration C_{sat}, and a saturation dose $M_{sat} = h_{dep} \times C_{sat}$ is extremely useful (7,8,34,35). The concept derives from a picture of the upper stratum corneum as a relatively permeable desquamating layer into which topically applied permeants are rapidly deposited (7). The C_{sat} parameter imposes a solubility limit of the permeant in the stratum corneum, and the ratio of applied dose to M_{sat}—the reduced dose M_r—distinguishes a large dose from a small one. According to the convention in Ref. 7, a small dose is described by $M_r \leq 1$ and is designated as Case 1. A large dose, described by $M_r > 1$, is designated as Case 2. Large doses show qualitatively different behavior than small doses, as may be seen from Figure 3. Solubility limitations

TABLE 2 Formulas for Stratum Corneum Transport Parameters for Partially Hydrated Skin.

Parameter	Units	Formula or Value	Eq. #
Defining relationship		$\dfrac{\partial C}{\partial t} = \dfrac{\partial}{\partial z}\left(D_{sc}\dfrac{\partial C}{\partial z}\right),\ 0 \leq C \leq C_{sat}$	(1)
h_{sc}	cm	0.0013365	(2)
H_{lat}		3	(3)
H_{trans}		3	(4)
MW_r		MW / 100	(5)
D_{lip}	cm²/sec	$\left[1.24 \times 10^{-7} MW_r^{-2.43} + 2.34 \times 10^{-9}\right]/H_{lat}$	(6)
k_{trans}	cm/sec	$0.1884 \cdot \left[\exp\left(-8.465 \cdot MW_r^{1/3}\right)\right]/H_{trans}$	(7)
K_{lip}		$0.43 \cdot \left(K_{oct}\right)^{0.81}$	(8)
D_{cor}^{free}	cm²/sec	$2.793 \times 10^{-6} MW_r^{-1.011}$	(9)
K_{cor}^{free}		$10 \wedge \left(-0.444 - 0.0655 \cdot MW_r - 0.00273 \cdot MW_r^2 + 0.000534 \cdot MW_r^3\right)$	(10)
σ		$D_{lip}K_{lip}/(D_{cor}^{free}K_{cor}^{free})$	(11)
R		$7.04642 \cdot k_{trans}/D_{lip}$	(12)
P_{sc}	cm/sec	$\dfrac{D_{lip}K_{lip}}{h_{sc}\left(0.8979 \cdot \sigma + 5.536 \times 10^5 / R\right)}$ for $R \geq 100$.	(13)
K_{sc}		$0.040\left(K_{oct}\right)^{0.81} + 0.359 + 4.057 \cdot \left(K_{oct}\right)^{0.27}$	(14)
D_{sc}	cm²/sec	$P_{sc}h_{sc}/K_{sc}$	(15)
h_{dep}	cm	$0.1 \cdot h_{sc}$	(16)
C_{sat}	g/cm³	$K_{sc}S_w$	(17)
M_{sat}	µg/cm²	$C_{sat}h_{dep} \times 10^6$	(18)

Source: From Refs. 7, 24–26.

(C_{sat}) and skin capacity limitations (M_{sat}) are among the reasons that finite dose skin absorption problems are inherently more difficult than steady-state permeability calculations. Another is that the math is harder.

Experimentally based calculation

If an experimental value of the steady-state permeability coefficient from aqueous solution is available, an alternative means of calculating stratum corneum transport properties should be used. This method comprises the following steps (8):

1. Start with the measured skin permeability coefficient k_p. Calculate the hydrated stratum corneum permeability P_{sc} (hydrated) as

$$\frac{1}{P_{sc}(\text{hydrated})} = \frac{1}{k_p} - \frac{h_{ed}}{D_{ed}K_{ed}} - \frac{1}{K_{de}(D_{de}k_{de})^{1/2}} \tag{19}$$

   where the epidermis and dermis parameters are taken from Tables 3 and 4. Unless the compound is highly lipophilic, this correction may be omitted and P_{sc} (hydrated) $\cong k_p$. Note that the series resistance model leading to Equation (19) follows from the steady-state analysis in Reference 13 and is also discussed in Reference 14.

2. Calculate the partially hydrated skin permeability P_{sc} as

$$P_{sc} = P_{sc}(\text{hydrated}) \cdot \frac{P_{sc}^{model}(\text{partially hydrated})}{P_{sc}^{model}(\text{hydrated})} \tag{20}$$

   where the ratio on the right corrects the experimental value to the partially hydrated state using the model calculation (25). As the model is presently parameterized (Table 2), this ratio is essentially 1:3 (8).

3. Calculate the remaining stratum corneum parameters according to Equations (14) to (18) (Table 2).

   Independent of whether the model-based calculation or the experimentally based calculation of stratum corneum properties is employed, one further correction is advised. The permeant solubility in stratum corneum, C_{sat}, and the related saturation dose, M_{sat}, are key parameters in the transient diffusion calculation. C_{sat} is estimated from water solubility S_w and stratum corneum/water partition coefficient K_{sc}, according to Equation (17). This approach of equating a partition coefficient, K_{sc} (which is defined for infinitely dilute solutions), to a solubility ratio, C_{sat}/S_w, works

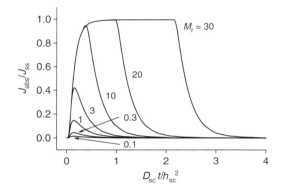

FIGURE 3 Transient absorption flux for a moderately volatile permeant (7). The reduced dose M_r = applied dose/M_{sat} determines the boundary between small and large doses. For small doses ($M_r \leq 1$), the absorption curves have the same shape and are dose-proportional.

well for poorly soluble permeants but can lead to substantial errors for more soluble permeants whose presence affects the structure of either stratum corneum or water. It is our experience that C_{sat} may be significantly overestimated by Equation (17) for very soluble permeants (34). In the absence of a better approximation than Equation (17), we recommend imposing a limit on C_{sat} based on experimental evidence. The current limit for our calculations for all permeants except water is $C_{sat} = 0.300$ g/cm³, which is the measured value for ethanol in stratum corneum containing 30% water (35). For water, C_{sat} may be as high as 0.79 (31). Imposition of these limits avoids the mistake of calculating skin absorption based on unrealistically high stratum corneum concentrations. Therefore, for all permeants except water, Equation (17) is modified to

$$C_{sat} = \min(K_{sc}S_w, 0.300 \text{ g/cm}^3) \tag{21}$$

If the 0.300 g/cm³ limit for C_{sat} is selected, a revised K_{sc} is then calculated as

$$K_{sc} = C_{sat} / S_w \tag{22}$$

effectively replacing Equation (14).

Dermis

The dermis is a fibrous matrix that is largely acellular. Collagen and elastin fibers hinder the diffusion of macromolecules, and the glycosaminoglycans, which fill much of the interfiber spaces, hinder transport of both large and small molecules due to their fine herringbone structure. There is a vascular plexus approximately 1 mm deep in the skin, which gives rise to a system of capillary loops that extend nearly to the dermal-epidermal junction. This system has been described in detail by Braverman (36).

A microscopic model for transport in the dermis may be derived by considering a system of capillary loops (Fig. 4). Mathematical analysis of solute diffusion and absorption by the capillaries (27,37) shows that the system may be modeled as a homogeneous matrix with a uniform clearance in the upper dermis. This analogy has been described in some detail (14), and the effective partitioning, diffusivity, and clearance values for mammalian dermis have been estimated (14). The latter analysis suggests that both partitioning and diffusivity of small lipophilic permeants in dermis are functions of noncovalent binding to extravascular serum proteins. They may be related to the ionization state of the permeant f_{non} (fraction nonionized at pH

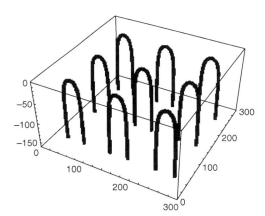

FIGURE 4 Three-dimensional array of capillary loops forming the basis of the dermal microtransport model described in Ref. 27.

TABLE 3   Formulas for Dermis Transport Parameters (14)

Parameter	Units	Formula or Value	Eq. #
Defining relationship	–	$\dfrac{\partial C}{\partial t} = D_{de}\dfrac{\partial^2 C}{\partial z^2} - k_{de}C$	(23)
h_{de}	cm	0.20	(24)
K_{free}	–	0.6	(25)
$K_{de}{}^a$	–	$K_{free}\left(0.68 + 0.32/f_u + 0.001f_{non}K_{oct}\right)$	(26)
D_{free}	–	$10^{\wedge}(-4.15 - 0.655\,\log MW)$	(27)
D_{de}	cm²/sec	$D_{free}/(0.68 + 0.32/f_u + 0.001f_{non}K_{oct})$	(28)
k_{free}	sec⁻¹	0.0022ᵇ	(29)
k_{de}	sec⁻¹	$K_{free}/\left(0.68 + 0.32/f_u + 0.001f_{non}K_{oct}\right)$	(30)

ᵃEq. 26 expresses K_{de} with respect to a pH 7.4 aqueous solution (i.e., $K_{de/pH\,7.4}$). To express K_{de} relative to a solution in which it is completely nonionized, the corresponding formula is (14)
ᵇValue assumes blood-flow limited clearance and is derived from data for rat (14)

$$K_{de/non} = K_{free}\left[(0.68 + 0.32/f_u)/f_{non} + 0.001K_{oct}\right] \qquad (31)$$

7.4) and to $1/f_u$, where f_u is the fraction unbound in a 2% albumin solution as shown in Equations (24) to (27) (Table 3). Steric and charge exclusion are also factors, leading to partition coefficients less than unity for small hydrophilic permeants (e.g., glucose (38)) and considerably smaller values for macromolecules such as albumin (15). For low MW moderately lipophilic compounds, the relationships in Table 3 serve as a working model for transport in dermis. The defining transport relationship for the distributed clearance model is given in this table as Equation (23).

The unique part of this relationship is the parameter k_{de} representing capillary clearance. The value of k_{de} is comprised of an intrinsic clearance k_{free}, which applies to freely diffusing permeant, and a binding factor identical to that for diffusivity [Equation (28)]. For small lipophilic compounds the intrinsic clearance k_{free} is approximately constant as it is limited by blood flow.

Viable Epidermis

The viable epidermis is the thin cellular epithelial layer sandwiched between the dermis and the stratum corneum. Its thickness in humans varies from about 50 to 100 μm due to the articulated nature of the dermis. Less is known about the transport properties of this layer than either stratum corneum or dermis because it is difficult to isolate. Due to its cellular structure, it presents a set of obstacles to solute transport different from those of dermis. In particular, hydrophilic solutes that do not easily cross cell membranes are confined to the tortuous extracellular space and experience longer diffusion pathways than do lipophilic solutes. This problem may be modeled using an extracellular fluid diffusivity modified by a tortuosity factor and void fraction (39) or, alternatively, with an effective medium approach. The latter is more easily generalized to cover both hydrophilic and lipophilic solutes as tortuosity and void fraction are functions of membrane permeability.

There is not yet a microscopic model for epidermal transport on which to base an effective medium model. There are, however, experimental diffusivity and permeability values for hydrophilic solutes in other cellular tissues (39,40) and an experimental value for glucose diffusivity in epidermis from our laboratory (38). Schultz and Armstrong (39) found the permeabilities of extracellular solutes in a rat diaphragm to be about 1/30 to 1/50 of their values in water. Although they modeled this in terms of a tortuous diffusion model, the effective medium approach would assign most of this reduction to an effective diffusivity D_{ed}. We determined the upper and lower limits for glucose diffusivity in epidermis to be 1/8 and 1/200th of aqueous diffusivity using a combination of desorption and permeability measurements (38). Considering both of the above results, it is evident that Equations (27) to (28), which yield diffusivity values 1/5 to 1/20 of aqueous diffusivity (14), are a reasonable starting point for epidermal diffusivity estimation. This is a working approximation until better estimates are developed. With a comparable level of uncertainty, we choose to represent K_{ed} with Equations (25) to (26), developed for dermis. As a comparison, the calculated value for K_{ed} for glucose according to Equations (25) to (26) is 0.6 versus a measured value of 0.81 ± 0.06 (38). The working values for transport parameters in the viable epidermis are summarized in Table 4.

EVAPORATIVE LOSS MODEL

Volatile permeants are lost from the skin surface at a rate governed by their vapor pressure, density, thermodynamic activity, and mass transfer coefficient at the skin–air interface. The working model for this calculation is summarized in Table 5. Thermodynamic activity is taken to be unity for a pure liquid or solid residing on the skin surface (Case 2) and $C(0,t)/C_{sat}$ for permeant dissolved in the upper stratum corneum (Case 1). Here, $C(0,t)$ is the concentration just below the skin-air interface, and C_{sat} is the solubility of the permeant in the stratum corneum (cf. Table 2). For Case 2, M_{surf} is the mass of permeant residing on the skin surface. The gas phase mass transfer coefficient k_g [Eq. (37)] is taken from the chemical spills literature (42) as per the suggestion of N-Dri-Stempfer and Bunge (42), as discussed in Ref. 7. The overall mass transfer coefficient $k_{evap} \times \rho$ is then calculated by assuming liquid-vapor equilibrium and ideal gas behavior at the skin-air interface [(Eq. 38)]. This has been termed the Raoult-Dalton model for evaporative loss (43).

IMPLEMENTATION OF TRANSPORT MODEL

The relationships shown in Tables 2 to 5, combined with appropriate boundary conditions (7,13) and the physical properties inputs from Table 1, constitute a well-posed system of partial differential equations describing transient transport of volatile substances applied to skin. To produce numbers from these relationships, the simultaneous equations [Eqs. (1), (23), and (32)] must be solved. A wide variety of tools including commercial software programs are available for this task. We have developed

TABLE 4 Formulas for Viable Epidermis Transport Parameters (14)

Parameter	Units	Formula or Value	Eq. #
Defining relationship	–	$\dfrac{\partial C}{\partial t} = D_{ed}\dfrac{\partial^2 C}{\partial z^2} - k_{ed}C$	(32)
h_{ed}	cm	0.0100	(33)
K_{ed}	–	Eqs. (25)–(26) (Table 3)[a]	–
D_{ed}	cm²/sec	Eqs. (27)–(28) (Table 3)[a]	–
k_{ed}	sec⁻¹	0 (in the absence of skin metabolism)	(34)

[a]These relationships are placeholders until a more complete analysis is available.

TABLE 5 Formulas for Evaporative Loss Calculation (7,8,34)

Parameter	Units	Formula or value		Eq. #
Defining relationships		$D_{sc} \left. \dfrac{\partial C}{\partial x} \right|_{x=0} = k_{evap} \cdot \dfrac{\rho}{C_{sat}} \cdot C(0,t)$	Case 1	(35)
		$-\dfrac{dM_{surf}}{dt} = k_{evap} \cdot \rho + D_{sc} \left. \dfrac{\partial C}{\partial x} \right|_{x=h_{dep}}$	Case 2	(36)
k_g	cm/sec	$1.756\, u^{0.78} / MW^{1/3}$		(37)
k_{evap}	cm/sec	$k_g \dfrac{P_{vp} MW}{(0.76 \times 10^6)\, \rho RT}$		(38)

TABLE 6 Physical Properties and Derived Skin Transport Parameters for Benzyl Alcohol. The Temperature for All Calculations Has Been Taken as 32°C

Parameter	Units	Value		
Input properties				
MW	Da	108		
$\log K_{oct}$	–	1.10		
S_w	g/cm^3	0.0429		
P_{vp}	torr	0.18		
ρ	g·cm^3	1.04		
f_u		0.37[a]		
f_{non}		1		
Experimental skin transport properties				
k_p (hydrated)	cm/sec	4.69×10^{-6}		
Derived properties		*Model based*	*Experimental based*	
P_{sc} (hydrated)	cm/sec	$[1.01 \times 10^{-6}]^b$	4.69×10^{-6}	
P_{sc}	cm/sec	0.32×10^{-6}	1.74×10^{-6}	
D_{sc}	cm^2/sec	0.49×10^{-10}	3.32×10^{-10}	
K_{sc}		8.71	6.99	
h_{sc}^2/D_{sc}	hours	10.1	1.77	
C_{sat}	g·cm^{-3}	0.374	0.300	
M_{sat}	µg·cm^{-2}	49.9	40.1	
D_{ed}	cm^2/sec	2.15×10^{-6}		
K_{ed}	–	0.93		
D_{de}	cm^2/sec	2.15×10^{-6}		
K_{de}	–	0.93		

[a]Calculated from the model of Yamazaki and Kanaoka (28).
[b]Calculated as in Ref. 25. For comparison, the value calculated from the Potts-Guy equation (44) is 0.66×10^{-6} cm/sec.

our own computer code using the finite difference approach discussed in Ref. 7. Essentially, the Visual Basic code for stratum corneum + vehicle from Ref. 7 was modified by adding the viable epidermis and dermis layers. The calculation is implemented as an add-in operating under Microsoft Excel®, with an associated spreadsheet to calculate the various properties and output results as tables and graphs.

EXAMPLE CALCULATIONS FOR A FRAGRANCE INGREDIENT

The nature of the solution to the problem depicted in Figure 1 and described by Equations (1) to (38) can be illustrated by considering the skin disposition of a fragrance ingredient applied to skin either neat or from a highly volatile solvent. We choose as an example benzyl alcohol, applied as a dilute solution in ethanol. This compound has been studied in our laboratory, both in vitro (2,8) and in vivo (4). Its physical properties, experimental skin permeability, and derived skin transport properties are listed in Table 6. For the following calculations, we choose the experimentally based skin transport parameters listed in Table 6. Thus, the saturation dose (M_{sat}) is taken to be 40.1 µg/cm². Doses less than 40.1 µg/cm² dissipate in a dose-proportional manner, whereas larger doses do not (cf. Fig. 3).

Figure 5 shows the overall disposition of a small applied dose (0.9 µg/cm², M_r = 0.022) and a large applied dose (127 µg/cm², M_r = 3.17) as a function of wind velocity above the skin surface. The evaporated fraction increases with wind velocity, as intuitively expected. For a given value of the wind velocity, the fractional absorption of the small dose (Fig. 5A) is higher than that of the larger dose (Fig. 5B). How may this be explained?

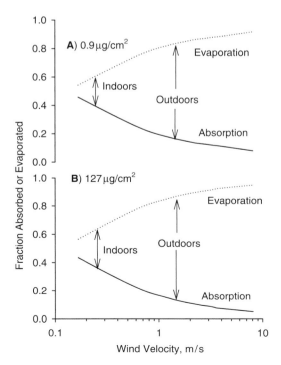

FIGURE 5 Calculated effect of wind velocity (u) on skin disposition of benzyl alcohol. (**A**) Small dose (M_r = 0.022; Case 1); (**B**) large dose (M_r = 3.17; Case 2). Arrows mark recommended choices for indoor and outdoor exposure scenarios. The fractional absorption is higher for the small dose because more of the dose is initially deposited into the upper skin layers. For highly volatile solvents, the difference is larger (34). Note added in proof: For calculation of k_g according to Equation (37) our updated recommendation is to use u = 0.165 m/sec for indoor exposures and u = 0.72 m/sec for outdoor exposures. These values result in more conservative estimates of the evaporation rates than those shown in the figure.

The answer lies in the deposition depth h_{dep} (cf. Fig. 1). According to this concept, small doses of skin permeants are rapidly deposited into the upper stratum corneum. The evaporation rate from the deposition layer is slower than that from the surface because the compound must diffuse back to the surface before it can be released. The deposition layer concept is supported by detailed analyses of the skin disposition of DEET (33) and benzyl alcohol (8) and by ongoing work in our laboratories on volatile solvents. Based on in vitro absorption studies with ethanol and benzene (34), the deposition layer appears to be particularly important to understanding solvent absorption, which is higher than might be expected from finite dose models lacking this feature [cf. Ref. 45 and Eqs. (29)–(35) of Ref. 7].

Figure 6 shows representative transient absorption profiles for benzyl alcohol applied to the skin. The model curves are compared with in vitro human skin absorption data from Ref. 8. The small doses (Fig. 5A) are better described by the model than the large doses (Fig. 5B), for which the absorption rate is underpredicted. This discrepancy can be corrected by employing a concentration-dependent diffusivity for benzyl alcohol in stratum corneum, as described in Ref. 8. By allowing the diffusivity to increase threefold between low concentrations and the solubility limit C_{sat}, the agreement is substantially improved (inset to Fig. 5B). This skin penetration enhancement effect is also evident in the dose dependence for benzyl alcohol (8) and DEET (32) absorption, which goes opposite to that shown in Figure 6. A model for predicting such skin permeability enhancement effects is clearly needed to obtain

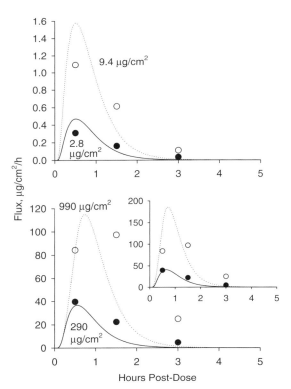

FIGURE 6 Absorptive flux of benzyl alcohol applied to human skin in vitro. (**A**) Small doses; (**B**) large doses. The experimental data were taken from Ref. 8 and the theoretical curves from the model described in this chapter using a wind velocity of 1.5 m/sec. Absorption rates for the larger doses are underpredicted due to skin permeability enhancement by benzyl alcohol as described in Ref. 8. This can be corrected (*Inset*) by allowing a concentration-dependent diffusivity for the permeant in the stratum corneum as described in the text.

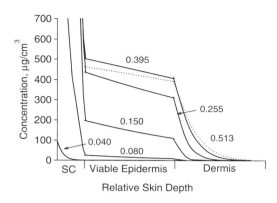

FIGURE 7 Calculated concentration profiles in lower skin layers for benzyl alcohol following topical application of 127 µg/cm² in ethanolic solution at a skin temperature of 32°C and a wind velocity of 0.25 m/sec. The numbers on the graph reflect hours post-dose. Layer thicknesses are scaled for better visibility. According to the calculation, a maximum mid-epidermal concentration (C_{max}) of 450 µg/cm³ was achieved at a time (t_{max}) of 0.395 hours.

quantitative agreement with absorption data for compounds like benzyl alcohol. We would anticipate similar findings for many other skin permeation enhancers.

Figure 7 shows an additional way in which the transient absorption/evaporation model may be employed. Concentration profiles within each skin layer throughout the course of the absorption are automatically generated during the calculation. For some problems, these skin concentrations are more important than systemic absorption estimates. For example, the efficacy of topical drug or the allergenicity of a fragrance ingredient or a preservative is likely to be related to skin concentrations. The computer model allows one to estimate peak concentration (C_{max}) and time-to-peak concentration (t_{max}) at an arbitrary depth in the tissue. The utility of such calculations in interpreting contact allergy dose–response data has recently been discussed (46).

SUMMARY

Volatile compounds in cosmetic formulations rarely, if ever, achieve steady-state absorption profiles following application to the skin. Their disposition is governed by physical properties (MW, lipophilicity, solubility, vapor pressure, and density) and environmental factors (temperature and wind velocity) as well as the dose and the formulation in which they are applied. A working model to calculate this disposition from simple formulations has been presented. Some of the model components are not yet completely characterized and require additional research. In particular, the extent to which small molecules affect their own permeation rates through the stratum corneum is generally unknown. Key features that make the present computational model potentially more useful than other transient skin absorption models are (1) microscopically based components for stratum corneum and dermis, (2) the incorporation of hydration effects and solubility limits in the stratum corneum, and (3) the concept of a deposition depth and an associated saturation dose that defines the transition from small to large doses of permeant on the skin.

ACKNOWLEDGMENTS

Support from the U.S. National Institute for Occupational Safety and Health, the U.S. National Science Foundation, Procter & Gamble Company's International Program for Animal Alternatives, and COLIPA for the development of these methods is gratefully acknowledged.

REFERENCES

1.   Kasting GB, Saiyasombati P. A physico-chemical properties based model for estimating evaporation and absorption rates of perfumes from skin. Int J Cosmet Sci 2001; 23:49–58.
2.   Saiyasombati P, Kasting GB. Disposition of benzyl alcohol following topical application to human skin in vitro. J Pharm Sci 2003; 92(10):2128–2139.
3.   Saiyasombati P, Kasting GB. Two-stage kinetic analysis of fragrance evaporation and absorption from skin. Int J Cosmet Sci 2003; 25:235–243.
4.   Saiyasombati P, Kasting GB. Evaporation of benzyl alcohol from human skin in vivo. J Pharm Sci 2004; 93(2):515–520.
5.   Saiyasombati P, Kasting GB. Prediction of fragrance headspace concentrations from physicochemical properties. Perfum Flavor 2004; 29(5):38–47.
6.   Kasting GB. Estimating the absorption of volatile compounds applied to skin. In: Riviere JE, ed. Dermal Absorption Models in Toxicology and Pharmacology. New York: Taylor and Francis, 2005:175–188.
7.   Kasting GB, Miller MA. Kinetics of finite dose absorption through skin 2. Volatile compounds. J Pharm Sci 2006; 95(2):268–280.
8.   Miller MA, Bhatt V, Kasting GB. Absorption and evaporation of benzyl alcohol from skin. J Pharm Sci 2006; 95(2):281–291.
9.   Cleek RL, Bunge AL. A new method for estimating dermal absorption from chemical exposure. 1. General approach. Pharm Res 1993; 10(4):497–506.
10.   Anissimov YG, Roberts MS. Diffusion modeling of percutaneous absorption kinetics: 2. Finite vehicle volume and solvent deposited solids. J Pharm Sci 2001; 90:504–520.
11.   Kasting GB. Kinetics of finite dose absorption 1. Vanillylnonanamide. J Pharm Sci 2001; 90(2):202–212.
12.   Cross S, Magnusson BM, Winckle G, Anissimov YG, Roberts MS. Determination of the effect of lipophilicity on the in vitro permeability and tissue reservoir characteristics of topically applied solutes in human skin layers. J Invest Dermatol 2003; 120:759–764.
13.   Kretsos K, Kasting GB, Nitsche JM. Distributed diffusion-clearance model for transient drug distribution within the skin. J Pharm Sci 2004; 93(11):2820–2835.
14.   Kretsos K, Miller MA, Zamora-Estrada G, Kasting GB 2007. Partitioning, diffusivity and clearance of skin permeants in mammalian dermis. Int J Pharm in press, doi:10.1016/ j.ijpharm.2007.06.020.
15.   Maxwell JC. A Treatise on Electricity and Magnetism. Vol. I. Oxford: Clarendon Press, 1892:440–441.
16.   Rayleigh L. On the influence of obstacles arranged in rectangular order upon properties of a medium. Phil Mag (Fifth Ser) 1892; 34:481–502.
17.   Brenner H, Edwards DA. Macrotransport Processes. Boston: Butterworth-Heinemann, 1993.
18.   Scheuplein RJ. Mechanism of percutaneous absorption: II. Transient diffusion and the relative importance of various routes of skin penetration. J Invest Dermatol 1967; 48(1):79–88.
19.   Pirot F, Kalia YN, Stinchcomb AL, Keating G, Bunge A, Guy RH. Characterization of the permeability barrier of human skin in vivo. Proc Nat Acad Sci USA 1997; 94: 1562–1567.
20.   Kalia YN, Pirot F, Guy RH. Homogeneous transport in a heterogeneous membrane: water diffusion across human stratum corneum in vivo. Biophys J 1996; 71:2692–2700.
21.   Frasch HF, Barbaro AM. Steady-state flux and lag time in the stratum corneum lipid pathway: results from finite element models. J Pharm Sci 2003; 92(11):2196–2207.
22.   Barbero AM, Frasch HF. Modeling of diffusion with partitioning in stratum corneum using a finite element model. Ann Biomed Eng 2005; 33:1281–1292.
23.   Barbero AM, Frasch HF. Transcellular route of diffusion through stratum corneum: results from finite element models. J Pharm Sci 2006; 95(10):2186–2194.
24.   Wang T-F, Kasting GB, Nitsche JM. A multiphase microscopic model for stratum corneum permeability: I. Formulation, solution and illustrative results for representative compounds. J Pharm Sci 2006; 95(3):620–648.
25.   Wang T-F, Kasting GB, Nitsche JM. A multiphase microscopic model for stratum corneum permeability: II. Estimation of physicochemical parameters and application to a large permeability database. J Pharm Sci 2007; 96(11):3024–3051.

26. Nitsche JM, Wang T-F, Kasting GB. A two-phase analysis of solute partitioning into the stratum corneum. J Pharm Sci 2006; 95(3):649–666.

27. Kretsos K, Kasting GB. A geometrical model of dermal capillary clearance. Math Biosci 2007; 208(2):430–453.

28. Yamazaki K, Kanaoka M. Computational prediction of the plasma protein-binding percent of diverse pharmaceutical compounds. J Pharm Sci 2004; 93(6):1480–1494.

29. Talreja PS, Kleene NK, Pickens W, Wang T-F, Kasting GB. Visualization of lipid barrier and measurement of lipid path length in human stratum corneum. AAPS PharmSci 2001; 3(2):Article 13.

30. Johnson ME, Berk DA, Blankschtein D, Golan DE, Jain RK, Langer RS. Lateral diffusion of small compounds in human stratum corneum and model lipid bilayer systems. Biophys J 1996; 71(November):2656–2668.

31. Kasting GB, Barai ND. Equilibrium water sorption in human stratum corneum. J Pharm Sci 2003; 92(8):1624–1631.

32. Kasting GB, Barai ND, Wang T-F, Nitsche JM. Mobility of water in human stratum corneum. J Pharm Sci 2003; 92(11):2326–2340.

33. Santhanam A, Miller MA, Kasting GB. Absorption and evaporation of *N,N*-diethyl-*m*-toluamide (DEET) from human skin in vitro. Toxicol Appl Pharmacol 2005; 204:81–90.

34. Ray Chaudhuri S. Mathematical modeling of percutaneous absorption of volatile compounds following transient liquid-phase exposures. PhD thesis, University of Cincinnati, Cincinnati, 2007.

35. Berner B, Juang R-H, Mazzenga GC. Ethanol and water sorption into stratum corneum and model systems. J Pharm Sci 1989; 78(6):472–476.

36. Braverman IM. The cutaneous microcirculation: ultrastructure and microanatomical organization. Microcirculation 1997; 4(3):329–340.

37. Kretsos K. Transport phenomena in the human skin. PhD thesis, State University of New York, Buffalo, 2003.

38. Khalil E, Kretsos K, Kasting GB. Glucose partition coefficient and diffusivity in the lower skin layers. Pharm Res 2006; 23(6):1227–1234.

39. Schultz JS, Armstrong W. Permeability of interstitial space of muscle (rat diaphragm) to solutes of different molecular weights. J Pharm Sci 1978; 67(5):696–700.

40. Jain RK. Interstitial Transport in Tumors: Barriers and Strategies for Improvement. American Association for Cancer Research 96th Annual Meeting, 2005.

41. Peress J. Estimate evaporative losses from spills. Chem Eng Prog 2003; (April):32–34.

42. N-Dri-Stempfer B, Bunge AL. How Much Can Evaporation of Dermally Absorbed Chemical Reduce the Systemically Absorbed Dose? Occupational and Environmental Exposure of Skin to Chemicals, Stockholm, Sweden, 2005.

43. Lyman WJ, Reehl WF, Rosenblatt DH. Handbook of Chemical Property Estimation. New York: McGraw-Hill, 1982.

44. Potts RO, Guy RH. Predicting skin permeability. Pharm Res 1992; 9(5):663–669.

45. Frasch HF, Barbaro AM. The Transient Dermal Dose Problem, Occupational and Environmental Exposures of Skin to Chemicals, Stockholm, Sweden, 2005.

46. Basketter DA, Casati S, Cronin MTD, et al. Skin sensitisation and epidermal disposition. The relevance of epidermal bioavailability for sensitisation hazard identification/risk assessment. Altern Lab Anim 2007; 35:137–154.

24 Efficacy, Absorption, and Safety of Essential Oils

Ulrich F. Schäfer
Biopharmaceutics and Pharmaceutical Technology, Saarland University, Saarbruecken, Germany

Jürgen Schneele, Sonja Schmitt, and Jürgen Reichling
Department of Biology, Institut of Pharmacy and Molecular Biotechnology, University of Heidelberg, Heidelberg, Germany

INTRODUCTION

Essential oils are produced by blossoms, leaves, and fruits of different plants and stored in special tissues such as glandular hairs, oil cells, oil receptacles, and oil ducts. For commercial use, essential oils are derived from plant material by extraction or steam distillation. Each essential oil is a complex aromatic-smelling volatile mixture of many different compounds having low molecular weights and diverse chemical structures (see Dweck, this volume, for chemical details). Predominant compounds are monoterpene hydrocarbons, sequiterpene hydrocarbons, their corresponding oxidized products (e.g., alcohols, aldehydes, ethers, ketones, and phenols), homologues of phenylpropanoids, as well as minor amounts of diterpenoids and miscellaneous volatile organic compounds (1). Normally, essential oils are characterized by their plant origin and in some cases by predominating chemical components. For essential oils, antibacterial, antifungal, anti-inflammatory, antirheumatic, antitussive, antiviral, expectorant, immunomodulatory, sedative, and blood-circulation-enhancing effects have been described. They are able to improve the odor of cosmetic preparations, and they may act on cognition, memory, and mood (2). It is commonly accepted that the biological activity of an essential oil is the result of both its active and inactive substances. Inactive substances may influence resorption, skin penetration, rate of reaction, or bioavailability of the active compounds. In addition, several active compounds may have a synergistic effect. Furthermore, the biological activity of a given essential oil may also be influenced by factors related to the medicinal plant (e.g., genotype, chemotype, and geographical origin) as well as to environmental and agronomic conditions. The means of application depends on the pathophysiology, the desired outcome, safety, and toxicity data, as well as cultural preferences. For treating respiratory symptoms and nervous disorders, inhalation may be the best means of application, whereas topical application is the best way for treating skin diseases. Oral administration is not common, except in the case of inflammation of the oral cavity and the pharynx. For dermal application, which together with inhalation is the most common application of essential oils, percutaneous absorption is of great interest. Among the local effects, the amount of a substance remaining on the surface of the body is very decisive. Many substances are able to penetrate into the different layers of the skin and even into the bloodstream. The extent of skin permeation may be the reason why essential oils often have systemic side effects or systemic bioavailability following dermal application. Another problem concerning the cutaneous use of essential oils is the degree of skin and mucous membrane irritation. Essential oils applied undiluted may cause irritation and toxic erythema. Therefore, it is recommended that essential oils are used only in diluted forms for external application.

EFFICACY OF ESSENTIAL OILS
Antibacterial Activity
Numerous studies have demonstrated the broad antibacterial activity of essential oils against gram-positive and gram-negative bacteria (3–8). In addition, antifungal properties of essential oils have been documented (9). Essential oils are reported to differ in their biological activity against various bacterial species (Table 1). The different susceptibility of bacteria to essential oils may be due not only to the variable chemical composition of the essential oils, but also to variations in the cell wall structure, lipid and protein composition of the cytoplasmic membrane, and specific physiological processes of the different bacterial species.

As shown in Table 1, the gram-negative bacterium *Pseudomonas aeruginosa* was not inhibited by most of the essential oils tested. This finding is in good agreement with results obtained by other researchers (10). With this in mind, it is of interest that the outer membrane of *Escherichia coli* and *P. aeruginosa* was reported to present a relatively hydrophilic barrier, protecting the cytoplasmic membrane and the cytoplasm against an attack by lipophilic compounds. On the other hand, it has also been demonstrated that raising the permeability of the outer membrane of *P. aeruginosa* using EDTA led to an increased antibacterial activity of tea tree oil (TTO) (10).

Mode and Mechanism of Antibacterial Action
While the antibacterial activity of essential oils is well documented, their mode and mechanism of action are not yet fully understood. Current research work on this topic suggests that there are different target sites and modes of action. At present, it

TABLE 1 Antibacterial Activity of Essential Oils Against Gram-Positive and Gram-Negative Bacteria—a Selection

Bacteria	Clove oil	Lemon balm oil	Peppermint oil	Rosemary oil	Thyme oil
Gram-positive					
Bacillus subtilis	0.2	0.1	0.2	0.2	0.1
Enterococcus durans	0.2	0.5	0.5	2.0	0.2
Listeria monocytogenes	0.1	0.06	0.06	0.2	0.1
Staphylococcus aureus	0.1	0.1	0.1	0.5	0.1
Gram-negative					
Escherichia coli	0.2	0.5	2.0	4.0	0.2
Helicobacter pylori	Not tested	0.015	0.015	0.015	0.03
Pseudomonas aeruginosa	0.2	4.0	4.0	4.0	4.0
Shigella flexneri	0.1	0.06	0.2	4.0	0.1

(header spanning: Minimum inhibitory concentration (MIC))

Note: MIC values given in % v/v. *Source*: From Refs. 4 and 5.

is commonly accepted that essential oils and some of their components act mainly on microbial cytoplasmic membranes.

For example, TTO not only increased the leakage of K^+ ions from cells of *Staphylococcus aureus* and *E. coli*, but also inhibited cell respiration of both strains of bacteria. Furthermore, it is known that oxidized monoterpenes, such as alcohols, aldehydes, and phenols, will increase cytoplasmic membrane fluidity and permeability, disturb the order of membrane-embedded proteins, inhibit cell respiration, and alter ion transport processes. Sites of action other than the cytoplasmic membrane also exist (Table 2).

Antiviral Activity

There is considerable evidence, from both in vitro studies and controlled clinical trials, of the potential of plant-derived phytoantiviral agents for the treatment of viral infections (25). Many essential oils have been evaluated for antiviral activity. Most were tested against enveloped RNA and DNA viruses, such as Herpes simplex virus type 1 and type 2 (DNA viruses), Dengue virus (RNA virus), human immunodeficiency virus type 1 (RNA virus), influenza virus (H1N1; RNA virus), Junin virus (RNA virus), and Newcastle disease virus (RNA virus (26–33), whereas only few essential oils (e.g., oregano oil and clove oil) were tested against nonenveloped RNA and DNA viruses, such as Adenovirus type 3 (DNA virus), Poliovirus (RNA virus), and Coxsackie virus B-1 (RNA virus) (26,27). The antiviral activity of the essential oils tested was clearly demonstrated for enveloped viruses of both the DNA and RNA type. On the contrary, the nonenveloped viruses were not susceptible to essential oils.

Mode and Mechanism of Antiviral Action

To learn more about the effect of essential oils on enveloped viruses, we investigated the antiviral activity of anise oil, hyssop oil, thyme oil, dwarfpine oil, citrus oil, manuka oil, ginger oil, camomile oil, and sandalwood oil against HSV-1 and HSV-2 in vitro (34). The replication cycle of Herpes simplex virus is characterized by a complex sequence of different steps that offer opportunities for antiviral agents to intervene. To determine the mode of action, essential oils were added to host cells and viruses at different stages during viral infection.

1. Host cells (African green monkey kidney cells) were pretreated for 1 hour with essential oils prior to inoculation with herpes viruses (pretreatment of cells).
2. Herpes viruses were incubated with essential oils for 1 hour prior to infection of host cells (pretreatment of virus).
3. Herpes viruses were mixed with essential oils and added to the host cells immediately (adsorption).
4. Host cells were incubated with essential oils after penetration of herpes viruses into the cells (intracellular replication).

Inhibition of HSV replication was measured by a plaque reduction assay. In this assay, the number of plaques of drug-treated cells and viruses [plaque-forming unit (pfu)] was expressed as percent (% v/v) of the untreated control (number of plaques formed by viruses in the absence of essential oil). In all assays, the maximum noncytotoxic concentrations of the essential oils tested (0.0006–0.01%) were used.

TABLE 2 Targets and Physiological Effects of Selected Essential Oils and Individual
Oil Components

Targets	Bacteria	Substances	References
Cell morphology			
Forming elongated filamentous forms after treatment with essential oil; normal cells: 3–5 μm in length; elongated cells: 10–25 μm in length	*E. coli*	Palmrose oil; peppermint oil	(11)
Alteration of cell shape: cells of wild type exhibit a flask-shaped morphology, whereas TTO-treated strains form ovoid or round cells	*M. pneumoniae*	TTO	(12)
Cytoplasmic membrane (alteration of integrity and permeability)			
Inhibition of cell respiration	*E. coli; S. aureus*	TTO	(13,14)
Inhibition of oxygen uptake, respiratory electron flow, and oxidative phosphorylation	*R. sphaeroides*	Thymol, carvacrol, other monoterpene alcohols	(15)
K$^+$ leakage	*E. coli; S. aureus*	TTO; TTO, farnesol, nerolidol	(13,14,16)
Depletion of intracellular ATP concentration	*E. coli, L. monocytogenes; E. coli*	Oregano oil, cinnamon oil, savory oil; carvacrol, thymol	(17,18)
Formation of multilamellar mesosome-like structures	*S. aureus*	TTO; terpinen-4-ol	(19,20)
Cell wall			
Formation of extracellular blebs	*E. coli*	TTO; lemongrass oil	(21,22)
Disintegration of outer membrane and outer-membrane-associated LPS release	*E. coli*	Thymol, carvacrol	(17)
Cell lysis	*S. pneumoniae; E. coli, B. subtilis*	Oregano oil, thyme oil; oregano oil, glove oil	(23,24)
Cell division			
Total inhibition of cell division	*S. aureus*	TTO	(20)
Cell cytoplasm/cytosol			
Formation of condensed filamentous electron-dense material in the cytoplasm/cytosol	*S. aureus*	TTO	(20)

Abbreviations: TTO, tea tree oil; *Bacillus subtilis, B. subtilis; Escherichia coli, E. coli; S. aureus, Staphylococcus aureus; S. pneumoniae, Streptococcus pneumoniae; R. sphaeroides, Rhodopseudomonas sphaeroides; L. monocytogenes, Listeria monocytogenes*; and *M. pneumoniae, Mycoplasma pneumoniae*.

Pretreatment of cells with essential oils 1 hour prior to virus infection did not reduce the virus plaque formation. This suggests that essential oils did not affect the adsorption of viruses to cell surface, indicating that essential oils did not interfere with virus binding by blocking cellular receptors. On the other hand, pretreatment of viruses with essential oils 1 hour prior to cell infection caused a significant reduction of plaques of 95% to 99% (pfu: 5% to 1%) for HSV-1 and of 70% to 98% (pfu: 30% to 2%) for HSV-2 (Fig. 1). When the test oils were added during the adsorption period of viruses to host cells, only dwarf pine oil and citrus oil reduced the plaque formation of about 80% for both HSV-1 and HSV-2. All other essential oils exhibited somewhat different antiviral effects with respect to HSV-1 and HSV-2.

In contrast, when essential oils were added to the overlay medium after penetration of the viruses into the host cells, only manuka oil significantly reduced the plaque formation of HSV-1 by about 40%. From dose–response assays, the IC_{50} (concentration of the test oil that inhibited plaque numbers by 50% when viruses were pretreated with the oil one hour prior to cell infection) and TC_{50} (cytotoxic concentration of the test oil that reduced viable cell numbers by 50%) values were calculated and summarized in Table 3. A clear dose-dependent antiviral activity was demonstrated for HSV-1 and HSV-2.

Increasing concentrations of essential oils at noncytotoxic concentrations induced a decline in viral replication. The most effective essential oils were camomile oil, ginger oil, hysop oil, and manuka oil, which all had high selectivity indices (SI values). The selectivity index (quotient of TC_{50} / IC_{50}) describes the relative difference between the cytotoxic concentration and inhibitory concentration of the selected oil. A large SI value indicates that the cytotoxic effect of an essential oil is low relative to its antiviral effect. With respect to therapeutic applications, it makes more sense to use essential oils with comparatively high SI values.

In conclusion, our results indicate that free viruses in particular are very sensitive to essential oils. Both types of herpes simplex virus are inactivated before adsorption or during adsorption to cell surfaces but not after penetration into cells, the typical mode of action of nucleoside analogues such as acyclovir. These data suggest that essential oils interfere with the virus envelope or mask the viral compounds that are necessary for adsorption or entry into host cells. Recently, an electron microscopic examination demonstrated that the envelope of HSV-1 was disrupted when treated with oregano oil and clove oil (26). Furthermore, eugenol (4-hydroxy-3-methoxy-allyl-benzene), the main component of clove oil, was shown to be very effective against HSV-1 and HSV-2 in vitro (35).

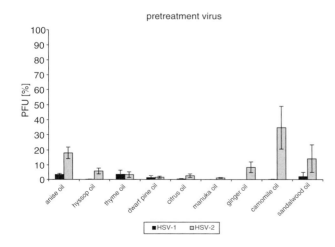

FIGURE 1 Mode of antiviral action of selected essential oils against HSV-1 and HSV-2. Data were expressed as percent (% v/v) of untreated control. *Abbreviation*: pfu, plaque-forming unit. *Source:* From Ref. 34.

TABLE 3 Antiviral Activity of Selected Essential Oils Against Herpes Viruses

Essential oil	Plant	Virus	TC_{50} [%]	IC_{50} [%]	SI
Anise oil	*Illicium verum*	HSV-1	0.016	0.004	4.0
		HSV-2	0.016	0.003	5.0
Camomile oil	*Matricaria recutita*	HSV-1	0.003	0.00003	100.0
		HSV-2	0.003	0.00015	20.0
Citrus oil	*Citrus limon*	HSV-1	0.0045	0.0015	3.0
		HSV-2	0.0045	0.0015	3.0
Ginger oil	*Zingiber officinale*	HSV-1	0.004	0.0002	20.0
		HSV-2	0.004	0.0001	40.0
Hyssop oil	*Hyssopus officinalis*	HSV-1	0.0075	0.0001	75.0
		HSV-2	0.0075	0.0006	13.0
Manuka oil	*Leptospermum*	HSV-1	0.0035	0.0001	35.0
	scoparium	HSV-2	0.0035	0.00009	39.0
Sandalwood oil	*Santalum album*	HSV-1	0.0015	0.0002	7.5
		HSV-2	0.0015	0.0005	3.0
Thyme oil	*Thymus vulgaris*	HSV-1	0.007	0.001	7.0
		HSV-2	0.007	0.0007	10.0
Dwarf pine oil	*Pinus mugo*	HSV-1	0.004	0.0007	5.7
		HSV-2	0.004	0.0007	5.7

Abbreviations: IC50, 50% inhibitory concentration; TC50, 50% cytotoxic concentration; SI, selectivity index = TC50 / IC50.

DERMAL ABSORPTION

One of the main routes of human exposure to essential oils in cosmetics and therapeutics is via the dermal route. It is well known that the rate of absorption is dependent on the integrity of the skin. Shaving with a razor blade, for example, may damage skin resulting in a higher absorption than through intact skin (36). It is also well known that absorption rates can be affected by occlusion. Occlusion of the skin usually results in a higher rate and extent of absorption when compared to nonoccluded skin (37). The reasons for this could be the increased hydration of the stratum corneum (SC), increased surface skin temperature, or reduced evaporation of the test permeant. This factor should always be considered when evaluating the skin permeability of essential oil components because it is not unusual to cover treated skin with clothes after the application of such products.

The ingredients of essential oils have lipophilic properties, and they are soluble in lipophilic media. Therefore essential oils are not only well absorbed through the mucosal membranes of the oral cavity, the nose, the pharynx, and the gastrointestinal tract but also through the skin. In 1940, Strähli et al. (38) demonstrated that, following dermal application of essential oils, the components of these oils appeared in respired air after a certain time. Despite the significant importance of understanding the behavior of essential oil-containing products applied to the skin, there are only a few current reports on skin absorption. The majority of the information reviewed suggests that lipophilic ingredients of essential oils are well absorbed.

There are different methods available to investigate the permeation of substances through skin. A common technique is to use excised skin from laboratory animals whose skin has a similar behavior to human skin. Another possibility is to examine permeation through human skin. In the latter case, the experiments may be performed either in vivo with subsequent examination of blood levels or using excised human skin from patients who undergo abdominal plastic surgery. This chapter summarizes some of the existing literature regarding the percutaneous absorption of essential oils and their ingredients with the main focus on different experimental systems.

Human Studies

The first investigations to obtain information on the permeation behavior of volatile substances were carried out in humans. In this case, an essential oil-containing formulation was applied to a defined area and the amount of substance penetrated was determined in blood samples.

A very common formulation for essential oils is massage oil because its ingredients are able to increase blood circulation and, moreover, essential oils often have sedative effects. A group from Austria investigated the systemic absorption of topically applied carvone (39). (-)-*R*-carvone is found in various plants, of which the oil of spearmint leaves has the highest concentration. Although some data on the absorption of carvone from animal models exist, there were no data on human skin. Massage oil containing 20% (-)-*R*-carvone in peanut oil was applied on a defined skin area of the lower abdomen. A normal massage, a massage with an occlusion wrap and an irradiation massage with orange light, were employed. Blood samples were taken from the left cubital vein at selected time intervals, and the amount of carvone was determined using gas chromatography.

Carvone rapidly permeated the skin and could be detected in the blood samples 10 minutes after application and starting the massage. However, the mechanical treatment of the skin could also be a reason for the fast permeation of carvone. Dependent on the massage technique, the time to reach the peak (normal massage: $t_{max} = 25.81$ min; occlusion wrap: 36.65 min; irradiation: 23.49 min) and the blood levels (23.92, 32.56, and 28.31 ng/ml) for massage with an occlusion wrap were significantly longer than those for normal massage and the irradiation technique. In this study a plastic film was used to wrap the body tightly to cover the massaged skin area. Usually the treated area is covered with clothes, rather than a plastic film, and the absorption rate would not be as high; however, a higher absorption rate should be assumed for every day life. Similar effects were found using nanoparticles (40).

Because of their effects on microorganisms and their expectorant and antitussive qualities, essential oils are often used in cold rubs such as Pinimenthol®-S-Salbe. This ointment contains monoterpenes and is used in the treatment of diseases of the respiratory tract, especially chronic bronchitis and colds. After dermal application of the ointment, the monoterpenes are absorbed through the skin as well as via inhalation.

To investigate the extent of dermal absorption, test subjects were separated into two groups. In both groups Pinimenthol-S-Salbe was applied to the thorax. In the first group, the treated skin area was covered airtight, but in the other group the treated area was uncovered and the subjects were able to breathe in the essential oils (41). At set time intervals, blood samples were taken from the left cubital vein, and the amounts of the individual components were determined. The four monoterpenes measured (α-pinene, camphor, β-pinene, and 3-carene) could be detected in the blood five minutes after application (Fig. 2).

Most of the monoterpenes reached their highest blood concentration within five minutes following application with a lag time of around 0.6 minutes. These results suggest that the skin does not represent a major diffusion barrier for these

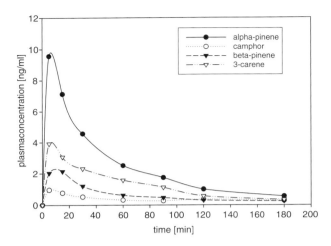

FIGURE 2 Time-dependent plasma concentration of different monoterpenes after application of Pinimenthol-S-Salbe. *Source*: From Ref. 41.

substances. In addition, statistical analysis of the pharmacokinetic factors showed that there were no differences with regard to gender and that inhalation of the monoterpenes did not add to the systemic load. However, subsequent investigations with laboratory animals have shown that the inhalation route cannot be completely neglected (42–44).

Use of Animal Skin

Although human in vivo experimentation generates realistic results, a major disadvantage is the invasive technique required to obtain the blood samples. Animal skin is, therefore, often used as a substitute. Excised animal skin was used, and the permeation studies were carried out in Franz diffusion cells. The skin or the membrane was positioned between the donor compartment, containing the drug preparation, and the acceptor compartment of the Franz diffusion cells. After predetermined time intervals, samples were taken from the receptor compartment and analyzed, e.g., using gas chromatography or high-performance liquid chromatography.

Porcine buccal mucosal membrane has been used to examine the in vitro permeation of *Salvia sclarea* L. essential oil from topical formulations (45). This type of membrane was used because its permeability is very similar to human buccal mucosal membrane. Of the *S. sclarea* L. essential oil components, the monoterpenes (1,8-cineole, linalool, and terpineol) had a higher permeability coefficients (K_p) than the other components (linalyl acetate and methyl chavicole). Terpenic components are often used as skin penetration enhancers.

In this study, three different formulations (gel, microemulsion, and gelled microemulsion), with varying concentrations of essential oil, were compared to pure oil to determine the influence of formulation on permeation. In comparison to pure oil, there was a considerable increase in the permeability coefficient of each component in all formulations. The gelled microemulsions gave the highest permeability coefficients for the components. For example, the permeability coefficients for linalool were $16.49 \pm 0.76 \times 10^{-3}$ cm/hr (gelled microemulsion 5%), $7.6 \pm 1.05 \times 10^{-3}$ cm/hr (microemulsion 5%), and $8.5 \pm 0.53 \times 10^{-3}$ cm/hr (gel 5%).

Human Skin (In Vitro)

The preferred choice of membrane for in vitro permeation studies is excised human skin. Usually, excised skin from Caucasian patients undergoing abdominal or breast reduction surgery is used. Immediately after excision, the subcutaneous fatty tissue is removed using a scalpel, and the skin is stored in polyethylene bags in a freezer at -26°C until use. Previous experiments have shown that neither the penetration characteristics nor the thickness of the SC are affected after a freezing period of up to six months (46). For permeation experiments, full thickness, dermatomed, or heat-separated human epidermis (HSE) may be used. HSE, prepared according to the method of Kligman et al. (47), is preferred when determining the skin permeation of the lipophilic constituents of essential oils.

Essential oils have a wide range of use both in cosmeceutical and pharmaceutical preparations. With regard to pharmaceutical preparations, the absorption of the essential oil and its various ingredients is very important. Most substances only have a therapeutic effect after reaching a certain concentration at the target site.

Reichling et al. (48) investigated the capability of terpinen-4-ol to permeate human skin. Terpinen-4-ol is the main component (30–40%) of Australian TTO, an essential oil derived by steam distillation of the leaves of the Australian native tea tree *Melaleuca alternifolia* (Myrtaceae). TTO is a component of skin care products where it is used for cleaning, healing, and relieving itch, hotspots, abrasions, and other minor rashes and irritations. In the last few years, TTO has become more important as topical antimicrobial (49,50) or antiviral preparations (51,52) such as a 5% semisolid oil-in-water (O/W) emulsion and cream or as a 6% gel formulation (51).

We have investigated the effect of formulation on the human skin permeation of terpinen-4-ol from TTO preparations (48). Before starting the skin permeation experiments, the influence of the formulation on the liberation of terpinen-4-ol was investigated using an ointment, a cream, and a semisolid O/W emulsion, all containing 5% TTO. The cream had the lowest release rate, and the ointment had the highest. Because of the two phases in the cream system and the consequential complex diffusion pathway, the absorption route for terpinen-4-ol may be longer. Additionally, the incorporation of the lipophilic terpinen-4-ol into the lipoidal phase may play a role. However, the main purpose of this experiment was the investigation of the influence of different formulations on the skin permeation of terpinen-4-ol. Permeation of the TTO-containing formulations was tested and compared with pure TTO. The application formulation had a distinct influence on the permeation of terpinen-4-ol through HSE, as shown in Figure 3. The highest permeation was found for pure TTO followed by the semisolid O/W emulsion preparation, the ointment, and the cream.

Table 4 gives the flux values and the apparent permeation coefficients (according to Fick's first law of diffusion) of terpinen-4-ol. The flux value is in accordance with the slope of the linear portion of the graph of the cumulative amount penetrated as a function of time.

The apparent permeation coefficient is described by the quotient of the flux value and the content of terpinen-4-ol in the formulation or in pure TTO. Pure TTO exhibits the highest flux value but the lowest apparent permeation coefficient (P_{app}), which is due to the high content of terpinen-4-ol. The P_{app} is used to compare the formulations with pure TTO because this value is independent of the concentration of terpinen-4-ol. The P_{app} value of the cream is very similar to that of the native oil. The reason for this result may be the reduced release from the formulations due to their lipophilic properties. The semisolid O/W emulsion shows the highest P_{app}

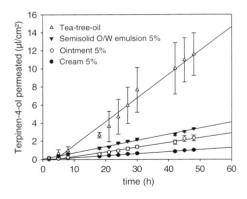

FIGURE 3 Permeation of terpinen-4-ol through heat-separated human epidermis from various preparations (mean ± SD, n = 3 to 4). *Source*: From Ref. 48.

value, which may be due to the high water content of this formulation, that is, the SC is probably fully hydrated (53). This hydration level could not be achieved over the corresponding time period with the cream and the ointment.

In a further experiment, we investigated the permeation of methyl eugenol, a prominent compound of the essential oil of *Rosa damascena* L. Rose oil is often used in aromatherapy and as a component of cosmetic and personal care products. Methyl eugenol is of great interest because it is thought to have negative side effects on the human body (54). The purpose of this study was to investigate the influence of different amounts of rose oil in cream preparations on the permeation of methyl eugenol through human skin and to observe the permeation of methyl eugenol from rose oil containing formulations under practical conditions.

To study the influence of different amounts of rose oil, different cream formulations were prepared containing 1%, 3%, and 5% rose oil. The experiments were carried out under infinite dose conditions, that is, the dose was large enough to maintain constant concentration of methyl eugenol during the course of the experiment.

The amounts of methyl eugenol permeated through HSE are shown in Figure 4. The values are dependent on both time and the concentration of rose oil in the cream. The higher the concentration of rose oil in the formulation, the higher the permeation of methyl eugenol.

Normally, substances are practically used under conditions different from those simulated under infinite dose conditions. In everyday use, most preparations are applied in thin layers to the skin (finite dose conditions). In the subsequent exper-

TABLE 4 Comparison of Release and Permeation Data of Terpinen-4-ol

Preparation	Content of terpinen-4-ol (µl/ml)	Release rate (µl/cm²/√hr) mean ± SE	Flux of terpinen-4-ol through HSE (µl/cm²/hr) mean ± SE	P_{app} of terpinen-4-ol (cm/sec) × 10⁻⁷ mean ± SE
Cream 5%	22.37	0.356 ± 0.010	0.022 ± 0.001	2.74 ± 0.06
Semisolid O/W emulsion 5%		0.659 ± 0.038	0.067 ± 0.001	8.41 ± 0.15
Ointment 5%		0.778 ± 0.017	0.051 ± 0.002	6.36 ± 0.21
Native TTO	447.4	n.d.	0.262 ± 0.019	1.62 ± 0.12

Abbreviations: HSE, human epidermis; n.d., not determined.
Source: From Ref. 48

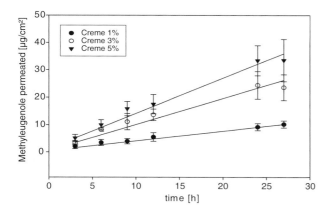

FIGURE 4 Permeation of methyl eugenol through heat-separated human epidermis (mean ± SD).

iments, the cream preparations were applied at doses of between 5 and 10 mg/cm^2. In this way, the extent of skin permeation of methyl eugenol from rose-oil-containing preparations under in-use conditions can be estimated. Furthermore, the amount of methyl eugenol in and on the surface of the SC was determined at the end of the experiment to determine mass balance.

Table 5 shows the percentage permeation of methyl eugenol over the course of the experiment. After 12 hours, about 80% of the applied dose of methyl eugenol had permeated the skin, which suggests that the skin is not a significant permeation barrier for this substance. The recovery of methyl eugenol averaged between 85% and 98% of the applied dose. These values are acceptable given that methyl eugenol is a volatile substance and, despite covering the donor compartment, evaporation cannot be completely avoided.

Penetration Enhancement and Distribution of Essential Oils in Skin Strata

In general, essential oils or their native compounds are often used for cosmetic and pharmaceutical purposes. They may act as fragrances, as therapeutic drugs, or solely as skin penetration enhancers. There are many reports on the penetration enhancement of both lipophilic and hydrophilic drugs by various terpenes, e.g., for 5-fluorouracil (55) and estradiol (56). As a result, it was clearly shown that, for the

TABLE 5 Methyl Eugenol Permeated Through Heat-Separated Epidermis After Various Time Intervals From Cream

Time (hours)	Methyl eugenol permeated (%) mean ± SD
3	32.30 ± 10.27
6	61.06 ± 13.16
9	72.98 ± 9.51
12	82.05 ± 11.21
24	77.49 ± 6.71
27	83.41 ± 9.32

hydrophilic drug, 5-fluorouracil hydrocarbon terpenes (e.g., D-limonene) were less potent than alcohol or ketone structures containing terpenes (e.g., 1,8-cineole), and the greatest enhancement activity was shown by the oxide terpenes and terpenoids. In contrast, hydrocarbon terpenes were the most effective enhancers for the steroidal drug estradiol. However, the data could not be generalized, and it appears that the action of terpenes as penetration enhancers may be specifically related to the drug in use. A summary of the use of different terpenes as penetration enhancers for various drugs is provided by Medi et al. (57). There are only a few reports on the use of the whole native essential oil for penetration enhancement. For example, Monti et al. (58) present data on the effects of melissa, cajput, cardamon, myrtle, niaouli, and orange essential oil, dissolved at 10% in propylene glycol, on the penetration of estradiol through hairless mouse skin. Niaouli oil showed the largest enhancement factor, whereas melissa and cardamon oil failed to improve the penetration rate. Comparing the four main terpene components of niaouli oil, 1,8-cineole, α-pinene, α-terpineol, and D-limonene (10% in propylene glycol) on skin permeation, separately, 1,8-cineole gave the largest enhancement factor (EF 33), but this was significantly lower than for the native niaouli oil (EF 52.1). Moreover, they found that a ternary mixture of 1,8-cineole (69.2%), α-pinene (22.5%), and D-limonene (8.3%) gave the same increase of permeation as the native niaouli oil. These results clearly demonstrate that the use of the whole essential oil may be superior to a single component of that oil. However, it cannot be concluded that other minor components of the oils do not significantly influence enhancing activity. Considering the enhancement capability of essential oils, one should be aware of potential enhanced delivery of other substances if essential oils or their components are incorporated into formulations for dermal applications. This may increase the risk of toxic effects and reduce the safety of such preparations.

Interesting effects for the essential oils, lavender oil (32% linalool and 35% linalyl acetate), TTO (30% terpinen-4-ol), juniper oil (41% α-pinene), and geranium oil (28% citronellol), incorporated in formulations or applied pure, on the distribution of the main component between SC and epidermis/dermis (ED) have been reported recently (59). When the essential oils were applied as pure oils, higher amounts of the constituent terpenes were found in the skin when compared to their application as part of dermal formulations (oil content 0.75%). There was no proportionality to the penetrant concentration, and the author reasoned that this was due to a limited capacity of the SC for the components. Comparing the SC/ED ratio for linalyl acetate and linalool from lavender oil to that of the pure substances, the partitioning was shifted to the SC, resulting in a fourfold larger accumulation in the SC. Formulation differences were observed. For example, when lavender oil was incorporated in an O/W emulsion or grape seed oil, similar concentrations for linalool and linalyl acetate in the SC and ED were observed. In contrast using the same formulations with TTO, terpinen-4-ol penetrated more rapidly when delivered as an oily solution. These findings demonstrated that the influence of formulation depends on the type of terpene or essential oil and their physicochemical characteristics.

In conclusion, components of essential oils penetrate the SC, the viable epidermis, and the dermis. The magnitude depends on the lipophilicity and hydrophilicity of the terpene itself and the formulation in which the substance is applied. Furthermore, there are differences in the penetration behavior between pure essential oils and their neat components. Therefore, conclusions from experiments with neat components of essential oils and the complex mixture of the essential oil itself should be treated with caution.

SAFETY
Topical Side Effects of Essential Oils

The most common application of essential oils is topical application to the skin or mucous membranes. Direct skin contact occurs from perfumes, cosmetic fragrances, and pharmaceuticals, whereas mucous membranes are exposed when using toothpastes, mouth fresheners, and feminine hygiene products or inhaling essential oils. Known clinical side effects occurring following topical application of essential oils are allergic contact dermatitis, skin and mucous membrane irritation, hyperpigmentation, and cytotoxic effects (1,60–62). To learn more about the side effects of essential oils when used topically, we investigated the potential irritation effects of essential oils on eyes and mucous membranes. Different in vivo and in vitro methods are available for testing eye and mucous membrane irritation potency of essential oils.

The Draize test

The Draize rabbit eye irritation test (Draize test) is the classical in vivo experiment to detect potential eye or mucous membrane irritation of substances (63).This test method is required by legislature worldwide to obtain data for the risk assessment of consumer products. To detect potential eye irritation, a test substance is applied directly into the conjunctival sac of the rabbit's eye. The irritation responses of the cornea (the area of corneal opacity), the iris (swelling, reaction to light, and hemorrhage), and the conjunctivae (redness and swelling with closing of lids) are scored depending on their severity. Ethical as well as scientific concerns have been raised on this test system because it is reported to be not only very painful for the animals, but also poorly reproducible (64). Against this background, in 1987, the OECD stated that there is no need for animal experiments if data are available from a generally accepted and validated alternative method (65).

The HET-CAM test

The hen egg test-chorioallantoic membrane (HET-CAM) test, described for the first time by Lüpke (66), is a non-animal test system that is accepted by the German regulatory authorities (67) to identify severe irritants. In this test system, the highly vascularized CAM of hen eggs is exposed to suspected irritants. Depending on the onset times of the different endpoints (hyperemia, hemorrhage, lysis, and coagulation), a scoring system was developed to classify different degrees of potential mucous membrane/eye irritation ranging from severe to not irritant (68).

Modified HET-CAM test

The HET-CAM test protocol (67) is not useful for detecting mucous membrane irritation potential of essential oils because they are known to be nonsevere irritants. According to our findings, pure essential oils cause only hemorrhage on the CAM. Therefore, we developed a modified test protocol in which hemorrhage is the ultimate endpoint. Furthermore, varying from the normal test protocol, we determine the irritation threshold concentration (ITC) of an essential oil. The ITC is defined as the lowest concentration of an irritant leading to clearly visible hemorrhage within five minutes of application, compared with the reaction of the CAM after exposure to 0.5% sodium dodecyl sulfate solution (69,70).

Using the modified HET-CAM test protocol, we analyzed the irritation potential of selected essential oils and compared their ITC to those of their corresponding
major constituents. The results are summarized in Figure 5. According to our findings, the essential oils tested revealed clear differences in their irritation potential to
the CAM. Based on the ITC values, the test oils can be ranked in three groups: ITC
< 30%, rose oil, clove oil, cinnamon oil, melissa oil, and eucalyptus oil; ITC ≤ 50%,
lemon grass oil, peppermint oil, sage oil, and caraway oil; and ITC ≤ 100%, anise
oil, orange carp oil, and lemon oil. Camomile oil did not irritate the CAM at any
concentration tested.

Because essential oils are known to be complex mixtures of different volatile
substances, the question arises as to whether the irritation potential of an essential
oil can be linked to one or more of its components. Therefore, we first determined
the ITC values of the main components of each essential oil. The results demonstrate
clearly that the irritation potential of an essential oil is based on its chemical components. In some cases, the ITC values of the main constituents fitted those of the corresponding essential oil (e.g., rose oil, clove oil, cinnamon oil, eucalyptus oil, and sage
oil). On the other hand, it was also shown that the minor components contributed
to the overall irritation potential and that synergistic and antagonistic effects were
possible (e.g., lemon grass oil, caraway oil, orange carp oil, and lemon oil).

In summary, our investigation has shown that essential oils that differ in their
irritation potential can be significantly discriminated by our modified HET-CAM
test. We believe that, based on the ITC values, essential oils can be ranked in three
categories: ITC ≤ 25% essential oil (strongly irritative to the CAM), ITC 30% to 70%

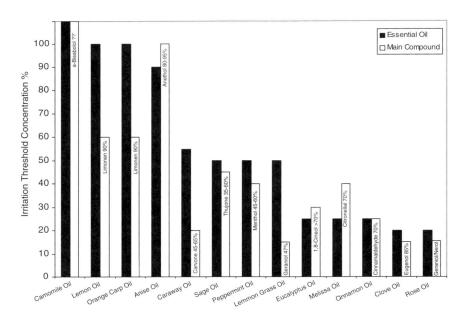

FIGURE 5   ITC of essential oils and their corresponding main constituents. Results are given in
% (v/v) or % (m/m). Black bars represent the ITC values of the test oils, whereas the white bars
depict the ITC values of the corresponding main compounds. The main individual compounds are
named in the white bars. *Abbreviation*: ITC, irritation threshold concentrations.

essential oil (moderately irritative to the CAM), and ITC 75% to ≤ 100% (slightly to nonirritative to the CAM). Although the extrapolation of in vitro data to the in vivo situation should always be treated with caution, the ITC values derived from the modified HET-CAM test confirm the experience of practitioners that essential oils should never be used undiluted on the skin and mucous membranes. Furthermore, our modified HET-CAM test may be helpful in discriminating between strongly irritative and slightly to nonirritative essential oils. In this context, it is of interest that clove oil is reported to be an irritant to eyes and skin (1,71) whereas camomile oil is known for its anti-inflammatory and nonirritative effect (1). As shown in Figure 5, the irritation potential of both of these essential oils can be discriminated clearly using the ITC values from our modified HET-CAM test.

REFERENCES

1. Lis-Balchin M. Aromatherapy Science. London: Pharmaceutical Press, 2006; Vol. 1.
2. Buchbauer G, Jirovetz L. Aromatherapy—use of fragrances and essential oils as medicaments. Flav Fragr J 1994; 9:217–222.
3. Reichling J. Plant-microbe interaction and secondary metabolites with antiviral, antibacterial and antifungal properties. In: Wink M, ed. Functions of Plant Secondary Metabolite and their Exploitation in Biotechnology. Annual Plant Review. Sheffield: Sheffield Acad. Press, 1999:187–273.
4. Weseler A, Geiss HK, Saller R, et al. A novel colorimetric broth microdilution method to determine the minimum inhibitory concentration (MIC) of antibiotics and essential oils against *Helicobacter pylori*. Pharmazie 2005; 60:498–502.
5. Reichling J, Harkenthal M, Saller R. In-vitro-Untersuchungen zur antimikrobiellen Wirkung ausgewählter ätherischer Öle. Erfahrungsheilkunde 1999; 48:357–366.
6. Yousef R, Tawil G. Antimicrobial activity of volatile oils. Pharmazie 1980; 35:698–701.
7. Dorman H-J, Deans SG. Antimicrobial agents from plants: antibacterial activity of plant volatile oils. J Appl Microbiol 2000; 88:308–316.
8. Takarada K, Kimizuka R, Takahashi N, et al. A comparison of the antibacterial efficacies of essential oils against oral pathogens. Oral Microbiol Immunol 2004; 19:61–64.
9. Hammer K, Carson CF, Riley TV. In-vitro activity of essential oils, in particular *Melaleuca alternifolia* (tea tree) oil and tea tree oil products against *Candida* ssp. Antimicrob Agents Chemother 1998; 42:591–595.
10. Longbottom C, Carson CF, Hammer KA, et al. Tolerance of *Pseudomonas aeruginosa* to *Melaleuca alternifolia* (tea tree) oil is associated with the outer membrane and energy dependent cellular processes. Antimicrob Agents Chemother 2004; 54:386–392.
11. Pattnaik S, Subramanyam VR, Rath CC. Effect of essential oil on the viability and morphology of *Escherichia coli* (SP-11). Microbios 1995; 84:195–199.
12. Harkenthal M, Lay-Schmitt G, Reichling J. Effect of Australian tea tree oil on the viability of the wall-less bacterium *Mycoplasma pneumoniae*. Pharmazie 2000; 55:380–384.
13. Cox S, Gustafson JE, Mann CM, et al. Tea tree oil causes K⁺ leakage and inhibits respiration in *Escherichia coli*. Lett Appl Microbiol 1998; 26:355–358.
14. Cox S, Mann CM, Bell HC, et al. The mode of antiviral action of the essential oil of *Melaleuca alternifolia* (tea tree oil). J Appl Microbiol 2000; 88:170–175.
15. Knobloch K, Weigand H, Weis N, et al. Action of terpenoids on energy metabolism. In: Brunke E, ed. Progress in Essential Oil Research. Berlin: Walter de Gruyter, 1986: 429–445.
16. Inoue Y, Shiraishi A, Hada T, et al. The antibacterial effects of terpene alcohols on *Staphylococcus aureus* and their mode of action. FEMS Microbiol Lett 2004; 237:25–331.
17. Helander I, Alakomi H-L, Lavata-Kala K, et al. Characterization of the action of selected essential oil components on gram-negative bacteria. J Agric Food Chem 1998; 46: 3590–3595.
18. Oussalah M, Caillet S, Lacroix M. Mechanism of action of Spanish oregano, Chinese cinnamon, and savory essential oils against cell membranes and walls of *Escherichia coli* O157:H7 and *Listeria monocytogenes*. Can J Food Prot 2006; 69:1046–1055.

19. Carson C, Mee BJ, Riley TV. Mechanism of action of *Melaleuca alternifolia* (tea tree) oil on *Staphylococcus aureus* determined by time-kill, lysis, leakage, and salt tolerance assays and electron microscopy. Antimicrob Agents Chemother 2002; 46:1914–1920.
20. Reichling J, Harkenthal M, Geiss HK, et al. Electron microscopic investigation on the antibacterial effects of Australian tea tree oil against *Staphylococcus aureus*. Curr Top Phytochem 2002; 5:77–84.
21. Gustafson J, Liew YC, Chew S, et al. Effects of tea tree oil on *Escherichia coli*. Lett Appl Microbiol 1998; 26:194–198.
22. Ogunlana E, Höglund G, Onawunmi G, et al. Effects of lemongrass oil on the morphological characteristics and peptidoglycan synthesis of *Escherichia coli*. Microbios 1987; 50:43–49.
23. Horne D., Holm M, Oberg DG, Antimicrobial effects of essential oils on *Streptococcus pneumoniae*. J Essential Oil Res 2001; 13:387–392.
24. Rhayour K, Bouchikhi T, Tantaoui-Elaraki A, et al. The mechanism of bactericidal action of oregano and clove essential oils and their phenolic major components on *Escherichia coli* and *Bacillus subtilis*. J Essential Oil Res 2003; 15:356–362.
25. Jassim S, Naji MA. Novel antiviral agents: a medicinal plant perspective. J Appl Microbiol 2003; 95:412–435.
26. Siddiqui Y, Ettayebi M, Hadlab AM, et al. Effect of essential oils on the enveloped viruses: antiviral activity of oregano and clove oils on herpes simplex virus type 1 and Newcastle disease virus. Med Sci Res 1996; 24:187–188.
27. Hayashi K, Kamiya M, Hayashi T. Virucidal effects of the steam distillate from *Houttuynia cordata* and its components on HSV-1, influenza virus, and HIV. Planta Med 1994; 61:237–241.
28. Schumacher A, Reichling J, Schnitzler P. Virucidal effect of peppermint oil on the enveloped viruses herpes simplex virus type 1 and type 2 in vitro. Phytomedicine 2003; 10:504–510.
29. Reichling J, Koch C, Stahl-Biskup E, et al. Virucidal activity of a beta-triketone-rich essential oil of *Leptospermum scoparium* (manuka oil) against HSV-1 and HSV-2 in cell culture. Planta Med 2005; 71:1123–1127.
30. Minami M, Kita M, Nakaya T, et al. The inhibitor effect of essential oils on Herpes simplex virus type-1 replication in vitro. Microbiol Immunol 2003; 47: 681–684.
31. Benencia F, Courreges MC. Antiviral activity of sandalwood oil against Herpes simplex viruses-1 and -2. Phytomedicine 1999; 6:119–123.
32. Garcia C, Talarico L, Almeida N, et al. Virucidal activity of essential oils from aromatic plants of San Luis, Argentina. Phytother Res 2003; 17:1073–1075.
33. De logu A, Loy G, Pellerano ML, et al. Inactivation of HSV-1 and HSV-2 and prevention of cell-to-cell virus spread by *Santolina insularis* essential oil. Antiviral Res 2000; 48:177–185.
34. Koch C. Antivirale Effekte ausgewählter ätherischer Öle auf behüllte Viren unter besonderer Berücksichtigung des Herpes simplex Virus Type 1 und 2. Thesis, University of Heidelberg, 2005.
35. Benencia F, Courreges MC. In vitro and in vivo activity of eugenol on human herpesvirus. Phytother Res 2000; 14:495–500.
36. Edman B. The influence of shaving method on perfume allergy. Contact Dermatitis 1994; 31(5):291–292.
37. Bronaugh RL, Stewart RF, Wester RC, et al. Comparison of percutaneous absorption of fragrances by humans and monkeys. Fd Chem Toxicol 1985; 23(1):111–114.
38. Strähli, W., Dissertation Bern 1940, ref. in Gildemeister, E., Hoffmann, Fr. - "Die Ätherischen Öle", Berlin: Akademie-Verlag 1956, Bd. I, 114.
39. Fuchs N, Jaeger W, Lenhardt A, et al. Systemic absorption of topically applied carvone: influence of massage technique. J Cosmet Sci 1997; 48(6):277–282.
40. Lademann J, Richter H, Schaefer UF, et al., Hair follicles—A long-term reservoir for drug delivery. Skin PharmPhys 2006; 19:232–236.
41. Schuster O, Haag F, Priester H. Transdermal absorption of terpenes from essential oils of Pinimenthol-S ointment. Med Welt 1986; 37(4):100–102.
42. Kovar KA, Gropper B, Friess D, et al. Blood levels of 1,8-cineole and locomotor activity of mice after inhalation and oral administration of rosemary oil. Planta Med, 1987; 53(4):315–318.

43. Buchbauer G, Jirovetz L, Jaeger W, et al. Aromatherapy: evidence for sedative effects of the essential oil of lavender after inhalation. Z Naturforsch. C, 1991; 46(11–12): 1067–1072.
44. Buchbauer G, Jaeger W, Jirovetz L, et al., Effects of valerian root oil, borneol, isoborneol, bornyl acetate and isobornyl acetate on the motility of laboratory animals (mice) after inhalation. Pharmazie 1992; 47(8):620–622.
45. Ceschel GC, Maffei P, Moretti MDL, et al. In vitro permeation through porcine buccal mucosa of *Salvia sclarea* L. essential oil from topical formulations. STP Pharma Sci 1998; 8(2): 103–106.
46. Schaefer H, Loth H. An ex-vivo model for the study of drug penetration into human skin. Pharm Res 1996; 13(9 Suppl.):S-366.
47. Kligman AM, Christophers E. Preparation of isolated sheets of stratum corneum. Arch Dermatol 1963; 88:702–705.
48. Reichling J, Landvatter U, Wagner H, et al. In vitro studies on release and human skin permeation of Australian tea tree oil (TTO) from topical formulations. Eur J Pharm Biopharm 2006; 64:222–228.
49. Syed TA, Qureshi ZA, Ali SM, et al., Treatment of toenail onychomycosis with 2% butenafine and 5% *Melaleuca alternifolia* (tea tree) oil in cream. Trop Med Int Health 1999; 4(4):284–287.
50. Bassett IB, Pannowitz DL, Barnetson RSC. A comparative study of tea-tree oil versus benzoylperoxide in the treatment of acne. Med J Aust 1990; 153(8):455–456.
51. Carson CF, Ashton L, Dry L, et al. *Melaleuca alternifolia* (tea tree) oil gel (6%) for the treatment of recurrent herpes labialis (5). J Antimicrob Chemother 2001; 48(3):450–451.
52. Schnitzler P, Schön, K, Reichling, J. Antiviral activity of Australian tea tree oil and eucalyptus oil against herpes simplex virus in cell culture. Pharmazie 2001; 56:343–347.
53. Wagner H, Kostka KH, Adelhardt W, et al. Effects of various vehicles on the penetration of flufenamic acid into human skin. Eur J Pharm Biopharm 2004; 58(1):121–129.
54. Iten F, Saller R, Reichling J. Sind Naturprodukte mit Methyleugenol kanzerogen? Dtsch Apoth Ztg 2004; 144:3192–3199.
55. Williams A, Barry BW. Terpenes and the lipid-protein-partitioning theory of skin penetration enhancers. Pharm Res 1991; 8:17–24.
56. Williams A, Barry BW. The enhancement index concept applied to terpene penetration enhancers for human skin and model lipophilic (oestradiol) and hydrophilic (5-fluoruracil) drugs. Int J Pharm 1991; 74:157–168.
57. Medi B, Singh S, Singh J. Assessing efficacy of penetration enhancers. In: Riviere J, ed. Dermal Absorption Models in Toxicology and Pharmacology. Boca Raton: Taylor & Francis, 2006:213–249.
58. Monti D, Chetoni P, Burgalassi S, et al. Effect of different terpene-containing essential oils on permeation of estradiol through hairless mouse skin. Int J Pharm 2002; 237:209–214.
59. Cal K. Skin penetration of terpenes from essential oils and topical vehicles. Planta Med 2006; 72:311–316.
60. de Groot AC, Frosch PJ. Adverse reactions to fragrances. A clinical review. Contact Dermatitis 1997; 36(2):57–86.
61. Monajemi R, Oryan S, Haeri-Roohani A, et al. Cytotoxic effects of essential oils of some Iranian citrus peels. Iranian J Pharm Res 2005; 4:183–187.
62. Ahmed A. Cytotoxic potentialities of essential oils. Mansoura J Pharm Sci 2001; 17:38–50.
63. OECD. Detailed Review on Classification Systems for Eye Irritation/Corrosion in OECD Member Countries. Paris, France: OECD Publication Office, 1999.
64. Weil CS, Scala RA. Study of intra- and interlaboratory variability in the results of rabbit eye and skin irritation tests. Toxicol Appl Pharmacol 1971; 19(2):276–360.
65. OECD. Guideline for Testing Chemicals No 405: "Acute Eye Irritation/Corrosion." Paris, France: OECD Publication Office, 1987.
66. Luepke NP. Hen's egg chorioallantoic membrane test for irritation potential. Food Chem Toxicol 1985; 23(2):287–91.
67. ECVAM. INVITTOX Protocol No 47 HET-CAM-Test. 1992.
68. NICEAM. Draft Background Review Document—Current status of in vitro test methods for identifying ocular corrosives and severe irritants: The HET-CAM-Test-Chorioallantoic Membrane (HET-CAM-Test Method). 2004.

69. Reichling J, Harkenthal M, Landvatter U, et al. Ätherische Öle im HET-CAM-Test. Dtsch Apoth Ztg 2000; 41:42–48.
70. Möller M, Suschke U, Nolkemper S, et al. Antibacterial, antiviral, antiproliferative and apoptosis-inducing properties of *Brackenridgea zanguebarica* (Ochnaceae). J Pharm Pharmacol 2006; 58:1131–1138.
71. Safety (MSDS) data for clove oil. (Accessed October 11, 2005, at www.sciencelab.com/xMSDS-Clove_oil-9927498), (2006).

Sunscreens: Efficacy, Skin Penetration, and Toxicological Aspects

Heather A. E Benson

School of Pharmacy, Curtin University of Technology, Perth, Western Australia, Australia

INTRODUCTION

Ultraviolet radiation (UVR) from the sun is divided into UVA (UVA1 340–400 nm and UVA2 320–340 nm), UVB (290–320 nm), and UVC (270–290 nm). UVC is filtered by ozone in the stratosphere, whereas UVA and UVB reach the earth's surface. UVA can penetrate deeper through the skin than UVB, is not filtered by glass, and it is estimated that approximately 50% of exposure to UVA occurs in the shade (1). Acute exposure to UVB causes effects such as erythema, edema, tanning, thickening of the epidermis and dermis, and vitamin D synthesis. Chronic exposure to UVB can result in photoaging, immunosupression, and photocarcinogenesis (2,3). Exposure to UVA is more efficient in inducing tanning and causes less erythema, but it is also involved in photoaging and acute and chronic photodermatoses (4). Both UVA and UVB are associated with immunosupression and carcinogenesis (5); therefore, there is a need for protection.

Consequently, significant effort has been applied to educate the public in the use of photoprotective measures. These include reducing sun exposure during peak UVR (11 am–3 pm), seeking shade, and wearing appropriate clothing, sunglasses, wide-brimmed hat, and a broad-spectrum topical sunscreen product (6). Indeed, the estimated retail value of sunscreen products in Europe is approximately €1.3 billion, with annual growth of 4%. This chapter is focused on the efficacy, formulation, skin absorption, and toxicity of sunscreen chemicals and products as applied to human skin.

TOPICAL SUNSCREEN PRODUCTS

Sunscreen actives are incorporated into a range of daily use personal care products, such as shampoos and conditioners, moisturizers, foundations, lipsticks, as well as the more traditional sunscreen creams, lotions, oils, and sprays. To be effective in preventing sunburn and protecting the skin from damage, sunscreens must work efficiently to prevent transmission of UVR to the viable skin tissues. Most sunscreens achieve this by dissipating UVR either by scattering or absorbing the energy and releasing it as less harmful energy. It is essential that the photophysical and photochemical pathways involved in energy dissipation do not lead to the formation of potentially harmful reactive species in viable tissues where they could cause damage to DNA. Sunscreen products must be photostable, should minimize access of UVA and UVB radiation to viable cells, and should be formulated to minimize penetration of active ingredients through the skin. In addition, a sunscreen should be water-resistant, tasteless, odorless, and cosmetically elegant.

Sunscreen products are classified according to their Sun Protection Factor (SPF) value:

TABLE 1 Sunscreen Agents Permitted as Active Ingredients by the Food and Drug Administration (United States), European Commission, and Therapeutic Goods Administration (Australia)

Sunscreen	INCI	Trade names	Maximum concentration permitted		
			USA	EU	Australia
Organic absorbers					
UVB filters					
PABA derivatives					
4-Aminobenzoic acid	PABA		15	5	15
Padimate O (octyl dimethyl PABA)	Ethylhexyl dimethyl PABA	Eusolex 6007, Escalol 507	8	8	8
Ethoxylated ethyl 4-aminobenzoic acid	PEG25 PABA	Uvinul P-25, Unipabol U-17		10	10
Cinnamates					
Octinoxate (octyl methoxycinnamate)	Ethylhexyl methoxycinnamate	Parsol MCX, Neo Heliopon AV, Eusolex 2292, Escalol 57, Tinosorb OMC, Uvinul MC 80	7.5	10	10
Cinoxate			3		6
Isopentenyl-4-methoxycinnamate (isoamyl 4-methoxycinnamate)	Isoamyl *p*-methoxycinnamate	Neo Heliopan E-1000		10	10
Salicylates					
Octisalate (octyl salicylate)	Ethylhexyl salicylate	Neo Heliopan OS, Eusolex OS, Escalol 587, Uvinul)-18	5	5	5
Homosalate		Eusolex HMS, Neo Helipon HMS	15	10	15
Trolamine salicylate (triethanolamine salicylate)			12		12
Isopropylbenzyl salicylate					TBD
Salicylic acid salts (potassium, sodium, trianethanolamine					TBD
N,N,N-Trimethyl-4-(oxoborn-3-ylidenemethyl)anilinium methyl sulfate					
Camphor derivatives					
3-(4-Methylbenxylidene)-D-1 camphor; (4-methylbenzylidene camphor)	4 Methylbenzylidene camphor	Eusolex 6300, Parsol 5000, Neo Heliopan MBC, Uvinul MBC 95		4	4
3 Benzylidene camphor	3 Benzylidene camphor	Mexoryl SDS 20, Unisol S 22		2	6

Chemical name	Common/INCI name	Trade names			
Polymer of N-{(2 and 4)-[(2-oxoborn-3-ylidene) methyl]benzyl]acrylamide	Polyacrylamidomethyl benzylidene camphor	Mexoryl SW	6	6	
Alpha-(2-oxoborn-3-ylidene)-toluene-4-sulfonic acid and its salts	Benzylidene camphor sulfonic acid	Mexoryl SL	6 (as acid)	6	
Others					
2-Cyano-3,3-diphenyl acrylic acid, 2-ethyl hexyl ester	Octocrylene	Parsol 340, Eusolex OCR, Neo Heliopan 303, Escalol 597, Uvinul N-539 T	10	10	10
Ensulizole (phenylbenzimidazole sulfonic acid)		Parsol HS, Eusolex 232, Neo Heliopan Hydro	4	8	4
2,4,6-Trianalino-(p-carbo-2'-ethylhexyl-1'oxy)1,3,5-triazine	Octyl triazone, Ethylhexyl triazone	Univul T 150	5	5	5
Benzoic acid, 4,4-((6-(((1,1-dimethylethyl)amino) carbonyl)phenyl)amino)1,3,5-triazine-2,4-diyl)diamino)bis,-bis-(2-ethylhexyl)ester)	Diethylhexyl butamido triazone	Uvasorb HEB	10	10	10
Dimethicodiethylbenzal malonate	Polysilicone 15	Parsol SLX	TBD	10	3
UVA filters					
Benzophenones					
Benzophenone					
Benzophenone-2					
Benzophenone-8 (dioxybenzone)			TBD		3
Others					
Avobenzone	Butyl methoxydibenzoyl methane	Parsol 1789, Eusolex 9020, Uvinul BMBM, Neo Heliopan 357	3	5	5
Meradimate (menthyl anthranilate)			5 √		
3,3'-(1,4-phenylenedimethylene) bis (7,7-di methyl-2-oxobicyclo-[2,2,1]hept-1-yl-meth anesulfonic acid) and its salts; ecamsule	Terephthalydene dicamphor sulfonic acid	Mexoryl SX	5	10	10
2,2'-(1,4-phenylene)bis-(1-H-benzimidazole-4, 6-disulfonic acid, monosodium salt)	Disodium phenyl dibenzimidazole tetrasulfonate	Neo Heliopan AP	10	10	10
Benzoic acid, 2-[-4-(diethylamino)-2-hydroxybenzoyl]-, hexylester	Diethylamino hydroxybenzoyl hexyl benzoate	Uninul A Plus	10	10	
Ecamsule	Terephthalylidene dicamphor sulfonic acid	Mexoryl SO	10	6	10

TABLE 1 (continued)

Sunscreen	INCI	Trade names	Maximum concentration permitted		
			USA	EU	Australia
UVA and UVB filters					
Oxybenzone	Benzophenone-3	Eusolex 4360, Neo Heliopan BB, Uvinal M40, Escalol 567, Tinosorb B3	6	10	10
Phenol,2-(2H-benzotriazol-2-yl)-4-methyl-62-methyl-3-[1,3,3,3-tetramethyl-1-[(trimethylsilyl)oxy]disoloxanyl]propyl	Dromatrizole trisiloxane	Mexoryl XL		15	15
Camphor benzalkonium methosulfate		Mexoryl SO	10	6	10
2-Hydroxy-4-methoxybenzophenone-5-sulfonic acid and its sodium salt	Benzophenone-4 (sulisobenzone) Benzophenone-5 (sulisobenzone sodium)	Uvinul MS 40, Escalol 577, Uvasorb S5		5	10
2,2'-Methylene-bis-6-(2H-benzotriazol-2yl)-4-(tetramethyl-butyl)-1,1,3-phenol	Methylene bis-benzotriazolyl tetramethylbutyl phenol	Tinosorb M		10	10
Bemotrizinol	Bis-ethylhexyloxyphenol methoxyphenyl triazine	Tinosorb S		10	10
Inorganic absorbers					
Titanium dioxide			25	25	25
Zinc oxide			25	No limit	No limit

Abbreviations: INCI, International Nomenclature of Cosmetic Ingredients; PABA, *para*-aminobenzoic acid; TBD, to be determined.

$$SPF = MED_{protected}/MED_{unprotected}.$$

That is, the UVR energy required to produce a minimal erythemal dose (MED) on protected skin (with 2 mg/cm^2 of the sunscreen) divided by the UVR energy required to produce a MED on unprotected skin (7). The MED is the smallest dose of UVR (J m^2) that produces redness with clearly defined borders at the exposure site: often measured as the exposure time required to cause erythema. As erythema is caused primarily by UVB, the SPF value provides an indication of the sunscreen products' effectiveness to prevent UVB-induced sunburn, but there is no assessment of its UVA protection. A number of methods to assess UVA effectiveness have been suggested, including the "Boots Star System" invented by Diffy (8). The European Commission has recently launched an initiative to improve the labeling of sunscreen products from 2007, including standardized labeling of UVA protection (9,10).

In the United States, the Food and Drug Administration (FDA) has approved 17 sunscreen agents as over-the-counter medications (7). European Union regulators permit the use of 28 sunscreens (11), and in Australia the Therapeutic Goods Administration has approved 28 sunscreen agents with a further 4 under review (12). The sunscreen actives available in each of these jurisdictions are listed in Table 1, and the major sunscreen manufacturers are listed in Table 2. All but two of the approved sunscreens are organic or chemical filters, with only titanium dioxide (TiO$_2$) and zinc oxide (ZnO) inorganic or physical filters. Organic sunscreens act through chemical excitation by UVR, whereby incident UVR is absorbed and then dissipated as longer wavelength energy, thereby protecting the skin from a potentially damaging dose of UVR. They are classified into either UVA or UVB filters, with some absorbing in both ranges (Table 1). Inorganic sunscreens block UVA/UVB sunlight through reflection and scattering but have also been shown to absorb considerable UVR. Sunscreen products are generally formulated with a combination of organic sunscreens and may also include an inorganic filter (13). In this way, the sunscreen product is effective in reducing skin exposure to a broad spectrum of UVR.

Organic UV Filters

UVB filters include the *para*-aminobenzoic acid (PABA) derivatives, cinnamates, salicylates, and camphor derivatives. PABA is a water-soluble UVB filter that has been in extensive use since the 1940s. It is now less frequently used as it stains clothing and is the most commonly reported contact and photoallergen in sunscreens

TABLE 2 Sunscreen Active Manufacturers and Common Trade Names

Trade name	Manufacturer
Mexoryl	L'Oreal
Eusolex	Merck
Neo Heliopan	Symrise (formerly Haarmann & Reimer)
Uvinul	BASF
Escalol	ISP
Tinosorb	Ciba
Parsol	Roche
Uvasorb	3V-Sigma
Unisol	Induchem

(14–17). Octyl dimethyl PABA (padimate O) is a UVB filter with a better safety record than PABA and is the most commonly used derivative.

Octyl methoxycinnamate is the most widely used UVB filter. It is a less effective UVB absorber than PABA and requires formulation with additional UVB filters to achieve a high SPF. Octyl methoxycinnamate is reported to degrade following exposure to sunlight, leading to a decrease in efficacy (18) and potential photocontact sensitization (19,20). It is generally formulated with other UV filters to enhance its photostability. Cinoxate is an infrequently used cinnamate derivative.

The salicylate sunscreens, octyl salicylate, homosalate, and trolamine salicylate are weak UVB absorbers, generally used in combination to augment the effect of other UVB filters. They may also be included to minimize the photodegradation of other sunscreen agents in the product. In addition, trolamine salicylate is water soluble and therefore can be easily washed off the skin.

Octocrylene is a UVB absorber with good photostability and is generally used in combination with other organic and inorganic filters to enhance the photostability of the final product. Most camphor derivatives are moderately effective UVB sunscreens, with the exception of tetraphthalylidene dicamphor sulfonic acid, which is a broad UVA filter.

Dimethicodiethylbenzal malonate (Parsol SLX) is a UVB filter recently introduced globally (except the United States) by DSM Nutritional Products, Switzerland. It is larger than conventional organic sunscreens, consisting of organic chromophores attached to a polysiloxane chain. The silicone chain has an affinity to the skin, thereby retaining the UV filter at the skin surface to reduce skin penetration while optimizing substantivity. It also photostabilizes avobenzone and is particularly useful in sun protectant hair products.

UVA filters include benzophenones, anthranilates, and dibenzoylmethanes. Oxybenzone is the most commonly used benzophenone, absorbing both UVA and UVB (although it has two λ_{max}: 288 and 325 nm, absorption is more efficient in the UVB region). It has the disadvantage that it is photolabile and can be rapidly oxidized leading to inactivation of antioxidant systems (21). It has also been shown to be absorbed systemically following topical application (22).

Butyl methoxydibenzoylmethane (avobenzone) provides broad spectrum UVA filtration (up to λ 380 nm) but quickly loses potency on the skin. Photoprotective capacity decreases by 50–60% after one hour of exposure to sunlight (23). Consequently oxybenzone and avobenzone are formulated with other filters to enhance their photostability (24). However, avobenzone was reported to enhance the degradation of octyl methoxycinnamate (25), therefore careful selection of UV filter combinations is required. Menthyl anthranilate is a weak UVA filter (26).

Some effective UVA filters, used in Europe, Australia and elsewhere, are not included in the 1999 FDA monograph. Of these, terephthalydene dicamphor sulfonic acid (ecamsule; Mexoryl SX) has recently been approved by the FDA (Jul 2006) and is the first new organic sunscreen in the United States for 18 years. It is a photostable, broad-spectrum UVA filter which has been shown to prevent UVA-induced histological changes associated with photoaging in the skin (27,28). It also provides more effective suppression of UVR-induced carcinogenesis in mice than a UVB filter alone (29). Drometriazole trisiloxane (Mexoryl XL) is a photostable UVA/UVB filter consisting of two chemical groups: 12-hydroxyphenylbenzotriazole, which is a UVR filter active, and a liposoluble silicone chain. It has been suggested that sunscreen products incorporating these Mexoryl filters may be more effective in preventing the induction of lesions in patients with photosensitive lupus erythematosus than products containing avobenzone and TiO_2 as the UVA filters (30).

Methylene-bis-benzotriazolyl tetramethylbutylphenol and bis-ethylhexyloxy-phenol methoxyphenol triazine are broad-spectrum UVA/UVB filters developed by Ciba Specialty Chemicals (Switzerland) under the trade names Tinosorb M and Tinosorb S, respectively. Tinosorb M combines the benefits of organic and inorganic filters and is reported to be more effective than other UVA filters (31). It is a large, photostable, organic molecule that is formulated as microfine particles in the aqueous phase of the sunscreen emulsion. It absorbs UVR and dissipates the energy in a similar mechanism to other organic filters, but also scatters and reflects UVR. Tinosorb S is an oil-soluble equivalent with similar photostability and broad spectrum UVR absorbing activity. Both are effective filters and can enhance the stability of other UV filters such as octyl methoxycinnamate and avobenzone (25). Due to their particle size, skin penetration of these organometallic sunscreens is unlikely. In addition, they do not possess intrinsic estrogenic/antiestrogenic or androgenic/antiandrogenic activity in vitro (32).

Inorganic UV Filters
Inorganic UV filters, zinc oxide and titanium dioxide act by scattering, reflecting and/or absorbing UVR (33,34) dependent on their refractive index, the size of the particles, dispersion in the emulsion and film thickness (35). The drawback of inorganic mineral sunscreens is that they are opaque on the skin. To improve cosmetic acceptability, particle size can be reduced to 20-50 nm, rendering them transparent to visible radiation (36), but this also reduces their ability to scatter and reflect UVR. The availability of microfine ZnO (for example Z-cote from BASF and Zin-Clear from Advanced Nanotechnology Ltd, Australia) and TiO_2 has increased the formulation of these inorganic filters in sunscreen products, thus permitting high SPF values and broad spectrum absorption, with reduced amounts of organic filters.

Formulation Approaches to Improve Photostability of UV Filters
Although the recently developed organic filters are photostable, many of the older organic filters, particularly avobenzone, octyl methoxycinnamate and padimate O, are photolabile. A number of approaches have been developed to improve photostability. This has involved judicious combinations with ZnO, TiO_2, octocrylene, the salicylates, methylbenzylidene camphor and Tinosorb. In order to protect these filters, novel formulation methods have been investigated including complexation with cyclodextrins (37,38), encapsulation in liposheres (39), nanoparticles (40,41) and microspheres (42). Oxonica (Oxfordshire, U.K.) has recently introduced Optisol, an ultrafine TiO_2 with 0.7% manganese in the crystal, which eliminates the potential of the TiO_2 to generate free radicals (43).

SKIN PERMEATION OF SUNSCREENS

Sunscreen products are applied to large areas of the skin repeatedly, in the case of beach application, or on a daily basis to the face and other areas of the skin in personal care and cosmetic products. To provide effective sun protection to the skin, sunscreens need to reside on or near the skin surface. There is no therapeutic requirement for systemic absorption of UV filters; therefore, determination of the skin absorption of sunscreens is essential in their risk assessment. Various factors, such as the nature of the formulation, can influence the skin absorption of topically applied chemicals, so it is essential that sunscreen skin absorption is measured in well-designed in vitro or in vivo studies (a summary of reported studies can be found in Table 3).

In Vivo Dermal Absorption Studies

Urinary excretion of oxybenzone and its metabolites was monitored for 48 hours following the administration of a commercial sunscreen product containing 6% oxybenzone to the forearms of healthy human volunteers for a 10-hour period (22). Approximately 1–2% of the applied dose was excreted in the urine, and there was considerable intersubject variability in skin absorption (Fig. 1). In this study, the product application rate was 12.4 mg/cm^2, which is considerably greater than the application rate recommended for SPF assessment (2 mg/cm^2). Benson et al. (44) demonstrated that oxybenzone absorption was up to four times greater through face skin than through back skin. Gustavsson Gonzalez et al. reported that about 10 mg (0.5% of the applied dose) of oxybenzone was recovered in the urine of healthy volunteers over 48 hours following the whole body application of an SPF 14 sunscreen lotion containing 4% oxybenzone (45). On repeated application of the sunscreen, morning and night, for five days, 1.2–8.7% (mean 3.7%) of the total amount of applied oxybenzone was excreted in urine over 10 days from the initial application (46). The authors concluded that absorption and accumulation in the body were substantial as the volunteers excreted oxybenzone up to five days after the last application. Oxybenzone has also been detected in human breast milk following topical application (47).

Feldman and Maibach (48) reported that 28% of the dose (4 µg/cm^2) of PABA applied to human skin was excreted in the urine over five days. The sunscreen was dissolved in acetone that evaporated to deposit the PABA on the skin surface, a method of application that is likely to overestimate absorption relative to application in a more conventional sunscreen product. Lower skin absorption rates were reported by Arancibia et al. (49), who applied 5% PABA in three different formulations to large body surface areas of six human male volunteers and monitored urinary excretion. They reported no difference in skin absorption from the three formulations (hydroalcoholic gel and oil-in-water emulsions at pH 4.2 and 6.5), but there was considerable variation between subjects, with 1.6% to 9.6% of the applied dose absorbed.

Dupuis et al. reported that a linear relationship exists between drug concentration in the stratum corneum, determined by tape stripping, and in vivo percutaneous absorption, determined by urinary excretion (50). Treffel and Gabard used the tape-stripping technique to assess the skin absorption of oxybenzone, octyl methoxycinnimate, and octyl salicylate from an emulsion gel and petroleum jelly (51). There were significantly greater amounts of all sunscreen actives in the stratum corneum at 0.5 hours post-application of the emulsion gel than the petroleum jelly (Fig. 2). These epidermal retention data were confirmed in a parallel in vitro study. Only oxybenzone was detected in appreciable quantities in the dermis and receptor fluid.

The systemic absorption of the new sunscreen terephthalylidine dicamphor sulfonic acid (Mexoryl SX) was determined following application to human skin in an emulsion formulation for four hours (52). Urinary recovery of 0.014% was obtained. In vitro absorption, following a similar four-hour application period, was 0.16% of the applied dose over 24 hours.

TABLE 3 Reported Human Skin Absorption of Sunscreen Actives

Sunscreen	Type of test	% dose absorbed	Exposure time (hours)	Flux ($\mu g/cm^2/hr$)	Vehicle	Other	References
PABA	In vivo	1.6 – 9.6	48		5% in hydroalcoholic gel o/w emulsion		(49)
	In vivo	28.37 urine	120		Solvent deposited solid radiolabel		(48)
Octyl dimethyl PABA	In vivo	Loss from donor	6	0.53	Propylene glycol	Permeability: 0.259 cm/hr	(74)
Octyl methoxy-cinnamate	In vitro	1.6–9.3	6		o/w emulsion gel and petrolatum	In skin only, none in receptor	(51)
Octyl methoxy-cinnamate	In vitro	10	16		o/w emulsion		(75)
Octyl methoxy-cinnamate	In vitro	7–17	8		Commercial formulations	In skin only, none in receptor	(58)
Isoamyl-*p*-methoxy-cinnamate	In vivo	Loss from donor	6	3.16	Propylene glycol	Permeability: 0.105 cm/hr	(74)
Octyl salicylate	In vitro	1.9–7.7	6		o/w emulsion gel and petrolatum	In skin only, none in receptor	(51)
Homosalate	In vitro	5–10 in receptor 4–12 in skin	8		Commercial formulations		(58)
4-Methylbenzyldene camphor	In vivo	Loss from donor	6	2.11	Propylene glycol	Permeability: 0.091 cm/hr	(74)
Oxybenzone	In vivo	Loss from donor	6	4.44	Propylene glycol	Permeability: 0.053 cm/hr	(74)
	In vitro	5.3–6.4	6		o/w emulsion gel and petrolatum		(51)
	In vivo	1–2% urine	10		Commercial formulation		(22)
	In vivo						(44)
	In vivo	0.5% urine	48 5 days, twice daily		Commercial formulation		(45)
	In vitro	1.2–8.7% urine			Commercial formulation		(46)
Tetraphyhalydene dicamphor sulfonic acid	In vivo	% dose absorbed	4		Commercial emulsion	0.014% in urine	(52)
Camphor benzalkonium methosulfate	In vitro	% dose dermis and receptor	4		Commercial emulsion	0.16% in 24 hours	(75)

Abbreviation: o/w, oil-in-water.

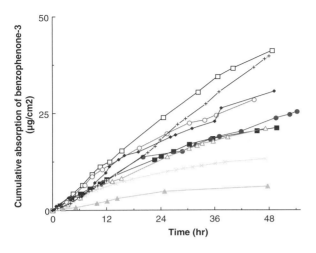

FIGURE 1 Skin absorption of oxybenzone following topical application in a commercial formulation. Data calculated from urinary recovery of the sunscreen agent and its metabolites. *Source*: From Ref. 22.

Lademann et al. (53) evaluated the penetration of TiO₂ microparticles into human stratum corneum and follicles using tape stripping, coupled with UV–VIS spectroscopic and X-ray fluorescence measurement, to determine distribution of TiO₂ throughout the stratum corneum. An oil-in-water emulsion containing the TiO₂ was applied to the volar forearm of volunteers in multiple doses over three days. The largest concentration of TiO₂ was located in the outer layers of the stratum corneum and in the pilosebaceous orifice regions. The authors concluded that no TiO₂ particles permeated through the intact stratum corneum, although there was some penetration into the hair follicles. Bennat and Müller-Goymann (54) also reported very little penetration of TiO₂ into the deeper layers of the stratum corneum from an aqueous dispersion, although deeper penetration into the skin occurred from an oily dispersion containing octyl palmitate. Further confirmation was provided by Pflucker et al. (55,56), who examined punch biopsies of the skin by optical and elec-

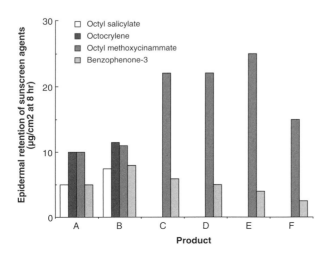

FIGURE 2 The amount of sunscreen agent recovered from human skin epidermal membranes following eight-hour exposure to several commercial sunscreen products designated as A–F. *Source*: From Ref. 58.

tron microscopy and reported that, regardless of the surface characteristics, particle size, or shape, the micronized TiO_2 was deposited on the outermost surface of the stratum corneum and could not be detected in deeper stratum corneum layers.

In vivo and in vitro studies have demonstrated that the more lipophilic organic sunscreen actives do not permeate into the dermis but remain in the stratum corneum and are likely lost by desquamation. The relatively polar PABA and oxybenzone (calculated log P 1.00 and 3.87 respectively (57)) are less tightly bound in the stratum corneum and can permeate through the epidermis to the systemic circulation.

In Vitro Dermal Absorption Studies

In vitro studies are useful in evaluating the influence of formulation on permeation, but the protocol should be carefully planned, particularly with regard to appropriate choice of receptor solution for assessing lipophilic compounds. Jiang et al. (58) assessed the penetration of five sunscreen actives, applied in commercial lotions, using isolated human epidermis. Significant amounts of oxybenzone, octyl methoxycinnimate, octocrylene, and octyl salicylate (up to 250 mg/m² or 14% of the applied dose) were absorbed into the epidermis at eight hours post-application (Fig. 2). Up to 10% of the applied dose of oxybenzone (80 mg/m²) penetrated to the receptor phase (4% BSA in buffer) over the eight-hour application period (Fig. 3). This absorption rate is similar to that observed in the in vivo assessment (22) of the same product (in vitro 80 mg/m² and in vivo 70 mg/m² at eight hours post-application). The other sunscreens evaluated did not penetrate to the receptor solution in quantifiable amounts.

Walters et al. (59) measured the permeation of ¹⁴C-labeled octyl salicylate across human epidermis in vitro using a receptor phase containing the nonionic surfactant polyethylene glycol oleyl ether (6% Volpo N20). A finite dose (5 mg/cm²) of two different formulations containing 5% octyl salicylate was applied. The permeation of octyl salicylate into the receptor phase over 48 hours was similar for the two formulations (1.58 µg/cm²), but sunscreen remaining in the epidermis at

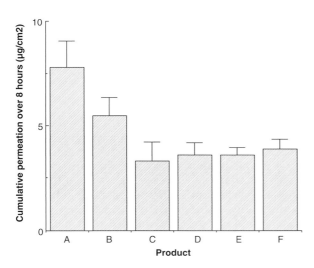

FIGURE 3 Amount of oxybenzone permeated through human skin epidermal membranes following eight-hour exposure to several commercial sunscreen products designated as A–F. *Source*: From Ref. 58.

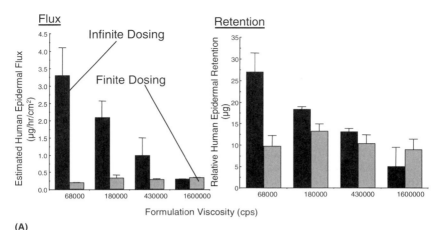

(A)

INFINITE DOSE (THICK FORMULATION)

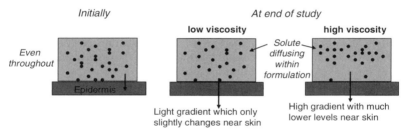

FINITE DOSE (THIN "IN USE" FORMULATION)

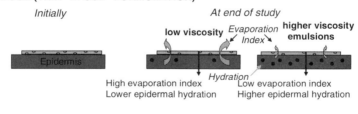

(B)

FIGURE 4 **(A)** Effect of formulation viscosity on epidermal flux and retention of oxybenzone. **(B)** Diagrammatic representation of possible processes involved. *Source*: From Ref. 62.

48 hours was higher for a hydroalcoholic solution than for an oil-in-water emulsion (32.77% and 17.18% of applied dose, respectively).

Gupta et al. (60) reported that the penetration of oxybenzone and octyl methoxycinnimate into and across micro-Yucatan pig skin was higher when the sunscreens were applied in combination than when each was applied alone. It has also been reported that the flux and permeability coefficient of oxybenzone is related to vehicle solubility parameter and that alcohol appears to enhance skin and membrane diffusivity (44,61). Increasing the viscosity of a vehicle decreased penetration flux under infinite dosing conditions but had the opposite effect on flux following in-use (or finite) doses (Fig. 4A) (62). The authors suggested that the reduced penetration in the infinite dosing case reflected a diminished diffusivity of sunscreen in the vehicle. In contrast, a high-viscosity product under in-use conditions was postulated to have promoted penetration via increased stratum corneum hydration (Fig. 4B). The results confirm that skin permeation studies should be conducted under in-use conditions to more closely represent the application conditions in practice. Risk assessment for a UV filter in the European Union is based on the application of 2 mg/cm^2 of a sunscreen product to the skin (63).

Microfine ZnO and TiO$_2$ were applied to porcine skin in vitro and penetration assessed by the analysis of receptor fluid, tape strips, and surface washes. Virtually all applied ZnO was recovered in the first five tape strips, and almost all applied TiO$_2$ was recovered in the washes (64). Cross et al. (65) recently reported that less than 0.03% of applied Zn penetrated the human epidermis, following in vitro application of ZnO as Zin-Clear (26–30 nm particles). No particles were detected in the lower stratum corneum or viable epidermis by electron microscopy.

Of concern is the potential of some sunscreen actives to act as penetration enhancers. Pont et al. reported that a number of sunscreen actives and the insect-repellent DEET enhanced the penetration of the herbicide 2,4-dichlorophenoxyacetic acid across hairless mouse skin in vitro (66,67). In a further study, incorporation of inorganic filters and change of vehicle were shown to counteract the penetration enhancement ability of organic UV filters (66). Although hairless mouse skin is known to be more sensitive to penetration enhancers, the authors suggested that similar effects were seen in human skin. Morgan et al. (68) reported that octyl salicylate increased testosterone skin permeation 6.3-fold and padimate O increased permeation of testosterone, estradiol, and progesterone by 2.4-, 3.5-, and 9.3-fold, respectively. Indeed, this has been used as the basis for a new transdermal delivery technology being developed by Acrux Pty. Ltd., Australia

BENEFITS AND RISKS OF TOPICAL SUNSCREENS

Acute toxic side effects of specific sunscreen agents include contact irritation, allergic contact dermatitis, phototoxicity, photoallergy, and staining of the skin (69). However, considering the widespread use of sunscreens, the incidence of side effects is small. Based on the in vitro and in vivo data, the amount of sunscreen that permeates the skin is minimal, even for oxybenzone, and negligible for the more lipophilic sunscreens and inorganic filters. Modern sunscreens must meet rigorous testing for photostability, acute, subchronic, and chronic toxicity, irritation, sensitization, phototoxicity, photosensitization, reproductive toxicity, genotoxicity, photogenotoxicity, and carcinogenicity prior to approval (6,63). Modern sunscreens are designed for skin retention and water resistance so that skin permeation is minimal. This is exemplified by the recently introduced Mexoryl and Tinosorb UV filters.

There have been some controversies regarding sunscreen use. Concerns regarding reduced vitamin D synthesis in long-term sunscreen use have been shown to be insignificant (70). Considerable media coverage followed the suggestion that UV filters, in particular octyl methoxycinnamate and 4-methylbenzylidene camphor, may have estrogenic activity (71). However the Scientific Committee of Cosmetic Products and Non-food Products, a European Commission advisory body, questioned the experimental protocols and concluded that the relative estrogenic potencies of the UV filters were about 1 million times less than that of the positive control substance estradiol (72).

Sunscreen products have been used extensively for many years with little clinical evidence of toxicity. They play a valuable role in reducing the risks associated with exposure to solar radiation such as sunburn, photoaging, and skin cancer. The most recently introduced UV filters have been specifically designed to improve efficacy and safety through broad UVR absorption, photostability, and skin binding. The risk/benefit assessment clearly favors the use of topical sunscreen products as part of our defense against UVR-induced skin damage.

CONCLUSIONS

Modern sunscreen products are designed to provide long-lasting protection from the absorption of UVA and UVB radiation to viable skin tissues. Whereas assessment of their ability to absorb UVB has been available for some time in the form of the SPF value, a rating for UVA efficacy has only recently been introduced. It has been suggested that an immune protection factor should also be included in the assessment of sunscreens. Hamilton Laboratories, an Australian sunscreen manufacturer, has recently introduced a product with enhanced protection from UV-induced immunosuppression, denoted the "Hamilton Optimal Enhanced Protection Sunscreen" (73). There is evidence that oxybenzone permeates the skin following administration in sunscreen products, but there is no evidence that this is related to toxic consequences. Permeation to viable tissues of the more lipophilic sunscreens and inorganic filters is negligible. All common sunscreens penetrate into the stratum corneum, but the extent to which permeation to deeper tissues occurs over time has not been established. The affinity of highly lipophilic sunscreens for the stratum corneum confers an ability to resist removal by water, which is important to ensure that a sunscreen product remains effective after swimming or sweating. One of the most significant health concerns is obesity, particularly the rapid increase in childhood obesity rates. Regular exercise in the outdoors is essential for a healthy lifestyle, yet there is clear evidence that exposure to UVR can cause acute and long-term skin damage. Topical sunscreen products are an effective part of the overall sun protection regimen. The continued development of UV filters with improved efficacy and safety is essential.

REFERENCES

1. Schaefer H, Moyal D, Fourtanier A. Recent advances in sun protection. Semin Cutan Med Surg 1998; 17:266–275.
2. Gil EM, Kim TH. UV-induced immune suppression and sunscreen. Photodermatol Photoimmunol Photomed 2000; 16:101–110.
3. Pearse AD, Gaskell SA, Marks R. Epidermal changes in human skin following irradiation with either UVB or UVA. J Invest Dermatol 1987; 88:83–87.
4. Moyal D, Fourtanier A. Acute and chronic effects of UV on skin. In: Rigel DS, Weiss RA, Lim HW, et al., eds. Photoaging. New York: Marcel Dekker Inc; 2004:15–32.
5. Phan TA, Halliday GM, Barnetson RS, et al. Spectral and dose dependence of ultraviolet radiation-induced immunosuppression. Front Biosci 2006; 11:394–411.
6. Kullavanijaya P, Lim HW. Photoprotection. J Am Acad Dermatol 2005; 52:937–958.
7. FDA. Part 352—Sunscreen drug products for over-the-counter-human use: final monograph. Fed Regist 1999; 64:27687–27693.
8. Lowe NJ. An overview of ultraviolet radiation, sunscreens, and photo-induced dermatoses. Dermatol Clin 2006; 24:9–17.
9. European Commission. Sunscreen products: what matters? MEMO/06/185 May 2006.

10. European Commission. Sunscreens: commission moves to improve labeling. IP/06/571 May 2006.
11. EU. List of UV filters which cosmetic products may contain, Council Directive 76/768 EEC, Annex VII. European Union 1976; and amendments inclusive to 2005/80/EC.
12. TGA. Sunscreening agents permitted as active ingredients in listed products. Therapeutic Goods Administration, Australia 2006 (Accessed September 26, 2007, at http://www.tga .gov.au/docs/pdf/argom_10.pdf).
13. Lademann J, Schanzer S, Jacobi U, et al. Synergy effects between organic and inorganic UV filters in sunscreens. J Biomed Opt 2005; 10:14008.
14. Horio T, Higuchi T. Photocontact dermatitis from *p*-aminobenzoic acid. Dermatologica 1978; 156:124–128.
15. Thune P, Jansen C, Wennersten G, et al. The Scandinavian multicenter photopatch study 1980–1985: final report. Photodermatology 1988; 5:261–269.
16. van Ketel WG. Allergic contact dermatitis from an aminobenzoic acid compound used in sunscreens. Contact Dermatitis 1977; 3:283.
17. Marmelzat J, Rapaport MJ. Photodermatitis with PABA. Contact Dermatitis 1980; 6:230–231.
18. Tarras-Wahlberg N, Stenhagen G, Larko O, et al. Changes in ultraviolet absorption of sunscreens after ultraviolet irradiation. J Invest Dermatol 1999; 113:547–553.
19. Kimura K, Katoh T. Photoallergic contact dermatitis from the sunscreen ethylhexyl-*p*-methoxycinnamate (Parsol MCX). Contact Dermatitis 1995; 32:304–305.
20. Schmidt T, Ring J, Abeck D. Photoallergic contact dermatitis due to combined UVB (4-methylbenzylidene camphor/octyl methoxycinnamate) and UVA (benzophenone-3/butyl methoxydibenzoylmethane) absorber sensitization. Dermatology 1998; 196:354–357.
21. Schallreuter KU, Wood JM, Farwell DW, et al. Oxybenzone oxidation following solar irradiation of skin: photoprotection versus antioxidant inactivation. J Invest Dermatol 1996; 106:583–586.
22. Hayden CG, Roberts MS, Benson HAE. Systemic absorption of sunscreen after topical application. Lancet 1997; 350:863–864.
23. Bouillon C. Recent advances in sun protection. J Derm Sci 2000; 23(Suppl. 1):S57–S61.
24. Pathak MA. Sunscreens: progress and perspectives on photoprotection of human skin against UVB and UVA radiation. J Dermatol 1996; 23:783–800.
25. Chatelain E, Gabard B. Photostabilization of butyl methoxydibenzoylmethane (Avobenzone) and ethylhexyl methoxycinnamate by bis-ethylhexyloxyphenol methoxyphenyl triazine (Tinosorb S), a new UV broadband filter. Photochem Photobiol 2001; 74:401–406.
26. Beeby A, Jones AE. The photophysical properties of menthyl anthranilate: a UV-A sunscreen. Photochem Photobiol 2000; 72:10–15.
27. Seite S, Moyal D, Richard S, et al. Mexoryl SX: a broad absorption UVA filter protects human skin from the effects of repeated suberythemal doses of UVA. J Photochem Photobiol B 1998; 44:69–76.
28. Seite S, Colige A, Piquemal-Vivenot P, et al. A full-UV spectrum absorbing daily use cream protects human skin against biological changes occurring in photoaging. Photodermatol Photoimmunol Photomed 2000; 16:147–155.
29. Fourtanier A. Mexoryl SX protects against solar-simulated UVR-induced photocarcinogenesis in mice. Photochem Photobiol 1996; 64:688–693.
30. Stege H, Budde MA, Grether-Beck S, et al. Evaluation of the capacity of sunscreens to photoprotect lupus erythematosus patients by employing the photoprovocation test. Photodermatol Photoimmunol Photomed 2000; 16:256–259.
31. Gelis C, Girard S, Mavon A, et al. Assessment of the skin photoprotective capacities of an organo-mineral broad-spectrum sunblock on two ex vivo skin models. Photodermatol Photoimmunol Photomed 2003; 19:242–253.
32. Ashby J, Tinwell H, Plautz J, et al. Lack of binding to isolated estrogen or androgen receptors, and inactivity in the immature rat uterotrophic assay, of the ultraviolet sunscreen filters Tinosorb M-active and Tinosorb S. Regul Toxicol Pharmacol 2001; 34:287–291.
33. Serpone N, Salinaro A. Terminology, relative photonic efficiencies and quantum yields in heterogeneous photocatalysis: Part I. Suggested protocol. Pure Appl Chem 1999; 71:303–320.

34. Salinaro A, Emeline A, Zhao J, et al. Terminology, relative photonic efficiencies and quantum yields in heterogeneous photocatalysis: Part II. Experimental determination of quantum yields. Pure Appl Chem 1999; 71:321–335.
35. Murphy GM. Sunblocks: mechanisms of action. Photodermatol Photoimmunol Photomed 1999; 15:34–36.
36. Serpone N, Dondi D, Albini A. Inorganic and organic UV filters: their role and efficacy in sunscreens and suncare products. Inorg Chim Acta 2007; 360(3):794–802.
37. Sarveiya V, Templeton JF, Benson HAE. Inclusion complexation of the sunscreen 2-hydroxy-4methoxy benzophenone (oxybenzone) with hydroxypropyl-b-cyclodextrin: effect on membrane diffusion. J Incl Phenomen Macrocyclic Chem 2004; 49:275–281.
38. Simeoni S, Scalia S, Benson HA. Influence of cyclodextrins on in vitro human skin absorption of the sunscreen, butyl-methoxydibenzoylmethane. Int J Pharm 2004; 280:163–171.
39. Scalia S, Tursilli R, Sala N, et al. Encapsulation in liposheres of the complex between butyl methoxydibenzoylmethane and hydroxypropyl-[beta]-cyclodextrin. Int J Pharm 2006; 320:79–85.
40. Wissing SA, Muller RH. Solid lipid nanoparticles as carrier for sunscreens: in vitro release and in vivo skin penetration. J Control Release 2002; 81:225–233.
41. Perugini P, Simeoni S, Scalia S, et al. Effect of nanoparticle encapsulation on the photostability of the sunscreen agent, 2-ethylhexyl-p-methoxycinnamate. Int J Pharm 2002; 246:37–45.
42. Yener G, Incegul T, Yener N. Importance of using solid lipid microspheres as carriers for UV filters on the example octyl methoxy cinnamate. Int J Pharm 2003; 258:203–207.
43. http://www.oxonica.com/materials/materials_optisol.php
44. Benson HAE, Sarveiya V, Risk S, et al. Influence of anatomical site and topical formulation on skin penetration of sunscreens. Ther Clin Risk Manag 2005; 1:209–218.
45. Gustavsson Gonzalez H, Farbrot A, Larko O. Percutaneous absorption of benzophenone-3, a common component of topical sunscreens. Clin Exp Dermatol 2002; 27:691–694.
46. Gonzalez H, Farbrot A, Larko O, et al. Percutaneous absorption of the sunscreen benzophenone-3 after repeated whole-body applications, with and without ultraviolet irradiation. Br J Dermatol 2006; 154:337–340.
47. Hany J, Nagel R. Detection of sunscreen agents in human breast milk. Dtsch Lebensmitt Rundsch 1995; 91:341–345.
48. Feldman R, Maibach HI. Absorption of some organic compounds through the skin in man. J Invest Dermatol 1970; 54:399–404.
49. Arancibia A, Borie G, Cornwell E, et al. Pharmacokinetic study on the percutaneous absorption of p-aminobenzoic acid from 3 sunscreen preparations. Farmaco 1981; 36:357–365.
50. Dupuis D, Rougier A, Lotte C, et al. An original predictive method for in vivo percutaneous absorption studies. Acta Derm Venereol Suppl 1987; 134:9–21.
51. Treffel P, Gabard B. Skin penetration and sun protection factor of ultra-violet filters from two vehicles. Pharm Res 1996; 13:770–774.
52. Benech-Kieffer F, Meuling WJ, Leclerc C, et al. Percutaneous absorption of Mexoryl SX in human volunteers: comparison with in vitro data. Skin Pharmacol Appl Skin Physiol 2003; 16:343–355.
53. Lademann J, Weigmann H, Rickmeyer C, et al. Penetration of titanium dioxide microparticles in a sunscreen formulation into the horny layer and the follicular orifice. Skin Pharmacol Appl Skin Physiol 1999; 12:247–256.
54. Bennat C, Müller-Goymann CC. Skin penetration and stabilization of formulations containing microfine titanium dioxide as physical UV filter. Int J Cosmet Sci 2000; 22: 271–283.
55. Schulz J, Hohenberg H, Pflucker F, et al. Distribution of sunscreens on skin. Adv Drug Deliv Rev 2002; 54(Suppl. 1):S157–S163.
56. Pflucker F, Wendel V, Hohenberg H, et al. The human stratum corneum layer: an effective barrier against dermal uptake of different forms of topically applied micronised titanium dioxide. Skin Pharmacol Appl Skin Physiol 2001; 14(Suppl. 1):92–97.
57. Watkinson AC, Brain KR, Walters KA, et al. Prediction of the percutaneous penetration of ultra-violet filters used in sunscreen formulations. Int J Cosmet Sci 1992; 14:265–275.

58. Jiang R, Roberts MS, Collins DM, et al. Absorption of sunscreens across human skin: an evaluation of commercial products for children and adults. Br J Clin Pharm 1999; 48:635–637.
59. Walters KA, Brain KR, Howes D, et al. Percutaneous penetration of octyl salicylate from representative sunscreen formulations through human skin in vitro. Food Chem Toxicol 1997; 35:1219–1225.
60. Gupta VK, Zatz JL, Rerek M. Percutaneous absorption of sunscreens through micro-yucatan pig skin in vitro. Pharm Res 1999; 16:1602–1607.
61. Jiang R, Benson HAE, Cross SE, et al. In vitro human epidermal and polyethylene membrane penetration and retention of the sunscreen benzophenone-3 from a range of solvents. Pharm Res 1998; 15:1863–1868.
62. Cross SE, Jiang R, Benson HAE, et al. Can increasing the viscosity of formulations be used to reduce the human skin penetration of the sunscreen oxybenzone? J Invest Dermatol 2001; 117:147–150.
63. Nohynek GJ, Schaefer H. Benefit and risk of organic ultraviolet filters. Regul Toxicol Pharmacol 2001; 33:285–299.
64. Gamer AO, Leibold E, van Ravenzwaay B. The in vitro absorption of microfine zinc oxide and titanium dioxide through porcine skin. Toxicol In Vitro 2006; 20:301–307.
65. Cross SE, Innes B, Roberts MS, et al. Human skin penetration of sunscreen nanoparticles: in-vitro assessment of a novel micronised zinc oxide formulation. Skin Pharmacol Physiol 2007; 20:148–154.
66. Pont AR, Charron AR, Brand RM. Active ingredients in sunscreens act as topical penetration enhancers for the herbicide 2,4-dichlorophenoxyacetic acid. Toxicol Appl Pharmacol 2004; 195:348–354.
67. Pont AR, Charron AR, Wilson RM, et al. Effects of active sunscreen ingredient combinations on the topical penetration of the herbicide 2,4-dichlorophenoxyacetic acid. Toxicol Ind Health 2003; 19:1–8.
68. Morgan TM, Reed BL, Finnin BC. Enhanced skin permeation of sex hormones with novel topical spray vehicles. J Pharm Sci 1998; 87:1213–1218.
69. Schauder S, Ippen H. Contact and photocontact sensitivity to sunscreens. Review of a 15-year experience and of the literature. Contact Dermatitis 1997; 37:221–232.
70. Farrerons J, Barnadas M, Rodriguez J, et al. Clinically prescribed sunscreen (sun protection factor 15) does not decrease serum vitamin D concentration sufficiently either to induce changes in parathyroid function or in metabolic markers. Br J Dermatol 1998; 139:422–427.
71. Schlumpf M, Cotton B, Conscience M, et al. In vitro and in vivo estrogenicity of UV screens. Environ Health Perspect 2001; 109:239–244.
72. Opinion on the Evaluation of Potentially Estrogenic Effects of UV-filters adopted by the SCCNFP during the 17th Plenary meeting of 12 June 2001.
73. http://www.hamiltonlabs.com.au.
74. Hagedorn-Leweke U, Lippold BC. Absorption of sunscreens and other compounds through human skin in vivo: derivation of a method to predict maximum fluxes. Pharm Res 1995; 12:354–1360.
75. Benech-Kieffer F, Wegrich P, Schwarzenbach R, et al. Percutaneous absorption of sunscreens in vitro: interspecies comparison, skin models and reproducibility aspects. Skin Pharmacol Appl Skin Physiol 2000; 13:324–335.

26 Efficacy and Safety of Tea Tree and Other Oils

Christine F. Carson and Kate A. Hammer
Department of Microbiology and Immunology, School of Biomedical, Biomolecular, and Chemical Sciences, Faculty of Life and Physical Sciences, The University of Western Australia, Crawley, Western Australia, Australia

Jesper B. Nielsen
Institute of Public Health, University of Southern Denmark, Odense C, Denmark

INTRODUCTION

Essential oils are incorporated into many products designed for cosmetic and dermatological uses. Their use is based on claimed efficacy against a wide variety of ailments and their potential as fragrances. Their safety, particularly at the low levels present in formulated products, is most frequently not questioned because of their long history of reasonably safe use and a low incidence of serious adverse side effects. However, in some instances, the level of evidence required from regulatory agencies to confirm safety has risen. In contrast, as long as claims are limited to cosmetic nontherapeutic indications, the thresholds for efficacy evidence set by regulatory agencies remain relatively low. Increasingly though, a more substantial and higher quality evidence of efficacy is becoming available for many essential oils. This chapter follows from Chapter 24 and emphasizes the provenance, use, and potential toxicity of tea tree, peppermint, eucalyptus, lavender, and chamomile essential oils. Where available, in vivo data with a relevant route of exposure based on complete oils have been used as such data give a functional assay with direct relevance for hazard and risk evaluations. When data on individual constituents are used or when data originate from in vitro studies, a critical assessment is needed. Thus, data from individual constituents ignore the potential for interaction (agonistic or antagonistic effects) and in vitro assay ignores the possibility that not all constituents may reach the target for toxicity due to differences in absorption, metabolism, or elimination.

TEA TREE OIL
Provenance, Composition, and Uses

Tea tree oil (TTO) is a complex mixture of terpene hydrocarbons and tertiary alcohols steam distilled almost exclusively from plantation stands of the Australian native plant *Melaleuca alternifolia* (Maiden and Betche) Cheel of the Myrtaceae family (1). The natural variation seen in this heterogenous mixture is tempered by an international standard for "Oil of *Melaleuca*, terpinen-4-ol type," which sets maxima and/or minima for 14 components of the oil (Table 1) (2). This is not to suggest that TTO that meets the prevailing international standard will be efficacious and without adverse effects. It does, however, highlight that compositional data are an absolute requirement for studies on complex natural products with inherent variation to assist correct interpretation of the results.

TABLE 1 Composition of *Melaleuca alternifolia* (Tea Tree) Oil

Component	ISO 4730 range (2)	Typical composition (3)
Terpinen-4-ol	≥30[a]	40.1
γ-Terpinene	10–28	23.0
α-Terpinene	5–13	10.4
1,8-Cineole	≤ 15[b]	5.1
Terpinolene	1.5–5	3.1
ρ-Cymene	0.5–12	2.9
α-Pinene	1–6	2.6
α-Terpineol	1.5–8	2.4
Aromadendrene	Traces–7	1.5
δ-Cadinene	Traces–8	1.3
Limonene	0.5–4	1.0
Sabinene	Traces–3.5	0.2
Globulol	Traces–3	0.2
Viridiflorol	Traces–1.5	0.1

[a]No upper limit is set, although 48% has been proposed.
[b]No lower limit set.

The efficacy of TTO primarily relates to its antimicrobial and anti-inflammatory properties (7). Based on these properties, TTO is used in liquid and bar soaps and skin washes, moisturizing creams and lotions, toothpastes, mouthwashes, dental floss and other oral care products, antiseptic and disinfectant products, and acne and blemish products. Although much oil is sold neat in small volumes (10–50 ml), formulated products for topical use usually contain 0.5–10%.

Systemic Toxicity
Experimental studies in rats and data from cases of human poisoning show that TTO can be toxic if ingested. The oral LD_{50} for TTO in a rat model is 1.9–2.6 ml/kg (4). Rats dosed with the lesser amount ≤1.5 g TTO/kg body weight appeared lethargic and ataxic and showed depressed activity levels 72 hours post dosing (5), but by day 4 all but one of 13 animals given this lower dose had regained all locomotor functions. As experimental studies with longer exposure times are presently missing, systemic toxicity can not be excluded. Target organs of relevance would be liver, kidney, and, potentially testes, and toxicity would be expected to be dose dependent.

Limited data are available describing the frequency of human poisoning with TTO (6). The American Association of Poison Control Centers surveillance system recorded 737 unintentional exposures to TTO in 2003, with 518 (66%) having occurred in children less than six years of age (7). In children, clinical symptoms may occur following oral intake of less than 10 ml 100% TTO and are most often attributed to central nervous system depression with recovery within 24 hours. A case of poisoning in an adult occurred when a patient drank approximately half a tea cup of TTO estimated to be a dose of 0.5–1.0 ml/kg body weight (8). The patient was comatose for 12 hours and semiconscious and hallucinatory for a further 36 hours. Symptoms of abdominal pain and diarrhea continued for approximately six weeks. No deaths due to TTO have been reported in the literature.

Apart from these reports, there are no data on the systemic toxicity of TTO in humans. However, the available knowledge clearly demonstrates that the toxicity of TTO following oral exposure and the intentional ingestion of neat TTO should be discouraged. Incorporation of TTO into toothpastes, mouthwashes, and other oral products leads to exposure that is considered topical since the products are expelled and not swallowed.

Dermal Toxicity

Studies on irritancy and allergy frequently exclude subjects with a previous history of allergies to cosmetic products, a history of active skin disease, or dark skin. This potentially excludes individuals that may be more susceptible to irritancy and allergy, which may lead to an underestimation of the true potential for TTO to cause dermal toxicity. Conversely, studies using outpatients visiting dermatological clinics may overestimate the true prevalence of allergy and irritancy. Accordingly, the study population needs to be considered when interpreting human studies on the toxicity of dermal exposure to TTO.

Irritant Reactions

The irritant potential of TTO has been investigated using a protocol based upon the Draize human sensitization test (9) with occlusive patch testing using Finn chambers (10,11). In the first of these studies, TTO at concentrations ranging from 5% to 100% in different formulations was applied in patch tests on the backs or upper arms of volunteers (10). After 24 hours, the patches were removed and the sites examined for any reactions. New patches were then applied to the same area and examined again at 24 hours. This process was repeated at 24-hour intervals for a total of 21 days. Of the 28 patients, 25 did not demonstrate any irritant reactions, but the remaining three showed allergic type reactions. The TTO component 1,8-cineole, which had a reputation as a skin irritant, was included in the tests at concentrations up to and including 28% and did not produce any irritant reactions (10). Using a similar protocol, Aspres and Freeman (11) tested 5%, 25%, and 100% TTO in cream, ointment, and gel bases on 311 volunteers. The mean irritancy scores for 306 evaluable subjects were very low, the highest being 0.25 for neat TTO (11). A smaller study with 20 patients patch-tested with 1% TTO found no irritant reactions (12). In a recent Danish study, 217 consecutive dermatology clinic patients were patch-tested with 10% TTO without any irritant reactions recorded (13). The same group of patients was also tested, with a lotion containing 5% TTO that caused weak irritant reactions in 44 (20%) patients. This part of the study was later repeated on 160 new patients exposed to four newly formulated lotions containing 5% TTO. In this second trial, only four had weak but apparently TTO-related irritant reactions (13). The latter trial in which the new formulations elicited no irritant reactions suggests a generic problem related to the formation of oxidized and potentially irritant products in most natural oils, a problem that relates not only to irritant reactions, but also to allergic reactions (see below) and should be addressed by oil producers, product formulators, and vendors.

Irritant reactions are generally concentration dependent and not reliant on prior exposure to the irritating agent. They may usually be avoided by using lower concentrations of the irritant, and this strengthens the argument for discouraging the use of 100% TTO and promoting the use of well-formulated products containing lower levels of TTO.

Contact Allergy

Contact allergy is defined as a cutaneous reaction caused by direct contact with an allergen to which the patient has previously been exposed and to which they have become sensitized (14). Once an allergic reaction to TTO has occurred, all subsequent exposures to TTO, regardless of concentration, are likely to elicit further allergic reactions. Numerous case reports of contact allergy due to topically applied TTO have been published (15–20). These reactions have occurred in response to 100% TTO as well as to lower concentrations of TTO in various formulations.

In general, higher and lower incidences of positive patch tests have occurred after a challenge with neat TTO and lower concentrations, respectively. For example, neat oil resulted in positive patch tests in 2–6% of patients tested (21,22), whereas 5% and 10% TTO yielded positive reactions in 0.3–2% of patients (13,23–25). Patch testing in healthy volunteers has also been conducted, with incidences of 1–3% positive patch tests (11).

In a few instances, patients with a history of contact allergy toward TTO have been investigated in detail, providing more insight into the components responsible for allergy and/or positive patch tests. The data suggest that oxidation products formed within TTO during prolonged or poor storage are the main allergens (26,27). Freshly distilled TTO appears to have a low sensitizing capacity, whereas TTO kept for prolonged periods is a moderate to strong sensitizer and has a significantly increased peroxide value (26). This same study also suggests that the most important allergens formed could be ascaridole, and 1,2,4-trihydroxymethane (26,27). However, the cause of allergy is still controversial, and no single allergen responsible for all allergies has been identified.

Ototoxicity

The antimicrobial profile of TTO has led to suggestions that it may be efficacious in the treatment of otitis media and externa. The ototoxicity of TTO has only been evaluated in a single study suggesting that concentrations of 2% TTO or less may be safe for otic use, whereas neat TTO applied to the round window for a relatively short time was at least partially ototoxic (28).

Fetotoxicity

No studies of the potential fetotoxicity of TTO have been published. However, a study of the embryo/fetotoxicity of α-terpinene, usually present at approximately 9% in TTO, showed significant fetotoxicity at 60 mg/kg in rats (29). The offspring of dams given 60 mg/kg from day 6 to day 15 of gestation had delayed ossification and skeletal malformations. At 30 mg/kg, no effects were seen on either dams or offspring. Considering that α-terpinene constitutes less than 10% of TTO, these limited data suggest that TTO is potentially embryo/fetotoxic if ingested at relatively high levels.

Genotoxicity

TTO was nonmutagenic in the bacterial reverse mutation assay using *Salmonella typhimurium* strains TA98 and TA100 (30,31) and *Escherichia coli* strain WP2*uvr* (30), both with and without activation. Furthermore, the following components were non-mutagenic in the *Salmonella* microsome (Ames) test or the *Bacillus subtilis* rec-assay: terpinen-4-ol (32), α-terpinene (33), 1,8-cineole (34–36), α-terpineol (34,37), cymene (38), limonene (37,39,40), α-pinene (33,37,38,40), β-pinene (37), linalool (34,38,41), and β-myrcene (33). In contrast, terpineol caused a slight but dose-related increase in the number of revertants with the TA102 tester strain both with and without S9 mixture (+/- metabolism). However, no significant effect was seen in the other three bacterial strains, indicating that terpineol induced a base pair substitution affecting an A–T base pair (36).

In tests with mammalian cells, γ-terpinene did not increase DNA strand breakage in human lymphocytes at 0.1 mM but did at 0.2 mM (42). Cineole, D-(+)-limonene, linalool, L-phellandrene, and β-pinene at concentrations ranging from 10 to 1000 µM did not increase the frequency of spontaneous sister–chromatid exchanges in Chinese hamster ovary cells (43). Another study showed linalool to be nonmutagenic using a Chinese hamster fibroblast cell line (41). β-Myrcene did not have mutagenic activity when tested with human lymphocytes (44) and was not genotoxic in bone marrow cells of rats administered β-myrcene orally (45). Overall, the available data on the mutagenicity of TTO and its individual constituents indicate low mutagenic potential, using both bacterial and mammalian test systems.

Risk Estimate

On the basis of present knowledge, it may be concluded that TTO is toxic when ingested in high doses, can cause skin irritation at high concentrations, and may cause allergic reactions in predisposed individuals. However, since data indicate that the toxicity of TTO is dose dependent, the majority of adverse events can be avoided through the use of lower concentrations. The exception to this is allergic reactions, which occur in only a small fraction of the human population and may be caused by oxidation products. There is little evidence to suggest that TTO or its components exhibit significant genotoxic potential, and available data suggest that TTO has a low potential for fetotoxicity.

As with many natural products, conclusions about the overall toxicity of TTO are complicated by the fact that it contains more than 100 components. In the absence of data for whole oil, insight on toxicity still needs to be gained partly from data for individual components. This lack of information is of less importance when evaluating observational studies on toxicity of TTO, but it will be a considerable challenge to toxicologists trying to identify specific perpetrators or potential health promoting substances within TTO as well as to regulators within different administrative organizations. More data in this area would lead to an increased understanding of not only which TTO components cause toxicity, but also those that cause positive health effects, which is the ultimate reason for its use. Lastly, if oxidation products can be avoided, the available literature suggests that TTO can be used topically in diluted form by most individuals without adverse effects.

PEPPERMINT OIL
Provenance, Composition, and Uses

Peppermint oil is obtained from the *Mentha piperita* plant and is a mixture of carbohydrates, with menthol (approximately 60%) and menthone (18–20%) as the dominating constituents. Other minor constituents include limonene (5%) and lower amounts of a range of other terpenes and sesquiterpenes (46).

Peppermint oil relaxes smooth muscle, relieves gastric pain and constipation, and has, beside a range of less well-defined ailments, been used orally for many years (47,48). Peppermint oil has also been used as a fragrance in a wide number of food items. The continued use of peppermint oil in cosmetics and as a fragrance component has accentuated the need for information on the efficacy of the oil and on unintended effects on the skin and on percutaneous penetration. Peppermint oil is used in rinse-off (<3% oil) as well as leave-on (<0.2% oil) formulations (48). Furthermore, indications of a virucidal effect of peppermint oil against herpes infections (49) may increase the potential for dermal exposure and the need for information on safety following dermal exposure.

Systemic Toxicity

The principal pharmacodynamic effect of peppermint oil following oral exposure is a dose-related spasmolytic effect on the smooth musculature due to the interference of menthol with the movement of calcium across cell membranes (50). Peppermint oil is relatively rapidly absorbed after oral administration and eliminated through the kidney or via the bile. The major biliary metabolite is menthol glucuronide, which undergoes enterohepatic circulation. The urinary metabolites result from hydroxylation and are excreted in part as glucuronic acid conjugates. Studies with tritiated I-menthol reported equal excretion in feces and urine (50).

In an experimental study, male rats received peppermint tea as the sole source of drinking water for 30 days (47). The dose was stated as 20 g/l, which would equal a daily dose of close to 1000 mg/kg. Minor degeneration of hepatocytes was observed (47), but there was no nephrotoxicity at this dose level (51). In a study on the subchronic (90 days of exposure) toxicity of peppermint oil in rats, histopathological changes consisting of cyst-like spaces in the white matter of cerebellum and signs of nephrotoxicity at a dose of 100 mg peppermint oil/kg were observed (52). These observations have, however, not been confirmed in published reports by other research groups.

Dermal Toxicity

In 1995, 12 cases of contact sensitivity to the flavoring agents menthol and peppermint oil in patients presenting with intraoral symptoms were reported (53). These observations are, however, contrasted by patch test screening of 73 patients from Finish dermatological clinics in which menthol and peppermint oil demonstrated no allergic or irritant reactions (54). In a more recent review on the sensitization potential of menthol, allergic contact dermatitis from peppermint oil and its principal constituent (menthol) was rated as rare (55), although casuistic reports may occur (21,56). Peppermint oil (8%) was not a sensitizer when tested using a maximization protocol (48).

Peppermint oil acts as a penetration enhancer for percutaneous penetration of 5-fluorouracil through rat skin (57). In accordance with this observation, topically applied peppermint oil was demonstrated to dose-dependently decrease the integrity of the skin (58). However, concomitant dermal exposure to low concentrations of peppermint oil reduced the percutaneous penetration of benzoic acid and tritiated water (58). The concentration where peppermint oil changes from being protective to being a penetration enhancer will probably depend on physicochemical properties of the specific penetrant.

Genotoxicity

Peppermint oil was not mutagenic in the *Salmonella*/microsomes assay (46,59). In human lymphocytes, peppermint oil was cytotoxic and induced chromosome aberrations, although only when inhibition of mitotic activity was 70% or higher (46). Peppermint oil has been classified as a "high-toxicity clastogen," which induces chromosome aberrations by a secondary mechanism associated with cytotoxicity

(60), and it has been suggested that such compounds do not react with DNA, are not genotoxic in vivo, and usually not carcinogenic (61). Earlier, however, menthone was shown to be genotoxic in *Drosophila melanogaster* (62). Peppermint oil was negative in the mouse lymphoma mutagenesis assay but gave equivocal results in a Chinese hamster fibroblast cell chromosome aberration assay (48). Peppermint oil is a mixture, and the different constituents apparently have different toxicological profiles in different in vitro test systems and in most cases only at high and cytotoxic doses. If effects on DNA occur only at these high doses in the presence of cytotoxicity, peppermint oil may be assumed to be safe at lower doses relevant to human dermal exposure, but more in vivo mammalian data are warranted.

Risk Estimate

Considering the traditional uncertainty factors applied in risk assessment and anticipating a reasonable rate of percutaneous penetration of peppermint oil, a no observed adverse effect level (NOAEL) based on the suggested changes in the cerebellum does not leave much room for the safe use of neat peppermint oil for dermal applications. The topical use of peppermint oil in rinse-off (<3% oil) as well as leave-on (<0.2% oil) formulations is, however, not considered a relevant risk for systemic toxicity. Sensitization to peppermint oil appears to be rare.

EUCALYPTUS OIL

Provenance, Composition, and Uses

Eucalyptus oil is obtained from *Eucalyptus globules*, and the dominant constituent of eucalyptus oil (75–80%) is eucalyptol, also known as 1,8-cineole. Eucalyptus oil is used as a folk remedy for various dermatological conditions. Recently, evidence has been presented that eucalyptol may show anti-inflammatory activity in asthma patients and thus may be of use as a mucolytic agent in upper and lower airway diseases (63).

Systemic Toxicity

Human intoxications following exposure to eucalyptol have been well documented. It usually occurs after oral administration of larger amounts of eucalyptus oil and includes symptoms such as nausea, vomiting, muscle weakness, ataxia, tachycardia, hypotension, and depression of respiration (64), although casuistic reports describe fatal intoxication following ingestion of as little as 5 ml (65). A single case of severe intoxication after dermal application has been described in a child suffering from urticaria who had eucalyptus oil distributed generously on the entire body. The child experienced the same symptoms as described following oral intoxications but made a full recovery within six hours (66).

The most recent review by The European Commission (67) states that eucalyptol undergoes oxidation in vivo with the formation of hydroxycineole, which is excreted as glucuronide. In rats, 2-hydroxycineole, 3-hydroxycineole, and 1,8-dihydroxycineol-9-oic acid were identified as the main urinary metabolites (68).

Hepatic microsomal enzyme activity was greatly enhanced in adult rats treated with eucalyptol both during and after pregnancy and was also increased in the fetal and newborn offspring of such rats. Administration of the oil to lactating mothers did not lead to any enzyme induction in the suckling rats. It thus appears that while eucalyptol is able to penetrate the placental barrier it is unable to cross the blood–milk barrier to any effective extent (69).

Groups of mice and rats were given up to 6000 mg eucalyptol/kg/day by gavage or in encapsulated form for 28 days. Statistically significant decreases in the terminal body weight and increased relative liver and kidney weights were found at doses above 600 mg/kg/day, whereas the relative brain weight was increased only in the highest dose groups. No macroscopic changes were seen. Only brain, liver, and kidneys were examined histopathologically, showing no changes in the brain and minor focal infiltration of mononuclear cells in the liver among all groups. In kidneys, a dose-related accumulation of eosinophilic protein droplets containing $\alpha2\mu$-globulin in the cytoplasm of proximal tubular epithelial cells was induced (67,70).

Eucalyptol was tested as a constituent of toothpaste in an oral long-term study with specific pathogen-free CFLP mice given 0, 8, and 32 mg eucalyptol/kg/day for 80 weeks followed by a observation period of 16–24 weeks. No treatment-related effects on body weight, food consumption, survival, weight of adrenals, kidneys, liver, lungs, or spleen on the microscopic appearance of brain, lungs, liver, and kidneys and on tumor incidence were observed (71).

Dermal Toxicity

Eucalyptol at a concentration of 5% enhanced the skin permeation of propranolol significantly (72), whereas a previous study demonstrated that it was a poor enhancer of the in vitro percutaneous absorption of diclofenac sodium (73). Eucalyptol was suggested to reduce the intensity of lipid-based reflections, which may be linked to a disruption of lipid packing within the bilayers and/or to a disturbance in the stacking of the bilayers (74). In vitro, eucalyptol was not detected in the receptor fluid following four-hour exposure of the human skin, but a significant temporary deposition was seen in the stratum corneum (75). These in vitro data indicate that the dermal absorption of eucalyptol is probably limited but that effects on the barrier integrity in the upper skin layers are possible.

Skin irritancy following occlusive patch testing was not detected in two studies on humans exposed to pure eucalyptol in concentrations ranging from 4% to 28% in soft paraffin (10,12). Among a group of humans without prior allergic reactions to cosmetic products, none gave a positive response when tested with up to 29% eucalyptol in a TTO mixture with terpinen-4-ol in the occlusive patch test (daily readings and replacement for 21 days) (10) nor could its sensitizing capacity be shown experimentally in guinea pigs exposed to 5% eucalyptol (27).

Genotoxicity

Eucalyptol was not mutagenic when evaluated by the *Salmonella*/microsome assay with and without addition of an extrinsic metabolic activation system (36,76). Eucalyptol, at concentrations ranging from 10 to 1000 μM, did not increase the frequency of spontaneous sister–chromatid exchanges in Chinese hamster ovary cells (43). Eucalyptol did not induce primary lung tumors in mice following 24 ip injections during an eight-week period with 24 weeks follow-up. The doses used were either maximal tolerated dose (MTD) or 20% of MTD (77).

Risk Estimate

The expected concentrations of eucalyptol in cosmetic products are 0.4% in soaps, 0.04% in detergents, 0.5% in creams and lotions, and 1.6% in perfume. Currently, eucalyptol is regarded as generally recognized as safe by Flavoring Extract Manufacturer's Association (1965) and is approved by the U.S. Food and Drug Administration (FDA) for food use. The FDA advisory review panel on over-the-counter drugs has concluded that eucalyptol is safe for a variety of products, such as lozenges taken every 0.5–1 h at 0.2–15 mg or taken every two hours at 1–30 mg of eucalyptol (FDA, 1976–1990). Neither animal nor human evidence indicates that eucalyptol is an irritant. Available information from animal and human exposure indicates that pure eucalyptol is not a sensitizer. Eucalyptol is not mutagenic in Ames test, but it is possibly a weak promoter but not carcinogenic in mice tested at MTD. Based on the studies on hepatic and renal toxicity, a NOAEL might be estimated as 300 mg/kg. Dermal exposure to eucalyptol following use of cosmetic products is not expected to cause systemic toxicity. However, the casuistic reports on severe toxicity following oral exposure warrant considerations as to the use of products with higher concentrations of eucalyptol.

LAVENDER OIL
Provenance, Composition, and Uses
The major botanical source of lavender oil is *Lavandula angustifolia* Miller (syn *L. officinalis* Chaix) (Lamiaceae). The oil is obtained by steam distillation of the fresh flowering tops. The components linalyl acetate and linalool constitute approximately 70–80% of the oil, with the remainder comprised of components such as terpinen-4-ol, 1,8-cineole, caryophyllene, myrcene, and α-terpineol (30,78,79). English and French lavender oils are derived from *L. angustifolia*, with the country name denoting the country of origin. However, *Lavandula dentata* has also been cited as a source of French lavender oil. Additional lavender oils are obtained from species, such as Spanish lavender from *L. stoechas* and spike lavender from *L. latifolia*. The major uses of lavender oil are as a fragrance, in perfumery, and, to a lesser extent, in aromatherapy. This would therefore include both leave-on and rinse-off products.

Lavender oil has shown antimicrobial (80) and antiallergic activity (81) in laboratory and animal studies, respectively, but clinical data are lacking. In contrast, the sedative and mood-altering properties of lavender oil have been the focus of a number of clinical studies. Lavender oil odor has been shown to induce transient mood changes such as relaxation, improved mood, and reduced anxiety (82–84). However, a contradictory study found no effect on anxiety in patients undergoing radiotherapy (85). Lavender oil has been postulated to act as a mild sedative on the basis of a study showing that lavender odor promoted deep sleep in young adults (86). Lavender oil odor has also been shown to affect cognitive function by impairing both working memory and reaction time (87).

Systemic Toxicity
The acute oral and dermal LD_{50} values for lavender oil in rats are in excess of 5000 mg/kg (88), indicating very low acute toxicity. Oral administration of coriander oil containing 72.9% linalool to rats for 28 days resulted in changes to the kidney and liver, including increased organ weight. From this same study, a NOAEL of 160 mg/kg for coriander oil was determined, equivalent to 117 mg/kg/day linalool. Rats administered linalool orally also had transiently elevated levels of hepatic cytochrome P-450 enzymes (68).

Administered orally, linalyl acetate is quickly metabolized in the stomach to linalool and acetic acid. The linalool then rapidly changes into α-terpineol (89). Linalool is presumed to be metabolized similarly to other tertiary alcohols by conjugation with glucuronic acid followed by urinary excretion and to a lesser extent elimination through air and feces (89). After administration of linalool, the metabolites 8-hydroxy-linalool and 8-carboxy-linalool were found in urine (68).

Dermal Toxicity

Following dermal exposure (1.5 g of oil massaged into an area of skin), both linalool and linalyl acetate were detected in the blood after five minutes, peaked after about 20 minutes, but decreased to virtually undetectable levels by 90 minutes (90). Equivalent to several other essential oils, lavender oil (91), and linalool (92,93) were both shown to enhance the penetration of compounds through skin.

Neat lavender oil is nonirritating when applied to the backs of hairless mice and swine, but it is slightly irritating when applied neat to intact or abraded rabbit skin under occlusion for 24 hours (88). Sixteen percent of lavender oil in petrolatum in closed patch tests for 48 hours with human volunteers did not produce any irritant reactions (88). Similarly, no reactions were seen when 16% of lavender oil was tested in human volunteers using a maximization test to investigate sensitization (88). Occlusive patch tests with 33% linalyl acetate applied to the backs of male volunteers for 48 hours did not show irritancy (94). Oxidation plays a very important role in sensitization as nonoxidized linalool did not show any sensitizing potential in the local lymph node assay whereas air-exposed linalool did (95). This means that studies where the oxidation status of the oil or component is not known may overestimate irritancy.

Individual cases of contact allergy to lavender oil have been reported (96–99). A large study investigated lavender oil allergy in 1483 patients with suspected cosmetic contact dermatitis using a two-day closed patch test with 20% lavender oil. The overall positivity rate was 4% over the period of 1990 to 1998, with rates for individual years ranging from 0% in 1994 to 14% in 1998. The rapid rise in positive reactions was attributed to the increased use of lavender oil in aromatherapy (100).

Genotoxicity

Lavender oil was not mutagenic using the bacterial reverse mutation assay with *Salmonella* (30). A recent review of the available data for linalool and linalyl acetate, generated in both bacterial and mammalian test systems, concluded that these compounds have negligible genotoxic potential (89).

Risk Estimate

The expected maximum concentrations of lavender oil in products are 1.2% in perfume and 0.3% in soap (88). Dermal systemic exposure to lavender oil components in cosmetic products has been calculated as 0.3 mg/kg/day for both linalool and linalyl acetate (89). Using the estimation that each component represents 50% of whole oil, this gives an estimated dermal systemic exposure of approximately 0.6 mg/kg/day, which is well below the NOAEL of 50 mg/kg/day based on available toxicological data for linalool and some of its related esters (89). As such, systemic toxicity due to topical lavender oil application is highly unlikely.

CHAMOMILE OIL
Provenance, Composition, and Uses
The term chamomile essential oil generally refers to one of two compositionally distinct oils derived from *Chamaemelum nobile* or *Matricaria recutita* L. (both Compositae, syn. Asteraceae), commonly known as Roman and German chamomile, respectively.

German chamomile oil is produced by steam distillation or solvent extraction of the flower heads of *Matricaria recutita* (101,102), synonyms of which include *Matricaria chamomilla* or *Chamomilla recutita* (103). The essential oil contains up to 60% (-)-α-bisabolol, an unsaturated monocyclic sesquiterpene alcohol, and α-bisabololoxides A and B (101,104,105).

Chamomile oil is used in foodstuffs, cosmetics, toiletries (106), and over-the-counter medicaments chiefly for its flavoring, aromatic, anti-inflammatory, and sedative properties. The range of products available results in exposure by topical and oral routes.

Dermal Toxicity
In keeping with its place in the Compositae (Asteraceae) family, individuals with known Compositae sensitivity must be particularly wary of products containing chamomile extracts (107). Numerous incidents of irritancy and allergy to chamomile extracts have been reported, although the provenance and composition of the extracts and the components responsible are not always clear (108). Contact reactions or positive patch tests to chamomile extracts (21, 108–116) or their components (21,117,118) appear to be the most frequently reported adverse reaction, although anaphylaxis after the consumption of chamomile tea has also been reported (119). Although the exact components responsible remain unknown in most cases, the sesquiterpene lactones present in chamomile extracts are the suspected culprits (102,109).

Systemic Toxicity and Genotoxicity
Systemic toxicity due to nonsensitizing mechanisms or genotoxicity following exposure to chamomile oils has not been described in the literature.

REFERENCES

1. Carson CF, Hammer KA, Riley TV. *Melaleuca alternifolia* (tea tree) oil: a review of antimicrobial and other properties. Clin Microbiol Rev 2006; 19:50–62.
2. International Organisation for Standardisation. ISO 4730:2004, Oil of *Melaleuca*, terpinen-4-ol type (tea tree oil). Geneva, Switzerland: International Organisation for Standardisation; 2004.
3. Brophy JJ, Davies NW, Southwell IA, et al. Gas chromatographic quality control for oil of *Melaleuca* terpinen-4-ol type (Australian tea tree). J Agric Food Chem 1989; 37:1330–1335.
4. Russell M. Toxicology of tea tree oil. In: Southwell I, Lowe R, eds. Tea Tree: The Genus *Melaleuca*. Amsterdam:Harwood Academic Publishers, 1999:191–201.
5. Kim D, Cerven DR, Craig S, et al. American Chemical Society National Meeting, Orlando, Fla, USA, April 7, 2002. p114-MEDI Part 112.
6. Hammer KA, Carson CF, Riley TV, et al. A review of the toxicity of *Melaleuca alternifolia* (tea tree) oil. Food Chem Toxicol 2006; 44:616–625.
7. Watson WA, Litovitz TL, Klein-Schwartz W, et al. 2003 Annual report of the American Association of Poison Control Centers toxic exposure surveillance system. Am J Emerg Med 2004; 22:335–404.
8. Seawright A. Tea tree oil poisoning—Comment. Med J Aust 1993; 159:831.

9. Draize JH. Procedures for the appraisal of the toxicity of chemicals in foods, drugs and cosmetics: VIII. Dermal toxicity. Food Drug Cosmet Law J 1955; 10:722–731.
10. Southwell IA, Freeman S, Rubel D. Skin irritancy of tea tree oil. J Essential Oil Res 1997; 9:47–52.
11. Aspres N, Freeman S. Predictive testing for irritancy and allergenicity of tea tree oil in normal human subjects. Exogenous Dermatol 2003; 2:258-261.
12. Knight TE, Hausen BM. Melaleuca oil (tea tree oil) dermatitis. J Am Acad Dermatol 1994; 30:423–427.
13. Veien NK, Rosner K, Skovgaard G. Is tea tree oil an important contact allergen? Contact Dermatitis 2004; 50:378–379.
14. Hensyl WR. Stedman's Medical Dictionary. 25th ed. Baltimore: Williams and Wilkins, 1990.
15. Apted JH. Contact dermatitis associated with the use of tea-tree oil [letter]. Australas J Dermatol 1991; 32:177.
16. de Groot AC, Weyland JW. Systemic contact dermatitis from tea tree oil. Contact Dermatitis 1992; 27:279–280.
17. van der Valk PG, de Groot AC, Bruynzeel DP, et al. Allergic contact eczema due to 'tea tree' oil. Ned Tijdschr Geneeskd 1994; 138:823–825.
18. Selvaag E, Eriksen B, Thune P. Contact allergy due to tea tree oil and cross-sensitization to colophony. Contact Dermatitis 1994; 31:124–125.
19. de Groot AC. Airborne allergic contact dermatitis from tea tree oil. Contact Dermatitis 1996; 35:304–305.
20. Bhushan M, Beck MH. Allergic contact dermatitis from tea tree oil in a wart paint. Contact Dermatitis 1997; 36:117–118.
21. Lisi P, Meligeni L, Pigatto P, et al. The prevalence of sensitivity to *Melaleuca* essential oil. Ann Ital Dermatol Clin e Sper 2000; 54:141–144.
22. Coutts I, Shaw S, D. O. Patch testing with pure tea tree oil—12 months experience. Br J Dermatol 2002; 147(Suppl. 62):70.
23. Belsito DV, Fowler Jr. JF, Sasseville D, et al. Delayed-type hypersensitivity to fragrance materials in a select North American population. Dermatitis 2006; 17:23–28.
24. Rutherford T, Nixon R, Tam M, et al. 39th Annual Scientific Meeting of the Australasian Society of Dermatology, Melbourne, Victoria, 2006:A21.
25. Pirker C, Richter HG, Kinaciyan T, et al. Increase of sensitization to tea tree oil. Contact Dermatitis 2000; 42(suppl):59–60.
26. Hausen BM, Reichling J, Harkenthal M. Degradation products of monoterpenes are the sensitizing agents in tea tree oil. Am J Contact Dermatitis 1999; 10:68–77.
27. Hausen BM. Evaluation of the main contact allergens in oxidized tea tree oil. Dermatitis 2004; 15:213–214.
28. Zhang SY, Robertson D. A study of tea tree oil ototoxicity. Audiol Neurootol 2000; 5:64–68.
29. Araujo IB, Souza CA, De-Carvalho RR, et al. Study of the embryofoeto-toxicity of alpha-terpinene in the rat. Food Chem Toxicol 1996; 34:477–482.
30. Evandri MG, Battinelli L, Daniele C, et al. The antimutagenic activity of *Lavandula angustifolia* (lavender) essential oil in the bacterial reverse mutation assay. Food Chem Toxicol 2005; 43:1381–1387.
31. Fletcher JP, Cassella JP, Hughes D, et al. An evaluation of the mutagenic potential of commercially available tea tree oil in the United Kingdom. Int J Aromather 2005; 15:81–86.
32. Fletcher JP, Cassella JP, Hughes D, et al. An evaluation of the mutagenic potential of commercially available tea tree oil in the United Kingdom. Int J Aromather 2005; 15:81–86.
33. Gomes-Carneiro MR, Viana MES, Felzenszwalb I, et al. Evaluation of β-myrcene, α-terpinene and (+)- and (-)-α-pinene in the *Salmonella*/microsome assay. Food Chem Toxicol 2005; 43:247–252.
34. Oda Y, Hamano Y, Inoue K, et al. Mutagenicity of food flavors in bacteria. Shokuhin Eisei Hen 1978; 9:177–181.
35. Yoo YS. Mutagenic and antimutagenic activities of flavoring agents used in foodstuffs. J Osaka City Med Center 1985; 34:267–288.

36. Gomes-Carneiro MR, Felzenszwalb I, Paumgartten FJR. Mutagenicity testing of (±)-camphor, 1,8-cineole, citral, citronellal, (−)-menthol and terpineol with the *Salmonella*/microsome assay. Mutat Res 1998; 416:129–136.
37. Florin I, Rutberg L, Curvall M, et al. Screening of tobacoo smoke constituents for mutagenicity using the Ames test. Toxicology 1980; 15:219–232.
38. Rockwell P, Raw I. A mutagenic screening of various herbs, spices, and food additives. Nutr Cancer 1979; 1:10–15.
39. Watabe T, Hiratsuka A, Ozawa N, et al. A comparative study on the metabolism of d-limonene and 4-vinylcyclohex-1-ene by hepatic microsomes. Xenobiotica 1981; 11:333–344.
40. Connor TH, Theiss JC, Hanna HA, et al. Genotoxicity of organic chemicals frequently found in the air of mobile homes. Toxicol Lett. 1985; 25(1):33–40.
41. Ishidate MJ, Sofuni T, Yoshikawa K, et al. Primary mutagenicity screening of food additives currently used in Japan. Food Chem Toxicol 1984; 22:623–636.
42. Aydin S, Basaran N, Basaran AA. The effects of thyme volatiles on the induction of DNA damage by the heterocyclic amine IQ and mitomycin C. Mutat Res 2005; 581:43–53.
43. Sasaki YF, Imanishi H. Modifying effects of components of plant essence on the induction of sister-chromatid exchanges in cultured Chinese hamster ovary cells. Mutat Res 1989; 226:103–110.
44. Kauderer B, Zamith H, Paumgartten FJR, et al. Evaluation of the mutagenicity of beta-myrcene in mammalian cells in vitro. Environ Mol Mutag 1991; 18:28–34.
45. Zamith HP, Vidal MN, Speit G, et al. Absence of genotoxic activity of beta-myrcene in the in vivo cytogenetic bone marrow assay. Braz J Med Biol Res 1993; 26:93–98.
46. Lazutka JR, Mierauskiene J, Slapsyte G, et al. Genotoxicity of dill (*Anethum graveolens* L.), peppermint (*Mentha piperita* L.) and pine (*Pinus sylvestris* L.) essential oils in human lymphocytes and *Drosophila melanogaster*. Food Chem Toxicol 2001; 39:485–492.
47. Akdogan M, Ozguner M, Aydin G, et al. Investigation of biochemical and histopathological effects of *Mentha piperita* Labiatae and *Mentha spicata* Labiatae on liver tissue in rats. Hum Exp Toxicol 2004; 23:21–28.
48. Nair B. Final report on the safety assessment of *Mentha piperita* (peppermint) oil, *Mentha piperita* (peppermint) leaf extract, *Mentha piperita* (peppermint) leaf, and *Mentha piperita* (peppermint) leaf water. Int J Toxicol 2001; 20(Suppl 3):61–73.
49. Schuhmacher A, Reichling J, Schnitzler P. Virucidal effect of peppermint oil on the enveloped viruses herpes simplex virus type 1 and type 2 in vitro. Phytomedicine 2003; 10:504–510.
50. Grigoleit HG, Grigoleit P. Pharmacology and preclinical pharmacokinetics of peppermint oil. Phytomedicine 2005; 12:612–616.
51. Akdogan M, Kilinc I, Oncu M, et al. Investigation of biochemical and histopathological effects of *Mentha piperita* L. and *Mentha spicata* L. on kidney tissue in rats. Hum Exp Toxicol 2003; 22:213–219.
52. Spindler P, Madsen C. Subchronic toxicity study of peppermint oil in rats. Toxicol Lett 1986; 32:147–152.
53. Morton CA, Garioch J, Todd P, et al. Contact sensitivity to menthol and peppermint in patients with intra-oral symptoms. Contact Dermatitis 1995; 32:281–284.
54. Kanerva L, Rantanen T, Aalto-Korte K, et al. A multicenter study of patch test reactions with dental screening series. Am J Contact Dermatitis 2001; 12:83–87.
55. Dharmagunawardena B, Takwale A, Sanders KJ, et al. Gas chromatography: an investigative tool in multiple allergies to essential oils. Contact Dermatitis 2002; 47:288–292.
56. Wilkinson S, Beck, MH. Allergic contact dermatitis from menthol in peppermint. Contact Dermatitis 1994; 30:42–43.
57. Abdullah D, Ping, QN, Liu, GJ. Enhancing effect of essential oils on the penetration of 5-fluorouracil through rat skin. Yao Xue Xue Bao 1996; 31:214–221.
58. Nielsen JB, Nielsen F. Topical use of tea-tree oil reduces the dermal absorption of benzoic acid and methiocarb. Arch Dermatol Res 2006; 297:395–402.
59. Andersen P, Jensen NJ. Mutagenic investigation of peppermint oil in the Salmonella/mamalian-microsome test. Mutat Res 1984; 138:1720.
60. Kirkland D. Chromosome aberration testing in genetic toxicology—past, present and future. Mutat Res 1998; 404:173–185.

61. Galloway SM. Cytotoxicity and chromosome aberrations in vitro: experience in industry and the case for an upperlimit on toxicity in the aberration assay. Environ Mol Mutagen 2000; 35:191–201.
62. Karpouhtsis I, Pardali E, Feggou E, et al. Insecticidal and genotoxic activities of oregano essential oils. J Agric Food Chem 1998; 46:1111–1115.
63. Juergens UR, Dethlefsen U, Steinkamp G, et al. Anti-inflammatory activity of 1,8-cineol (eucalyptol) in bronchial asthma: a double-blind placebo-controlled trial. Respir Med 2003; 97:250–256.
64. Ernst E. Adverse effects of herbal drugs in dermatology. Br J Dermatol 2000; 143:923–929.
65. De Vincenzi M, Silano M, De Vincenzi A, et al. Constituents of aromatic plants: eucalyptol. Fitoterapia 2002; 73:269–275.
66. Darben T, Cominos B, Lee CT. Topical eucalyptus oil poisoning. Aust J Dermatol 1998; 39:265–267.
67. European Commission. Opinion of the scientific committee on food on eucalyptol. Brussels; 2002 17 April 2002. Report No.: SCF/CS/FLAV/flavour/20 Add2 Final.
68. Chadha A, Madyastha KM. Metabolism of geraniol and linalool in the rat and effects on liver and lung microsomal enzymes. Xenobiotica 1984; 14:365–374.
69. Jori A, Briatico G. Effect of eucalyptol on microsomal enzyme activity of foetal and newborn rats. Biochem Pharmacol 1973; 22:543–544.
70. Kristiansen E, Madsen C. Induction of protein droplet (alpha 2m-globulin) nephropathy in male rats after short-term dosage with 1,8-cineole and L-limonene. Toxicol Lett 1995; 80:147–152.
71. Roe FJ, Palmer AK, Worden AN, et al. Safety evaluation of toothpaste containing chloroform. I. Long-term studies in mice. J Environ Pathol Toxicol 1979; 2:799–819.
72. Amnuaikit C, Ikeuchi I, Ogawara K, et al. Skin permeation of propranolol from polymeric film containing terpene enhancers for transdermal use. Int J Pharm 2005; 289:167–178.
73. Arellano A, Santoyo S, Martin C, et al. Enhancing effect of terpenes on the in vitro percutaneous absorption of diclofenac sodium. Int J Pharm 1996; 130:141–145.
74. Cornwell PA, Barry BW, Bouwstra JA, et al. Modes of action of terpene penetration enhancers in human skin; differential scanning calorimetry, small-angle X-ray diffraction and enhancer uptake studies. Int J Pharm 1996; 127:9–26.
75. Cal K, Kupiec, K, Sznitowska, M. Effect of physicochemical properties of cyclic terpenes on their ex vivo skin absorption and elimination kinetics. J Dermatol Sci 2006; 41:137–142.
76. Haworth S, Lawlor T. *Salmonella* mutagenicity test results for 250 chemicals. Environ Mutagen 1983; 5(Suppl 1):1–142.
77. Stoner GD, Shimkin MB, Kniazeff AJ, et al. Test for carcinogenicity of food additives and chemotherapeutic agents by the pulmonary tumor response in strain A mice. Cancer Res 1973; 33:3069–3085.
78. Daferera DJ, Ziogas BN, Polissiou MG. GC-MS analysis of essential oils from some Greek aromatic plants and their fungitoxicity on *Penicillium digitatum*. J Agric Food Chem 2000; 48:2576–2581.
79. Shellie R, Mondello L, Marriott P, et al. Characterisation of lavender essential oils by using gas chromatography-mass spectrometry with correlation of linear retention indices and comparison with comprehensive two-dimensional gas chromatography. J Chromatogr A 2002; 970:225–234.
80. Hammer KA, Carson CF, Riley TV. Antimicrobial activity of essential oils and other plant extracts. J Appl Microbiol 1999; 86:985–990.
81. Kim HM, Cho SH. Lavender oil inhibits immediate-type allergic reaction in mice and rats. J Pharm Pharmacol 1999; 51:221–226.
82. Dieterle WE, Wetzel U. Olfactory stimulated change in state of mood and heart rate: effects of essential peppermint and lavender oil. J Psychophysiol 2004; 18:219–220.
83. Lehrner J, Marwinski G, Lehr S, et al. Ambient odors of orange and lavender reduce anxiety and improve mood in a dental office. Physiol Behav 2005; 86:92–95.
84. Itai T, Amayasu H, Kuribayashi M, et al. Psychological effects of aromatherapy on chronic hemodialysis patients. Psychiatry Clin Neurosci 2000; 54:393–397.

85. Graham PH, Browne L, Cox H, et al. Inhalation aromatherapy during radiotherapy: results of a placebo-controlled double-blind randomized trial. J Clin Oncol 2003;21: 2372–2376.
86. Goel N, Kim H, Lao RP. An olfactory stimulus modifies nighttime sleep in young men and women. Chronobiol Int 2005; 22:889–904.
87. Moss M, Cook J, Wesnes K, et al. Aromas of rosemary and lavender essential oils differentially affect cognition and mood in healthy adults. Int J Neurosci 2003; 113:15–38.
88. Opdyke DL. Lavender oil. Food Chem Toxicol 1976; 14:451.
89. Bickers D, Calow P, Greim H, et al. A toxicologic and dermatologic assessment of linalool and related esters when used as fragrance ingredients. Food Chem Toxicol 2003; 41:919–942.
90. Jäger W, Buchbauer G, Jirovetz L, et al. Percutaneous-absorption of lavender oil from a massage oil. J Soc Cosmet Chem 1992; 43:49–54.
91. Thacharodi D, Rao KP. Transdermal absorption of nifedipine from microemulsions of lipophilic skin penetration enhancers. Int J Pharm 1994; 111:235–240.
92. Vaddi HK, Ho PC, Chan YW, et al. Terpenes in ethanol: haloperidol permeation and partition through human skin and stratum corneum changes. J Control Release 2002; 81:121–133.
93. Kunta JR, Goskonda VR, Brotherton HO, et al. Effect of menthol and related terpenes on the percutaneous absorption of propranolol across excised hairless mouse skin. J Pharm Sci 1997; 86:1369–1373.
94. Motoyoshi K, Toyoshima Y, Sato M, et al. Comparative studies on the irritancy of oils and synthetic perfumes to the skin of rabbit, guinea pig, rat, miniature swine and man. Cosmet Toiletries 1979; 94:41–48.
95. Sköld M, Borje A, Harambasic E, et al. Contact allergens formed on air exposure of linalool. Identification and quantification of primary and secondary oxidation products and the effect on skin sensitization. Chem Res Toxicol 2005; 17:1697–1705.
96. Brandao FM. Occupational allergy to lavender oil. Contact Dermatitis 1986; 15:249–250.
97. Maddocks-Jennings W. Critical incident: idiosyncratic allergic reactions to essential oils. Complement Ther Nurs Midwifery 2004; 10:58–60.
98. Coulson IH, Khan ASA. Facial 'pillow' dermatitis due to lavender oil allergy. Contact Dermatitis 1999; 41:111.
99. Rademaker M. Allergic contact-dermatitis from lavender fragrance in Difflam(R) gel. Contact Dermatitis 1994; 31:58–59.
100. Sugiura M, Hayakawa R, Kato Y, et al. Results of patch testing with lavender oil in Japan. Contact Dermatitis 2000; 43:157–160.
101. Mann C, Staba EJ. The chemistry, pharmacology, and commercial formulations of chamomile. In: Craker LE, Simon JE, eds. Herbs, Spices, and Medicinal Plants: Recent Advances in Botany, Horticulture, and Pharmacology. Phoenix: Oryx Press, 1986:235–280.
102. Balazs T. Research reports. Int J Aromather 2000; 10:68–71.
103. Applequist WL. A reassessment of the nomenclature of *Matricaria* L. and *Tripleurospermum* Sch. Bip. (*Asteraceae*). Taxon 2002; 51:757–761.
104. Isaacs J. Essential oils have a fragrant history. American Druggist, 1998; 215:46–48.
105. Tully JG, Rose DL, McCoy RE, et al. *Mycoplasma melaleucae* sp. nov., a sterol-requiring mollicute from flowers of several tropical plants. Int J Syst Bacteriol 1990; 40:143–147.
106. Cusack C, Buckley C. Compositae dermatitis in a herbal medicine enthusiast. Contact Dermatitis 2005; 53:120–121.
107. Paulsen E, Andersen KE. Colophonium and Compositae mix as markers of fragrance allergy: Cross-reactivity between fragrance terpenes, colophonium and Compositae plant extracts. Contact Dermatitis 2005; 53:285–291.
108. McGeorge BCL, Steele MC. Allergic contact dermatitis of the nipple from Roman chamomile ointment. Contact Dermatitis 1991; 24:139–140.
109. Pereira F, Santos R, Pereira A. Contact dermatitis from chamomile tea. Contact Dermatitis 1997;36:307.
110. Rodríguez-Serna M, Sánchez-Motilla JM, Ramón R, et al. Allergic and systemic contact dermatitis from *Matricaria chamomilla* tea. Contact Dermatitis 1998; 39:192–193.
111. Rycroft M. Recurrent facial dermatitis from chamomile tea. Contact Dermatitis 2003; 48:229.

112. Beetz VD, Cramer HJ, Mehlhorn HC. Zur Häufigkeit der epidermalen Allergie gegenüber Kamille in kamillenhaltigen Arzneimitteln und Kosmetika. Dermatol Monatsschr 1971; 157:505–510.
113. Bruynzeel DP, van Ketel WG, Young E, et al. Contact sensitization by alternative topical medicaments containing plant extracts. Contact Dermatitis 1992; 27:278–279.
114. García-Bravo B, Bernal AP, García-Hernández MJ, et al. Occupational contact dermatitis from anethole in food handlers. Contact Dermatitis 1997; 37:38.
115. Rudzki E, Grzywa Z, Bruo WS. Sensitivity to 35 essential oils. Contact Dermatitis 1976; 2:196–200.
116. Selvaag E, Holm J-O, Thune P. Allergic contact dermatitis in an aroma therapist with multiple sensitizations to essential oils. Contact Dermatitis 1995; 33:354–355.
117. Balato N, Lembo G, Nappa P, et al. Allergic chelitis to azulene. Contact Dermatitis 1985; 13:39–40.
118. Wilkinson SM, Hausen BM, Beck MH. Allergic contact dermatitis from plant extracts in a cosmetic. Contact Dermatitis 1995; 33:58–59.
119. McKay DL, Blumberg JB. A review of the bioactivity and potential health benefits of chamomile tea (*Matricaria recutita* L.) Phytother Res 2006; 20:519–530.

Safety Assessments Based on Exposure, Skin Permeation, and Toxicity Considerations

William E. Dressler
Shelton, Connecticut, U.S.A.

Kenneth A. Walters
An-eX Analytical Services Ltd., Cardiff, U.K.

INTRODUCTION

Safety assessments for cosmetics and cosmeceutical products need to integrate information on the external exposure permeants of the skin surface with relevant data on percutaneous absorption in order to estimate their systemic availability and/or their penetration into skin compartments (see Chapter 1). The systemic availability under conditions of use can then be related to no-adverse-effect levels (NOAELs) determined from preclinical toxicology evaluations in order to estimate a margin of safety (MOS).

Percutaneous absorption is influenced by a variety of factors including: the physicochemical characteristics of the permeating molecule, the concentration of the permeating molecule in the vehicle or matrix in which it is applied, the nature of the application vehicle, the amount applied and the method of application, the site of application and area of contact, the condition of the skin (e.g., normal, compromised) as well as external factors such as temperature, humidity and UV exposure. Mathematical modeling and the use of quantitative structure permeation relationships can provide estimates of the rate of diffusion of molecules across the skin (1) and generate predictions of the maximum rate of flux of a given compound (2). Such predictive tools can play an important role in the early stages of research and development but they are of little use in rational risk assessment and the generation of margins of safety because they take no account of exposure during normal product usage (3).

EXPOSURE CONSIDERATIONS

Exposure conditions can vary considerably and are often nonquantifiable. For example, in occupational settings an agricultural worker may be exposed to concentrated liquid pesticide while preparing a dilution for application; a painter may be exposed to a variety of solvents on a regular basis. Several studies have been conducted in attempts to improve quantification of dermal exposure. For example, Api et al. (4) attempted to measure the dermal hand transfer of three fragrance materials (cinnamic aldehyde, D-limonene, and eugenol) from scented candles. The candles were uniformly handled and the fragrance materials from each hand were recovered using isopropyl alcohol wipes. The residue/transfer from the candles to the hands was below the limit of detection for d-limonene and very low for the other two fragrances (0.26 µg/cm^2 for cinnamic aldehyde and 0.28 µg/cm^2 for eugenol). Others have attempted to establish default values for hand exposure (5) and used tape-stripping techniques to quantify dermal exposures to dusts and powders (6,7).

A European dermal exposure study aimed at improving the understanding of the nature and range of dermal exposures to hazardous substances collected exposure measurements to determine whether a predictive model could be developed for regulatory risk assessment purposes (8). There was a high level of variability observed in the results within each work task (mixing, spraying, and wiping) but the majority of dermal exposure was to the hands. It was suggested that dermal exposure was partly dependent on human behavior and on the occurrence of accidental contact with contaminated surfaces. The authors concluded that interpretation of the results for predictive risk assessment purposes was difficult.

Although the majority of occupational dermal exposure is via the hands, the usual advice to wear gloves is often ignored. Work by Cherrie et al. (9), who used a conceptual model of dermal exposure to analyze how the skin may become exposed while wearing gloves, proposed a glove workplace protection factor that was based on the ratio of the estimated uptake of chemicals through the hands without gloves to the uptake through the hands while wearing protective gloves. Their mathematical simulations demonstrated that the glove protection factor was unlikely to be constant for a given glove type and was strongly influenced by the work situation and the duration of the exposure. This has important consequences for the selection of protective gloves. However, gloves that provide adequate protection are usually too expensive to be considered disposable and are often reused. Without effective decontamination, this may result in secondary exposure and injury but decontamination may alter the physical and/or chemical properties of the glove material, which may subsequently cause variations in breakthrough time and steady-state permeation rate. To evaluate this, Gao et al. (10) used neoprene, butyl rubber, and nitrile synthetic rubber glove materials and challenged the material with toluene and acetone. Permeation was measured in a closed loop system and, following the permeation tests, the materials were thermally decontaminated. After each exposure and decontamination cycle, breakthrough time and steady-state permeation rate were measured for up to 10 cycles. It was concluded that, except for the butyl/toluene combination, thermal decontamination was an effective method in removing the solvents from the matrix of selected glove materials, and it was suggested that multiple reuses of some protective gloves could be considered safe if effective decontamination methods were used and the glove materials did not have significant degradation. However, although this may be the case for some selected gloves and solvent materials, it did not consider protection against less volatile chemicals that may accumulate in protective gloves on re-use. The uncertain exposure levels associated with the use of personal protective equipment has an adverse effect on the calculation of margins of safety following dermal exposure.

On the other hand, cosmetics and personal care products are applied at reasonably well-defined amounts to specific areas of the skin for known periods of time without the use of protective materials and thus allow more reliable predictions of margins of safety. For the purpose of exposure assessments for cosmetic ingredients, there is historical precedence for the use of default assumptions for estimating the amount and frequency of product usage. Examples of such assumptions for a variety of product types are given in Table 1, which shows estimates of the skin surface areas exposed by the use of a variety of product types as given by the U.S. Environmental Protection Agency (EPA) (11) and the Dutch authority, RIVM (RijksInstituut voor Volksgezondheld & Milieu) (12). The skin areas exposed are a function of both the product type and the mode of application. For example, hair dyes, bleaches, and permanent solutions are typically applied to the scalp with gloved hands. In contrast shampoo use would expose the whole hand surface whereas a styling gel/conditioner would mostly contact the palmar surface. The estimates published by the two groups are notably similar and, in some cases, identical. Only the RIVM provided estimates of exposure for eye area, nail, deodorant, and toilet water/perfume exposures. These estimates of the exposed skin surface areas together with estimates or measurements of the usual amounts applied (Table 2) can be used to calculate realistic application rates (gm of product applied/cm^2 of skin surface) for percutaneous absorption studies.

Table 2 compiles historical default values for single application rates (13) as well as daily exposures estimated by COLIPA, The European Cosmetic Toiletry and Perfumery Association. These are shown together with data from more recent studies conducted in the United States by the Cosmetics, Toiletries and Fragrance Association (CTFA) [(15) and L. Loretz, "Exposure Data for Cosmetic Products; Facial Cleanser, Hair Conditioner, and Eye Shadow," (personal communication)]

TABLE 1 Body Regions and Skin Surface Areas Exposed to Cosmetics and Personal Care Products

| Exposed regions | Skin surface area (cm^2) | | Products |
	RIVM 2005	EPA 1997	
Scalp (1/2 head)	580	590	Hair dyes
			Hair permanent lotion
			Hair bleach
Face (1/4 head male)	305	325	Shave cream
			After shave
Face (1/2 head female)	565	555	Face cream
			Facial make-up
			Facial cleanser
			Skin whitening cream
			Hair Spray
			Face pack
			Peeling/scrubbing gel
Hands	860	840	Hand wash (liquid/solid)
Feet	1170	1120	Foot antiperspirant
			Foot antifungal
Legs	5530	5460	Depilatory
Hands and scalp	1440	1430	Shampoo
			Hair conditioner
Hands (1/2) and scalp	1010	1010	Hair styling gel/mousse
Body (less head)	16340	NA	Bath oil/foam/salt
Body (less head-female)	15670	NA	Body lotion
			Body Pack
Body (total)	17500	19400	Sunscreen lotion/cream
			Showering soap
Eye Area	50	NA	Eye makeup remover
	24	NA	Eye shadow
	3.2	NA	Eyeliner
	1.6	NA	Mascara
Nails	11	NA	Nail polish remover
	4	NA	Nail polish
Underarm	100	NA	Deodorant stick/roller/spray
Unspecified	200	NA	Eau de toilette spray
	100	NA	Perfume spray

Abbreviations: RIVM, RijksInstituut voor Volksgezondheld & Milieu; EPA, Environmental Protection Agency.
Sources: From Refs. 11 and 12.

and in Europe by CREMe (Central Risk and Exposure Modeling e-solution) (16). For the more detailed CTFA data, mean use amounts per application, frequency of application, and corresponding daily product exposures are shown in **bold.** When typical product use frequency is considered, there is reasonable agreement between the ECETOC (European Centre for Ecotoxicology and Toxicology of Chemical) and COLIPA default values for application/exposure rates. Similarly, in most instances there is reasonable agreement between experimentally measured values from independent studies conducted in the US and Europe. In turn, these measured values are typically in accord with the historical default figures. For solid antiperspirants, measured values appeared to be about twofold higher in Europe as compared with the United States and were higher than the historical default value. A similar pattern was noted with lipstick data. Such cultural differences in product use, including temporal variations over time, are not unanticipated.

Note that for rinse-off/rinse-out products, "Retention Factors" have been given by the Scientific Committee on Consumer Products (SCCP) (17). This is to acknowledge that most of the applied material is rinsed off or out shortly after exposure and more protracted exposure is associated with residual material remaining in contact with the skin. For some product ingredients such as preservatives, daily exposures from multiple products may need to be considered in the risk assessment. The SCCP has calculated a global daily exposure value of 17.8 gm for a worst-case scenario for a person using multiple products on a single day (exclusive of sunscreen use).

In addition to the mean values cited here, the published CTFA data also provides information on the nature of the distributions of product usage. In many cases log-normal distributions were noted and geometric means are presented together with 50th (median), 90th and 95th and intermediate percentile values (data not given in Table 2). Under certain circumstances, this information may be desired or useful in the calculations of the MOS. The reports emphasize the wide variation in usage patterns that was not unanticipated. Such variation may reflect factors such packaging, preference, and cost as well as climate/geography. For most, but not all, studies the subjects' preferred product was provided. This might minimize preference factors but accentuate packaging considerations.

External exposures to chemicals of interest can be estimated from such data based on representative use concentrations in such formulations. The cosmetic data (14) was obtained using lipstick, body lotion, and face cream. Three hundred and sixty women were recruited at ten different geographical locations within the U.S. The number of recruits was chosen to ensure a minimum of 300 completes per product type. Subjects were provided with prototype test products, and kept diaries and recorded detailed daily usage information over a two-week period. Products were weighed at the start and completion of the study in order to determine the total amount of product used. Statistical analysis of the data was conducted to derive summary distribution of use patterns. For the "personal care" products, six widely used product types were used (15). Five were cosmetics (spray perfume, hairspray, liquid foundation, shampoo, body wash) and one was a cosmetic/over-the-counter drug product (solid antiperspirant). The number of recruits and locations were as for the earlier study. Products of their own preference and selection were weighed at the start and completion of the study in order to determine the total amount of product used. Statistical analyses of the data were conducted to derive summary distributions of use patterns. Both studies provide current exposure information for commonly used products that will be useful for risk assessment purposes.

TABLE 2 Dermal Exposure to Leave-On and Rinse-Off/Out Cosmetic and Personal Care Products. Reported Default and Experimentally Measured Values.

		gm/application	(x) applications/day (=)	daily exposure-gm/day				
Product type	Product	ECETOC default value	CTFA measured	ECETOC default value	CTFA measured	CREMe measured	COLIPA default value	Retention factor
Leave-on	Body Lotion	7.5	0.26–2.1[a]	**4.4**	**8.7**	7.8	8	
	Sunscreen	8					18[b]	
	Hair spray-pump	10	1.5	**3.6**	**5.2**			
	Hair spray-aerosol	10	1.5	**2.6**	**3.6**			
	Spray deodorant	3				6.5		
	Talcum powder	2.5						
	Face cream	0.8	1.8	**1.2**	**2.1**	1.5	1.6	
	Toilet water	0.75						
	Solid antiperspirant	0.5	1.3	**0.61**	**0.78**	1.5	0.5	
	Liquid foundation		1.2	**0.54**	**0.67**			
	Perfume spray		1.7	**0.33**	**0.53**			
	Lipstick	0.01	2.4	**0.01**	**0.02**	0.06	0.04	
	Eye shadow	0.01	1.2	**0.03**	**0.04**		0.02	
	Eyeliner	0.005					0.005	
	Eye mascara	0.025					0.025	
Rinse-off	Hair conditioner	14	1.1	**13.1**	**13.8**	10.5	4	0.01
	Shampoo	12	1.1	**11.8**	**12.8**		8	0.01
	Body wash	10	1.4	**11.3**	**14.5**		10	0.01
	Facial cleanser	2.5	1.6	**2.6**	**4.1**		5	0.1
	Hair dye-oxidative	50					100[c]	0.1
	Hair dye-direct	30					35	0.1
	Shave cream	2						
Rinse out	Toothpaste	1.5				2.7	2.8	0.05–0.17
	Mouthwash	12					30	0.1

[a] Range of use frequency for individual body part (hands, arms, feet, legs, back, other).
[b] SCCP estimate.
[c] After mixing.

Abbreviations: CTFA, Cosmetics, Toiletries, and Fragrance Association; ECETOC, European Centre for Ecotoxicology and Toxicology of Chemical; CREMe, Central Risk and Exposure Modeling e-solution; COLIPA, The European Cosmetic Toiletry and Perfumery Association; SCCP, Scientific Committee for Consumer Products. *Source*: From Refs. 13, 14–16, 17, and 18.

In some circumstances, such as for hair care or hair color products, exposure to skin and the potential for percutaneous absorption may be merely an unavoidable consequence of product usage rather than an intentional exposure. In addition to those factors influencing absorption cited in the Introduction, local habits and practices might play an important role in determining exposure type and frequency. Certain cosmetic products such as those used for cleansing skin and hair may be used in "rinse-off" rather than" leave-on" applications. In these circumstances exposure conditions, rather than the inherent permeation of the material under consideration, may be the rate-limiting determinant for systemic availability. Permeants of interest for cosmetic safety often include ingredients (or potential constituents and contaminants of ingredients) with broad applicability across a range of product types, such as preservatives or surfactants. Some materials in cosmetic formulations may also be utilized as excipients in therapeutic dermatologicals and therefore of similar interest from a safety perspective.

SKIN PERMEATION CONSIDERATIONS

It is important to design in vitro skin permeation experiments such that they mimic in-use scenarios. This is exemplified in the European Union SCCP 6th Revision of the Notes of Guidance for the Testing of Cosmetic Ingredients and their Safety Evaluation (17), which state:

> "The aim of the *in vitro* dermal/percutaneous absorption study is to determine the amount of topically applied substance that may cross the stratum corneum and to enter into deeper skin layers. This amount is subsequently considered as relevant for safety evaluation (calculation of the Margin of Safety), if the application was performed mimicking in-use conditions. The amount is expected to enter the circulatory system unless irreversible binding in the epidermis and/or dermis is demonstrated."

However, the Notes for Guidance highlight what the SCCP consider to be contentious issues, despite the fact that there is reasonable agreement between skin permeation scientists on most of these points. The Guidance continues:

> "There are a number of points that require special attention
>
> 1. The design of the diffusion cell (technicalities and choice between static and flow through system)
> 2. The choice of the receptor fluid (solubility and stability of chemical in receptor fluid should be demonstrated, no interference with skin/membrane integrity, analytical method, etc.)
> 3. The skin preparations should be chosen and treated with care (human skin from an appropriate site remains the gold standard)
> 4. Skin integrity is of key importance and should be verified
> 5. Skin temperature has to be ascertained at normal human skin temperature
> 6. The test substance has to be rigorously characterized and should correspond to the substance that is intended to be used in the finished cosmetic products
> 7. Dose and vehicle/formulation should be representative for the in-use conditions of the intended cosmetic product
> 8. Dose, volume and contact time with the skin have to mimic in-use conditions
> 9. Regular sampling is required over the whole exposure period
> 10. Appropriate analytical techniques should be used.
> 11. The test compound is to be determined in all relevant compartments:
>
>   11.1. skin surface (product excess),
>   11.2. stratum corneum,

11.3. living epidermis,
11.4. dermis,
11.5. receptor fluid.

12. Mass balance analysis and recovery data are to be provided
13. Variability/validity/reproducibility of the method should be discussed.
14. The amounts measured in the dermis, epidermis (without stratum corneum) and the receptor fluid will be considered as dermally absorbed and taken into account for further calculations. If results are derived from an inadequate *in vitro* study, the default value of 100% absorption could be applied.

In case an insufficient number of skin samples have been tested, the highest absorption value will be taken into account; otherwise the mean value ± 2 SD (standard deviation of the mean) will be used for further calculations."

Some of these identified points are no longer contentious. For example, there is a general agreement between skin permeation scientists that flow-through and static diffusion cells will produce the same data if other established criteria are followed (18). It is discomforting, and somewhat alarming, to note the statement "If results are derived from an inadequate in vitro study, the default value of 100% absorption could be applied." Upon who's shoulders will the decision about the adequacy of a study fall? It is also interesting to note that "amounts [of permeant] measured in the dermis, epidermis (without stratum corneum) and the receptor fluid will be considered as dermally absorbed and taken into account for further calculations." There has been considerable debate about the inclusion or exclusion of the amount of permeant in the stratum corneum in the total systemic dose.

At present the amount of permeant remaining in the stratum corneum at the end of an experiment is excluded from the systemic load for cosmetic products but, for other risk assessment purposes, this amount may be considered as a reservoir for a systemic dose. Analyses have confirmed that desquamation significantly reduces the absorption of applied substances for highly lipophilic and high molecular weight compounds (19,20). Data obtained using polycyclic musks and rat skin in vivo confirmed this observation for lipophilic materials (21), and desquamation was also observed to slightly increase the percutaneous absorption of N-methyl-2-pyrrolidone across rat skin (22). Yourick et al. (23) reported studies on the fate of several compounds following dermal application. Of the three compounds studied (dihydroxyacetone, DHA; 7-(2H-naphtho(1,2-d)triazol-2-yl)-3-phenylcoumarin, 7NTPC; Disperse Blue 1, DB1), two (DHA and DB1) formed epidermal reservoirs and the authors concluded that the amount remaining in the skin should not be considered as absorbed material. On the other hand, the data for 7NTPC indicated that this material was spread throughout the epidermis and dermis and, as such, could not be justifiably excluded from the total absorbed dose without further experimentation.

Point 7 of the SCCP Guidance emphasizes the importance of dosage and suggests that this should be representative for the in-use conditions of the intended cosmetic product. Thus a product, such as a hair dye, which is rinsed off the skin following a defined exposure period should be rinsed from the skin in a diffusion cell at the same time point as would occur in use. For example, Kraeling et al.(24) evaluated the in vitro human skin permeation of lawsone (2-hydroxy-1,4-naphthoquinone). Lawsone is the principal color ingredient in henna, a hair color additive approved with limitations by the U.S. FDA. However, in 2002, the Scientific Committee for Consumer Products (SCCP) evaluated the safety of lawsone and concluded that it was mutagenic and not suitable for use as a hair coloring agent. Lawsone skin absorption was determined from two hair coloring products and two shampoo products, all containing henna. The products were applied to dermatomed, nonviable human skin mounted in flow-through diffusion cells and remained on the skin for five minutes (shampoos) and one hour (hair color paste). For all evaluated products, the majority of the applied lawsone was washed from the surface of the skin (83–102%) at the end of the exposure period. For the hair paste products, 0.3% and 1.3% of the applied dose permeated the skin in 24 hours while 2.2% and 4.0% remained in the skin. Similar levels permeated from the shampoo products (0.3% of the applied dose at 24 hours) with 3.6% and 6.8% remaining in the skin. Extended absorption studies indicated that the majority of the lawsone remained in the skin with only a small increase (for three out of four products) in receptor fluid values. The authors concluded that receptor fluid values would provide a good estimate of lawsone absorption for an exposure estimate and that skin levels of lawsone need not be included.

MARGIN OF SAFETY AND TOXICITY CONSIDERATIONS
Noncancer (Threshold) Endpoints
The margin of safety (MOS) is estimated for non-cancer (threshold) effects as the ratio of the NOAEL to the systemic exposure dose (SED). The critical value for an acceptable MOS is typically 100, based on 10-fold uncertainty factors applied to account for both species differences and human variability. Each of these uncertainty factors reflects both kinetic and dynamic variations.

NOAEL: The NOAEL is usually derived from a repeat dose subchronic or reproductive study using the most conservative value if multiple studies exist, while exposure may be estimated from in vivo or in vitro studies using human or animal skin. It is important to recognize that the NOAEL is a discontinuous variable and is in large part a function of dosage selection and spacing. The challenge in the design of toxicology studies is to use range-finding or other data to choose a low dose that is expected to cause no effect, or no adverse effect, a mid dose that will produce some effect, and a high dose that will, if feasible, produce toxicity and identify target organs. Depending on the results, the true NOAEL may, in fact, be higher than the observed value. In some circumstances the use of a low effect (e.g., lower 95% confidence limit for 10% response dose) "benchmark dose" interpolated or extrapolated from within or near the experimental range is taken as equivalent to a NOAEL for a more realistic estimate of the MOS. The NOAEL units are expressed as mass (e.g., mg, µg)/kg/day.

SED: Exposure, on the other hand is a continuous variable, measured experimentally. It is preferably expressed as mass/unit area (i.e., cm^2)/day. It is sometimes given as a percentage which is a function of the dose applied experimentally and may be misleading or ambiguous if the true applied use levels and experimental values differ, especially as may occur for rinse-off products. It also appears preferable that the experimental exposure conditions mimic the actual in-use conditions as close as possible rather than to apply arbitrary retention factors to account for rinse-off exposures. Care needs to be exercised such that arbitrary retention factors not be applied to experimental skin absorption data derived from use simulations where the observed amounts absorbed already reflect the effects of retention over the measurement period.

One area of continuing scientific debate is the appropriateness of including/excluding amounts measured in skin compartments in in-vitro studies for the estimation of the SED. It is generally agreed that dermal amounts be included, (if dermis is indeed present in the tissue preparation) and that amounts in (or adhering to) the stratum corneum be excluded. As discussed earlier, for cosmetic ingredients, the SCCP (17,25) defaults to inclusion of the epidermal compartment below the stratum corneum in the absorbed dose. It is acknowledged that skin amounts may be lost by desquamation processes that are not operative in vitro and that, in some instances, substantial amounts, greatly exceeding receptor fluid levels are found. However, to date, there are no clearly articulated criteria for inclusion or exclusion of these amounts in the SED. As mentioned earlier, Yourick et al. (23) cited experimental data for a number of chemicals in studies conducted from 24 to 72 hours using viable human and fuzzy rat skin in the U.S. Food and Drug Administration (FDA) laboratories. For dihydroxyacetone, a skin binding rationale was use to justify the exclusion of the substantial amounts found in the viable tissue (as well as the stratum corneum) from the systemic dose. For Disperse Blue 1, a hair dye, little additional absorption was seen between 24 and 72 hours, also justifying exclusion of skin amounts. For other substances such as musk xylol (26), phenanthracine, benzo(a)pyrene, and di(2-ethylhexyl) phthalate (27), as well as brevetoxin (28) in vitro data showed continued availability or agreed more closely with in vivo data. Justification has also been given for excluding skin amounts for diethanolamine (29) and for catechol (30) based on kinetics seen in extended time studies.

Cancer (Nonthreshold) Effects

Conservative estimates for cancer risks consider that even low doses of a cancer-causing chemical are associated with some finite risk, though such risk might be small. Different approaches have been taken by international regulatory agencies to estimate low exposure cancer risks. For example, the U.S. EPA utilizes a "linearized multistage model" in which the 95% upper bound confidence limit of doses associated with de minimus risks (e.g., 1 in 1,000,000) usually extrapolated from chronic rodent cancer bioassays are taken as a Virtually Safe Dose (VSD). Other local agencies (US California Proposition 65) consider a 1:100,000 cancer risk de minimus. In Europe a "T_{25} Method" is used whereby a chronic animal dose that will produce a 25% increase in tumors over the spontaneous rate in a particular tissue is calculated and scaled to a equivalent human dose (HT_{25}) based on body weight. The lifetime cancer risk is then calculated as the daily $SED/(HT_{25}/0.25)$. Another approach uses a TD_{50} defined as a lifetime dose that would cause tumors in half the animals. Although different methods are utilized for cancer risk assessment, typical agreement among these approaches with respect to an overall decision about a particular chemical's appropriateness for use in a particular exposure scenario is reassuring.

Toxicokinetics and Metabolism

The most appropriate measurement of a dermal exposure MOS for long term systemic toxicity would compare the bioavailability after dermal exposure in humans (or human skin) with that following oral administration in subchronic or chronic preclinical studies. In this regard, it is important to recognize that that the blood/plasma profile via these two routes is dissimilar, with the typical peak following an oral bolus dose absent in the dermal profile, which shows a more protracted rise. There is a presumption that the systemic toxicity in long-term studies relates to the net exposure rather than peak effects. Further, the NOAEL from toxicity studies presumes 100% availability by the oral route, which may be nonconservative if the toxicity were actually manifested at levels below the orally administered dose.

Differences in the metabolic fate (extent and type of metabolism) between the oral and topical routes may also influence the reliability of the calculated MOS. Of much importance is whether the metabolic processes are saturable and result in detoxification or activation, as well as whether the contribution of "first pass" metabolism varies with the route of administration. Reduced first-pass hepatic metabolism could result in greater exposure to the parent compound following topical application as compared to oral absorption. On the other hand, decreased systemic exposure to the parent compound could occur if it were more extensively or more rapidly metabolized following topical application. For example topical application of ^{14}C-radiolabeled hair dye precursors p-aminophenol (PAP) and p-phenylenediamine (PPD) to rats resulted in systemic exposure to their N-acetylated metabolites and not to the parent arylamines (31). The N-acetylated metabolite of PAP is paracetamol, a widely used oral analgesic drug. Such detoxification, presumably by N-acetyltransferase-1 in the skin, converts the parent amine to amides that are less likely to be activated by cytochrome P-450 to DNA reactive and, presumably mutagenic or carcinogenic, metabolites.

Consideration of toxicokinetics may, therefore, become important for those chemicals with a marginally acceptable MOS and where ancillary data on the material or related chemicals suggest a potential for differences in the nature and/or extent of metabolism between the oral and dermal routes of administration.

Furthermore, in some circumstances, the nature of the compound of interest may undergo changes during the exposure period, sometimes prior to penetration into the skin. For example, lower molecular weight oxidative (permanent) hair dye precursors complex within the hair shaft, as well as on and in the stratum corneum, to form higher molecular weight dimeric and trimeric colored species. Thus the driving concentration of the precursor is reduced as less absorbable reaction products are formed.

THE THRESHOLD OF TOXICOLOGICAL CONCERN

The threshold of toxicological concern (TTC) is an emerging approach for characterizing risk that may be applied to both noncancer and cancer endpoints (32). It has already gained acceptance for chemicals that may migrate into food and for flavoring agents. The TTC is based on the premise that if the structure is known, and exposure is sufficiently low, risk (or lack thereof) can be inferred from related chemicals and no toxicology data are needed. In part it is intended to help conserve scientific, technical and animal resources that would be needed to specifically test each chemical.

The chemical of interest is assigned to one of three structural classes based on the presence or absence of alerting groups. Thresholds of concern have been previously established by applying a 100-fold uncertainty factor to a 5th percentile NOAEL calculated from chronic toxicity data on a large number of representative chemicals in each class. On this basis, cut points for estimated oral intakes of 1800, 540, and 90 μg/day, corresponding respectively, to 30, 9 and 1.5 μg/kg/day, based on a 60 kg body weight have been established for those materials lacking structural alerts for genotoxicity (33). If the internal exposure were determined to be lower than these values, the substance would not be expected to pose a safety concern. For those chemicals with structural alerts for genotoxicity, a highly conservative threshold corresponding to an exposure below 0.15 µg/60 kg person/day (0.0025 µg/kg/day) is used, below which the cancer risk would be considered negligible (less than 1 in 1,000,000). The paradigm provides for certain chemical structures that are inappropriate for a TTC analysis because of high potency or lack of representation in the toxicology database. These would require compound-specific data.

The TTC has recently been proposed for use with cosmetic products applied to skin (34). In this regard it relates to systemic effects only and not local skin effects at the application site. An expert group, organized by COLIPA, the European cosmetic trade association, has advocated the utility of the TTC approach for estimating risks for systemic toxicity of topically applied ingredients (and impurities). This was done after careful consideration of their similarity to structures represented in the toxicology database from which NOAELs were derived and the potential differences in toxicokinetics following oral administration and dermal application. They described a stepwise procedure for applying the TTC approach for cosmetic ingredients and have developed or recommended default adjustment factors for estimating the systemic exposure of leave-on, rinse-off, and intermittent use products. These are summarized briefly below and the reader is referred to the panel report for more detailed information.

Default Assumptions

In the EU, the Scientific Committee on Consumer Products (SCCP) has historically advocated that, in the absence of experimental data, a default value of 100% be used for percutaneous absorption (17,25). However based on a theoretical consideration of the relationships of the maximum flux (J_{max}) of chemicals across skin with molecular weight, log P, and the degree of saturation of the chemical in the formulation, and data available on 62 chemicals in the open literature, alternate default factors based on worst-case assumptions were recommended by the panel as follows:

J_{max} (µg/cm2/hr)	Default % dose absorbed per 24 hours
Non-reactive chemicals with MW 1000	Negligible
$J_{max} < 0.1$	10
$0.1 < J_{max} < 10$	40
$J_{max} > 10$	80

In their stepwise approach the panel included adjustments based on the default retention factors of 0.01 or 0.1 (i.e., 1% or 10%) as recommended by the SCCP for certain rinse-off products. For intermittent use products the panel proposed that the estimated intake be decreased by a default of threefold for ingredients used only once a week and 10-fold for products used less frequently unless the data supported a smaller or larger margin between acute and multiple dose toxicities. They recognized that aggregate exposure to an individual cosmetic ingredient (e.g., a preservative, a common excipient) from concurrent use of multiple products might also have to be considered in estimating total daily exposure for comparison to the TTC.

It is important to recognize that viability of the TTC panel recommendations in the regulatory environment for cosmetics, particularly in the EU, awaits confirmation, but the scientific approach appears reasonable and is consistent with current resource conservation and animal welfare initiatives impacted by regulatory requirements for safety substantiation. Mathematical calculations not withstanding, many of the cancer risk assessment methods allow for (or require) consideration of how ancillary data such as toxicokinetics may modulate the cancer risk or its reliability.

CONCLUSIONS

The ability to more accurately estimate and predict exposure levels of materials accidentally or deliberately applied to the skin will allow a better definition of any associated risk. With cosmetic products, studies underway in the US and Europe attempt to better quantify exposures based on the habits and practices of consumers in varying cultural environments. Data from these studies will help refine historical default estimates of exposure. However, exposure per se does not necessarily suggest that the compound of interest will become systemically available to any great extent. Actual determination of rates and amounts of skin penetration, distribution and permeation using human skin provides a realistic and quantifiable measurement against which more precise risk assessments can be made. In the absence of skin absorption data default estimates of 100% absorption may be unreasonably over-conservative. Based on an understanding of the influence of physical/chemical parameters on the flux of chemicals across skin, extant data suggests lower default factors may be appropriate and still reflect worst-case scenarios. Similarly, an understanding of the associations between chemical structure and toxicity suggests that daily systemic exposure levels below thresholds established on the basis of existing long-term data on representative chemicals should not give rise to toxicity concerns. Such scientifically based approaches will help reduce the impact of regulatory requirements for the safety substantiation of chemicals on valuable animal and technical resources.

REFERENCES

1. Fitzpatrick D, Golden D, Corish J. Modelling skin permeability in risk assessment. In: Roberts MS, Walters KA, eds. Dermal Absorption and Toxicity Assessment. 2nd ed. New York: Informa Inc., 2007.
2. Magnusson BM, Anissimov YG, Cross SE, et al. Molecular size as the main determinant of solute maximum flux across the skin. J Invest Dermatol 2004; 122:993–999.
3. Kroes R, Kleiner J, Renwick A. The threshold of toxicological concern concept in risk assessment. Toxicol Sci 2005; 86:226–230.
4. Api AM, Bredbenner A, McGowen M, et al. Skin contact transfer of three fragrance residues from candles to human hands. Regul Toxicol Pharmacol 2007; 48:279–283.
5. Marquart H, Warren ND, Laitinen J, et al. Default values for assessment of potential dermal exposure of the hands to industrial chemicals in the scope of regulatory risk assessments. Ann Occup Hyg 2006; 50:469–489.
6. Fent KW, Jayaraj K, Gold A, et al. Tape-strip sampling for measuring dermal exposure to 1,6-hexamethylene diisocyanate. Scand J Work Environ Health 2006; 32:225–240.
7. Liljelind IE, Michel I, Damm M, et al. Development, evaluation and data acquired with a tape-stripping technique for measuring dermal exposure to budesonide at a pharmaceutical manufacturing site. Ann Occup Hyg 2007; 51:407–413.
8. Hughson GW, Aitken RJ. Determination of dermal exposures during mixing, spraying and wiping activities. Ann Occup Hyg 2004; 48:245–255.
9. Cherrie JW, Semple S, Brouwer D. Gloves and dermal exposure to chemicals: proposals for evaluating workplace effectiveness. Ann Occup Hyg. 2004; 48:607–615.
10. Gao P, El-Ayouby N, Wassell JT. Change in permeation parameters and the decontamination efficacy of three chemical protective gloves after repeated exposures to solvents and thermal decontaminations. Am J Ind Med 2005; 47:131–143.

11. US EPA Exposure Factors Handbook Doc EPA/600?P-95/002Fa Office of Research and Development, US Environmental Protection Agency, Washington, D.C., 1997.
12. Bremmer HJ, Prud'Homme de Lodder LCH, van Engeolen JGM. Cosmetics fact sheet to assess risks for the consumer; updated version for ConsExpo4. RIVM Report 320104 oo1/2005, 2005.
13. ECETOC Percutaneous Absorption. Monograph No. 20 European Centre for Ecotoxicology and Toxicology of Chemical, Brussels, Belgium, 1993.
14. Loretz LJ, Api AM, Barraj LM, et al. Exposure data for cosmetic products: lipstick, body lotion, and face cream. Food Chem Toxicol 2005; 43:279–291.
15. Loretz L, Api AM, Barraj L, et al. Exposure data for personal care products: hairspray, spray perfume, liquid foundation, shampoo, body wash, and solid antiperspirant. Food Chem Toxicol 2006; 44:2008–2018.
16. CREMe, Central Risk and Exposure Modeling e-solution European consumer exposure to cosmetic products-data analysis Final Draft Report, 17th September 2005.
17. SCCP: The SCCP Notes of Guidance for the Testing of Cosmetic Ingredients and Their Safety Evaluation, 6th Revision, 2006.
18. Kielhorn J, Melching-Kollmuss S, Mangelsdorf I. WHO Environmental Health Criteria No. 235. Dermal Absorption, 2006.
19. Reddy MB, Guy RH, Bunge AL. Does epidermal turnover reduce percutaneous penetration? Pharm Res 2000; 17:1414–1419.
20. O'Connor J, Cage S, Fong L. In vitro skin absorption—can it be used in isolation for risk assessment purposes? In: Brain KR, Walters KA, eds. Perspectives in Percutaneous Penetration Volume 9a. Cardiff: STS Publishing, 2004:92.
21. Ford RA, Hawkins DR, Schwarzenbach R, et al. The systemic exposure to the polycyclic musks, AHTN and HHCB, under conditions of use as fragrance ingredients: evidence of lack of complete absorption from a skin reservoir. Toxicol Lett 1999; 111:133–142.
22. Payan JP, Boudry I, Beydon D, et al. Toxicokinetics and metabolism of N-((14)C)N-methyl-2-pyrrolidone in male Sprague-Dawley rats: in vivo and in vitro percutaneous absorption. Drug Metab Disp 2003; 31:659–669.
23. Yourick JJ, Koenig ML, Yourick DL, et al. Fate of chemicals in skin after dermal application: does the in vitro skin reservoir affect the estimate of systemic absorption? Toxicol Appl Pharmacol 2004; 195:309–320.
24. Kraeling ME, Bronaugh RL, Jung CT. Absorption of lawsone through human skin. Cutan Ocul Toxicol 2007; 26:45–56.
25. SCCP: Opinion on Basic Criteria for the In Vitro Assessment of Dermal Absorption of Cosmetic Ingredients, updated March 2006.
26. Hood HL, Wickett RR, Bronaugh RL. *In vitro* percutaneous absorption of the fragrance ingredient musk xylol. Food Chem Toxicol 1996; 34:483–488.
27. Chu I, Dick D, Bronaugh RL, et al. Skin reservoir formation and bioavailability of dermally administered chemicals in hairless guinea pigs. Food Chem Toxicol 1996;34:267–276.
28. Kemppainen BW, Reifenrath WG, Stafford RG, et al. Methods for in vitro skin absorption studies of a lipophilic toxin produced by red tide. Toxicology 1991; 66:1–18.
29. Kraeling ME, Yourick JJ, Bronaugh RL. In vitro human skin penetration of diethanolamine. Food Chem Toxicol. 2004; 42:1553–1561.
30. Jung CT, Wickett RR, Desai PB, et al. In vitro and in vivo percutaneous absorption of catechol. Food Chem Toxicol 2003; 41:885–895.
31. Dressler WE, Appelqvist T. Plasma/blood pharmacokinetics and metabolism after dermal exposure to *para*-aminophenol and *para*-phenylenediamine. Food Chem Toxicol 2006; 44:371–379.
32. Kroes R, Renwick AG, Cheeseman M, et al. Structure based thresholds of toxicological concern (TTC): guidance for application to substances present at low levels in the diet. Food Chem Toxicol 2004; 42:65–83.
33. Munro IC, Ford RA, Kennepohl E, et al. Correlation of structural class with no-observed effect levels: a proposal for establishing a threshold of concern. Food Chem Toxicol 1996; 37:207–232.
34. Kroes R, Renwick AG, Feron AG, et al. Application of the threshold of toxicological concern (TTC) to the safety evaluation of cosmetic ingredients. Food Chem Toxicol 2007, Epub: doi 10.1016/j.fct2007.06.021.

28 Noninvasive Evaluation of Skin in the Cosmetic Industry

Carlos Galzote and Michael Suero
Johnson & Johnson, Asia Pacific Skin Testing Center, Parañaque City, Metro Manila, Philippines

Raman Govindarajan
Johnson & Johnson Singapore Research Center, Singapore

INTRODUCTION

Evaluation of the surface structure and functional properties of the skin for the purpose of making claims on the efficacy of skin care products is a key part of cosmetic product research and development. Other parts of this book have dealt with structure and properties of the skin. This chapter will deal with instrumental and expert methods to evaluate skin as used by the cosmetics industry. The principles governing clinical trials in the consumer products industry are much the same as in therapeutic drug clinical trials. Thus, safety and ethical clearance of products, procedures to be used, investigator training, and monitoring and auditing of trials are considered important for both the safety of the subjects enrolled into trials and for the validity of the results obtained. Choice of subjects, skin properties, ethnicity, age, sex, absence of other confounding factors, disease, drug ingestion, etc. that will invalidate the results are taken cared of by careful crafting of inclusion and exclusion criteria.

Trials fall into two major categories: proof of principle trials and full clinical trials. The former are generally small studies of 10 to 15 subjects aimed to determine feasibility of the study protocol, to evaluate a new measurement technique, and also to determine if products show any directional effects. Full clinical studies are larger, consist of 25–50 subjects per cell where head-to-head comparisons can be made, can be sequential or crossover, or more complex in design. Table 1 outlines the contents of a well-designed and written clinical protocol, and Table 2 gives suggested ethical considerations for clinical studies. Measurements are made using instruments detailed later in this chapter and using expert grading and self-assessment. Grading scales are used.

The functional, structural, and beauty parameters that are generally measured in the cosmetic industry are the following:

1. Skin health: water content (hydration), rate of water loss (a measure of barrier integrity), and skin pH
2. Skin surface properties: texture, scaling/desquamation, friction, sebum, close-up view (macrophotography) and image analysis, confocal microscopy, laser Doppler perfusion, transcutaneous oxygen and carbon dioxide, spectrofluorimetry, and elasticity
3. Skin color (for skin lightening, darkening, and inflammation)

TABLE 1

Contents of a good clinical protocol

Names of investigators and qualifications
Rationale and objective
        Business justification
Details of conduct of study
        Outline of the study
        What questions will be answered by what measurements
        Number of panelists/rationale for this number—pilot study/statistician recommendation
            based on sensitivity and reproducibility of the measurement method
Inclusion/Exclusion criteria
Proposed start and end dates
Recruiting methods
Procedures and potential hazards/distress
        Safety clearance for the procedures
Products and possible side effects
        Safety clearance for the products
        Precautions and labeling
Duration of the study
Instrumentation and specifications of instruments
Data collection forms
Record keeping and confidentiality
Study location and how it is qualified to be an approved site
Adverse event reporting forms
Medical cover provision, investigator and doctor contact numbers
Informed consent, information sheet for volunteers
Compensation to be given to participants
Previous studies/similar studies
Regulatory considerations if any
End of study participation forms
Usefulness of the study—investigator to intimate the ethics committee on how the study was useful

TABLE 2

Ethical considerations

- Are there appropriate authorizations?
- Are the products to be used and the procedure safety cleared?
- Are the numbers of subjects statistically justified?
- Are age and sex of subjects appropriate for the end point—not minor unless specifically justified?
- Is the procedure ethical?
- Is medical cover in place?
- Is compensation commensurate with the effort/involvement (this will be location specific)?
- Is the informed consent clear and accurate—has all the information been shared (if necessary in local language) and have subjects been able to ask and clear their doubts?
- Is the clinical site adequate, comfortable, safe, and well equipped (e.g., lighting, instruments, sanitary facilities, and ventilation)?
- Is privacy of subjects protected and mechanisms in place to guard the data obtained?
- Is documentation adequate?
- Is there an adverse event management procedure in place?
- Are the study personnel adequately trained?
- Will the study add real value?

SKIN HEALTH: HYDRATION, RATE OF WATER LOSS, AND pH
Skin Hydration
As discussed in Chapter 7, the water content of the stratum corneum influences other skin characteristics like barrier formation, drug penetration, and mechanical properties (softness, elasticity, etc.). There are three main methods used to evaluate skin moisture using noninvasive instruments: capacitance, conductance, and impedance.

Capacitance
The measurement principle is based on the physical principle of a common capacitor, which is a complex of two plates, insulated by a medium that acts as a dielectric. A capacitor has the capability to store electrical charge when a charged field comes into close proximity. More specifically, the measurement is based on the very different dielectric constant of water (81) and other substances (mostly <7). This means that most materials increase the capacity of a capacitor by a factor of 7, whereas water increases the capacity by a factor of around 81. Hence, this means that the capacitance is directly proportional to the moisture content of the samples: the higher the moisture, the higher the capacitance [1].

Instruments using the capacitance method include the Corneometer® (Courage & Khazaka GmbH, Germany). According to the manufacturer, an advantage of capacitance measurements versus impedance measurements is that there is no galvanic relation between the device and measuring object or polarization, hence chemical substances or slats of products that are applied on the skin do not influence the readings [2].

Conductance
The conductance method is based on the changes in the electrical properties of the stratum corneum. Dry stratum corneum has weak electrical conduction, whereas hydrated stratum corneum is more sensitive to the electric field, inducing an increase of dielectric constant. The electrical properties of skin are expressed in terms of resistance (ohms), conductance (current/resistance, mho, or Siemens), or impedance (ohms at a fixed frequency). An increase in the dielectric constant leads to a decrease in impedance and increased conductance and capacitance [1].

As briefly mentioned above, impedance measurements have shortcomings in that they do not provide accurate information on the electrical and physical properties of the stratum corneum because it is easily influenced by external factors that act on the stratum corneum. For example, at high frequencies, it is impossible to measure resistance and capacitance accurately. In addition, at high frequencies, impedance provides information not only on the stratum corneum, but also on the deeper layers of the skin [1].

The conductance method of Skicon® 200 (I.B.S. Company, Japan) overcomes these pitfalls. Using a frequency of 3.5 MHz, the closely spaced electrodes of the probe maintain the electric field in the superficial portion of the skin, leading to a noninvasive measurement of water content [3].

Impedance
Other variations to the above methods include the Nova™ Dermal Phase Meter and the Surface Characterizing Impedance Monitor. In Nova Dermal Phase Meter, measurements at different frequencies of the applied alternating current are integrated, which allows impedance-based capacitance readings. Samples are measured along a controlled rise time up to 1 MHz. This is the main difference versus Corneometer,

which uses variable frequencies at a lower range (40 to 75 kHz) or the Skicon 200, which uses a fixed frequency (3.5 MHz). In Surface Characterizing Impedance Monitor, electrical impedance, both magnitude and phase, are measured at 31 frequencies to five selectable depths under the probe. This allows electrical impedance spectroscopy of selected layers of the skin (1).

Transepidermal Water Loss

Transepidermal water loss (TEWL) refers to the total amount of water vapor lost through the skin. It can be used to characterize the water barrier function of the stratum corneum both in physiological and pathological conditions to perform predictive irritancy tests and to evaluate the efficacy of therapeutic treatments on diseased skin. TEWL can only be representative of the stratum corneum function if there is no sweat gland activity (4). In vivo measurements of TEWL can be measured according to three different techniques. Distante and Berardesca (4) described the three techniques as the following:

1. **Closed-chamber method:** This consists of a capsule applied to the skin, collecting water vapor from the skin surface. The relative humidity inside the capsule is recorded with an electronic hygrosensor. The change in vapor loss concentration is initially flat and decreases proportionally as the humidity approaches 100%. The closed-chamber method does not permit recording of continuous TEWL because, when the air inside the chamber is saturated, skin evaporation ceases.
2. **Ventilated-chamber method:** A chamber in which a gas of known water content passes through is applied on the skin. The water is picked up by the gas and measured through a hygrometer. This method allows the continuous measurement of TEWL, but if the carrier gas is too dry, it artificially increases evaporation.
3. **Open-chamber method:** The open-chamber method has the skin capsule open to the atmosphere. TEWL is calculated from the slope provided by two hygrosensors precisely oriented in the chamber. Air movement and humidity are the greatest drawbacks of this method when in vivo studies are performed. This method is currently used in commercially available devices (4).

Since TEWL measurements follow diffusion laws, the TEWL results would then depend directly on the ambient relative humidity, the stratum corneum barrier integrity, the temperature, and inversely on the stratum corneum thickness, which determines penetrability.

Instruments that measure TEWL include the Tewameter® (Courage & Khazaka GmbH), Servo Med Evaporimeter (Servo Med AB, Sweden), and Vapometer (Delfin Technologies, Finland) (5,6).

Skin pH

The skin is covered by an acid mantle, which is formed through secretion from the sweat and sebaceous glands. It provides skin protection via chemical buffering, detoxifying, and bacteriostatic functions. The normal pH range of the acid mantle is from 4.5 to 6.5. This is maintained by a lactate–bicarbonate buffer system that can neutralize small amounts of acids or alkali encountered during work and leisure activities. However, repeated application of acid or alkali causes the buffering capacity to decline. Significant changes in pH may give rise to bacterial invasion, sensitization, and various forms of dermatitis. The measurement of pH uses electro-chemical interface processes between metal or glass and solutions. Changes in the potential of the measuring electrode can be evaluated by determining the potential difference between this electrode and a standard electrode with constant potential. This reference electrode is made of Ag/AgCl in a KCl solution, whereas the active electrode consists of a glass membrane filled with a buffer solution. After contact with water, the glass membrane swells and develops a gel layer that is able to release or take up hydrogen ions, depending on the pH of the external solution, i.e., moist skin. The resulting potential difference between the outer and inner layer of the glass membrane is then compared with the constant potential of the reference electrode and is converted by the pH meter to pH values. Temperature can affect pH measurements because both the electrode properties and H^+ concentration are temperature dependent. Redox reactions or uptake of ions other than H^+ can also lead to erroneous readings (7).

SKIN SURFACE PROPERTIES: TOPOGRAPHY, SEBUM, SCALING, FRICTION, MACROIMAGING AND ELASTICITY, CONFOCAL MICROSCOPY, LASER DOPPLER PERFUSION IMAGING, TRANSCUTANEOUS OXYGEN, AND CARBON DIOXIDE LEVELS
Skin Surface Topography/Roughness

There are several methods to analyze roughness of the skin. The first method is mechanical profilometry. Instruments using this method normally have three components: a receiver, a transducer, and an expenditure instrument. The receiver is a sensing instrument (normally in stylus form) driven linearly and with constant speed over the surface. The transducer converts the vertical movements of the stylus into an electrical signal. An amplifier and a standard bypass filter cut off disturbances by boosting electrical signal to a useful level before calculating roughness parameters. Vertical resolution (which may be within 1 mm) is limited by background mechanical vibrations, electronic influences, and the dimensions of the stylus. The horizontal resolution depends on the dimensions of the stylus.

The advantage of using this method is that all U.S. national roughness standards are based upon it. Disadvantages include bulk, complexity, fragility, and limitation to a section of a surface resulting in long measuring times. Furthermore, the process of surface evaluation is susceptible to mechanical damage of the stylus and the object being measured. Negative influences on the measuring results are caused by a feedback system between the stylus tip and the object being measured.

Recently, optical methods have been developed to avoid the above problems. In the light-cutting technique, surface profile cuts are generated via a plane of light or shadow cutting the surface at an angle. The emerging cutting curve can be observed through a microscope. In the throwing-shadows technique, the length of the shadows caused by slanted lighting characterizes the peak heights of a surface. This technique has been used for many years now in electron microscopy, and it is only recently that this was introduced to the field of image processing. In interference methods, a light wave is sent out by a light source and split into two equal, same-phase parts. Depending on the surface of the object, when the light reunifies, the light can be amplified or extinguished or somewhere in between. Hence, an image of interference can reproduce the spatial order of an object.

Light microscopy and holography are fairly similar to the above interference method but use lasers instead of visible light. In laser profilometry, which has a similar principle as mechanical profilometry, but instead of a stylus, a laser beam is used to read the surface, resulting in a contactless assessment of the skin. Adequate lateral and vertical resolutions are obtained (<0.1 μm). Advantages of this method are the contactless operation and the resolution. Disadvantages include interpretation of results in terms of optical surface parameters and correlation with surface photography.

Lastly, there is transmission profilometry, which requires the use of blue silicon with special colored absorption coefficient and low viscosity. The replica is perpendicularly illuminated with a parallel light source and the transmitted light detected by a CCD camera. Silicon replicas with known parameters are used as standards. The measuring principle is based on Bouger–Lambert's law of absorption. Known differences in the height of the standards allow calculation of the absorption constant of the silicon. Gray values are then analyzed using image analysis software, and absolute values and standard profilometric parameters according to DIN norms are calculated (8,9).

Skin surface topography can be analyzed using replicas (normally silicone replicas) or by imaging systems (contact or noncontact). Examples of imaging systems include the Visioscan (Courage & Khazaka GmbH) and the PRIMOS (GFM, Germany).

Visioscan
An example of contact imaging is the Visioscan. The Visioscan is a UVA light video camera with a black-and-white high-resolution video sensor chip. Two halogen lights, arranged on opposite sides, illuminate the skin area (6 × 8 mm) uniformly. The image of the skin is taken by a built-in CCD camera. The accompanying software called Surface Evaluation of Living Skin provides image processing functions and provides calculations like texture parameters, height and width of lesions, etc. (10).

PRIMOS
PRIMOS is an optical three-dimensional in vivo noncontact skin-measuring system which uses digital micromirror devices to project stripes on the surface of the skin and a high-velocity camera that is capable of recording the stripe projection patterns for the measurement of the topography of the skin. The accompanying software has the ability to match images (i.e., orient post-treatment images exactly as the baseline image) for a more accurate analysis. The software then analyzes specific attributes like roughness, lesion size, etc. An advantage of noncontact imaging measurements is that it does not in any way affect the topography, unlike contact imaging which may affect the topography of skin if the pressure is too great (11).

Friction
Most friction instruments today fall within the three basic instrument types used for the measurement of skin friction: the sled, the spinning drum or spool, and the rotating disk. Both static and dynamic friction can be calculated using the above methods. The three methods operate mainly on the same principle: dragging or spinning or rotating the edge against the skin and the resistance encountered by the machine is measured. This would give the friction value of the skin (12). Instruments include the M.T. Skin Friction Instrument (Measurement Technologies, California, U.S.A.) and the Frictiometer (Courage & Khazaka GmbH) (13).

Desquamation

Dry skin leads to excessive scaling and premature desquamation. The shedding of corneocytes from the skin surface can be quantified by separating a portion of the stratum corneum from the underlying tissue and subsequently measuring light-absorbing properties or detecting endogenous or exogenous components by chemical/biochemical analysis. Imaging of the tapes/discs obtained can be carried out with suitable magnification, and such images are amenable to image analysis. Macrophotography will also directly visualize the affected area, and quantification can be carried out by image analysis. Pressure-sensitive adhesive discs have been developed specifically for harvesting stratum corneum samples easily and reproducibly. The discs are made from a very clear grade of polyester support film and an aggressive, superclear adhesive that forms an intimate mechanical bond with the stratum corneum surface under applied pressure. This film–adhesive combination results in very high contrast between the optical properties of the adhering corneocytes and the sampling medium (14).

Macrophotography and Image Analysis

This now simple and efficient tool has many uses. A good skin testing laboratory must have the necessary equipment and expertise to carry out high-quality macrophotography—images obtained are now in digital format and amenable to image analysis using several commercial software tools. One must remember the "GIGO" rule (garbage in, garbage out)—if the image is bad, so are the results. The ability to change features of images is no substitute for good lighting and sharp images of high resolution. In fact, some purists believe that image should not be manipulated at all prior to image analysis. Various modes of lighting–tungsten, halogen, fluorescent, UV, and cross and parallel polarized light–can all be used, and the experienced photographer will choose the right lighting or play with the options he/she has to obtain the best images for analysis.

Spectrofluorimetry is a valuable tool to characterize fluorescing constituents, or fluorophores, in the skin. Fluorescence bands may originate from the amino acids tryptophan, tyrosine, and phenylalanine (excitation between 280 and 295 nm), as well as cross-links in collagen (335 and 350 nm) and elastin (360 and 370 nm). Irritation, aging, and photoaging have been associated with alterations in the fluorescing patterns of these intrinsic fluorophores in skin. Therefore, spectrofluorimetry may be applied to product evaluation and claim support studies (15).

Skinskan (SPEX, New Jersey, U.S.A.) is a spectrofluorimeter specifically designed for noninvasive fluorescence measurements on the skin. It consists of a xenon arc light source that is filtered through a double monochromator that is scanned across the excitation spectrum from 290 to 450 nm, and the light is transmitted to the skin through the excitation fibers of a bifurcated fiber optic bundle. Remitted light from the skin (containing both reflected and fluorescence signals) is captured with the emission fibers of the fiber optic bundle and is separated by a second double monochromator that is separately scanned across the emission spectrum (340–500 nm). The height of the fluorescence signals indicates the condition of the fluorophores in the skin and how they change with topical treatments.

Confocal microscopy has been developed to minimize the blur created by out-of-focus planes of a thick sample such as skin. In confocal microscopy, light from a laser source passes through a pinhole aperture, which is focused in turn into the sample, forming an illuminated point of equal diameter. The light from the bright spot in the sample is then focused at a conjugate point through a second aperture in front of the detector. Light that lies out of focus is excluded from the detector because it is transferred through the lens system inefficiently. Therefore, confocal microscopy allows sampling in depth with minimum interference of the overlying and underlying structures. In vivo confocal microscopy is an imaging device that can be used in a clinical setting and provides surface and depth information. Epidermal thickness, shape of epidermal cells, melanin contained in various layers of the epidermis, the distribution of melanin granules, and the structure of the superficial dermis can all be visualized, compared, and analyzed (16).

Sebum

Sebum is a semiliquid mixture of lipids and cellular debris excreted by the sebaceous glands, which are found in highest concentrations on the face and scalp. The function of sebum can only be speculated upon. It does have some mild bactericidal and antifungal properties, but it probably does little in maintaining the skin's barrier function. Sebum production is largely controlled by endogenous hormone levels. Levels are highest during the teenage years, falling off in women after menopause and remaining relatively unchanged into old age in men. Excess sebum production can contribute to packing of horny cells at the follicle surface, leading to an occlusive plug or comedone. This is why its quantification and suppression are of great interest to dermatologists and cosmetic scientists.

Sebumeter

The measuring principle of this instrument is based on the observation that a ground glass plate of a certain opacity becomes translucent when its surface is covered by lipids. The translucency or light transmission increase is proportional to the amount of lipids on the surface (17). The Sebumeter uses a disposable opaque plastic tape in lieu of the glass plate. This tape is wound up in a plastic film cassette and runs through a protruding head that facilitates sebum collection. The head is pressed against the skin for 30 seconds with a fixed pressure. The film becomes transparent due to the absorbed sebum, and the resulting increase in transparency is measured via an optoelectronic method. The reading on the liquid crystal display corresponds to the sebum amount on the skin surface in micrograms per square centimeter. The Sebumeter is convenient to use since there is no need to clean the sampling surface and new tape is made available with a simple turn of a dial. However, it cannot give accurate readings when a site is measured several times since the method involves the removal of sebum from the skin's surface.

Skin Elasticity

The skin can be described as a complex material with elastic and viscous characteristics. Under a constant, continuous stress, its deformation increases slowly, and if the stress is removed, it does not immediately return to its original state and remains slightly deformed. These viscoelastic properties of the skin are due to the components of the dermis: collagen and elastin fibers impregnated in a ground substance of proteoglycans. Collagen limits the extensibility of the skin, elastin provides a return spring system allowing the collagen fibers to return to their original position after deformation, and proteoglycans contribute to the plastic behavior of skin (18).

Cutometer

The principle of the instrument is the application of a vacuum perpendicular to the skin surface and the measurement of the resulting deformation. A variable vacuum is applied on the skin through the opening of the probe. Skin deformation is measured by an optical system that detects the diminution of intensity of an infrared light beam caused by the penetration of the skin (18). The device consists of a main unit and a handheld probe. The main unit contains the vacuum pump, which can generate a vacuum between 50 and 500 mbar, the electronic circuit to control the pump, and the analog/digital data conversion. The standard probe, attached to the main unit with two rubber tubes, has a 2-mm circular opening for suction and is fitted with a spring to ensure that constant pressure is applied to the skin (19).

Under well-controlled experimental conditions where parameters such as load (vacuum), probe aperture, position, and pressure of application of the probe are kept constant, reproducible strain–time curves can be obtained.

Laser Doppler Perfusion

When skin tissue is illuminated by a coherent, monochromatic low-powered light (e.g., a low-power 670-nm solid-state laser beam), only a minor part is reflected back (around 3% to 7%). The remaining 93% to 97% of the incident radiation not returned by regular reflectance is partially absorbed by various structures and partially undergoes single or multiple scattering. A variable amount of this scattered light (>50% at 633 to 785 nm) is then remitted from the surface and is collected by a photodetector. The light recaptured by photodetector produces the raw signal, which is then converted mathematically to perfusion readings. The shifts in perfusion (either higher or lower) are interpreted depending on the product used or the objective of the study. Examples of instruments that use this technique include Periscan PIM II (Perimed, Sweden), Laserflo BPM (TSI, Minnesota, U.S.A.), MPM 3S (Oxford Optronix, Oxford, U.K.), and MBF3 series (Moor Instruments, Axminster, U.K.) (20,21).

Transcutaneous pO_2 and pCO_2

pO_2: With the Clark type pO_2 sensor, oxygen is measured amperometrically through reduction at a platinum (or gold) microcathode which is negatively polarized with respect to an Ag/AgCl reference electrode. The current measured is proportional to the oxygen partial pressure.

pCO_2: Based on the concept of Stow–Severinghaus, CO_2 molecules released from the skin diffuse through a hydrophobic membrane made of a highly gas-permeable material. The CO_2 then goes into a chamber inside a sensor filled with bicarbonate solution. Once CO_2 passes through the membrane, it becomes H_2CO_3 through slow reaction with water and then dissociates quickly into H^+ and CO_3^-. The H^+ ions create a potential in the Ag/AgCl glass electrode, which can be measured by a high-impedance voltmeter. Since potential is proportional to pH, the potential then is proportional to the logarithm of the CO_2 partial pressure. Some instruments that measure pO_2 and pCO_2 include TCM 3 (Radiometer Copenhagen, Denmark), Microgras 7650 (Kontron Instruments, Watford, U.K.), and Oxykapnomitor Servo Med SMK 365 and VICOM-sm SMU 612 (both from PPG Hellige GmbH, Germany) (22).

SKIN COLOR MEASUREMENTS

Changing the genetically determined color of skin by external topical agents is a very large consumer market worldwide. Much research is being carried out to understand the biologic basis of skin color and control points that can be manipulated by external treatments. To aid these efforts, methods to accurately and reproducibly measure skin color (as perceived by the consumer) and changes due to treatments, clinical and instrumental, are used. This section details various methods used commonly.

Visual cues are of primary importance for the accurate diagnosis of skin lesions or skin conditions in general (e.g., color). The human eye is extremely sensitive in grading different color intensities especially when there is a comparison available side by side. With an expert eye, a skin condition can be evaluated for size/area, color, degree of erythema and edema, roughness of the surface, etc. In addition, an expert grader automatically views a skin site stereoscopically by moving his/her head slightly and by varying both the observation and illumination angles to come to an "expert grading."

Clinical Grading: Ordinal scales are commonly used in clinical trials. Skin conditions are classified by degree of severity, e.g., none mild, moderate, severe, or evaluated by using a 10-point scale where a grade of 0 corresponds to the best or perfect condition and a grade of 9 to the worst or most severe condition (Figs. 1 and 2). This approach warrants the use of photo analogs to increase the objectivity and reproducibility of grading.

Nevertheless, although the human eye is very sensitive enough to distinguish subtle differences between two colors, the rating remains subjective. There are great differences in scoring between physicians, making it impossible to rate in a quantitative way the absolute difference between two colors. In addition, the human eye cannot memorize precisely a color. As such, comparison of two similar colors shown at different time periods is hard to perform. Since color perception is highly subjective (even with grading scales), nonlinear, and semiquantitative at best, noninvasive color-measuring devices have been developed and have become very popular in use in dermatocosmetic research. Majority of clinical research organizations

Attribute	0	1	2	3	4	5	6	7	8	9
Spot Lightening	No Pigmentation	Very Light Spots		Light Spots		Medium Dark Spots		Dark Spots		Very Dark Spots
Overall Fairness	Extremely Light	Very Light		Light		Medium Dark		Dark		Very Dark
Overall Evenness	Perfect Evenness	Very Slightly Blotchy		Slightly Blotchy		Medium Blotchy		Medium/ Severe Blotchy		Severe Blotchy

FIGURE 1 Typical scale commonly used in clinical trials.

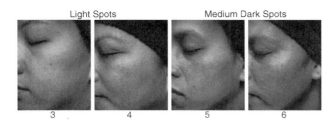

Light Spots   Medium Dark Spots

3   4   5   6

FIGURE 2 Photo analogs for a clinical grading scale.

or test centers normally have at least one of the instruments to complement clinical grading for a more holistic and accurate grading. Although it is impossible for any instrument to approach clinical evaluation, instrumental measurements do have its advantages. These include objectivity of the measurement and a linear response in detecting light, whereas the eye is a logarithmic detector. Instrumental evaluation thus gives out a number or a series of numbers that describe some aspects of skin appearance. Since instrumental results are normally continuous, more powerful and more sensitive statistical tools can be applied on the results, compared with the normally ordinal grading scale for expert grading.

Reflectance Measurements at Selected Bands

These instruments are based on the difference of absorption of melanin and hemoglobin. Hemoglobin has a peak light absorption at 560 nm (green light) and absorbs little light in the wavelength range of 650 to 700 nm (red light). The absorption spectrum of melanin is continuously decreasing from 450 to 700 nm. By selecting carefully the wavelength of incident light and measuring the reflected light, the respective contribution of hemoglobin and melanin to the total reflectance can be measured. An erythema index for hemoglobin and a melanin index for melanin can then be calculated from the intensity of the reflected light.

Top instruments using this measurement method include DermaSpectrometer (Cortex Technology, Hadsund, Denmark), erythema/melanin meter (DiasStron Ltd., Andover, U.K.), Mexameter® (Courage & Khazaka GmbH), UV-Optimize (Matik, Denmark). These instruments are popular since they are commercially available, simple to use, and usually have a convenient probe size. However, these methods have limitations in quantifying the relevant biological markers. This comes from the fact that absorption in the red part of the spectrum contains contributions from melanin and deoxyhemoglobin. The measurement also completely neglects the scattering effects on the measured reflectance. This allows no distinction between different types of hemoglobin or types of melanin. Another limitation is that color changes attributable to other chromophores, e.g., jaundice, cannot be measured (23–27).

CIE Colorimetry/The 'Tristimulus' System ($L^*a^*b^*$)

Westerhof describes the Commission Internationale de'l Eclairage (CIE) system as follows:

"The perceived color of objects depends on: (1) the nature of the illuminating light, (2) its modification by interaction with the object, and (3) the characteristics of the observer response." The CIE system defines these conditions as follows: "(1) The relative spectral energy distributions of various illuminants, known as CIE standard illuminants, are specified and available as published tables, (2) the modification of

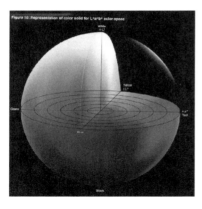

FIGURE 3 Color volume.

an illuminant by interaction with the object is measured with a reflectance spectrophotometer having an optical configuration that conforms to CIE recommendations, and provides a visible spectrum expressed as the fractions of incident light intensity reflected in the wavelength range 400–700 nm; (3) the nature of human color vision has been quantified for the purpose of color measurement in terms of three color matching functions x, y, z." (28).

The CIE system was modified in 1976 to a tristimulus system based on a psychophotometric method. In tristimulus analysis, intensity vs. wavelength data (i.e., spectral information) are converted into three numbers that indicate how a color of an object appears to a human observer, hence the psychophotometric characterization. All possible perceivable colors are represented in a three-dimensional space called "color volume" (Fig. 3).

The CIE $L^*a^*b^*$ has been developed to be closely and linearly correlated with the response of the human eye. The color is expressed in the following parameters:

L^* indicates light intensity and is related to the 'luminous reflectance' and takes values from 0 (black) to 100 (white). a^* and b^* are chromacity coordinates (hue of a color), with the a^* axis going from –60 for green to +60 for red and b^* axis going from –60 for blue to +60 for yellow.

Axes a^* and b^* cross the L^* axis at their zero values. Colors which are located at zero values for a^* and b^* are achromic, either gray, white, or black. In the study of skin color, only the positive sides of the a^* and b^* parameters are considered (i.e., red and yellow). The saturation of the color is described as the distance from the L^* axis to the point of the a^*–b^* plane (Fig. 4). The total color is described as using the respective $L^*a^*b^*$ color parameters or using the mathematical expression for E equal to

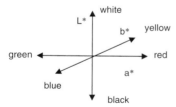

FIGURE 4 CIE $L^*a^*b^*$ color system.

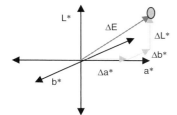

FIGURE 5   Color difference in the CIE $L^*a^*b^*$ space.

$$E = \sqrt{L^{*2} + a^{*2} + b^{*2}}$$

Changes in color or pigmentation can be calculated as

$$\Delta E = \sqrt{\Delta L^{*2} + \Delta a^{*2} + \Delta b^{*2}}$$

Erythema is often evaluated using the a^* parameter. Pigmentation is evaluated by the values of L^*, b^*, or combinations of them (Fig. 5) (28–31). Stamatas et al. (26) described the correlation of L^*, a^*, and b^* with reflectance measurements and factors affecting the measurements in the following manner:

a^* correlates closely with the erythema index of the narrow-band instruments. L^* and b^* show weak correlations with the melanin index. In particular, increases in hemoglobin concentrations can decrease both values of L^* and b^* in the absence of any change in melanin pigmentation. a^* values are influenced by melanin concentrations. In UVA-induced persistent pigment darkening, the b^* value was found to initially decrease and later increase as the yellow component of newly generated melanin becomes prominent.

In a three-dimensional $L^*a^*b^*$ space, all skin colors of light-complexioned subjects fall within a banana-shaped volume (skin color volume). Increases in skin pigmentation can be graphed as a shift on the L^*–b^* plane, whereas skin reddening (erythema reaction) is represented as a shift on the L^*–a^* plane" (26).

One calculated parameter based on the $L^*a^*b^*$ system is the individual typology angle (ITA) or alpha characteristic angle. This is defined as the vector direction in the L^*–b^* plane:

ITA° = (ArcTangent(L^* - 50) / b^*) × 180 / π

The ITA values are inversely related to skin pigmentation. According to ITA values, skin color can be classified into the following categories:

Very Light > 55° > Light > 41° > Intermediate > 28° > Tan > 10°

This parameter has been validated as an expression of skin pigmentation by analysis of diffuse reflectance measurements. ITA has its limitations though due to the effect of other chromophores other than melanin, which can visually simulate pigmentation. For example, an increase in local concentration of deoxyhemoglobin has a similar effect on ITA as increases in melanin pigmentation (32).

The $L^*a^*b^*$ system originally has been used in the paint and color reproduction industry. This system has been widely used in the study of skin color due in part to its ease of use and the commercial availability of instruments that calculate $L^*a^*b^*$ values, generally called as colorimeters. Some of the colorimeters manufactured include Labscan (Hunter Associates Inc., Pennsylvania, U.S.A.), Chromameter® (Minolta,

Osaka, Japan), Dr. Lange Micro Color (Dr. Bruno Lange GmbH, Dusseldorf, Germany) and Photovolt (UMM Electronics, Indianapolis, U.S.A). The sizes of the probes are not small due to the size of an internal integrating sphere necessary for the measurements. Hence, these instruments can be used on flat areas like the forearm, but not on areas of high curvature (e.g., under the eye, nasolabial fold, etc.). As mentioned above, another limitation of this type of measurement is the inability to differentiate which chromophores are contributing to the color that is seen (29).

Diffuse Reflectance Spectroscopy

The visual perception of skin color is the cumulative result of contributions of several chromophores found in varying concentrations in the skin. The most abundant skin chromophores are melanin, oxyhemoglobin and deoxyhemoglobin. The corresponding absorption profiles are shown in Fig. 6. In the visible region, oxyhemoglobin has two maxima at 542 and 577 nm (known as the alpha–beta or q-bands), whereas deoxyhemoglobin has one at 555 nm. These local maxima provide a convenient wavelength region (green–yellow) for the quantification of these absorbers. As for melanin, although it also has low absorption in longer wavelengths, its relative absorption is more prominent than that of oxyhemoglobin and deoxyhemoglobin. Thus, the red region can be used for pigmentation measurements (16).

Aside from absorption, another mode of interaction of light with skin is scattering, the changing of the direction of travel of light. Collagen and elastin, the extracellular matrix components of the dermis, are very strong scatterers.

Spectroscopic methods allow for the quantification of chromophores and scatterers in the skin. The contribution of melanin, oxyhemoglobin, deoxyhemoglobin, and scattering to skin color can be extracted from absorption spectra obtained via diffuse reflectance spectroscopy (DRS). DRS measurements are rapid, noninvasive, and quantitative, and the instrument is small and easy to use. The DRS instrument (Fig. 7) consists of a halogen light source, a bifurcated fiber bundle, a spectrometer, and a laptop computer. One leg of the fiber bundle is connected to the light source and the other to the spectrometer. Measurements are performed by placing the common end of the fiber bundle in contact with the skin site. The fiber bundle that collects the reflected light delivers it to an analyzer that disperses the light and gives a complete spectrum of the reflected light. This spectrum, which is a record of the intensity of the reflected light as a function of wavelength, can then be analyzed for the contributions of each chromophore. From the absorbance curve, melanin concentration is estimated as the slope of the fitted line over the range of 620–720 nm, whereas oxyhemoglobin and deoxyhemoglobin concentrations are estimated by the

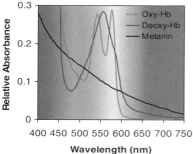

FIGURE 6   Chromophore absorption profiles.

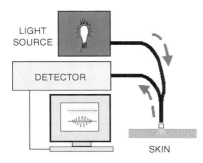

FIGURE 7 DRS instrument. *Abbreviation*: DRS, diffuse reflectance spectroscopy.

maxima in the range of 540–580 nm. The results are given as apparent concentrations for each chromophore (33).

Imaging

Digital photography provides a two-dimensional record of the appearance of the skin. It has an important advantage over other instrumental methods: It involves no direct contact with the skin and therefore does not interfere with the measurement of skin color e.g., blanching. Not only is it useful for documenting skin condition, it also allows for quantification of relevant parameters using advanced image analysis software. This combination–photography and image analysis–is an attempt to capture and reproduce what the eye–brain sees and grades in expert assessment.

An imaging system consists of an illumination source, the camera lens, the detector, and often filters in front of the source and/or lens. Proper calibration is essential to ensure color reproducibility. It is often done by taking an image of a gray card of known reflectivity and adjusting the camera or light source settings so that the intensities in the gray card image are consistent for the duration of an experiment.

Color digital cameras create color views of a scene by combining three images acquired simultaneously at three different spectral bands: red, green, and blue. These bands approximate the light sensitivity of the cones in the human eye. In the green channel image, erythema appears black and normal skin white. The blue channel is normally used for examining melanin since it absorbs light more in the UV-blue part of the spectrum. However, hemoglobin also absorbs in this region and must be considered during image analysis. The red channel can serve as an alternative for this purpose because melanin is the predominant chromophore in this region. Image analysis software is available which converts images from the red, green, and blue space to the $L^*a^*b^*$ space provided that the acquired images have been properly calibrated (26).

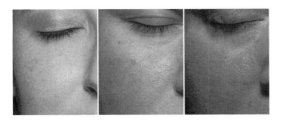

FIGURE 8 Sample pictures for polarized light photography.

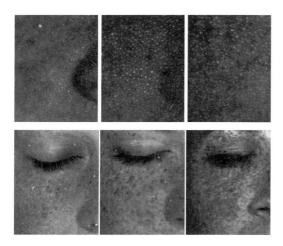

FIGURE 9 Sample pictures for fluorescence photography.

Specialized techniques such as polarized light and fluorescence photography have been introduced to supplement regular photography in documenting specific features. In polarized light photography, linear polarizing filters are used both on the camera lens and on the flash to selectively enhance surface features, such as fine lines and wrinkles, scales, and pores, or subsurface features, such as erythema, pigmentation, and capillaries (Fig. 8) (34).

In fluorescence photography, the flash is filtered to emit radiation in the long UVA (360–400 nm) and the camera is filtered to receive only radiation that is emitted by the skin (440–700 nm). This technique has been used to enhance the distribution of solar lentigines, *Propionibacterium acnes*, and open comedones (Fig. 9).

Spectral Imaging

A more accurate method to quantify chromophore distribution is to use a hyperspectral imaging system. In spectral imaging, a series of images of the same view are acquired. Each image represents the reflected light of the scene at a specific wavelength. This results in a three-dimensional array of images, where each pixel in the stack has a corresponding spectrum (Fig. 10). The acquired spectra can then be analyzed by using the same calculations used with the DRS to obtain chromophore values for each pixel. The end result is a distribution map of a particular chromophore. Fig. 11 is an example of an oxyhemoglobin map.

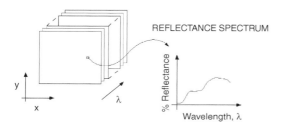

FIGURE 10 Spectral imaging.

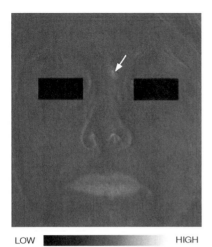

LOW　　　　　　　HIGH　　**FIGURE 11**　Oxyhemoglobin map.

CORRELATION OF INSTRUMENTS WITH EXPERT ASSESSMENT

Expert grading and self-assessment are carried out using semiobjective scales as given below for fine lines and wrinkles. Similar scales are used for other clinical end points. Photographic aids are used to train graders and as guides for self-assessment.

None	Very slight lines		Slight lines		Wrinkles form as skin moves		Wrinkles visible at all times		Severe & deep throughout
0	1	2	3	4	5	6	7	8	9

There have been numerous studies detailing the correlation of results from different kinds of color measurements vs. expert grading assessment. Generally, the instruments show good correlation with expert grading assessment. In one correlation assessment done on a clinical study on Chinese skin (Shanghai, China, September–October 2005), the following comparisons were made:

- Mexameter melanin index vs. expert grading of fairness
- Mexameter erythema index vs. expert grading of irritation/erythema
- Chromameter L^* value vs. expert grading of fairness
- Chromameter a^* value vs. expert grading of irritation/erythema
- Chromameter b^* value vs. expert grading of sallowness

In this study, it was concluded that dermatological assessment of sallowness and fairness is strongly correlated with instrumental measurements. In terms of erythema, there was a low to moderate correlation (Fig. 12).

As discussed in the previous sections, this does not mean that one method is wrong and the other is right, but a more probable cause of the results is the intrinsic shortcomings of each method (e.g., subjectivity of expert graders vis-a-vis incomplete capabilities of bioengineering instruments). Hence, this shows again the

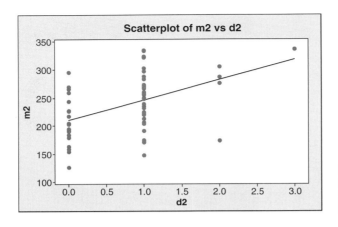

FIGURE 12 Correlation of Mexameter erythema index (m2) versus expert grading of erythema (d2).

importance of combining expert grading and instrumental measurement to obtain a holistic assessment of skin conditions (Galzote, unpublished data, 2005).

CONCLUSIONS

A typical dermatological examination relies primarily on the trained eyes of the physician. Together with one's mind, which contains a large library of images accumulated through the years, the eye–brain tandem is indeed a powerful tool for evaluating the skin. In addition, one's capability to view a skin site at different angles to minimize glare and maximize contrast makes it even more difficult for images and point measurements to approximate the information collected by the physician in its totality.

However, visual inspection remains subjective, semiquantitative at best. The assessment of one clinician will most likely be different from that of another due to a variety of factors such as room lighting conditions, years of professional experience, and even ethnocultural background of the evaluator and/or subject. In addition, even if the human eye is capable of differentiating between colors, it only works best with high contrast, i.e., pigmented lesion surrounded by normal skin, making it difficult to quantify color perception without the aid of instrumental means.

Thus, the best approach to obtain an objective and accurate evaluation of skin pigmentation is to incorporate both expert grading and instrumental measurements into the clinical trial.

REFERENCES

1. Distante F, Berardesca E. Hydration. In: Berardesca E, Elsner P, Wilhelm KP, et al, eds. Bioengineering of the Skin: Methods and Instrumentation. Boca Raton: CRC Press, 1995:5–12.
2. Corneometer® CM 825, Germany. Technical Information.
3. Skicon® 200, Japan, Technical Information.
4. Distante F, Berardesca E. Transepidermal water loss. In: Berardesca E, Elsner P, Wilhelm KP, et al, eds. Bioengineering of the Skin: Methods and Instrumentation. Boca Raton: CRC Press, 1995:1–4.
5. Tewameter® TM 210, Germany. Technical Information.
6. Vapometer®, Finland. Tehcnical Information.

7. Welzel J. pH and Ions. In: Berardesca E, Elsner P, Wilhelm KP, et al, eds. Bioengineering of the Skin: Methods and Instrumentation. Boca Raton: CRC Press, 1995:91–93.
8. Articus K, Khazaka G, Wilhelm KP. The skin visiometer—a photometric device for the measurement of skin roughness. In: Wilhelm KP, Elsner P, Berardesca E, et al, eds. Bioengineering of the Skin: Skin Surface Imaging and Analysis. Boca Raton: CRC Press, 1997:59–72.
9. Serup J. Skin imaging techniques. In: Berardesca E, Elsner P, Wilhelm KP, et al, eds. Bioengineering of the Skin: Methods and Instrumentation. Boca Raton: CRC Press, 1995: 65–69.
10. Visioscan, Germany. Technical Information.
11. PRIMOS, Germany. Technical Information.
12. Elsnau WH. Skin friction measurement. In: Berardesca E, Elsner P, Wilhelm KP, et al, eds. Bioengineering of the Skin: Methods and Instrumentation. Boca Raton: CRC Press, 1995:121–124.
13. Frictiometer, Germany. Technical Information.
14. Miller D. Sticky slides and tape techniques to harvest stratum corneum material. In: Serup J, Jemec GBE, eds. Handbook of Non-Invasive Methods and the Skin. Boca Raton: CRC Press, 1995:149–151.
15. Stamatas GN. Skinskan Standard Operating Procedures. 1999.
16. Kollias N, Stamatas GN. Optical non-invasive approaches to diagnosis of skin diseases. J Investig Dermatol Symp Proc 2002; 7:64–75.
17. Elsner P. Sebum. In: Berardesca E, Elsner P, Wilhelm KP, et al, eds. Bioengineering of the Skin: Methods and Instrumentation. Boca Raton: CRC Press, 1995:81–85.
18. Barel AO, Courage W, Clarys P. Suction method for measurement of skin mechanical properties. In: Serup J, Jemec GBE, eds. Handbook of Non-Invasive Methods and the Skin. Boca Raton: CRC Press, 1995:335–339.
19. Elsner P. Skin elasticity. In: Berardesca E, Elsner P, Wilhelm KP, et al, eds. Bioengineering of the Skin: Methods and Instrumentation. Boca Raton: CRC Press, 1995:53–57.
20. Bernardi L, Berardesca E. Measurement of skin blood flow by laser-Doppler flowmetry. In: Berardesca E, Elsner P, Wilhelm KP, et al, eds. Bioengineering of the Skin: Methods and Instrumentation. Boca Raton: CRC Press, 1995:13–28.
21. Periscan PIM II, Sweden, Technical Information.
22. Roszinski S. Transcutaneous pO_2 and pCO_2 measurements. In: Berardesca E, Elsner P, Wilhelm KP, et al, eds. Bioengineering of the Skin: Methods and Instrumentation. Boca Raton: CRC Press, 1995:95–104.
23. Babel AO. Measurement of the color changes of the skin. In: Barel, ed. Color Changes. pp451–469.
24. Takiwaki H, Serup J. Measurement of erythema and melanin indices. In: Serup J, Jemec GBE, eds. Handbook of Non-Invasive Methods and the Skin. Boca Raton: CRC Press, 1995:377–384.
25. Kollias N. The Physical Basis of Skin Color and Its Evaluation. New York: Elsevier Science Inc., 1995:365.
26. Stamatas GN, Zmudzka BZ, Kollias N, et al. Non-invasive measurements of skin pigmentation in situ. Pigment Cell Res 2004; 17:618–626.
27. Mexameter, Courage & Khazaka, Germany, Technical Information.
28. Westerhof W. CIE Colorimetry. In: Serup J, Jemec GBE, eds. Handbook of Non-Invasive Methods and the Skin. Boca Raton: CRC Press, 1995:377–384.
29. Minolta Chromameter CR-300, Japan, Technical Information.
30. Elsner P. Skin color. In: Berardesca E, Elsner P, Wilhelm KP, et al, eds. Bioengineering of the Skin: Methods and Instrumentation. Boca Raton: CRC Press, 1995:29–40.
31. Chardon A, Cretois I, Hourseau C. Skin color typology and suntanning pathways. Int J Cosmet Sci 1991; 13:191–208.
32. Choe YB, Jang SJ, Jo SJ, et al. The difference between the constitutive and facultative skin color does not reflect skin phototype in Asian skin. Skin Res Technol 2006; 12:68–72.
33. Stamatas GN, Kollias N. Visual versus spectroscopic analysis of skin color reactions: separation of contributing chromophores. Internal report, pp1–4.
34. Kollias N. Polarized light photography of human skin. In: Wilhelm KP, Elsner P, Berardesca E, et al, eds. Bioengineering of the Skin: Skin Surface Imaging and Analysis. Boca Raton: CRC Press, 1997:95–104.

Application of In Vivo Scanning Microscopy for Skin Analysis in Dermatology and Cosmetology

Lars E. Meyer and Juergen Lademann
Universitätsklinikum Charité, Klinik für Dermatologie, Venerologie und Allergologie, Berlin, Germany

INTRODUCTION

The skin is the largest organ of our body and the boundary to the environment. Analysis of skin structure is essential for dermatological diagnoses and therapy control, as well as for the investigation of cosmetic products. In recent years, laser scanning microscopy (LSM) has achieved substantial improvements in the imaging of dermal tissue in vivo. Nowadays, laser microscopic systems on the open market are either significantly reduced in size or are fiber-based with handheld scanning devices, allowing a simple in vivo application and evaluation of the skin on any region of the body (1–5).

In 1955, the first confocal laser scanning microscope was developed by Minsky for studying neuronal networks in the living brain (6). Recently, the technique of LSM has improved significantly. Although the general operating mechanism has remained the same, the apparatus is now smaller and therefore more flexible, cheaper, and has a higher resolution.

Using confocal LSM, laser light is focused onto a small spot within the dermal tissue. A recurring light signal from the focal plane is collected simultaneously and used to obtain a confocal image. A special optical system ensures that only the light returning directly from the focal point is detected. Prevention of any scattered and reflected light from out-of-focus planes increases the imaging contrast. Moving the focus deeper into the tissue allows different cell layers to be observed. The high-resolution images contain information on the histological structure of the epidermis and the upper parts of the underlying dermis. The different epidermal layers (stratum corneum, stratum granulosum, stratum spinosum, and stratum basale) can be observed and distinguished by differences in their typical depth, cell size, and shape. Depending on the applied illumination wavelengths, it is also possible to analyze the capillary structure in the papillary dermis.

In contrast to conventional skin histology, where vertical images of the skin samples are obtained, LSM provides sectioning of thin horizontal tissue planes. The sampling plane can be adjusted and positioned below the skin surface to offer subsurface evaluation. Altogether, in vivo confocal imaging permits real-time scan sequences with images in microscopic resolution and in horizontal view (en face). In Figure 1, a vertical histology section illustrates the en face view received by confocal imaging. The corresponding laser scanning microscopic images were captured in different epidermal layers. The superficial stratum corneum and the deeper stratum spinosum, including bright papillae of the papillary dermis, can be analyzed.

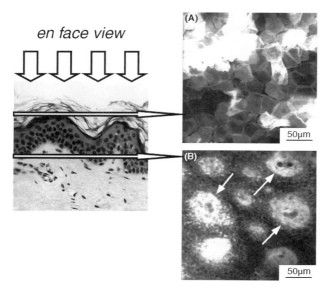

en face view

FIGURE 1 Comparison of a vertical histosection with the horizontal view by LSM on a dermal tissue sample. The superficial stratum corneum contains the corneocytes (**A**), whereas the deeper stratum spinosum (**B**) presents smaller epidermal cells (keratinocytes), embedding bright papillae with dark blood vessels (arrows). *Abbreviation*: LSM, laser scanning microscopy.

Different types of dermatological in vivo laser scanning microscopes are commercially available (7–9). Depending on the laser source, the detection mode, and the usage of a contrast dye, three different modes of in vivo confocal LSM have been established in dermatology: the reflectance, the Raman spectroscopic, and the fluorescence modes.

The reflectance mode is based on differences in the scattering properties of the various tissue microstructures. The laser beam is reflected irregularly by the heterogeneous dermal components. Only backscattered in-focus signals are captured for visualization. Generally, the greater the differences in the refractive index of the skin structures, the stronger the contrast of the images. In particular, melanin and keratin have high refractive indices, producing a bright contrast in the reflectance mode of LSM.

In the fluorescence mode, the application of a fluorescent dye is necessary. It can be applied topically and/or injected into the tissue. Thereafter, a laser is used to selectively excite the applied agent. The fluorescence emission is detected and exploited to create an imaging contrast. Subsequently, the distribution of the dye is analyzed by LSM. Because of the varying distribution patterns of the dye, cellular structures of the skin become visible.

Nevertheless, the clinical implementation of the fluorescence mode might be restricted in the case of scanning the deeper dermis or the injection of a fluorescent dye into malignant skin lesions. Generally, fluorescent measurements lead to a strong imaging contrast, allowing a precise identification of different skin structures. Reflection measurements are mostly carried out in the near-infrared range of the spectrum, where the penetration depth of the laser radiation is deeper than in the visible spectrum of the fluorescence light. Adversely, the contrast is less than with fluorescence measurements. Therefore experience is needed for the interpretation of the reflectance images.

Raman spectroscopic LSM is based on the detection of Raman spectra in the focal plane, which are characteristic of tissue molecules or of topically applied substances. Compared with fluorescence and reflection LSM, Raman microscopy does not deliver an image of the morphological structure but rather it provides chemical information with regard to the tissue.

Fluorescence and Raman spectroscopic laser scanning measurements are often used in cosmetics for the analysis of the distribution and the penetration process of topically applied fluorescent-labeled substances. In dermatology, in vivo LSM is used to distinguish between healthy and pathological cell structures for diagnoses and therapeutic procedures.

Typical commercially available confocal laser scanning microscopes are the Stratum® System (OptiScan, Ltd., Melbourne, Victoria, Australia), the near-infrared VivaScope® (Lucid, Inc., Henrietta, New Jersey, U.S.A.), and the Raman laser scanning microscope produced by River Diagnostics (Rotterdam, Netherlands). In the Stratum system, a single-line argon ion laser with a wavelength at 488 nm is used for scanning. The skin area under investigation is $250 \times 250\ \mu m^2$. Skin structures up to a depth of 200 μm can be analyzed using this system. The Stratum operates in the fluorescent and reflection mode. The VivaScope 1500 is a reflectance microscope working with a near-infrared laser at a wavelength of 830 nm. Skin structures can be examined up to a depth of 250–300 μm, and the single test field of view is $500 \times 500\ \mu m^2$. In Figure 2, images obtained by the laser scanning microscopes Stratum and VivaScope are compared for the stratum corneum and the stratum spinosum. In the fluorescence mode of the Stratum, single corneocytes located in the stratum

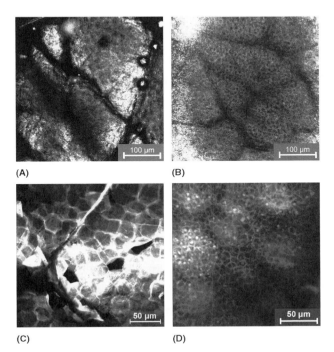

(A)   (B)

(C)   (D)

FIGURE 2 Images of the stratum corneum and the stratum spinosum taken by the laser scanning microscopes VivaScope (**A**, **B**) and Stratum (**C**, **D**).

corneum can be clearly recognized. Similar concrete images of the skin surface cannot be obtained by the VivaScope. The cell borders in deeper epidermal layers, such as the stratum spinosum, can be well observed with both LSM systems. The Raman microscope (River Diagnostics) is based on an argon ion pumped titanium–sapphire laser, which irradiates in the near-infrared spectrum at a wavelength of approximately 850 nm.

SKIN ANALYSIS IN COSMETOLOGY AND DRUG DELIVERY
Distribution of Topically Applied Drugs in the Skin
In the past, it was assumed that the intercellular route through the lipid layers surrounding the corneocytes was the main penetration pathway for topically applied substances. Recently, it was found that the hair follicles also represent an efficient penetration pathway through the skin barrier (10). A space-resolving online in vivo method is required for the analysis of the penetration and distribution of topically applied substances frequently used in dermatology and cosmetology. Confocal LSM is well suited for this. Using LSM, Otberg et al. (10) found that the reservoir in the hair follicles in different body regions is comparable to the reservoir of the stratum corneum for topically applied substances. Additionally, they demonstrated the distinction between open and closed hair follicles. Closed hair follicles are covered with a film of desquamated corneocytes and dried sebum (11), a cover that can be easily removed by washing or by soft peeling. Open follicles are more efficiently penetrable for topically applied substances into the follicular reservoir. The distribution of a dye-labeled drug in different depths of the hair follicles can be analyzed by fluorescent measurements. A typical example is shown in Figure 3.

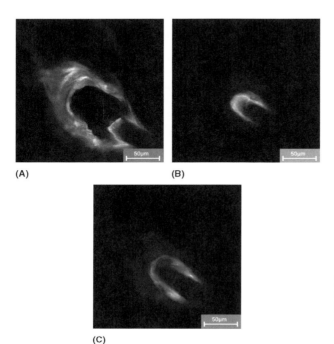

(A) (B)

(C)

FIGURE 3 In vivo LSM image of a fluorescent dye's distribution at different depths of the human hair follicle. *Abbreviation*: LSM, laser scanning microscopy.

Because LSM is a noninvasive process, it is possible to analyze the penetration kinetics of topically applied substances into the hair follicles and into the stratum corneum in vivo. Figure 4 shows the penetration of a topically applied formulation into the skin surface. Five minutes after the application, the formulation was located only in the superficial corneocyte layer. Ten minutes later, the fluorescent dye could also be detected in the fourth layer of the stratum corneum. The thin flat corneocytes are transparent for laser radiation, the penetration process can easily be followed, and deeper cell layers gradually become visible. Tape stripping or differential stripping should be used for the quantitative analysis of the dye's amount in the stratum corneum or the hair follicles (12).

Additionally, it is possible to investigate the homogeneity of distribution of topically applied formulations by using LSM. This is especially important in the field of sunscreen research, where the homogeneity of the distribution is directly correlated with the sun protection efficiency (13,14). A typical example of an inhomogeneous distribution of sunscreen on the skin is shown in Figure 5. The distribution of a dye-containing formulation in the lipid layers around the corneocytes can be noticed as a bright contrast. Furrows and wrinkles act as a reservoir, pooling a significant amount of the sunscreen (15). In the present figure, this phenomenon can be seen: a large fraction of the applied sunscreen (bright line) is detected in and around the furrow.

The application of nano- and microparticles is a new approach for an efficient drug delivery route through the skin barrier. Whereas particles of a size greater than 5 μm cover the skin surface homogeneously (Fig. 6A), nanoparticles at a size of about 100 nm can penetrate into the lipid layers and into the hair follicles (Fig. 6B). Surprisingly, it was found that nanoparticles at a size of 300 nm penetrate more efficiently into the hair follicles than nonparticulate substances (16). The reason for this effect could be the moving hair, acting as a geared pump, pushing the nanoparticles deeper into the follicles (17). In the follicle reservoir, they are stored for a longer time than in the stratum corneum. Therefore hair follicles represent an interesting

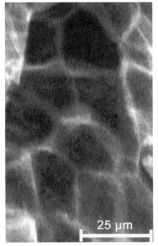
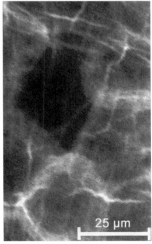

25 μm

25 μm

(A)   (B)

FIGURE 4 Penetration kinetics of a fluorescent-labeled dye into the stratum corneum: (**A**) 5 and (**B**) 15 minutes after application.

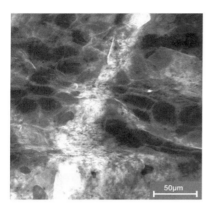

FIGURE 5 Distribution of a dye-containing sunscreen in the upper layer of the stratum corneum. The broad bright line represents a furrow, where significant amounts of sunscreen were located.

target for drug delivery, particularly because of the close neighborhood to the surrounding blood capillaries, hosted stem cells, and dendritic cells. The penetration effect stimulated by the moving hairs can be observed in vivo for nanoparticles only. To date, LSM is the sole method that allows such in vivo investigations to be carried out.

Penetration measurements based on the fluorescence mode of LSM need a combination of the dermatological or cosmetic product with a fluorescent dye. The disadvantage is that the formulation can have different penetration characteristics compared with the matrix. Therefore the direct detection of topically applied drugs in the skin is of great interest in research. Raman microscopic measurement enables the scanning of applied substances without an additional use of a fluorescent dye (18). Unfortunately, the chemical structure of some tissue compounds is often similar to topically applied substances. In such cases, it often becomes difficult to distinguish between the substances and the tissue. It has been demonstrated that Raman microscopic measurement is a good method for the determination of water distribution in different depths of the stratum corneum and the living epidermis (19,20). The analysis of water distribution in the skin is of great interest for the characterization of the barrier function of the skin and for therapy control. Additionally, it can be used to analyze the efficacy of moisturizing creams in cosmetology.

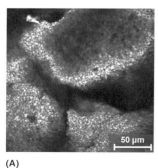

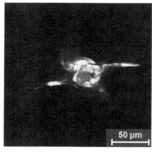

(A)   (B)

FIGURE 6 Particles smaller than 5 µm are located on the skin surface (**A**), whereas nanoparticles of a diameter of about 100 nm penetrate into the hair follicles (**B**).

ANALYSIS OF SKIN STRUCTURE FOR DIAGNOSES AND THERAPY CONTROL
Investigation of Cell Membrane Properties

Subsurface imaging of the skin is possible using fluorescence LSM after an intradermal injection of a fluorescent dye (21,22). When imaging is performed continuously for several minutes after the dye's application, a diffusion of the dye from extra- to intracellular regions can be observed (Fig. 7). Five minutes after application, the dye was found around the epidermal cells, but after 20 minutes, the nuclei were stained and highlighted. The kinetics of the diffusion process characterizes the properties of the cell membranes. Diseases and treatment of the skin influence kinetic processes significantly.

Only fluorescence LSM permits such a functional investigation with microscopic resolution in vivo (23). The hydrophilic fluorescein and the lipophilic curcumin are highly suitable fluorescent dyes for the evaluation of cell membranes.

Analysis of Mycoses by LSM

Standard diagnostic procedures for fungal infections include light-microscopic analyses of scrapings, fungal cultivations, and skin biopsies. Diagnoses can therefore be time-consuming and invasive (24). The application of fluorescence and reflectance LSM shortens and simplifies the diagnostic procedure. It allows real-time imaging of fungal microstructures on the human skin in vivo (23). In Figure 8, a yeast colony of the ubiquitous genus *Malassezia* is presented in their native habitat using the Stratum, forming a part of the normal cutaneous microflora (25).

Application of LSM in Diagnoses and Therapy Control of Skin Cancer

Nonmelanomous skin cancer represents the most common malignant neoplasia in human skin. In such cancers, 65% are basal cell carcinomas (BCC) and 20% are spinal cell carcinomas (SCC). Additionally, actinic keratosis (AK) represents the most common dermal precancerous condition. Eighty percent of all elderly adults with skin types I or II suffer from this disease (26). This explains the considerable importance of diagnostic research in dermatology. Diagnosis is usually performed by examining skin biopsies. The LSM represents a promising approach for noninvasive diagnosis and therapy control in skin cancer treatment. For example, Dietterle (27) demonstrated that fluorescence LSM could be used successfully for therapy control in the treatment of BCCs with imiquimod.

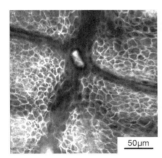

(A)

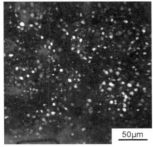

(B)

FIGURE 7 LSM fluorescence images obtained (**A**) 5 and (**B**) 20 minutes after application of a dye-containing formulation; immediately after application, the dye is located in the intercellular space; after 20 minutes, the dye has penetrated into the cells, staining the nuclei. *Abbreviation*: LSM, laser scanning microscopy.

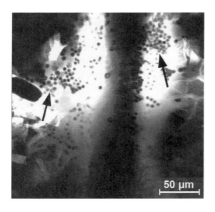

FIGURE 8 Laser scanning microscopic image obtained from healthy scalp skin. Small oval yeasts colonize a hair on the skin surface.

It is well known from histological investigations that BCC, SCC, and AK lesion are characterized by several joint morphological structures. BCC, SCC, and AK show hyperkeratosis as well as parakeratosis. Damage to the stratum granulosum can be detected in the case of AK only. Horizontal vascular loops are characteristic in the case of BCC. Pleomorphic nuclei can be detected in the case of AK and SCC, whereas BCC shows elongated cell nuclei. These differences in morphology can be used to distinguish between BCC, SCC, and AK using LSM. Typical examples are presented in Figure 9 (27).

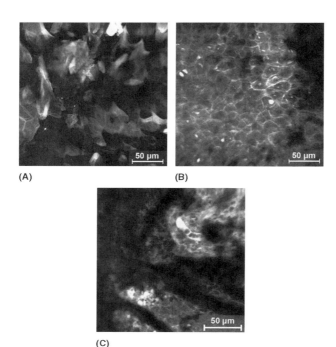

FIGURE 9 Changes in the morphological structures in the case of AK, SCC, and BCC. (**A**) AK: hyperkeratosis; (**B**) SCC: damage of the stratum granulosum (atypical pleomorphic cells and nuclei, loss of the regular architecture of the epidermis); (**C**) BCC, enlarged papillae with elongated blood vessels (cellular atypia, widened papillae, including elongated bright blood vessels with dark blood cells). *Abbreviations*: AK, actinic keratosis; SCC, spinal cell carcinoma; BCC, basal cell carcinoma.

The application of a fluorescent dye allows the detection of a pathological skin structure. Similar results can be observed in the reflectance mode of LSM, although the imaging contrast is not as good (3). Raman LSM was used to discriminate basal cell carcinoma from the surrounding tissue by identifying different chemical compositions in healthy tissue and basal cell carcinoma (28).

SUMMARY

In conclusion, three different types of LSM are commercially available for pharmacological purposes and physiological investigations. The fluorescence LSM can be used for penetration and distribution studies of topically applied substances labeled with a contrast dye. Additionally, morphological structures can be seen after an intradermal injection of a fluorescent agent. The necessity of a dye represents the main limitation for this method; dye-labeling of medical or cosmetic skin agents is a complicated process and dye injections are not always appropriate, such as in malignant skin lesions.

LSM measurement in the reflectance mode does not have such limitations. Nevertheless, the imaging contrast is less compared with the fluorescence LSM measurements. The field of application of the reflectance LSM covers histometric analyses of skin parameters, as well as comparisons between the healthy aspect and the pathological state of living skin.

The Raman LSM is generally the first choice for the detection of chemical compounds in the skin. One of the main applications of Raman LSM is the analysis of the water distribution in the stratum corneum and deeper skin layers.

Finally, the considerable developments and improvements for LSM in the light source, computer technology, and optical system (e.g., flexible fiber-based devices) offer new possibilities in the fields of dermatological and cosmetic research. The confocal systems became smaller, cheaper, and achieve a higher resolution. The noninvasive character of these methods guarantees an increased use in skin studies in the future.

REFERENCES

1. Zheng P, Kramer CE, Barnes CW, et al. Noninvasive glucose determination by oscillating thermal gradient spectrometry. Diabetes Technol Ther 2000; 2:17–25.
2. Nouveau-Richard S, Monot M, Bastien P, et al. In vivo epidermal thickness measurement: ultrasound vs. confocal imaging. Skin Res Technol 2004; 10:136–140.
3. Sauermann K, Gambichler T, Wilmert M, et al. Investigation of basal cell carcinoma [correction of carcionoma] by confocal laser scanning microscopy in vivo. Skin Res Technol 2002; 8:141–147.
4. Caspers PJ, Lucassen GW, Puppels GJ. Combined in vivo confocal Raman spectroscopy and confocal microscopy of human skin. Biophys J 2003; 85:572–580.
5. Lademann J, Meyer LE, Otberg N, et al. New insights into the skin—application of a dermatological laser scanning microscope in skin physiology. Skin Res Technol 2004; 10:8.
6. Minsky M. Microscopy apparatus. U.S. Patent 3013467, November 7, 1957, 1961.
7. McLaren W, Anikijenko P, Barkla D, et al. In vivo detection of experimental ulcerative colitis in rats using fiberoptic confocal imaging (FOCI). Dig Dis Sci 2001; 46:2263–2276.
8. Gambichler T, Sauermann K, Altintas MA, et al. Effects of repeated sunbed exposures on the human skin. In vivo measurements with confocal microscopy. Photodermatol Photoimmunol Photomed 2004; 20:27–32.
9. Caspers PJ, Lucassen GW, Wolthuis R, et al. In vitro and in vivo Raman spectroscopy of human skin. Biospectroscopy 1998; 4:S31–S39.

10. Otberg N, Richter H, Schaefer H, et al. Variations of hair follicle size and distribution in different body sites. J Invest Dermatol 2004; 122:14–19.
11. Otberg N, Richter H, Knuettel A, et al. Laser spectroscopic methods for the characterization of open and closed follicles. Laser Phys Lett 2004; 1:46–49.
12. Teichmann A, Jacobi U, Ossadnik M, et al. Differential stripping: determination of the amount of topically applied substances penetrated into the hair follicles. J Invest Dermatol 2005; 125:264–269.
13. Lademann J, Rudolph A, Jacobi U, et al. Influence of nonhomogeneous distribution of topically applied UV filters on sun protection factors. J Biomed Opt 2004; 9:1358–1362.
14. Weigmann HJ, Schanzer S, Herrling J, et al. Spectroscopic characterization of the sunscreen efficacy—basis of a universal sunscreen protection factor. SÖFW J 2006; 9:2–10.
15. Lademann J, Weigmann HJ, Schanzer S, et al. Optical investigations to avoid the disturbing influences of furrows and wrinkles quantifying penetration of drugs and cosmetics into the skin by tape stripping. J Biomed Opt 2005; 10:054015.
16. Lademann J, Richter H, Schaefer UF, et al. Hair follicles—a long term reservoir for drug delivery, Skin Pharm Physiol 2006; 19:232–236.
17. Lademann J, Richter H, Teichmann A, et al. Nanoparticles—an efficient carrier for drug delivery into the hair follicles. Eur J Pharm Biopharm 2007 May; 66(2):159–164.
18. Noonan KY, Beshire M, Darnell J, et al. Qualitative and quantitative analysis of illicit drug mixtures on paper currency using Raman microspectroscopy. Appl Spectrosc 2005; 59:1493–1497.
19. Caspers PJ, Lucassen GW, Puppels GJ, Combined in vivo confocal Raman spectroscopy and confocal microscopy of human skin. Biophys J 2003; 85:572–580.
20. Caspers PJ, Lucassen GW, Carter EA, et al. In vivo confocal Raman microspectroscopy of the skin: noninvasive determination of molecular concentration profiles. J Invest Dermatol 2001; 116:434–442.
21. Meyer LE, Otberg N, Sterry W, et al. In vivo confocal scanning laser microscopy: comparison of the reflectance and fluorescence mode by imaging human skin. J Biomed Opt 2006; 11:044012.
22. Meyer LE, In vivo investigation of normal and pathological human skin by confocal laser scanning microscopy. Doctoral thesis, Charité-Universitätsmedizin Berlin, 2007.
23. Meyer LE, Otberg N, Richter H, et al. New prospects in dermatology: fiber-based confocal scanning laser microscopy. Laser Phys 2006; 16:758–764.
24. Rajadhyaksha M, Gonzáles S, Zavislan JM, et al. In vivo confocal scanning laser microscopy of human skin II: advances in instrumentation and comparison with histology. J Invest Dermatol 1999; 113:293–303.
25. Swindle LD, Thomas SG, Freeman M, et al. View of normal human skin in vivo as observed using fluorescent fiber-optic confocal microscopic imaging. J Invest Dermatol 2003; 121:706–712.
26. Junqueira LC, Carneiro J. Histologie. 6th ed. Heidelberg Springer, 2005.
27. Dieterle S, Laser scanning microscopic investigations of non-melanoma skin cancer. Doctoral thesis, Charité-Universitätsmedizin Berlin, 2007.
28. Nijssen A, Bakker Schut TC, Heule F, et al. Discriminating basal cell carcinoma from its surrounding tissue by Raman spectroscopy. J Invest Dermatol 2002;119:64–69.

30 Chemical Penetration Enhancement: Possibilities and Problems

Adrian C. Williams

Reading School of Pharmacy, University of Reading, Reading, U.K.

Kenneth A. Walters

An-eX Analytical Services, Cardiff, U.K.

INTRODUCTION

> "Skin permeability is increased by contact with a variety of liquids. Excluding highly corrosive chemicals, e.g. concentrated acids and alkalis, there remain many substances which, although they do no great permanent damage, can markedly alter skin permeability" (1).

Scheuplein wrote these words in 1977, reviewing a decade's work on the effects of solvents and surfactants on permeation. The interaction between stratum corneum hydration and permeation had been explored in a series of articles by Blank et al. (2–3), Feldman and Maibach (4), and Scheuplein (5). However, the first systematic report of using an exogenous chemical to enhance flux through human skin appeared in 1964 in a series of papers from Stoughton and Fritsch (6), Horita and Weber (7), and Jacob et al. (8), employing dimethyl sulfoxide (DMSO). Some 40 years and over 2000 research articles later, DMSO is still being used in research laboratories to enhance transdermal drug delivery (9).

The promise of widespread small molecule delivery through the skin, facilitated by penetration enhancers, has yet to materialize; rationally designed enhancers such as Azone (laurocapram or 1-dodecylaza-cycloheptan-2-one) gave impetus to this field of study, but commercial exploitation did not follow. To date, materials with penetration-enhancing properties appear in many topical and transdermal preparations, such as surfactants in creams or solvents in patches. Indeed, an ever-expanding list of chemicals that act as permeation promoters is being generated, with mechanisms of action being probed. However, at present, commercial formulations do not specifically include accelerants to increase delivery of poorly permeable active ingredients. Thus, with chemical penetration enhancers, the possibilities remain. So what is the problem?

ENHANCERS AND SKIN STRUCTURE

The efficacy and potential modes of action of enhancers have been recently reviewed (10) and it is not the intention here to survey which enhancers work for which drugs in which skin membranes. Rather, some of the reasons why penetration enhancers have not achieved their promise will be considered.

In most studies examining the use and modes of action of skin penetration enhancers, the membrane is typically regarded as a physical barrier, albeit a rather heterogeneous complex one. Indeed, the focus for mechanistic studies is the stratum

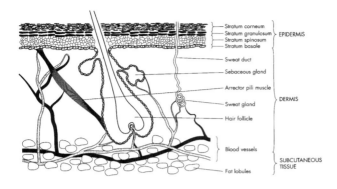

FIGURE 1 Diagrammatical representation of transverse section through human skin. *Source*: From Ref. 12.

corneum with its densely keratinized cells embedded in a multiply bilayered lipid matrix (Fig. 1). However, it is worth noting that the stratum corneum, the most superficial layer of the skin, is about 20 μm thick in normal tissue, whereas the remaining epidermal and dermal tissue is in the order of 5000 μm deep, i.e., the stratum corneum provides around 0.4% of the tissue thickness. There is therefore a lot of "biology" underlying the primary barrier to transdermal drug delivery and divorcing the physical properties of the membrane from its biological activity invites problems and may be a contributing factor in the poor exploitation of penetration enhancer research. Again, considering the oldest enhancer, DMSO is well known to be irritant at high concentrations and can cause erythema and wheals; 40 years ago, Kligman applied 90% DMSO to 20 volunteers twice daily and found, perhaps not surprisingly for a powerful aprotic solvent, erythema, scaling, contact uticaria, stinging, and burning sensations while 10% of the volunteers also developed systemic symptoms (11).

However, if we disregard biological factors and concentrate largely on the physicochemical basis for enhancement, numerous schemes have been developed to explain potential mechanisms of action of penetration enhancers within the human stratum corneum. The description of this model as a brick and mortar wall, described by Michaels et al. (13), endures today (Fig. 2).

Interaction (Disordering) of Intercellular Lipids

Essentially, permeation promoters can disrupt the intercellular packing motif within the multiple bilayers of lipids. Since permeants traversing the bulk of the stratum corneum must cross intercellular domains (irrespective of whether they also pass through or around the corneocytes) then disruption of these lipid bilayers may promote permeation.

However, the lipid domains themselves are heterogeneous with numerous packing motifs. For example (loosely termed), gel phase domains may be separate from liquid crystalline domains, not to forget interfacial areas between domains. Furthermore, components within the lipid bilayers are not homogeneously distributed giving regions where, for example, specific ceramides may predominate whereas other locations may be triglyceride-rich. Add to the mix other cellular remnants such as elements from desmosomes, proteins/enzymes, or natural moisturising factors and the simple models for skin/enhancer interactions appear naive. It is thus not surprising that, of the many enhancers that have some interaction with intercellular lipid bilayers, there appears to be no common structural feature to define

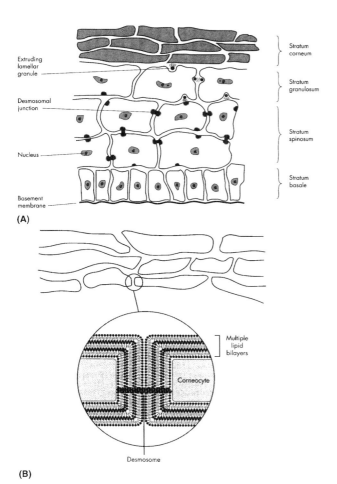

FIGURE 2 (**A**) Representation of human epidermis indicating cellular differentiation; (**B**) expansion of the stratum corneum showing "brick and mortar." *Source*: From Ref. 12.

their efficacy. Materials with fatty chains appear to work well, with examples such as oleic acid or Azone, and can be conceptualized as the fatty chains inserting into the bilayer structure. Alternatively, the enhancer may exist as a separate domain within the lipid bilayers, thus providing a fluid channel or offering porous interfaces with the endogenous lipids in the bilayers. Such a concept appears less likely for nonfatty enhancers such as DMSO or terpenes, which have also been shown to interact with the lipid domains. Again, we can hypothesize that they sit between the head groups of the lipid bilayers to distort the packing. Examples of potential interactions between some lipid-disruption permeation enhancers and human stratum corneum–bilayered lipids are given in Figure 3; it is interesting to note that the chemical structures and functional groups of the enhancers vary greatly.

Action Within Corneocytes
While much research is directed at chemicals that perturb intercellular lipid domains, other enhancers are well known to exert some influence on the relatively

Potential interaction of 1,8-cineole with intercellular lipids

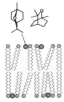

Potential interaction of oleic acid with intercellular lipids

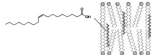

Potential interaction of sodium lauryl sulphate with intercellular lipids

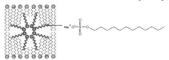

Potential interaction of laurocapram with intercellular lipids

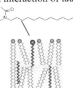

FIGURE 3 Diagram indicating potential mechanisms of interactions of some penetration enhancers with intercellular lipid domains of the stratum corneum.

dense corneocytes. In particular, keratolytic agents such as urea have been shown to enhance transdermal drug delivery, albeit (typically) to a lesser extent than agents that disrupt the lipid domains. Yet it is widely accepted that intracellular permeation (i.e., through the corneocytes with subsequent partitioning into and diffusion through the surrounding lipid matrix before partitioning into and diffusion through the next hydrated corneocyte, etc.) is probably of minor importance to transdermal permeation of most drugs and, as indicated above, even if a permeant alternatively partitions into and diffuses through lipophilic then hydrophilic domains, the principle barrier still resides within the intercellular lipid bilayers. The question arises, "why do keratolytic materials assist transdermal permeation?" There may be some advantage in promoting diffusivity in the corneocytes, but enhancers within the skin are not restricted to a single simple mode of action. Urea may also affect the lipid packing. DMSO can change the conformational state of keratin within the corneocytes and also act on lipid domains. Anionic surfactants can uncoil keratin fibers and also modify water binding within the tissue.

Alteration of Partitioning
Improved partitioning into the stratum corneum generally improves delivery through the membrane; what goes in usually comes through. To this end, solvents applied to the skin, which partition well into the tissue, can act as a "sink" for drug

partitioning. Such a reservoir effect has been shown for pyrrolidones and also for commonly used solvents such as propylene glycol and Transcutol (diethyleneglycol monoethyl ether). Of course, the solvent may also be useful for increasing the amount of another enhancer, such as oleic acid within the membrane, thus highlighting the importance of topical vehicle selection. Indeed, some standard "bases" for topical preparations contain significant quantities of enhancers, such as Arachis (peanut) oil, which typically contains 35–72% oleic acid.

Solvents at High Concentrations

As well as acting on the intercellular bilayers of the stratum corneum, high doses of potent solvents may have more drastic effects. Such solvents can damage the desmosomes responsible for cell adhesion, leading to fissuring of the intercellular lipid and splitting of the stratum corneum layers. Also, high levels of solvent can partition into the corneocyte, disrupting the keratin and even forming vacuoles. Clearly these dramatic effects would be unacceptable to regulatory agencies.

Metabolic Manipulations

One further option for increasing transdermal drug delivery is to interfere with the metabolic processes for the synthesis, assembly, activation, or processing of the intercellular lipid domains of the stratum corneum (14). As the authors state, such an approach poses significant regulatory problems but does serve to highlight the importance of considering skin biology alongside the physicomechanical properties of the tissue.

In developing penetration enhancers and evaluating their mechanism of action, one further issue is the selection of skin membranes. It is well established that many animal models, and in particular rodent models, poorly represent the structure and barrier properties of the human skin. It is thus difficult to extrapolate findings on these model membranes to the situation in human tissue in vivo.

ENHANCER SELECTION

From the above, it is axiomatic that penetration enhancer mechanisms of action are complex and, typically, an enhancer may be expected to act by a variety of the above schemes; DMSO may alter lipid packing, affect drug partitioning into the membrane, and also act on the keratin fibers. More recently, the multiplicity of actions has been tailored in generating a series of mixed enhancers that offer greater degrees of permeation promotion. While synergistic effects between enhancers and vehicles (such as oleic acid or terpenes with propylene glycol) are well described, the rational combination of enhancers to exploit differing modes of action has only been recently explored (15,16). Using a rational screening approach, the research generated synergistic combinations of penetration enhancers with considerable potency. Non- (or low-) irritant combinations were identified, which increased skin permeability to both small conventional and macromolecular agents including heparin, leutinizing hormone releasing hormone, and an oligonucleotide by up to two orders of magnitude. Interestingly, the two most successful combinations, sodium laureth sulfate with phenyl piperazine and a combination of *N*-lauroyl sarcosine with sorbitan monolaurate, are not widely regarded as potent enhancers in their own right.

PENETRATION ENHANCER POSSIBILITIES

Without a doubt, penetration enhancers can promote transdermal delivery of both hydrophilic and hydrophobic small molecule drugs. Thus the possibilities identified over 40 years ago remain today. Indeed, with a rational design of synergistic enhancer combinations, it may even be feasible to deliver larger therapeutic molecules such as heparin through human skin.

To some extent, materials with penetration-enhancing activity are already well accepted in numerous formulations, both for topical and transdermal delivery. Examples such as Arachis oil with high levels of oleic acid, or the use of ethanol in patches, show that enhancement is used, but these effects are coincidental to the main functions of these excipients as vehicles and solvents. Table 1 illustrates some of the major solvents used in topical and transdermal formulations and gives a brief summary of the enhancing activities of these solvents. The widespread use of these enhancing excipients also gives some confidence of their safety over the long-term and widespread use. Thus the principle of commercial use of penetration enhancement is well established but this may not allow other penetration enhancers to be used in novel formulations.

TABLE 1 Commonly Used Solvents in Topical and Transdermal Formulations, and Their Potential Enhancing Activity

Solvent	Enhancement activity
Water	Skin hydration increases transdermal delivery of most drugs.
Alcohols	Can modify the barrier nature of the stratum corneum. May get supersaturation.
Ethanol	Concentration-dependent effects on skin barrier and drug delivery. Readily absorbed through the skin. Listed as an inactive ingredient by FDA.
Isopropyl alcohol	Can disrupt stratum corneum. Listed as an inactive ingredient by FDA.
Benzyl alcohol	Minimal enhancing activity alone. Usually used as a cosolvent with other solvents.
Lanolin alcohols	Enhancement activity, but potential allergic responses.
Fatty alcohols	Penetration enhancing effects have been reported.
Glycols	Low enhancement activity alone, but act synergistically with other solvents to enhance permeation.
Propylene glycol	Readily absorbed through skin, widely used, and at high concentrations. Acts synergistically with other solvents to enhance permeation.
Polyethylene glycols	Not reported as an enhancer, not readily absorbed through skin.
Oils and waxes	May act by occlusion of skin or directly on stratum corneum lipids.
Mineral oils	Minimal enhancing effects other than occlusion.
Paraffins	Occlusive. Polycyclic aromatic hydrocarbon impurities can sensitize skin.
Other solvents	Not as widely used as the above materials. Varied materials for specific applications.
Isopropyl myristate	Readily absorbed through skin. Mild enhancement activity alone, but acts synergistically with other solvents.
Oleic acid	Potent penetration enhancer. Has been used as a component of Arachis oil.

Abbreviation: FDA, Food and Drug Administration

PENETRATION ENHANCER PROBLEMS

Though "safe" enhancers have been described in the literature, and materials are claimed to be nonirritating, it is difficult conceptually to see how any material that partitions into the stratum corneum to disrupt the natural organization of the barrier layer can have no adverse effects. Indeed, in order to enhance transdermal drug delivery, it is intuitive that some disruption of skin homeostasis is necessary. Thus enhancers may have "low" or "acceptable" risks associated with them, but even the most "inert" of enhancers, water, can adversely affect skin structure. Naturally, the risks should be correlated with those of competing delivery routes such as hepatic metabolism and consequent side effects or adverse effects on gastrointestinal epithelia, etc. However, the perception that enhancers are inherently damaging remains an obstacle to overcome.

With this perception, mechanistic data are often sought for penetration enhancers, and it is difficult to provide conclusive proof that a simple mechanism of action operates. From the above, it is apparent that many enhancers act via different modes in the stratum corneum, and when accelerants are combined to produce synergistic enhancement then the mechanisms operating become even more complex. This lack of clarity causes regulatory unease; without a mechanism, it is also difficult to show how the barrier repairs/restores over time with no long-term consequences. The widespread use of enhancing agents in formulations has not been accepted as evidence that other enhancers can be designed and included into formulations.

One further area that constitutes a "problem" is the lack of extrapolation of enhancement activities to biological effects. If considered at all, the gross structure of the skin may be viewed by researchers, but the effects of enhancers on biochemical cascades, inflammation, immunology, etc. are seldom cited. Feeding back into regulatory unease, such studies may show that the risks associated with penetration enhancement are equivalent to those when agents are applied to other bodily membranes.

One final obstacle, particularly within academic research into enhancer development and mechanistic understandings, is that the topic appears to have fallen out of favor. Over the last 20 years, transdermal drug delivery research has seen periods of high activity followed by lulls in research, evidenced by research paper publications shown in Figure 4. Clearly these data are approximate as more scientists now work in the general area of transdermal drug delivery than 25 years ago, but the plot shows an interesting cyclical trend. On top of a steady stream of activity, enhancers have been in and out of fashion, stimulated occasionally by new materials being

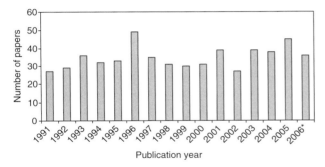

FIGURE 4 Annual number of publications describing skin penetration enhancers since 1991. Searched using the ISI Web of Science database with the terms penetration enhancer and skin. *Data for 2006 doubled from publications to end of June.

developed such as Azone or the application of biophysical methods such as infrared spectroscopy to probe mechanisms, before falling behind to other enhancement modes such as iontophoresis (which itself has cycled in and out of fashion). Presently, enhancer research appears to be waning and is competing with other modes for delivering materials through the stratum corneum, such as microneedles. Indeed, such new technologies also offer other significant advantages over enhancers, such as a capability to deliver large macromolecules, including genes, as well as conventional small organic therapeutic molecules. Perhaps these newer technologies will also fall out of favor or, more likely, combinations of enhancement strategies (as was seen with iontophoresis, electroporation and penetration enhancer combinations) will prevail.

REFERENCES

1. Scheuplein RJ. Permeability of the skin. In: Lee DHK, Falk HL, Murphy SD, Geiger SR, eds. Handbook of Physiology, Section 9: Reactions to Environmental Agents. Bethesda, Md, USA: American Physiological Society, 1977; Chapter 19:229–323.
2. Blank IH. Factors which influence the water content of the stratum corneum. J Invest Dermatol 1952; 18:433–440.
3. Blank IH. Further observations on factors which influence the water content of the stratum corneum. J Invest Dermatol 1953; 21:259–269.
4. Feldman RJ, Maibach HI. Penetration of ^{14}C hydrocortisone through normal skin. Arch Dermatol 1965; 91:661–666.
5. Scheuplein RJ. Mechanism of percutaneous absorption: I. Routes of penetration and the influence of solubility. J Invest Dermatol 1965; 45:334–346.
6. Stoughton RB, Fritsch WC. Influence of dimethyl sulphoxide on human percutaneous absorption. Arch Dermatol 1964; 90:512–517.
7. Horita A, Weber LJ. Skin penetrating property of drugs dissolved in dimethyl sulphoxide (DMSO) and other vehicles. Life Sci 1964; 3:1389–1395.
8. Jacob SW, Bischel M, Herschler RJ. Dimethyl sulphoxide: effects on the permeability of biologic membranes (preliminary report). Curr Ther Res 1964; 6:193–198.
9. Bugaj A, Juzeniene A, Juzenas P, et al. The effect of skin permeation enhancers on the formation of porphyrins in mouse skin during topical application of the methyl ester of 5-aminolevulinic acid. J Phytochem Photobiol 2006; 83:94–97.
10. Williams AC, Barry BW. Penetration enhancers. Adv Drug Deliv Rev 2004; 56:603–618.
11. Kligman AM. Topical pharmacology and toxicology of dimethyl sulfoxide. J Am Med Assoc 1965; 193:796–804.
12. Williams AC. Transdermal and Topical Drug Delivery; From Theory to Clinical Practice. London: Pharmaceutical Press, 2003; 3–10.
13. Michaels AS, Chanderasekaran SK, Shaw JE. Drug permeation through human skin; theory and in vitro experimental measurement. AIChE J 1975; 21:985–996.
14. Elias PM, Tsai J, Menon GK, Holleran WM, Feingold KR. The potential of metabolic interventions to enhance transdermal drug delivery. J Investig Dermatol Symp Proc 2002; 7:79–85.
15. Karande P, Jain A, Mitragotri S. Discovery of transdermal penetration enhancers by high-throughput screening. Nat Biotechnol 2004; 22:192–197.
16. Karande P, Jain A, Ergun K, Kispersky V, Mitragotri S. Design principles of chemical penetration enhancers for transdermal drug delivery. Proc Natl Acad Sci USA 2005; 102:4688–4693.

31 Multicomponent Formulations of Chemical Penetration Enhancers

Pankaj Karande, Amit Jain, and Samir Mitragotri

Department of Chemical Engineering, University of California, Santa Barbara, California, U.S.A.

INTRODUCTION

The transdermal route of drug administration offers several advantages, such as reduced first-pass drug metabolism, no gastrointestinal degradation, long-term delivery (>24 hours), and control over delivery and termination. However, only few drug molecules have been formulated into transdermal patches because of the low permeability of the skin (1). The outermost layer, the stratum corneum (SC), forms a barrier against permeation of drugs into the body. This barrier must be altered to maximize the possibilities of transdermal drug delivery. This problem has engaged pharmaceutical scientists, dermatologists, and engineers alike in research over the last few decades (2). High research activity in this field has led to the introduction of a variety of techniques, including formulation-based approaches (3), iontophoresis (4), electroporation (5,6), acoustic methods (7), microneedles (8), jet injection (9), and thermal poration (10) (see Chapter 1). Each of these techniques has its benefits and specific applications.

Formulation-based approaches have a number of unique advantages, such as design simplicity as well as flexibility and ease of application over a large area (11). The last 20 years have seen extensive research in the field of chemical enhancers, which form the core component of formulation-based strategies for transdermal drug delivery. More than 200 chemicals have been shown to enhance skin permeability to various drugs. These include molecules from a diverse group of chemicals, including fatty acids (12–14), fatty esters (15), nonionic surfactants (16), anionic surfactants (17), and terpenes (18,19). However, identification of safe and potent permeation enhancers has proved to be challenging. To date, only few chemicals are found in currently marketed transdermal products.

Although individual chemical penetration enhancers (CPEs) have found limited applications, combinations of CPEs represent a huge opportunity that has been sparsely tapped. Several reports have indicated that combinations of CPEs offer better enhancements of transdermal drug transport as compared with their individual constituents (20,21). However, such combinations do not necessarily yield safer enhancers. It should be feasible, in principle, to use CPEs as building blocks to construct new microstructures and novel formulations that offer enhancement without irritation. However, the challenge now shifts to screening the potency of enhancer combinations. Random mixtures of CPEs are likely to exhibit additive properties; that is, their potency and irritancy are likely to be averages of corresponding properties of their individual constituents. Occurrence of truly synergistic combinations is likely to be rare. In the absence of capabilities to predict the occurrence of such rare mixtures, one has to rely on a brute-force screening approach. Starting with a pool of more than 200 CPEs, millions of binary and billions of higher-order formulations can be designed. Screening of these mixtures is a mammoth task.

Screening of chemical enhancers can be performed in vitro and in vivo. In vivo experiments are likely to yield more relevant results; however, several issues, including variability, cost, and practicality, limit their applications for screening a large database of enhancers. Accordingly, in vitro screening based on excised tissue (human or animal) presents a more practical alternative (22). A number of models to predict in vivo pharmacokinetics based on in vitro data exist (23–27). The use of in vitro models for screening is also supported by the fact that SC, the principal site of enhancer action, shows similar behavior in vivo and in vitro except for the extent of metabolic activity (28). Most in vitro studies on transdermal drug transport have been performed using Franz diffusion cells (FDCs). The throughput of this traditional setup of a diffusion chamber is very low: not more than 10 to 15 experiments at a time. These permeation studies are time consuming and resource expensive because analytical methods such as high-pressure liquid chromatography and radiolabeled drugs for liquid scintillation counting are expensive. Automated in-line flow-through diffusion cells have been developed to increase the throughput of skin permeation experiments (29,30). Although these methods have facilitated the experiments, throughput has not been significantly improved. Furthermore, these methods are also cost prohibitive. Accordingly, standard FDCs still dominate the screening of CPEs.

The urgent need to increase experimental throughput has led to the development of high-throughput screening methods. Although still in their early stages, these methods have already shown promise in discovering novel formulations for transdermal drug delivery. A high-throughput assay to be used for screening of transdermal formulations should meet the following requirements:

1. Ability to screen a large number of formulations: Increasing the throughput by at least two to three orders of magnitude would result in a significant reduction in the effort and time spent in the very first stage of formulation development (31).
2. Use of a surrogate end point that is quick, easy, and independent of the physicochemical properties of the model permeant: Permeation experiments using radiolabeled (32), fluorescent (33), high-pressure liquid chromatography–detectable (23), or radioimmunoassay-/ELISA-detectable (34,35) markers necessitate extensive sample handling and sample analysis. These accentuate the cost of sample analysis and overall time spent in characterizing the efficacy of formulations. Furthermore, current state-of-the-art fluidics systems place a fundamental limit on the number of samples that can be handled in a given time. Permeation of a model solute across the skin in the presence of an enhancer is dependent not only on the inherent capacity of the enhancer to permeabilize skin but also on the physicochemical interactions of the enhancer with the model solute (36–38). An end point to characterize the effect of an enhancer on skin permeability should be able to decouple these two effects to ensure the generality of the results.
3. Low incubation times to further increase the throughput and hence time efficiency: FDC experiments typically use incubation times of 48 to 96 hours, thereby reducing the throughput of permeation experiments. Low incubation times favor high turnover frequencies for assay use.
4. Minimal use of test chemicals and efficient use of model membranes, such as animal skin: FDCs typically require application of 1 to 2 mL of enhancer formulation over approximately 3 to 4 cm^2 of skin per experiment. This makes it cost-

prohibitive to include candidates that are expensive in the test libraries and to screen a large number of formulations.

5. Adaptability to automation to reduce human interference: The typical FDC setup requires manual sampling with little opportunities for process automation (29).

6. Use of a common model membrane to represent human skin: In the transdermal literature, it is common to find a variety of models used to represent human skin, including rat skin (39), pig skin (40), snake skin (41), and excised human skin, among others. Although human skin is difficult to procure on a large scale, animal models show permeability characteristics different from human skin (39,42,43). In addition, results on one model cannot be directly translated to another.

7. Use of consistent thermodynamic conditions for enhancer formulations: The permeation enhancement efficacy of a CPE is a function of its chemical potential (44,45), temperature (46,47), and cosolvent (48,49), among other thermodynamic parameters. These thermodynamic conditions need to be standardized for all the enhancers that are being tested to create direct comparison of their efficacies in increasing skin permeation.

This chapter focuses on a specific high-throughput screening method called INSIGHT, IN vitro Skin Impedance–Guided High-Throughput, screening that was recently introduced (50). This method is described in detail with respect to its fundamentals, validation, and outcomes.

INSIGHT SCREENING

INSIGHT screening offers improvement in screening rates of transdermal formulations that is greater than 100-fold (50). This improvement in efficiency comes from two factors. First, INSIGHT screening, in its current version, can perform up to 50 tests per square inch of skin, as compared with approximately 2 cm^2 of skin per test in the case of FDCs (Fig. 1). Approximately 100 formulations can be screened per INSIGHT array. Second, INSIGHT screening uses skin impedance as a surrogate marker for skin permeability.

Skin impedance has been used to (*i*) assess skin integrity for in vitro dermal testing (51–53), (*ii*) evaluate the irritation potential of chemicals in a test known as Skin Integrity Function Test (54), and (*iii*) monitor skin barrier recovery in vivo after the application of current during iontophoresis (55,56). Because it is evident from the literature that skin impedance can be used to confirm skin integrity, it is logical to hypothesize that alterations in skin barriers caused by chemical enhancers can be used as an in vitro surrogate marker for permeability. Scattered literature data support this hypothesis. Studies by Yamamoto and Yamamoto (57,58) showed that total skin impedance reduced gradually with tape stripping and that skin impedance approached the impedance value of deep tissues after 15 strips. However, quantitative relationships between skin impedance and permeability in the presence of chemical enhancers and their validity for a wide range of markers have only been recently documented.

Skin Impedance–Skin Permeability Correlation

The SC is a composite of proteins and lipids in which protein-rich corneocytes are surrounded by lipid bilayers (59). Approximately 7 to 10 bilayers are stacked between two corneocytes (60,61). Because of its architecture, the SC is relatively nonconductive and possesses high electrical impedance (62). Skin impedance (alternating current) can be measured either by applying a constant current and

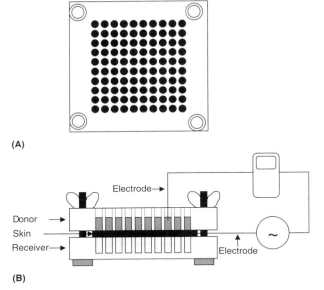

(A)

(B)

FIGURE 1 Schematic of the INSIGHT screening apparatus. The INSIGHT screen is made up of a donor array (*top*) and a symmetrical receiver array (*bottom*). A single screen can screen 100 formulations at one time. The skin is sandwiched between the donor (Teflon) and the receiver (polycarbonate), and the formulations contact the SC from the donor array. Conductivity measurements are made with one electrode inserted in the dermis and a second electrode moved sequentially in the donor wells. Figure parts **(A)** and **(B)** are the top and side views of the IN-SIGHT apparatus, respectively.

measuring the potential across the skin or by measuring the transepidermal current after the application of a constant alternating current potential. Data reported in this chapter are based on measurements of the transepidermal current after the application of a constant potential [100 mV (rms)]. Frequency of the applied potential is also an important parameter. Because of the capacitive components of the skin, the measured electrical impedance of the skin decreases with increasing frequency (57). Although the use of higher frequencies facilitates measurements because of decreased impedance, the correlation between electrical impedance and solute permeability is stronger at lower frequencies. Thus, an optimal frequency must be chosen. All experiments reported in this chapter were performed at a frequency of 100 Hz.

INSIGHT screening is founded on the relationship between the skin's electrical impedance (reciprocal of skin conductance) and solute permeability. There is a dearth of literature on the relationship between skin impedance (conductivity) and permeability, and, moreover, in most of the studies, this relationship was used to elucidate the mechanism of transport of hydrophilic molecules across the skin under the influence of temperature (63), hydration (64), electric current (65,66), or ultrasonic waves (67,68). Therefore, existing data cannot be used to generalize the relationship between skin impedance and permeability. Accordingly, a large data set was first generated to assess the correlation between skin impedance and permeability to small (mannitol) and macromolecule (inulin) hydrophilic solutes in the presence of different chemical enhancer formulations.

Skin permeability has been related to skin impedance through the porous pathway theory. The fundamental underlying assumption of the porous pathway theory is that solutes and ions migrate through the SC via the same pathways. According to the porous pathway theory, solute skin permeability, P, can be related to skin impedance, R, as follows:

$$\log P = \log C - \log R \qquad (1)$$

where C is a constant whose value depends on the solute radius and SC structure. Equation (1) provides a general equation to theoretically describe the diffusion of a solute across the skin. Relationships between skin permeability and impedance were evaluated for four molecules: mannitol, inulin, corticosterone, and estradiol. Equation (1) was fitted separately for each enhancer formulation. High r^2 values were found for the hydrophilic solutes mannitol and inulin (0.8 ± 0.1 and 0.8 ± 0.14, respectively). For the hydrophobic solutes corticosterone and estradiol, r^2 values were significantly lower (0.49 ± 0.14 and 0.53 ± 0.22, respectively) than those for hydrophilic solutes but were still reasonably good.

All data points are shown in Figure 2. The impedance reduction is calculated with respect to the data point, chosen from the entire set, corresponding to the highest impedance value (usually control). Permeability enhancement is calculated with respect to the permeability value corresponding to the same data point. There is a reasonable scatter in these data, which is inherent in biological systems, such as the skin, that exhibit high variability. In addition, the measurements reported in Figure 2 represent an aggregate of experiments performed on several animals and anatomical regions. The statistics of these correlations is discussed subsequently. The correlation between skin permeability and impedance can be clearly seen in Figure 3, in which data in Figure 2 are replotted after averaging over approximately 5-kW/cm^2 intervals ($r^2 = 0.97$, 0.98, 0.97, and 0.97 for mannitol, inulin, corticosterone, and estradiol, respectively). The last one or two points corresponding to high impedance were excluded from the fitted equation. This follows the fact that the correlation between impedance and permeability is somewhat chaotic under conditions close to the control (as is visually clear in Fig. 3A). Inclusion of these points in the fitted equation somewhat reduced the r^2 values to 0.94, 0.98, 0.92, and 0.94 for mannitol, inulin, corticosterone, and estradiol, respectively. High r^2 values for mannitol and inulin are understandable because these molecules have been shown to follow the porous pathway theory. However, the high degree of correlation for corticosterone and estradiol is surprising. It must be noted, however, that the error within each bin is significantly higher for hydrophobic solutes. It is not clear whether permeability-impedance relationships for hydrophobic solutes have a fundamental basis in the porous pathway theory. In other words, it is not clear whether hydrophobic solutes indeed follow the same path as do ions in the presence of chemical enhancers. It is likely that the relationship between the two is a coincidence in the sense that the pathways for ionic and solute transports in the presence of chemical enhancers are distinct but simultaneously affected by enhancers.

The correlation between permeability and impedance can be used to judge the "permeability status" of the skin. Quantitative predictions of permeability from impedance measurements require the development of equations of the type shown in Equation (1). However, the qualitative correlations shown in Figures 2 and 3 may suffice to rank the formulations in terms of their potencies. Implicit in this ranking is a statement that if a formulation enhances skin permeability to a given drug, it will also enhance permeability to other drugs. This statement is supported by the data in Figure 3. However, this statement does not assume that a given formulation will provide the same enhancement for all drugs. The accuracy of such ranking is depicted in Figure 4A, in which the percentile ranking of formulations (binned into 10% regions) judged based on their electrical conductivity is compared with that made based on mannitol permeability. The two rankings exhibit excellent correlation ($r^2 = 0.97$). Comparable results were obtained for other solutes.

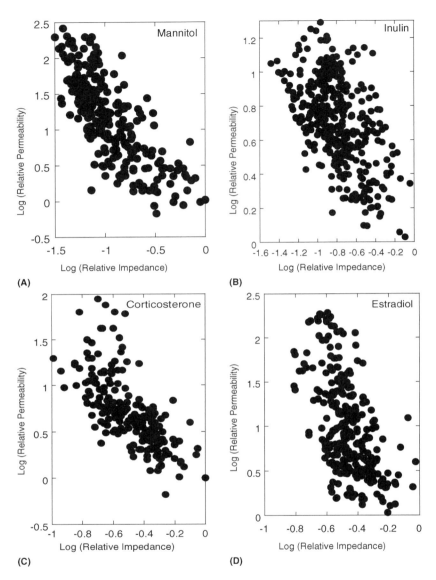

FIGURE 2 Relationships between skin permeability to mannitol (**A**), inulin (**B**), corticosterone (**C**), and estradiol (**D**) and skin impedance ($n=266$ for mannitol, $n=390$ for inulin, $n=218$ for corticosterone, and $n=279$ for estradiol).

Figure 4B shows the feasibility of using skin impedance to compare two formulations for mannitol permeability head to head and choose the more potent formulation. Two random points were selected from the data in Figure 2A (rounded off to 1 kΩ/cm^2), and the formulation yielding a lower impedance value was deemed more potent. It was then determined whether the formulation with lower impedance value

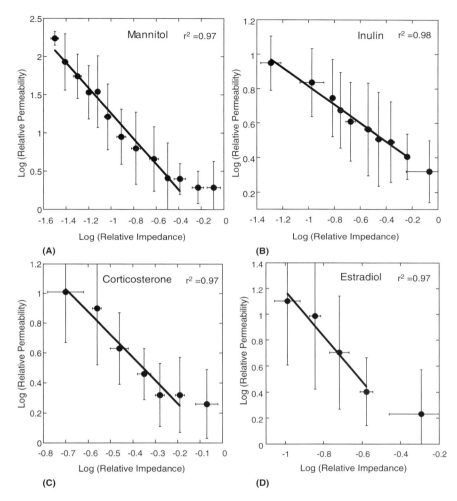

FIGURE 3   Relationships between skin permeability to mannitol (**A**), inulin (**B**), corticosterone (**C**), and estradiol (**D**) after binning the data in Figure 2.

was indeed the one with higher permeability. The rounding-off procedure implies that impedance cannot be used to choose the correct formulation if the difference between impedance values is less than 1 $k\Omega/cm^2$. These calculations were repeated for all possible pairs and then averaged (Fig. 4B). The probability of making a correct decision based on skin impedance depends on the difference between the impedance values of two formulations. If the difference is very large (>20 $k\Omega/cm^2$), then the probability of correctly picking a potent formulation from a pair of formulations is 100% (Fig. 4B). The accuracy of this decision decreases with decreasing difference between the impedance values. Ultimately, when the difference between skin impedance values exposed to formulations drops to below 1 $k\Omega/cm^2$, the accuracy of the decision is 50%, corresponding to a random guess. Nearly identical results were obtained for other solutes.

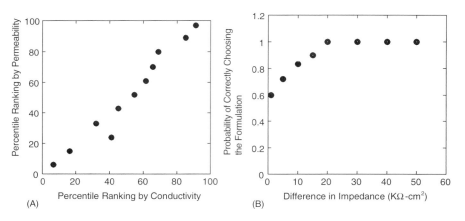

FIGURE 4   **(A)** The ranking of the percentile of formulations based on mannitol permeability plotted versus the percentile ranking based on conductivity. Data are first truncated to 1-kΩ/cm^2 impedance values and then over five consequent formulations. **(B)** The probability of choosing a potent mannitol formulation by comparing the impedance values of two formulations. Beyond a difference of 20 kΩ/cm^2, the decision is 100% correct. At 1 kΩ/cm^2, the accuracy is 60%.

APPLICATIONS OF INSIGHT SCREENING
Discovery of Rare Formulations

INSIGHT screening can be used to screen huge libraries of chemicals within a short span of time. Many current single enhancers are also potent irritants to the skin at concentrations necessary to induce meaningful penetration enhancement. Attempts to synthesize novel chemical enhancers, such as Azone, have been made; however, achieving sufficient potency without irritancy has proved to be challenging, especially for macromolecules. A number of studies have shown that formulations made up of combinations of chemical enhancers are more potent than their individual components (20,50,69). The addition of components increases the number of formulations exponentially. However, the use of INSIGHT screening allows one to tackle this challenge in a more cost-effective way as compared with FDCs. In addition, synergies between CPEs not only lead to new transdermal formulations but also potentially offer insight into mechanisms by which CPEs enhance skin permeability. Prediction of synergies from the first principles is challenging. INSIGHT screening offers an effective tool for identifying synergies (positive or negative) between the CPEs.

A library of chemical enhancers was first generated from 32 chemicals chosen from a list of more than 250 chemical enhancers belonging to various categories to identify SCOPE (synergistic combinations of penetration enhancers) formulations. Random pairing of CPEs from various categories led to 496 binary chemical enhancer pairs. For each pair, 44 chemical compositions were created, with the concentration of each chemical enhancer ranging from 0% to 2% w/v, yielding a library of 25,000 candidate SCOPE formulations. Approximately 20% of this library (5040 formulations) was screened using INSIGHT screening, the largest ever-cohesive screening study reported in the transdermal literature. Each formulation was tested at least four times in more than 20,000 experiments (50). Using the traditional tools for formulation screening to do these many experiments would have taken more than 7 years. With INSIGHT screening, the same task was accomplished in approximately 2 months, with a screening rate of 500 to 1000 experiments per day. Binary formulations exhibited a wide range of enhancement. The percentage of randomly generated enhancer combinations that exhibit enhancement ratio (ER) above a certain threshold decreases rapidly with increasing threshold. The inset shows a section of the main figure corresponding to high ER values. Less than 0.1% of formulations exhibited an enhancement of skin conductivity that is greater than 60-fold. Discovery of such rare formulations by brute-force experimentation is contingent on the throughput of the experimental tool. INSIGHT screening opens up the possibility of discovering such rare formulations.

Generation of Database for Quantitative Understanding
Looking beyond the search for potent combinations of enhancers, the sheer volume of information generated via INSIGHT screening on the behavior of a wide variety of penetration enhancers will provide, for the first time, a platform on which to build further investigations of the fundamental aspects of enhancer-skin interactions. Quantitative descriptions of structure-activity relations for CPEs, which have had limited success in the past (70,71), may lead to better outcomes in light of the availability of large volumes of data collected in a consistent manner. This information should help in generating hypotheses relating the chemistry of CPEs to their potencies. For working hypotheses, this knowledge can then help refine our selection rules for designing next-generation transdermal formulations. Repeating the experiment-hypothesis loop over a vast but limited number of candidate penetration enhancers will provide the missing pieces in solving a vast multivariate problem. In addition, this knowledge should significantly reduce the cost and effort of designing therapeutics for use on skin in the future.

REFERENCES

1. Barry BW. Novel mechanisms and devices to enable successful transdermal drug delivery. Eur J Pharm Sci 2001; 14:101–114.
2. Mitragotri S. Breaking the skin barrier. Adv Drug Deliv Rev 2004; 56:555–556.
3. Williams AC, Barry BW. Penetration enhancers. Adv Drug Deliv Rev 2004; 56:603–618.
4. Kalia YN, Naik A, Garrison J, Guy RH. Iontophoretic drug delivery. Adv Drug Deliv Rev 2004; 56:619–658.
5. Weaver JC, Vaughan TE, Chizmadzhev Y. Theory of electrical creation of aqueous pathways across skin transport barriers. Adv Drug Deliv Rev 1999; 35:21–39.
6. Prausnitz MR. A practical assessment of transdermal drug delivery by skin electroporation. Adv Drug Deliv Rev 1999; 35:61–76.
7. Mitragotri S, Kost J. Low-frequency sonophoresis: a review. Adv Drug Deliv Rev 2004; 56:589–601.
8. Prausnitz MR. Microneedles for transdermal drug delivery. Adv Drug Deliv Rev 2004; 56:581–587.
9. Hingson RA, Figge FH. A survey of the development of jet injection in parenteral therapy. Curr Res Anesth Analg 1952; 31:361–366.
10. Sintov AC, Krymberk I, Daniel D, Hannan T, Sohn Z, Levin G. Radiofrequency-driven skin microchanneling as a new way for electrically assisted transdermal delivery of hydrophilic drugs. J Control Release 2003; 89:311–320.
11. Prausnitz MR, Mitragotri S, Langer R. Current status and future potential of transdermal drug delivery. Nat Rev Drug Discov. 2004; 3:115–124.
12. Jain AK, Panchagnula R. Transdermal drug delivery of tricyclic antidepressants: effect of fatty acids. Methods Find Exp Clin Pharmacol 2003; 25:413–421.

13. Golden GM, McKie JE, Potts RO. Role of stratum corneum lipid fluidity in transdermal drug flux. J Pharm Sci 1987; 76:25–28.
14. Aungst BJ, Blake JA, Hussain MA. Contributions of drug solubilization, partitioning, barrier disruption, and solvent permeation to the enhancement of skin permeation of various compounds with fatty acids and amines. Pharm Res 1990; 7:712–718.
15. Chukwumerije O, Nash RA, Matias JR, Orentreich N. Studies on the efficacy of methyl esters of *n*-alkyl fatty acids as penetration enhancers. J Invest Dermatol 1989; 93:349–352.
16. Lopez A, Llinares F, Cortell C, Herraez M. Comparative enhancer effects of Span20 with Tween20 and Azone on the in vitro percutaneous penetration of compounds with different lipophilicities. Int J Pharm 2000; 202:133–140.
17. Nokhodchi A, Shokri J, Dashbolaghi A, Hassan-Zadeh D, Ghafourian T, Barzegar-Jalali M. The enhancement effect of surfactants on the penetration of lorazepam through rat skin. Int J Pharm 2003; 250:359–369.
18. Williams AC, Barry BW. Terpenes and the lipid-protein-partitioning theory of skin penetration enhancement. Pharm Res 1991; 8:17–24.
19. Jain AK, Thomas NS, Panchagnula R. Transdermal drug delivery of imipramine hydrochloride. I. Effect of terpenes. J Control Release 2002; 79:93–101.
20. Mitragotri S. Synergistic effect of enhancers for transdermal drug delivery. Pharm Res 2000; 17:1354–1359.
21. Thomas NS, Panchagnula R. Combination strategies to enhance transdermal permeation of zidovudine (AZT). Pharmazie 2003; 58:895–898.
22. Priborsky J, Muhlbachova E. Evaluation of in-vitro percutaneous absorption across human skin and in animal models. J Pharm Pharmacol 1990; 42:468–472.
23. Wu PC, Huang YB, Chang JJ, Chang JS, Tsai YS. Evaluation of pharmacokinetics and pharmacodynamics of captopril from transdermal hydrophilic gels in normotensive rabbits and spontaneously hypertensive rats. Int J Pharm 2000; 209:87–94.
24. Naito SI, Tsai YH. Percutaneous absorption of indomethacin from ointment bases in rabbits. Int J Pharm 1981; 8:263–276.
25. Guy RH, Hadgraft J, Maibach HI. A pharmacokinetic model for percutaneous bsorption. Int J Pharm 1982; 11:119–129.
26. Ogiso T, Ito Y, Iwaki M, Atago H. A pharmacokinetic model for the percutaneous absorption of indomethacin and the predication of drug disposition kinetics. J Pharm Sci 1989; 78:319–323.
27. Takayama K, Nagai T. Simultaneous optimization for several characteristics concerning percutaneous absorption and skin damage of ketoprofen hydrogels containing Dlinomene. Int J Pharm 1991; 74:115–126.
28. Chang P, Rosenquist MD, Lewis RW 2nd, KealyGP. A study of functional viability and metabolic degeneration of human skin stored at 4 degrees C. J Burn Care Rehabil 1998; 19:25–28.
29. Cordoba-Diaz M, Nova M, Elorza B, Cordoba-Diaz D, Chantres JR, Cordoba-Borrego M. Validation protocol of an automated in-line flow-through diffusion equipment for in vitro permeation studies. J Control Release 2000; 69:357–367.
30. Bosman IJ, Lawant AL, Avegaart SR, Ensing K, de Zeeuw RA. Novel diffusion cell for in vitro transdermal permeation, compatible with automated dynamic sampling. J Pharm Biomed Anal 1996; 14:1015–1023.
31. Karande P, Mitragotri S. High throughput screening of transdermal formulations. Pharm Res 2002; 19:655–660.
32. Rosado C, Cross SE, Pugh WJ, Roberts MS, Hadgraft J. Effect of vehicle pretreatment on the flux, retention, and diffusion of topically applied penetrants in vitro. Pharm Res 2002; 20:1502–1507.
33. Ogiso T, Niinaka N, Iwaki M. Mechanism for enhancement effect of lipid disperse system on percutaneous absorption. J Pharm Sci 1996; 85:57–64.
34. Magnusson BM, Runn P. Effect of penetration enhancers on the permeation of the thyrotropin releasing hormone analogue pGlu-3-methyl-His-Pro amide through human epidermis. Int J Pharm 1999; 178:149–159.
35. Xing QF, Lin S, Chien YW. Transdermal testosterone delivery in castrated Yucatan minipigs: pharmacokinetics and metabolism. J Control Release 1998; 52:89–98.

36. Auner BG, Valenta C, Hadgraft J. Influence of lipophilic counter-ions in combination with phloretin and 6-ketocholestanol on the skin permeation of 5-aminolevulinic acid. Int J Pharm 2003; 255:109–116.

37. Lee SJ, Kim SW. Hydrophobization of ionic drugs for transport through membranes. J Control Release 1987; 6:3–13.

38. Takács-Novak K, Szász G. Ion-pair partition of quaternary ammonium drugs: the influence of counter ions of different lipophilicity, size, and flexibility. Pharm Res 1999; 16:1633–1638.

39. Schmook FP, Meingassner JG, Billich A. Comparison of human skin or epidermis models with human and animal skin in in-vitro percutaneous absorption. Int J Pharm 2001; 215:51–56.

40. Sekkat N, Kalia YN, Guy RH. Biophysical study of porcine ear skin in vitro and its comparison to human skin in vivo. J Pharm Sci 2002; 91:2376–2381.

41. Itoh T, Xia J, Magavi R, Nishihata T, Rytting JH. Use of shed snake skin as a model membrane for in vitro percutaneous penetration studies: comparison with human skin. Pharm Res 1990; 7:1042–1047.

42. Auner BG, Valenta C, Hadgraft J. Influence of phloretin and 6-ketocholestanol on the skin permeation of sodium-fluorescein. J Control Release 2003; 89:321–328.

43. Panchagnula R, Stemmer K, Ritschel WA. Animal models for transdermal drug delivery. Methods Find Exp Clin Pharmacol 1997; 19:335–341.

44. Shokri J, Nokhodchi A, Dashbolaghi A, Hassan-Zadeh D, Ghafourian T, Barzegar Jalali M. The effect of surfactants on the skin penetration of diazepam. Int J Pharm 2001; 228:99–107.

45. Francoeur ML, Golden GM, Potts RO. Oleic acid: its effects on stratum corneum in relation to (trans)dermal drug delivery. Pharm Res 1990; 7:621–627.

46. Ongpipattanakul B, Burnette RR, Potts RO, Francoeur ML. Evidence that oleic acid exists in a separate phase within stratum corneum lipids. Pharm Res 1991; 8:350–354.

47. Narishetty ST, Panchagnula R. Transdermal delivery of zidovudine: effect of terpenes and their mechanism of action. J Control Release 2004; 95:367–379.

48. Yamane MA, Williams AC, Barry BW. Terpene penetration enhancers in propylene glycol/water co-solvent systems: effectiveness and mechanism of action. J Pharm Pharmacol 1995; 47:978–989.

49. Larrucea E, Arellano A, Santoyo S, Ygartua P. Combined effect of oleic acid and propylene glycol on the percutaneous penetration of tenoxicam and its retention in the skin. Eur J Pharm Biopharm 2001; 52:113–119.

50. Karande P, Jain A, Mitragotri S. Discovery of transdermal penetration enhancers by high-throughput screening. Nat Biotechnol 2004; 22:192–197.

51. Davies DJ, Ward RJ, Heylings JR. Multi-species assessment of electrical resistance as a skin integrity marker for in vitro percutaneous absorption studies. Toxicol In Vitro 2004; 18:351–358.

52. Fasano WJ, Manning LA, Green JW. Rapid integrity assessment of rat and human epidermal membranes for in vitro dermal regulatory testing: correlation of electrical resistance with tritiated water permeability. Toxicol In Vitro 2002; 16:731–740.

53. Lawrence JN. Electrical resistance and tritiated water permeability as indicators of barrier integrity of in vitro human skin. Toxicol In Vitro 1997; 11:241–249.

54. Heylings JR, Clowes HM, Hughes L. Comparison of tissue sources for the skin integrity function test (SIFT). Toxicol In Vitro 2001; 15:597–600.

55. Turner NG, Kalia YN, Guy RH. The effect of current on skin barrier function in vivo: recovery kinetics post-iontophoresis. Pharm Res 1997; 14:1252–1257.

56. Curdy C, Kalia YN, Guy RH. Post-iontophoresis recovery of human skin impedance in vivo. Eur J Pharm Biopharm 2002; 53:15–21.

57. Yamamoto T, Yamamoto Y. Electrical properties of the epidermal stratum corneum. Med Biol Eng 1976; 14:151–158.

58. Yamamoto T, Yamamoto Y. Dielectric constant and resistivity of epidermal stratum corneum. Med Biol Eng 1976; 14:494–500.

59. Madison KC, Swartzendruber DC, Wertz PW, Downing DT. Presence of intact intercellular lipid lamellae in the upper layers of the stratum corneum. J Invest Dermatol 1987; 88:714–718.

60. Elias PM, McNutt NS, Friend DS. Membrane alterations during cornification of mammalian squamous epithelia: a freeze-fracture, tracer, and thin-section study. Anat Rec 1977; 189:577–594.

61. Elias PM. Epidermal lipids, barrier function, and desquamation. J Invest Dermatol 1983; 80(Suppl.):44s–49s.

62. Lackermeier AH, McAdams ET, Moss GP, Woolfson AD. In vivo ac impedance spectroscopy of human skin. Theory and problems in monitoring of passive percutaneous drug delivery. Ann NY Acad Sci. 1999; 873:197–213.

63. Peck KD, Ghanem AH, Higuchi WI. The effect of temperature upon the permeation of polar and ionic solutes through human epidermal membrane. J Pharm Sci 1995; 84:975–982.

64. Tang H, Blankschtein D, Langer R. Prediction of steady-state skin permeabilities of polar and nonpolar permeants across excised pig skin based on measurements of transient diffusion: characterization of hydration effects on the skin porous pathway. J Pharm Sci 2002; 91:1891–1907.

65. Li SK, Ghanem AH, Peck KD, Higuchi WI. Characterization of the transport pathways induced during low to moderate voltage iontophoresis in human epidermal membrane. J Pharm Sci 1998; 87:40–48.

66. Sims SM, Higuchi WI, Srinivasan V. Skin alteration and convective solvent flow effects during iontophoresis: I. Neutral solute transport across human skin. Int J Pharm 1991; 69:109–121.

67. Tang H, Mitragotri S, Blankschtein D, Langer R. Theoretical description of transdermal transport of hydrophilic permeants: application to low-frequency sonophoresis. J Pharm Sci 2001; 90:545–568.

68. Tezel A, Sens A, Mitragotri S. Description of transdermal transport of hydrophilic solutes during low-frequency sonophoresis based on a modified porous pathway model. J Pharm Sci 2003; 92:381–393.

69. Tezel A, Sens A, Tuchscherer J, Mitragotri S. Synergistic effect of low-frequency ultrasound and surfactants on skin permeability. J Pharm Sci 2002; 91:91–100.

70. Moss GP, Dearden JC, Patel H, Cronin MT. Quantitative structure-permeability relationships (QSPRs) for percutaneous absorption. Toxicol In Vitro 2002; 16:299–317.

71. Walker JD, Rodford R, Patlewicz G. Quantitative structure-activity relationships for predicting percutaneous absorption rates. Environ Toxicol Chem 2003; 22:1870–1884.

Part VIII: Improving Therapeutic Outcomes Using Physical Techniques

32 Iontophoresis

Narayanasamy Kanikkannan
Tyco Healthcare Mallinckrodt, Webster Groves, Missouri, U.S.A.

Michael Bonner
School of Pharmacy, University of Bradford, Bradford, West Yorkshire, U.K.

Jagdish Singh
Department of Pharmaceutical Sciences, College of Pharmacy, North Dakota State University, Fargo, North Dakota, U.S.A.

Michael S. Roberts
School of Medicine, University of Queensland, Princess Alexandria Hospital, Woolloongabba, Queensland, Australia

INTRODUCTION

Iontophoresis, one of a number of techniques to promote percutaneous absorption (see Chapter 1), enables the administration of ionic therapeutic agents across a membrane, such as skin, by the application of a low-level electric current. Water-soluble ionic drugs, including peptides, may be effectively delivered through the intact skin by iontophoresis. Transdermal iontophoresis allows high control of delivery rate in a preprogrammed manner (1,2). Since the rate of drug delivery is proportional to the applied current, intersubject and intrasubject variability is considerably reduced in iontophoresis (1,3). Drugs of various therapeutic categories, including analgesics, anti-inflammatory agents, central nervous system agents, antihypertensive agents, peptides, and oligonucleotides, have been transported effectively by transdermal iontophoresis. This chapter presents an overview of transdermal iontophoresis, its current therapeutic applications, and dermal toxicity caused by this technique. The recent advances in the area of transdermal iontophoretic delivery have also been discussed.

FACTORS AFFECTING IONTOPHORESIS

Iontophoresis increases the transport of solutes by three main mechanisms (4):

1. Charged solutes are transported primarily by electrical repulsion from the electrode.
2. The flow of electric current may enhance the permeability of skin.
3. Electro-osmosis may alter the transport of unionized molecules and large polar peptides.

The factors affecting transdermal iontophoresis include current density, pH, ionic strength, concentration of drug, molecular size, and method of current application (continuous or pulse current). Iontophoretic delivery is affected by pH because of the varying degree of solute ionization and the permselectivity of the skin. Yoshida and Roberts (5) showed that the choice of the donor solution was critical in that the addition of other buffer ions led to ion competition for the applied current. The transport of uncharged solutes can be enhanced by the process of electro-osmosis. The transport of small cationic drugs from the anode is generally favored because the skin carries a net negative charge at physiological pH that renders it permselective to cations under the imposition of an electric field (6). For positively charged solutes, the relative contribution of electro-osmosis (compared with the electrorepulsive effect) becomes increasingly significant with increasing molecular weight, such that it is probably the primary mechanism for the iontophoretic transport of peptides and small proteins (7).

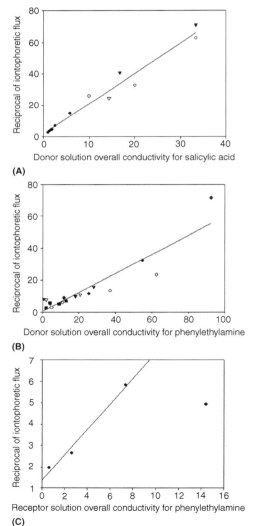

(A)

(B)

(C)

FIGURE 1 Relationship between the reciprocal of iontophoretic flux, J_{ss}, and overall conductivity of (A) donor solution ($k_{s,d}$) for salicylic acid, (B) donor solution ($k_{s,d}$) for phenylethylamine, and (C) receptor solution ($k_{s,r}$) for phenylethylamine.

Epidermal iontophoresis for solutes from a range of solutions can be described by an integrated ionic mobility–pore model that takes into account solute size (defined by MV, MW, or radius), solute mobility, solute shape, solute charge, Debye layer thickness, total current applied solute concentration, fraction ionized, presence of extraneous ions (defined by solvent conductivity), and epidermal permselectivity (8). The model incorporates partitioning rates to account for interaction of unionized and ionized lipophilic solutes with the wall of the pore, as well as electroosmosis. This model has been applied to describe the transport of local anesthetics (9) and more generally other solutes (10). This work has highlighted the importance of solute conductivity in solution and the desirability to exclude other ions that may compete with the solute as part of the overall current. Figure 1, adapted from that work, shows that there is a linear relationship between inverse flux for salicylic acid and phenylethylamine and overall conductivity of the donor solution. Additionally, at low concentrations of phenylethylamine, a linear relationship was observed between receptor conductivity and inverse flux (Fig. 1C). An observed outlier at high NaCl receptor concentration was attributed to ionic interactions. The contribution of electro-osmosis to flux of the species was assumed to be low. The model indicated

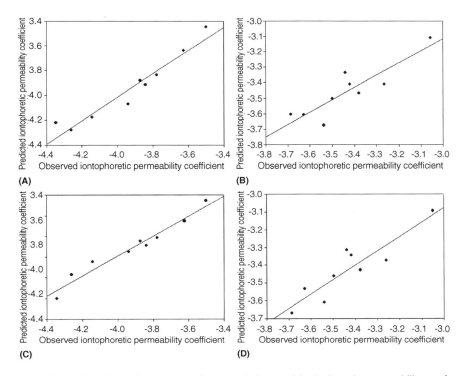

FIGURE 2 Correlation between predicted and observed iontophoretic permeability coefficients ($PC_{j,iont}$) for local anesthetics under varying pH donor and receptor conditions. Predicted data in (**A**) and (**B**) are generated using molecular volume and log ionic mobility, whereas predicted data in (**C**) and (**D**) are generated using molecular weight and log ionic mobility. For (**A**) and (**C**), donor and receptor pH values are both 4.5, whereas for (**B**) and (**D**) donor pH is 4.5 and receptor pH is 7.4.

that a linear relationship between flux and donor solution conductivity would only be found if donor conductivity was much larger than receptor conductivity (again if electro-osmosis was negligible).

The ionic mobility–pore model was then applied to the iontophoretic transport of anesthetics, which are commonly delivered in this manner (9). Figure 2 illustrates some correlations between predicted fluxes, obtained from solute size and conductivity, and observed iontophoretic fluxes. Optimal correlations were obtained when both donor and receptor were at the same pH value. Thus, it was found that the model was applicable to a range of drug molecules.

ROUTES OF PENETRATION OF DRUGS BY IONTOPHORESIS

The routes through which drugs can permeate the skin by passive diffusion are transcellular, intercellular, and transappendageal. There is a strong experimental evidence to show that iontophoretic transport of drugs across the skin occurs through transappendageal and intercellular pathways (11). Transappendageal pathways such as sweat glands and hair follicles have been suggested as the primary routes of drug transport by iontophoresis. Most small solutes are transported through a pore with radii of 6.8 to 17 A° (12). Although lateral iontophoretic transport may be possible, this is unlikely in vivo due to the effects of the skin microcirculation (10). Using a vibrating probe electrode, Cullander and Guy (13) showed that iontophoretic currents were primarily carried by residual hairs in hairless mouse skin.

Iontophoretic studies using human epidermal membrane showed that significant new pore induction (electroporation) occurs, resulting in an increase in the permeability of the membrane (14). Essa et al. (15) compared the anodal iontophoretic flux of estradiol and mannitol through human epidermal membrane and a human skin sandwich made from overlaying the stratum corneum from a given skin donor on top of an epidermal membrane from the same donor, in effect blocking the shunt route in both the upper stratum corneum and lower epidermis. A current density of 0.5 mA/cm^2 was used for five hours, and the ratio of sandwich to iontophoretic molecule flux was measured. In theory, if shunts were the only route of permeation, flux would be effectively abolished, whereas if their contribution to penetration was minimal flux would be reduced by 50% (due to a doubling of the stratum corneum barrier thickness). The investigators found fluxes reduced by 78% and 85% for estradiol and mannitol, respectively. They concluded that, whereas physical shunts had a role to play in the iontophoretic delivery of both drugs, penetration through new aqueous pathways created by the application of the constant current (as opposed to a constant driving force that would be produced under controlled voltage iontophoresis) could not be ruled out.

The pathway of iontophoretic transport of mercuric chloride in pig skin was studied (16). The mercuric salts were deposited in the intercellular space of the stratum corneum as observed by high-resolution transmission microscopy. Lee et al. (11) examined the iontophoretic pathways using hairless mouse skin and cultured skin models (EpiDerm™, MatTek Corporation Massachusetts, U.S.A. and Skin2™, Advanced Tissue Sciences, California, U.S.A.). The authors reported that hair follicles are the predominant transport path in hairless mouse skin, and for cultured skin models, which have no appendages, intercellular pathways are the paths of least resistance to ions permeating the skin. The transcellular pathway is also expected to be less important in the presence of low-resistance pores. The relative importance of each pathway may depend on several factors such as solubility, molecular weight, p*K*a, and the binding nature of the solute to the tissue (17–19). Hair follicles appeared to be the significant pathway for electro-osmotic flow (20).

CURRENT THERAPEUTIC APPLICATIONS OF IONTOPHORESIS AND IONTOPHORETIC DEVICES

Iontophoresis has gained growing acceptance for local therapy. Iontophoresis has been used in the diagnosis of cystic fibrosis (21). This test was first introduced by Gibson and Cooke (22) and received Food and Drug Administration (FDA) approval in 1983. The perspiration of the cystic fibrosis patients contains a substantially higher concentration of sodium and chloride ions (23), and the assay of the chloride ions is the basis for the diagnostic test. Macroduct® and Nanoduct® (Discovery Diagnostics, Canada) are the iontophoretic devices marketed by Wescor, Inc (Logan, Utah, U.S.) for sweat stimulation and collection in cystic fibrosis patients. Pilocarpine is used for sweat stimulation and is incorporated in a gel reservoir (Pilogel® discs, Alcon Laboratories, Hertfordshire, U.K.).

Tap water iontophoresis has been a method of choice for the treatment of palmoplantar hyperhidrosis (24,25). Drionic, a battery-operated device (General Medical Co., Los Angeles, California, U.S.A.) that is connected to free-floating felt pads, has been used in the treatment of hyperhidrosis. Iontocaine®, an iontophoretic lidocaine-epinephrine system (Iomed, Salt Lake City, Utah, U.S.), has been used to induce local anesthesia. This device consists of a microprocessor-controlled battery-powered DC current generator and electrodes. The anode chamber is filled with lidocaine or epinephrine prior to use. Noninvasive delivery of local anesthetics by iontophoresis has been particularly useful in pediatric patients, providing rapid and effective anesthesia before dermal procedures such as intravenous injections and blood withdrawal. LidoSite® (Vyteris, Inc., Fair Lawn, New Jersey, U.S.A.) is another lidocaine iontophoretic device recently approved by the FDA. It is the first prefilled iontophoretic product, designed to induce local anesthesia before medical procedures such as insertion of intravenous catheters and needle sticks for blood withdraws and other dermatological surgical procedures. LidoSite combines fast onset of action with an easy-to-use, preprogrammed design (26). The unit consists of a monolithic patch containing Ag-AgCl electrodes with 10% lidocaine and 0.1% epinephrine dispersed throughout a hydrogel matrix formulation at the anode.

GlucoWatch® Biographer, a glucose-monitoring device based on the principle of reverse iontophoresis (27), was developed by Cygnus, Inc, (Redwood City, California, U.S.A.) and approved by the FDA in 2001. It consists of a wrist-worn device that continuously extracts glucose by iontophoresis, and it measures by an electrochemical enzymatic sensor over a period of 13 hours. The correlation between glucose concentrations measured with this unit and blood concentrations has been demonstrated in both pediatric and adult patients, making it suitable for home use.

The FDA has recently approved IONSYS™ (fentanyl iontophoretic transdermal system, Ortho-McNeil, Inc., New Jersey, U.S.), the first needle-free, patient-activated analgesic system (28). IONSYS is indicated for the short-term management of acute postoperative pain in adult patients requiring opioid analgesia during hospitalization. IONSYS is the first product to incorporate the proprietary E-TRANS® iontophoretic transdermal drug delivery system developed by Alza Corporation (Mountain View, California, U.S.). When pain medication is needed, the patient double-clicks the dosing button, which delivers a preprogrammed, 40-mcg dose of fentanyl through the skin. Each dose is delivered over a 10-minute period. IONSYS should be applied to intact, nonirritated, and nonirradiated skin on the chest or upper outer arm. The product is expected to be available in the market in 2007. In January 2006, the European Commission approved the use of IONSYS in the 25 member states of the European Union.

Iontophoretic devices have been used in many other therapeutic areas. Iontophoresis has been widely used in physical therapy for the delivery of ionic drugs for local effects while minimizing their systemic levels. Corticosteroids such as dexamethasone sodium phosphate and methylprednisolone sodium succinate have been extensively employed as topical anti-inflammatory agents for the treatment of musculoskeletal conditions such as tendonitis, where they can be combined with lidocaine (29,30). The Phoresor® (Iomed), a handheld device for applying a small electric current, was approved exclusively as a device for use in humans. The user is required to fill the electrode with a drug solution immediately prior to use. Electrodes such as IOGEL®, TransQFlex™, TransQE™, and Numby Stuff® (Iomed) offer a variety of sizes and shapes to treat various anatomical sites. Life Tech, Inc (Houston, Texas, U.S.) and Empi, Inc (St. Paul, Minnesota, U.S.A.) also supply iontophoretic devices (Microphor® and Dupel®) and electrodes (Meditrode®, Dupel B.L.U.E®) for the application of ionic drugs to a localized area of the body.

Iontophoresis has also been used in dentistry. Three basic applications in dentistry are treatment of hypersensitive dentine using fluoride, therapy of oral ulcers and herpes orolabialis lesions using corticosteroids and antiviral drugs, respectively, and local anesthesia (29,31).

IONTOPHORETIC DELIVERY OF NONPEPTIDE DRUGS

Iontophoresis has been employed for the systemic delivery of a number of drugs from several therapeutic categories including analgesic, anti-inflammatory, cardiovascular, and antiviral agents. A number of reviews have been published on transdermal iontophoresis (1,26,32,33). Therefore, we have discussed here briefly the iontophoretic delivery of nonpeptide drugs. Iontophoresis of hydromorphone has been studied in pigs using hydrogel patches (34). A good correlation was observed between the plasma hydromorphone levels during both iontophoresis and constant IV infusion. The iontophoretic delivery of four nonsteroidal anti-inflammatory agents (salicylic acid, ketoprofen, naproxen, and indomethacin) was studied in Sprague–Dawley rats (35). A positive correlation was observed between lipophilicity and skin concentrations of nonsteroidal anti-inflammatory drugs, whereas plasma concentrations decreased with increasing lipophilicity. The effect of iontophoresis on the systemic pharmacokinetics and the local drug distribution of sodium diclofenac in the skin and underlying tissues were studied (36). Iontophoresis facilitated local and systemic delivery of diclofenac sodium compared with passive diffusion. The iontophoretic delivery of bupreonorphine was greater than the passive administration in weanling Yorkshire swine (37). Steady-state levels were achieved rapidly, and therapeutic amounts of bupreonorphine were reported to be delivered.

The iontophoretic delivery of atenolol, pindolol, metoprolol, acebutolol, oxprenolol, and propranolol was studied in vivo in Sprague-Dawley rats to determine the relationship between iontophoretic transport and drug lipophilicity (38). The concentrations of the drugs in the skin generally increased as a function of lipophilicity, whereas drug transport from the skin to the cutaneous vein was inversely proportional to log P. The effect of iontophoretic delivery of timolol maleate on the inhibition of isoprenaline-induced tachycardia was investigated in rabbits (39). Pretreatment of skin with Azone increased the delivery of timolol maleate, and the effect was similar to that with intravenous delivery of timolol (30 mcg/kg). In another study, pulsed-mode constant current (0.5 mA) iontophoretic delivery of metoprolol to rabbits made hypertensive by methoxamine IV infusion induced a decrease in systolic and diastolic pressures within two hours (40).

Iontophoretic delivery of apomorphine was studied both in vitro with human stratum corneum and in vivo in patients with Parkinson's disease (41–43). These studies showed that the delivery of apomorphine is feasible and furthermore that the rate of delivery can be controlled by variation of the current densities. Luzardo-Alvarez et al. (44) studied the effect of iontophoresis on the transdermal delivery of anti-parkinsonian drug ropinirole hydrochloride in vivo in hairless rats. The authors concluded that iontophoresis can deliver therapeutic amounts of ropinirole hydrochloride.

IONTOPHORETIC DELIVERY OF PEPTIDES

Most of the peptide drugs are currently administered parenterally, which has inherent disadvantages. The transdermal route is promising for the delivery of peptides because skin is easily accessible, has a large surface area with many possible sites for delivery, and readily recovers from minor injury (45). Transdermal iontophoretic delivery of peptides has been reviewed previously (46,47). Generally, peptides with high isoelectric point (>10) are suitable candidates for iontophoretic delivery (48). These peptides have a positive charge at physiological pH. The delivery of these peptides is further facilitated by electro-osmotic flow, which moves from anode to cathode. If the solution has a low pH (<4), the charge on the skin may be neutralized (49) and diminished or even reverse electro-osmotic flow is possible.

Clinical studies indicate that small peptides could be successfully delivered in humans by iontophoresis. Therapeutic doses of leuprolide, a nonapeptide leutinizing hormone-releasing hormone (LHRH) analogue, have been delivered to 13 human volunteers using iontophoretic patches (50). This study found that passive patches did not produce elevations in serum luteinizing hormone, whereas the active patches resulted in increased levels, comparable to those with subcutaneous injection. Iontophoretic delivery of LHRH in Yorkshire pigs in vivo was monitored via the plasma levels of follicle-stimulating hormone and luteinizing hormone, showing that pharmacologically active peptide had been delivered (51). In vitro studies with human epidermis have suggested that a pulsed direct current profile may be more efficient than a simple constant current application for delivering LHRH and its analog nafarelin (52). Iontophoretic delivery of growth-hormone-releasing hormone in hairless guinea pigs in vivo achieved steady-state plasma levels comparable to those after intravenous and subcutaneous injections (53).

Green (47) reported that the plasma concentration–time profile resulting from six hours of iontophoresis was found to be similar to that from intravenous infusion, but the appearance of the calcitonin analogue (molecular weight approximately 3000) in plasma following iontophoresis was slower than during intravenous infusion. Other iontophoretic studies have been performed with salmon calcitonin (54,55). Pulsatile iontophoretic delivery of human parathyroid hormone, a pharmacologically active fragment, to ovariectomized Sprague-Dawley rats produced an increase in bone mineral density similar to daily subcutaneous injections (56).

Transdermal delivery of insulin has been extensively investigated in vitro (57–59) and in small laboratory animals. In many of the studies, some kind of pretreatment of the skin (e.g., shaving, application of depilatory cream, or use of chemical penetration enhancers) has been done prior to iontophoresis (60,61). In many of these studies, a therapeutic dose of insulin was delivered by iontophoresis. Iontophoretic delivery of monomeric insulins has been shown to be better than the regular insulin (62,63). However, it must be noted that the dose of insulin required for human use is much higher and it will be difficult to deliver the human dose using an iontophoretic patch of reasonable size and current strength (64).

Iontophoretic transport of drugs across the skin has been shown to be inversely proportional to their molecular size (65,66). Turner et al. (67) studied the effect of iontophoresis (0.5 mA/cm^2 for up to 16 hours) on the delivery of a series of fluorescently labeled poly-L-lysines with three different molecular weights (4, 7, and 26 kDa). Iontophoresis greatly increased the penetration of the 4-kDa analogue, slightly elevated the delivery of the 7-kDa analogue but had no effect on the transport of the larger 26-kDa analogue. It appears that transdermal iontophoresis may not be suitable for the delivery of larger peptides (>7000 Da) across intact skin.

DELIVERY OF OLIGONUCLEOTIDES

The iontophoretic transport of oligonucleotides through excised, full-thickness hairless mouse skin was found to decrease with increasing size, with the 10-mer being transported at a rate about six times faster than the 30-mer and twice as fast as the 20-mer (68). A small six-base oligonucleotide (molecular weight 1927) was reported to permeate hairless mouse skin with little or no degradation in an in vitro study (69). Vlassov et al. (70) demonstrated measurable tissue concentration of oligonucleotides in mice after iontophoresis in vivo. Brand et al. (71) reported that the iontophoretically delivered phosphorothioate oligonucleotides could reach concentrations sufficient to induce changes in specific target enzymes in vivo in rats. However, Li et al. (72) reported that it would be difficult to deliver a human dose of pharmacologically active oligonucleotides using a reasonable patch size and current parameters. Iontophoresis of an antisense oligonucleotide directed against the 3′-untranslated region of mouse IL-10 mRNA induced an inhibitory effect on the production of IL-10, which is involved in the pathogenesis of atopic dermatitis, and an improvement of the skin lesions was observed in treated mice (73). An ophthalmic investigation in rats reported the iontophoretic penetration of oligonucleotide into all the corneal layers, without any detectable ocular damage (74). Many of the studies on the iontophoretic delivery of oligonucleotides have been conducted in vitro or in small laboratory animals. Further studies are needed to determine the application of transdermal iontophoresis for the delivery of oligonucleotides.

IONTOPHORETIC DELIVERY USING HYDROGELS

In comparison to solution formulations, semisolid formulations would be easier to incorporate and retain in the iontophoretic patch during the shelf life period. In the recently approved fentanyl iontophoretic transdermal system, the drug is incorporated as a hydrogel formulation. The iontophoretic delivery of insulin, calcitonin, and vasopressin was investigated using hydrogels of polyacrylamide, polyhydroxyethylmethacrylate, and carbopol 934 (32). The release of drug from the hydrogel formulation under iontophoresis was found to follow zero-order kinetics. The permeability coefficients for these peptides across hairless rat skin were found to be inversely related to their molecular size. Gupta et al. (75) employed gels containing sodium cromoglycate for in vitro transdermal iontophoretic delivery across hairless guinea pig skin. Hydrogels of ionic polymers decreased the flux of sodium cromoglycate, but nonionic polymers such as hydroxypropyl cellulose and polyvinyl alcohol did not affect the flux.

Gelatin containing microemulsion-based organogels were used for the iontophoretic transport of a model compound (sodium salicylate) across pig skin (76). These gels showed substantially higher release rates for sodium salicylate with passive diffusion, and fluxes were proportional to the drug concentration and the current density. Microemulsion-based organogels also appear to offer improved microbial resistance in comparison to aqueous solution or hydrogels. Hydrogels of poloxamer, methylcellulose, and polyvinyl pyrrolidone have been used successfully for transdermal iontophoretic delivery of lidocaine, enoxacin, and methotrexate (77–79). Bender et al. (80) reported that the iontophoresis of etofenamate using a gel formulation in patients with low back pain produced higher concentrations of drug in serum and synovial fluid.

Cathodal iontophoresis of piroxicam gel formulations increased the transport of piroxicam across porcine ear skin in vitro by approximately threefold compared with passive diffusion (81). Nair and Panchagnula (82) studied the effect of iontophoresis on the pharmacokinetic and pharmacodynamic activity of poloxamer gel formulation of arginine vasopressin. Iontophoresis produced a rapid onset of both pharmacokinetic and pharmacodynamic activity. The effect of iontophoresis on the transport of timolol maleate from hydroxypropyl cellulose gel across the combined polyflux membrane and pig stratum corneum was studied (83). Iontophoresis increased the transport of timolol maleate 13 to 15 times in comparison to passive transport.

Huang et al. (84) evaluated the effects of iontophoresis and electroporation on the transdermal delivery of nalbuphine benzoate and sebacoyl dinalbuphine ester from the solution and hydrogels of hydroxypropyl cellulose and carboxymethylcellulose. Application of iontophoresis or electroporation significantly enhanced the in vitro permeation of nalbuphine benzoate and sebacoyl dinalbuphine ester. The lipophilicity and molecular size of the drugs and the hydrogel compositions had significant effect on the delivery of nalbuphine benzoate and sebacoyl dinalbuphine ester. Because the delivery efficiency of iontophoretic transport of drugs from hydrogels would be less than that from solution formulations, hydrogels may not be suitable for expensive drugs.

IONTOPHORETIC DELIVERY IN COMBINATION WITH LIPID VESICLES

Li et al. (85) used an elastic lipid vesicle comprising polyoxyethylene and sucrose esters mixed with cholesterol sulfate to pretreat for three hours the stratum corneum and epidermal membranes. After this treatment, the iontophoresis of the anti-Parkinson's drug apomorphine was investigated. At a current density of $0.5 \, mA/cm^2$, the drug flux was increased by around 35% and 48% in the stratum corneum and epidermis, respectively. The authors correlated this flux enhancement with a decrease in electrical resistance of the skin after treatment with the lipid particles. Another study by Essa et al. (86) examined the in vitro transdermal iontophoretic delivery of estradiol encapsulated in specially tailored ultradeformable liposomes compared with saturated aqueous solution (control). As the liposomes bore a negative charge (bearing a zeta potential of approximately -29 mV), iontophoretic delivery was cathodal. Individually, both the use of the lipid vesicles and iontophoresis improved flux of the drug. When combined, the researchers found that iontophoresis of the vesicle at 0.5 mA/cm^2 encapsulating the estradiol could provide flux enhancements of approximately 15-fold, compared to the iontophoresis of the saturated solution. The authors concluded that iontophoresis of the lipid vesicle repelled it into the skin where its phospholipids adhered and fused with the stratum corneum, causing increased permeability while concurrently the applied current was disorganizing the lipid layer stacking. Consequently, phospholipids and electric current could synergistically enhance the estradiol flux, and the iontophoretic driving force may aid the deformability of the vesicle and enable the liposomes to squeeze through the temporarily impaired barrier.

Iontophoresis of a cationic liposome has been described by Han et al. (87). Using wax-depilated rat skin, liposomes including 1,2-dioleoyl-3-trimethyl-ammonium propane were prepared incorporating adriamycin. Applying anodal iontophoresis for 20 minutes, they obtained up to threefold penetration enhancement of the drug into the membrane, compared with topical application of the drug alone. Delivery to the follicles was highlighted as excellent in this work.

IONTOPHORESIS IN COMBINATION WITH MICROPROJECTION ARRAYS

In an in vivo study on hairless guinea pigs, a group of workers employed the Alza Macroflux® microprojection patch array to the delivery of antisense oligonucleotides (88). A 2-cm^2 array with 30-μm stainless steel projections at a density of 240/cm^2 was applied to the animals, and the delivery of a tritiated 20-mer oligonucleotide from a reservoir below it was evaluated. Skin biopsies were sectioned, and nucleotide content was assayed by scintillation counting. Following four hours of iontophoresis at 0.1 mA/cm^2, the flux of the compound was approximately 100-fold greater than that produced by the electrical treatment alone. The biopsies also indicated that drug concentrations within the tissue remained relatively constant at depths up to 700–800 μm when iontophoresis was applied to the array. Under iontophoresis alone, the compound was at concentrations approximately 1000-fold smaller at these depths. The authors concluded that the patch represented a delivery option for large hydrophilic molecules that could currently only be administered by injection.

REVERSE IONTOPHORESIS

An interesting application of iontophoresis is the noninvasive sampling for the diagnostic measurement of blood substrates. The noninvasive and minimally invasive methods for transdermal glucose monitoring have been recently reviewed (89). The approval of GlucoWatch Biographer for the noninvasive sampling of glucose in patients with diabetes has generated considerable interest in possible new applications of reverse iontophoresis. Prostaglandins E2 generated in response to transdermally applied drug irritants have been monitored noninvasively in vivo by reverse iontophoresis (90). Noninvasive sampling of phenylalanine by reverse iontophoresis was successfully performed in vitro using dermatomed porcine skin (91).

Delgado-Charro and Guy (92) have reported that transdermal reverse iontophoresis has the potential for the noninvasive therapeutic monitoring of valproate. Reverse iontophoresis has been reported to be a potentially useful and noninvasive tool for monitoring phenytoin and lithium (93,94). Further research on reverse iontophoresis may yield interesting findings that would be helpful in the noninvasive measurement of clinically important molecules in the body.

DERMATOTOXICITY FROM IONTOPHORESIS

Iontophoretic parameters that affect the skin safety include current intensity, length of application, electrode type in addition to pH of the formulation, permeant type, region of administration, and ethnicity (95,96). Despite several developments in the area of iontophoresis, there are concerns about the effects of iontophoresis on skin safety in humans, including skin barrier perturbation and irritation.

Skin irritation covers many manifestations of provoked nonimmunologic cutaneous responses in living tissue by the application of stimuli (97). Irritation reduces the efficiency of stratum corneum barrier function and results in an increase in transepidermal water loss. Hence, a high transepidermal water loss generally indicates barrier perturbation (98,99). Mild irritation due to brief clinical applications of iontophoresis with low-voltage electrodes has been reported (100). Skin irritation (e.g., erythema, edema, pain, itching, and heat) is the observed response at the delivery or contact site. The skin irritation mechanism involves the release of inflammatory mediators and their migration to the exposed area leading to erythema and edema.

Erythema may result from microscopic cellular damage at sites of high current density leading to cytokine and prostaglandin release and local vasodilatation (101). The possibility of direct electric stimulation of erythema also exists (102). Cutaneous stimuli can provoke the release of substance P and calcitonin-gene-related peptide at nerve endings in the epidermis (103,104). Calcitonin-gene-related peptide is a potent vasodilator, which is responsible for a localized erythema lasting several hours. Its release may therefore be a reason for the erythematous responses seen with iontophoresis.

There are differences in clinical effectiveness and toxicity of drugs among ethnic groups. Therefore, it is possible that differences in dermal toxicity among ethnic groups may exist in response to iontophoresis. Singh et al. (104) studied the racial differences on skin barrier function and skin irritation in response to iontophoresis. The effect of iontophoresis on the mean and significance (p values) erythema scores in four ethnic groups (i.e., African, Asian, Caucasian, and Hispanic) is shown in Table 1. Edema was not observed in any of the ethnic groups. However, there was a mild erythema in all of the four ethnic groups due to four-hour iontophoresis at 0.2 mA/cm^2 current density, which was resolved 24 hours after termination of iontophoresis. Table 2 depicts the summary of iontophoresis effect on clinical changes in four ethnic groups.

The human skin displays remarkable regional variation in percutaneous absorption of different molecules (105,106). Singh et al. (98) found regional variation in dermal toxicity in response to iontophoresis. Erythema as a reaction to iontophoresis was observed at all the body sites. Iontophoresis is shown to induce significantly higher erythema both at the anode and the cathode ($p < 0.01$) at the abdomen, upper arm, and chest, but these scores resolved 24 hours after termination of iontophoresis except at the chest under the anode (98). Thus, the chest was more sensitive because the erythema score was greater than at the upper arm or abdomen after 24 hours of the termination of iontophoresis. Figure 3 shows the effect of iontophoresis on Draize scores (107) for erythema at different sites of the body under anode and cathode, respectively. There was no edema at any of the studied body sites.

TABLE 1   Effect of Iontophoresis on Mean Values and Significance (*P* values) of Erythema Scores in Ethnic Groups

	Anode					Cathode				
					Time (min)					
Ethnic group	-10	0	60	120	1440	-10	0	60	120	1440
Caucasian	0	1	1	0.9	0.3	0	1.2	1	0.8	0.2
		P < 0.001	*P* < 0.001	*P* < 0.001	*P* > 0.05		*P* < 0.001	*P* < 0.001	*P* < 0.001	*P* > 0.05
African	0	0.7	0.7	0.3	0.2	0	1	0.6	0.6	0.1
		P > 0.05	*P* > 0.05	*P* > 0.05	*P* < 0.05		*P* < 0.001	*P* > 0.05	*P* > 0.05	
Hispanic	0	1	1.33	1.2	0.4	0	1.3	1.11	1.2	0.3
		P > 0.05	*P* < 0.001	*P* < 0.001	*P* < 0.05		*P* < 0.01	*P* < 0.001	*P* < 0.001	*P* > 0.05
Asian	0	0.09	1	0.9	0	0	1.5	1.2	1.1	0
		P < 0.01	*P* < 0.001	*P* < 0.01	*P* > 0.05		*P* < 0.001	*P* < 0.001	*P* < 0.001	*P* > 0.05

Time -10 minutes is the measurement taken before application of the patch (baseline). *Source:* From Ref. 104.

TABLE 2 Summary of Clinical Changes Due to Iontophoresis in Four Ethnic Groups

Clinical parameters	Anode	Cathode
TEWL	There was a significant difference between groups at baseline at the anode. However, there were no significant group effects after iontophoresis, indicating no effects due to iontophoresis at the anode. Iontophoresis did not produce any meaningful clinical changes at the anode.	A significant gender by ethnic group interaction was found after 1 hour of iontophoretic patch removal. Since neither the gender main effect nor the group main effect was significant and the effect was not present in the time contrast analyses, this was probably a spurious result with no scientific significance. Therefore, iontophoresis did not produce any meaningful clinical changes at the cathode.
Skin temperature	None	None
Skin capacitance	None	None
Draize score	Iontophoresis led to erythema at active anodes, which almost disappeared after 24 hours of patch removal. No edema was observed.	Iontophoresis led to erythema at active Cathode, which almost disappeared after 24 hours of patch removal. No edema was observed.

Abbreviation: TEWL, transepidermal water loss. *Source*: From Ref. 104.

However, Li et al. (108) reported that iontophoresis induced slight erythema and edema (Draize score of 1) compared with the control. Pretreatment of skin with a surfactant formulation (laureth-3 ethyloxylene ether/laureth-7 ethyloxylene ether/ sodium sulfosuccinate in a molar ratio of 0.7:0.3:0.05) caused slightly greater skin erythema and edema (Draize score of 1 or 2) in comparison to iontophoresis alone

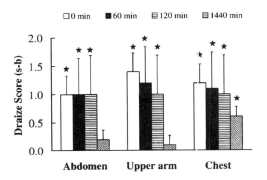

FIGURE 3 Effect of iontophoresis on visual scores at the anode sites. Values plotted are the mean $[(vs_{at} - vs_{ct})\ (vs_{a0} - vs_{c0})]$ for each time t after termination of iontophoresis, where vs_{at} and vs_{ct} are the measured visual scores at the active and control sites at time t, respectively. These contrasts of measurements recorded at time t, $(vs_{at} - vs_{ct})$, with the baseline measurements $(vs_{a0} - vs_{c0})$, define the iontophoresis effect on visual scores at each time t after the termination of iontophoresis. * indicates statistical significance ($p < 0.05$) in comparison to the background. *Source*: From Ref. 98.

(108). This study also emphasizes that skin irritation can be affected by not only iontophoretic parameters but also formulation components.

Iontophoresis may also result in skin reactions such as papules, rashes, tingling/warm sensations, and others. Papules are very small fluid-filled elevations on the skin and may be caused by the release of histamine from dermal mast cells, localized dermal cellular infiltrates, or localized hyperplasia of dermal or epidermal cellular elements. In some individuals, the application of current can cause increased redness and the release of histamine in the skin, and this can lead to the appearance of an allergic reaction even though the patient is not allergic. It is shown that iontophoresis, even at a low current density, results in skin papules (98,100,104). These skin reactions depend on the type of skin, site on the body, in addition to the iontophoresis parameters. Unusual skin reactions were reported in a subject following iontophoresis with skin rash developed on day 2 following iontophoresis and with dotty-like lesions by day 4 (108). The reactions disappeared by day 10. However, the exact nature of the skin reaction was unknown. Thus, the effect of iontophoresis on skin barrier function and cutaneous irritation depends on the site of the application on the body, type of skin (ethnicity), sensitivity of the skin, in addition to the iontophoretic parameters and formulation composition. The acceptance and further development of this technique depend on ensuring that it does not provoke unacceptable side effects.

FUTURE CONSIDERATIONS

Transdermal iontophoresis has gained growing acceptance for the topical delivery of drugs. The application of iontophoresis has been recently extended to systemic delivery. Transdermal iontophoretic delivery offers a unique opportunity for noninvasive, convenient, effective, and patient-controlled delivery of drugs. This technique may be particularly useful for the delivery of small peptide drugs and for the treatment of difficult-to-treat diseases such as skin cancer (basal cell carcinoma), psoriasis, dermatitis, venous ulcers, keloid, and hypertrophic scars. Reverse iontophoresis also has a great potential for the noninvasive sampling and monitoring of clinically important molecules in the body. The major challenge in the development of iontophoretic delivery systems is to design an easily used and relatively inexpensive system while maintaining the physical and chemical stability of the drug during shelf life. The safety of the long-term use of iontophoresis also needs to be studied thoroughly.

REFERENCES

1. Singh J, Roberts MS. Transdermal delivery of drugs by iontophoresis: a review. Drug Des Deliv 1989; 4:1–12.
2. Sage BH. Iontophoresis. In: Swarbrick J, Boylan JC, eds. Encyclopedia of Pharmaceutical Technology, Vol.8, New York: Marcel Dekker, 1993:217–247.
3. Burnette RR, Ongpipatanukul B. Characterization of the permselective properties of excised human skin during iontophoresis. J Pharm Sci 1987; 76:765–773.
4. Barry BW. Novel mechanisms and devices to enable successful transdermal drug delivery. Eur J Pharm Sci 2001; 14:101–114.
5. Yoshida NH, Roberts MS. Prediction of cathodal iontophoretic transport of various anions across excised skin from different vehicles using conductivity experiments. J Pharm Pharmacol 1995; 47:883–890.

6. Naik A, Kalia YN, Guy RH. Transdermal drug delivery: overcoming the skin's barrier function. Pharm Sci Technol Today 2000; 3:318–326.
7. Guy RH, Kalia YN, Delgado-Charro MB, et al. Iontophoresis: electrorepulsion and electroosmosis. J Control Release 2000; 64:129–132.
8. Roberts MS, Lai PM, Anissimov YG. Epidermal iontophoresis: I. Development of the ionic mobility-pore model. Pharm Res 1998; 15(10):1569–1578.
9. Lai PM, Roberts MS. Epidermal iontophoresis: II. Application of the ionic mobility-pore model to the transport of local anesthetics. Pharm Res 1998; 15(10):1579–1588.
10. Lai PM, Anissimov YG, Roberts MS. Lateral iontophoretic solute transport in skin. Pharm Res 1999; 16(1):46–54.
11. Lee D, White HS, Scott ER. Visualization of iontophoretic transport pathways in cultured and animal skin models. J Pharm Sci 1996; 85:1186–1190.
12. Lai PM, Roberts MS. An analysis of solute structure-human epidermal transport relationships in epidermal iontophoresis using the ionic mobility: pore model. J Control Release 1999; 58(3):323–333.
13. Cullander C, Guy RH. Sites of iontophoretic flow into the skin: identification and characterization with the vibrating probe electrode. J Invest Dermatol 1991; 97:55–64.
14. Zhu H, Peck KD, Li SK, et al. Quantification of pore induction in human epidermal membrane during iontophoresis: the importance of background electrolyte selection. J Pharm Sci 2001; 90:932–942.
15. Essa EA, Bonner MC, Barry BW. Human skin sandwich for assessing shunt route penetration during passive and iontophoretic drug and liposome delivery. J Pharm Pharmacol 2002; 54(11):1481–1489.
16. Monteiro-Riviere NA, Inman AO, Riviere JE. Identification of the pathway of transdermal iontophoretic drug delivery: light and ultrastructural studies using mercuric chloride in pigs. Pharm Res 1994; 11:251–256.
17. Riviere JE, Heit MC. Electrically-assisted transdermal drug delivery. Pharm Res 1997; 14:687–697.
18. Hirvonen J, Murtomaki L, Kontturi K. Experimental verification of the mechanistic model for transdermal transport including iontophoresis. J Control Release 1998; 56:169–174.
19. Turner NG, Guy RH. Iontophoretic transport pathways: dependence on penetrant physicochemical properties. J Pharm Sci 1997; 12:1385–1389.
20. Bath BD, Scott ER, Phipps JB, et al. Scanning electrochemical microscopy of iontophoretic transport in hairless mouse skin analysis of the relative contributions of diffusion, migration, and electro osmosis to transport in hair follicles. J Pharm Sci 2000; 46:281–305.
21. Panus P, Banga AK. Iontophoresis devices: clinical applications for topical delivery. Int J Pharm Comp 1997; 1:420–424.
22. Gibson LE, Cooke RE. A test for concentration of electrolytes in sweat in cystic fibrosis of the pancreas utilizing pilocarpine by iontophoresis. Pediatrics 1959; 23:545–549.
23. Huang YY, Wu SM, Wang CY. Response surface method as an approach to optimization of iontophoretic transdermal delivery of pilocarpine. In J Pharm 1996; 129:41–50.
24. Reinauer SA, Neusser G, Schauf G, et al. Iontophoresis with alternating current and direct current offset (AC DC iontophoresis): a new approach for the treatment of hyperhidrosis. Br J Dermatol 1993; 129:166–169.
25. Togel B, Greve B, Raulin C. Current therapeutic strategies for hyperhidrosis: a review. Eur J Dermatol 2002; 12:219–223.
26. Kalia YN, Naik A, Garrison J, et al. Iontophoretic drug delivery. Adv Drug Del Rev 2004; 56:619–658.
27. Glikfeld P, Hinz RS, Guy RH. Noninvasive sampling of biological fluids by iontophoresis. Pharm Res 1989; 6:988–990.
28. Gupta SK, Sathyan G, Phipps B, et al. Reproducible fentanyl doses delivered intermittently at different time intervals from an electrotransport system. J Pharm Sci 1999; 88:835–841.
29. Costello CT, Jeske AH. Iontophoresis: applications in transdermal medication delivery. Phys Ther 1995; 75:554–563.
30. Lark MR, Gangarosa LP. Iontophoresis: an effective modality for the treatment of inflammatory disorders of the temporomandibular joint and myofascial pain. Cranio 1990; 8:108–119.

31. Gangarosa LP. Iontophoresis for surface local anesthesia. J Am Dent Assoc 1974; 88:125–127.
32. Banga AK, Chien YW. Hydrogel-based iontotherapeutic delivery devices for transdermal delivery of peptide/protein drugs. Pharm Res 1993; 10:697–702.
33. Kanikkannan N. Iontophoresis-based transdermal delivery systems. BioDrugs 2002; 16:339–347.
34. Padmanabhan RV, Phipps JB, Lattin GA, et al. In vitro and in vivo evaluation of transdermal iontophoretic delivery of hydromorphone. J Control Release 1990; 11:123–135.
35. Tashiro Y, Shichibe S, Kato Y, et al. Effect of lipophilicity on in vivo iontophoretic delivery: I. NSAIDS. Biol Pharm Bull 2001; 24:278–283.
36. Hui X, Anigbogu A, Singh P, et al. Pharmacokinetic and local tissue disposition of [^{14}C] sodium diclofenac following iontophoresis and systemic administration in rabbits. J Pharm Sci 2001; 90:1269–1276.
37. DeNuzzio J, Boericke K, Sutter D, et al. Iontophoretic delivery of bupreonorphine. Proceedings of the International Symposium on Controlled Release of Bioactive Materials, Controlled Release Society Inc, Minneapolis, Minn, 1996; vol 23:285.
38. Tashiro Y, Sami M, Shichibe S, et al. Effect of lipophilicity on in vivo iontophoretic delivery. II. Beta-blockers. Biol Pharm Bull 2001; 24:671–677.
39. Kanikkannan N, Singh J, Ramarao P. Transdermal iontophoretic delivery of timolol maleate in albino rabbits. Int J Pharm 2000; 197:69–76.
40. Zakzewski CA, Li JKJ. Pulsed mode constant current iontophoretic transdermal metoprolol tartrate delivery in established acute hypertensive rabbits. J Control Release 1991; 17:157–162.
41. Li GL, Grossklaus A, Danhof M, et al. Iontophoretic R-apomorphine delivery in combination with surfactant pretreatment: in vitro validation studies. Int J Pharm 2003; 266:61–68.
42. Li GL, de Vries JJ, van Steeg TJ, et al. Transdermal iontophoretic delivery of apomorphine in patients improved by surfactant formulation pretreatment. J Control Release 2005; 101:199–208.
43. Junginger HE. Iontophoretic delivery of apomorphine: from in vitro modeling to the Parkinson patient. Adv Drug Deliv Rev 2002; 54(Suppl. 1):S57–S75.
44. Luzardo-Alvarez A, Delgado-Charro MB, Blanco-Mendez J. In vivo iontophoretic administration of ropinirole hydrochloride. J Pharm Sci 2003; 92:2441–2448.
45. Bronaugh RL, Maibach HI. Eds. Percutaneous absorption: drugs-cosmetics-mechanisms-methodology. New York: Marcel Dekker, 1999.
46. Parasrampuria D, Parasrampuria J. Percutaneous delivery of protein and peptides using iontophoresis techniques. J Clin Pharm Ther 1991; 16:7–17.
47. Green P. Iontophoretic delivery of peptide drugs. J Control Release 1996; 41:33–48.
48. Banga AK, ed. Electrically Assisted Transdermal and Topical Drug Delivery. Bristol: Taylor & Francis, 1998.
49. Bayon AMR, Guy RH. Iontophoresis of nafarelin across human skin in vitro. Pharm Res 1996; 13:798–800.
50. Meyer BR, Kreis W. Eschbach J. Successful transdermal administration of therapeutic doses of polypeptide to normal human volunteers. Clin Pharmacol Ther 1988; 44:607–612.
51. Heit MC, Williams PL, Jayes FL, et al. Transdermal iontophoretic peptide delivery: in vitro and in vivo studies with luteinizing hormone hormone releasing hormone. J Pharm Sci 1993; 82:240–243.
52. Raiman J, Koljonen M, Huikko K, et al. Delivery and stability of LHRH and Nafarelin in human skin: the effect of constant/pulsed iontophoresis. Eur J Pharm Sci 2004; 21:371–377.
53. Kumar S, Char H, Patel S, et al. In vivo transdermal iontophoretic delivery of growth hormone releasing factor GRF (1–44) in hairless guinea pigs. J Control Release 1992; 18:213–220.
54. Chang SL, Hofmann GA, Zhang L, et al. Transdermal iontophoretic delivery of salmon calcitonin. Int J Pharm 2000; 200:107–113.

55. Nakamura K, Katagai K, Mori K, et al. Transdermal administration of salmon calcitonin by pulse depolarization-iontophoresis in rats. Int J Pharm 2001; 218:93–102.
56. Suzuki Y, Nagase Y, Iga K, et al. Prevention of bone loss in ovariectomized rats by pulsatile transdermal iontophoretic administration of human PTH (1-34). J Pharm Sci 2002; 91:350–361.
57. Pillai O, Nair V, Panchagnula R. Transdermal iontophoresis of insulin: IV. Influence of chemical enhancers. Int J Pharm 2004; 269:109–120.
58. Rastogi SK, Singh J. Transepidermal transport enhancement of insulin by lipid extraction and iontophoresis. Pharm Res 2002; 19:427–433.
59. Rastogi SK, Singh J. Effect of chemical penetration enhancers and iontophoresis on the in vitro percutaneous enhancement of insulin through porcine epidermis. Pharm Dev Technol 2005; 10:97–104.
60. Kari B. Control of blood glucose levels in alloxan-diabetic rabbits by iontophoresis of insulin. Diabetes 1986; 35:217–221.
61. Siddiqui O, Sun Y, Liu JC, et al. Facilitated transdermal transport of insulin. J Pharm Sci 1987; 76:341–345.
62. Langkjaer L, Brange J, Grodsky GM, et al. Iontophoresis of monomeric insulin analogues in vitro: effects of insulin charge and skin pretreatment. J Control Release 1998; 51:47–56.
63. Kanikkannan N, Singh J, Ramarao P. Transdermal iontophoretic delivery of conventional and monomeric human insulin analogue. J Control Release 1999; 59:99–105.
64. Guy RH. Current status and future prospects of transdermal drug delivery. Pharm Res 1996; 13:1765–1769.
65. Yoshida NH, Roberts MS. Solute molecular size and transdermal iontophoresis across excised human skin. J Control Release 1993; 25:177–195.
66. Green PG, Hinz RS, Cullander C, et al. Iontophoretic delivery of amino acids and amino acid derivatives across the skin in vitro. Pharm Res 1991; 8:1113–1120.
67. Turner NG, Ferry L, Price M, et al. Iontophoresis of poly-L-lysines: the role of molecular weight? Pharm Res 1997; 14:1322–1331.
68. Oldenburg KR, Vo KT, Smith GA, et al. Iontophoretic delivery of oligonucleotides across full thickness hairless mouse skin. J Pharm Sci 1995; 84:915–921.
69. Brand RM, Iversen PL. Iontophoretic delivery of a telomeric oligonucleotide. Pharm Res 1996; 13:851–854.
70. Vlassov VV, Nechaeva MV, Karamyshev VN, et al. Iontophoretic delivery of oligo-nucleotide derivatives into mouse tumor. Antisense Res Dev 1994; 4:291–293.
71. Brand RM, Hannah TL, Norris J, et al. Transdermal delivery of antisense oligonucleotides can induce changes in gene expression in vivo. Antisense Nucleic Acid Drug Dev 2001; 11:1–6.
72. Li SK, et al. Iontophoretic transport of oligonucleotides across human epidermal mem-brane: a study of the Nernst-Planck model J Pharm Sci 2001; 90(7):915–931.
73. Sakamoto T, Miyazaki E, Aramaki Y. Improvement of dermatitis by iontophoretically delivered antisense oligonucleotides for interleukin-10 in NC/Nga mice. Gene Ther 2004; 11:317–324.
74. Berdugo M, Valamanesh F, Andrieu C, et al. Delivery of antisense oligonucleotide to the cornea by iontophoresis. Antisense Nucleic Acid Drug Dev 2003; 13:107–114.
75. Gupta SK, Kumar S, Bolton S, et al. Effect of chemical enhancers and conducting gels on iontophoretic transdermal delivery of cromolyn sodium. J Control Release 1994; 31:229–236.
76. Kantaria S, Rees GD, Lawrence J, et al. Gelatin-stabilized microemulsion-based organogels: rheology and application in iontophoretic transdermal drug delivery of cromolyn sodium. J Control Release 1999; 60:355–365.
77. Chen W, Frank SG. Iontophoresis of lidocaine H+ from polaxamer 407 gels (abstract). Pharm Res 1997; 14:S309.
78. Fang J-Y, Hsu L-R, Huang Y-B, et al. Evaluation of transdermal iontophoresis of enoxacin from polymer formulations: in vitro skin permeation and in vivo microdialysis using Wistar rat as animal model. Int J Pharm 1999; 180:137–149.
79. Alvarez-Figueroa MJ, Blanco-Mendez J. Transdermal delivery of methotrexate: iontophoretic delivery from hydrogels and passive delivery from microemulsions. Int J Pharm 2001; 215:57–65.

80. Bender T, Bariska J, Rojkovich B, et al. Etofenamate levels in human serum and synovial fluid following iontophoresis. Arztl Forsch 2001; 51:489–492.
81. Doliwa A, Santoyo S, Ygartua P. Transdermal iontophoresis and skin retention of piroxicam from gels containing piroxicam: hydroxypropyl-beta-cyclodextrin complexes. Drug Dev Ind Pharm 2001; 27:751–758.
82. Nair V, Panchagnula R. Poloxamer gel as vehicle for transdermal iontophoretic delivery of arginine vasopressin: evaluation of in vivo performance in rats. Pharmacol Res 2003; 47:555–562.
83. Stamatialis DF, Rolevink HH, Girones M, et al. In vitro evaluation of a hydroxypropyl cellulose gel system for transdermal delivery of timolol. Curr Drug Deliv 2004; 1:313–319.
84. Huang JF, Sung KC, Hu OY, et al. The effects of electrically assisted methods on transdermal delivery of nalbuphine benzoate and sebacoyl dinalbuphine ester from solutions and hydrogels. Int J Pharm 2005; 297:162–171.
85. Li GL, Danhof M, Bouwstra JA. Effect of elastic liquid-state vesicle on apomorphine iontophoresis transport through human skin in vitro. Pharm Res 2001; 18:1627–1630.
86. Essa EA, Bonner MC, Barry BW. Iontophoretic estradiol skin delivery and tritium exchange in ultradeformable liposomes. Int J Pharm 2002; 240:55–66.
87. Han I, Kim M, Kim J. Enhanced transfollicular delivery of adriamycin with a liposome and iontophoresis. Exp Dermatol 2004; 13:86–92.
88. Lin WQ, Cormier M, Samiee A, et al. Transdermal delivery of antisense oligonucleotides with microprojection patch (Macroflux) technology. Pharm Res 2001; 18(12):1789–1793.
89. Sieg A, Guy RH, Delgado-Charro MB. Noninvasive and minimally invasive methods for transdermal glucose monitoring. Diabetes Technol Ther 2005; 7:174–197.
90. Mize NK, Buttery M, Daddona P, et al. Reverse iontophoresis: monitoring prostaglandins E_2 associated with cutaneous inflammation in vivo. Exp Dermatol 1997; 6:298–302.
91. Merino V, Lopez A, Hochstrasser D, et al. Noninvasive sampling of phenylalanine by reverse iontophoresis. J Control Release 1999; 61:65–69.
92. Delgado-Charro MB, Guy RH. Transdermal reverse iontophoresis of valproate: a non-invasive method for therapeutic drug monitoring. Pharm Res 2003; 20:1506–1513.
93. Leboulanger B, Guy RH, Delgado-Charro MB. Noninvasive monitoring of phenytoin by reverse iontophoresis. Eur J Pharm Sci 2004; 22:427–433.
94. Leboulanger B, Fathi M, Guy RH. Reverse iontophoresis as a noninvasive tool for the lithium monitoring and pharmacokinetic profiling. Pharm Res 2004; 21:1214–1222.
95. Singh J, Bhatia K.S. Topical iontophoretic drug delivery: pathways, principles, factors, and skin irritation. Med Res Rev 1996; 16:285–296.
96. Banga AK, Bose S, Ghosh TK. Iontophoresis and electroporation: comparisons and contrasts. Int J Pharm 1999; 179:1–19.
97. Lammintausta K, Maibach HI. Contact dermatitis due to irritation. In: Adams EA, ed. Occupational Skin Disease. Philadelphia: W.B. Saunders, 1990.
98. Singh J, Gross M, Sage B, et al. Regional variations in skin barrier function and cutaneous irritation due to iontophoresis in human subjects. Food Chem Toxicol 2001; 39:1079–1086.
99. Sekkat N, Kalia YN, Guy RH. Biophysical study of porcine ear skin in vitro and its comparison to human skin in vivo. J Pharm Sci 2002; 91:2376–2381.
100. Camel E, O'Connell M, Sage B, et al. The effect of saline iontophoresis on skin integrity in human volunteers. I. Methodology and reproducibility. Fundam Appl Toxicol 1996; 32:168–178.
101. Ledger, WP. Skin biological issues in electrically enhanced transdermal delivery. Adv Drug Deliv Rev 1992; 9:289–307.
102. Myyra R, Dalpara M, Globerson J. Electrical erythema? Anesthesiology 1988; 69:440.
103. Dalsgaard CJ, Jernbeck J, Stains W, et al. Calcitonin gene-related peptide-like immuno-reactivity in nerve fibers in the human skin. Relation to fibers containing substance P, somatostatin- and vasoactive intestinalpolypeptide-like immunoreactivity. Histo-chemistry 1989; 91:35–38.
104. Singh J, Gross M, Sage B, et al. Effect of saline iontophoresis on skin barrier function and cutaneous irritation in four ethnic groups. Food Chem Toxicol 2000; 38:717–726.
105. Feldman RJ, Maibach HI. Regional variations in percutaneous penetration of ^{14}C cortisol in man. J Invest Dermatol 1967; 48:181–183.

106. Tsai JC, Lin CY, Sheu HM, et al. Noninvasive characterization of regional variation in drug transport into human stratum corneum in vivo. Pharm Res 2003; 20:632–638.
107. Draize J, Woodard G, Calvery H. Methods for the study of irritation and toxicity of substances applied topically to the skin and mucous membranes. J Pharmacol Exp Ther 1944; 82:377–390.
108. Li GL, Van Steeg TJ, Putter H, et al. Cutaneous side effects of transdermal iontophoresis with and without surfactant pretreatment: a single-blinded, randomized controlled trial. Br. J. Dermatol 2005; 153:404–412.

DNA Transfer in the Skin

Gaëlle Vandermeulen, Liévin Daugimont, and Véronique Préat

Unité de Pharmacie Galénique , Université Catholique de Louvain,
Avenue Emmanuel Mounier, 73 UCL, Brussels, Belgium

INTRODUCTION

The skin represents an attractive site for the delivery of nucleic-acid-based drugs for the treatment of topical or systemic diseases and immunization. However, attempts at therapeutic cutaneous gene delivery have been hindered by several factors. Usually, except for viral vectors, gene expression is transient and typically disappears with one to two weeks due to the continuous renewal of the epidermis. Moreover, DNA penetration is limited by the barrier properties of the skin, rendering topical application rather inefficient.

Therapeutic Use of DNA in the Skin

The potential use of DNA-based drugs in the skin are (1) gene replacement by introducing a defective or missing gene for the treatment of genodermatosis, (2) gene therapy by delivering a with a specific pharmacological effect or a suicidal gene, (3) wound healing, (4) immunotherapy with DNA encoding cytokines, and (5) DNA vaccine. The gene encoding the protein of interest can be inserted in a viral vector or a plasmid that carries this gene under the control of an appropriate eukaryotic promoter (e.g., the CMV promoter in most cases).

For gene therapy of inherited skin diseases, knowledge of the genome and identification of a mutation causing different hereditary diseases make it possible to consider a transfer of normal copies of the affected gene in the cells of the patient. Three types of pathologies have been particularly studied: epidermolysis bullosa (a group of blistering skin conditions), ichthyosis (a family of skin diseases causing a scaling of the skin), and xeroderma pigmentosum (a recessively inherited genodermatosis prone to UV-induced skin basal and squamous cell carcinomas) (1). Suitable animals models have demonstrated proof of concept for treating human genodermatosis (2).

In theory, secretion of therapeutic proteins for systemic therapy could be an application of gene transfer to the skin. However, due to the usually short-term expression of the gene when a nonviral method is used, other organs, in particular the muscle, are more appropriate for long-term expression of serum proteins. Wolff et al. showed that direct gene transfer into mouse muscle in vivo was possible and gave protein expression over several months (3).

Due to the little benefit of growth factors in the form of protein, gene transfer has been envisaged for the treatment of wound healing (4,5). Moreover, wound healing requires a transient increase in specific growth factors until the wound closure is achieved. This transient character makes local and transient gene therapy of particular interest. Recombinant growth factors are also much more expensive to produce compared with plasmid DNA. Delivery of plasmid DNA encoding, for example, keratinocyte growth factor-1 can improve cutaneous wound healing. However, gene delivery in this environment poses a particular challenge (5).

Another application of gene delivery in the skin is the transfer of gene encoding cytokines or cytokine inhibitors playing different roles in autoimmune and inflammatory diseases (6,7).

The skin is a target organ for vaccination. It acts as a physical barrier to prevent entrance of pathogens and is also an immunological barrier. Langerhans cells and dendritic cells are able to internalize allergens and infectious agents and stimulate innate and acquired immune responses. The rationale for DNA vaccine is easy to understand. DNA vaccine contains a gene that encodes an antigen. Following administration, the transfected cells express the antigen that can induce humoral and/or cellular immune response. In 1992, Tang et al. reported that an immune response could also be elicited by introducing the gene encoding a protein directly into mouse skin (8). After this proof-of-concept study, preclinical and clinical studies further confirmed the feasibility of cutaneous DNA vaccination (9).

Methods to Enhance DNA Delivery to the Skin

Effective gene therapy requires that a gene encoding a therapeutic protein must be administered and delivered to target cells, migrate to the cell nucleus, and be expressed to a gene product. DNA delivery is limited by (1) DNA degradation by tissues or blood nucleases, (2) low diffusion at the site of administration, (3) poor targeting to cells, (4) inability to cross membranes, (5) low cellular uptake, and (6) intracellular trafficking to the nucleus. Several approaches have been developed to overcome these barriers.

Local delivery reduces the risk of degradation by blood nucleases and provides a "passive" targeting of the skin, but the efficacy of naked DNA delivery is poor. The stratum corneum constitutes an impermeable barrier to hydrophilic or high molecular weight drugs. Hence, topical DNA delivery into the skin can only be achieved if the barrier function of the stratum corneum is broken by any method. The selection of the appropriate vector or method to promote the penetration of DNA through and/or into the skin has been shown to be paramount.

The continuous renewal and the compartmentalization of the skin are two challenges for efficient long-term gene therapy. The recent inability to sustain phenotypic correction of human genetic skin diseases due to loss of therapeutic gene expression in regenerated epidermal tissue has highlighted this limitation. Long-term expression would become possible only if transfer to stem cells was successful. However, besides immune response against the encoded proteins, gene inactivation, selective growth disadvantage for transduced stem cells, and gradual loss of these cells have been reported (2,10).

Epidermal gene transfer has been achieved with ex vivo approaches. Genes of interest have been introduced, mainly with viral vectors, in keratinocytes or fibroblasts and then grafted on nude mice or patients. Permanent expression can be achieved by this genetic manipulation of keratinocytes ex vivo followed by transplantation or local injection of viral vectors. In vivo approaches, which are more patient-friendly, less invasive, less time consuming, and less expensive, are more attractive and will gradually replace the ex vivo gene transfer protocols (2).

The methods developed for gene transfer into the skin are based on the methods developed for gene transfection in vitro and in other tissues in vivo and on methods developed to enhance transdermal drug delivery. They include (1) topical delivery, (2) intradermal injection, (3) mechanical methods, (4) physical methods, and (5) biological methods. These methods will be described, and their potential for

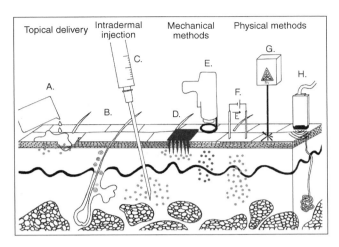

FIGURE 1   Nonviral methods to transfer DNA to the skin. (**A**) Topical delivery of naked DNA; (**B**) liposomes; (**C**) interdermal injection; (**D**) microneedles; (**E**) gene gun; (**F**) electrotransfer; (**G**) laser; and (**H**) ultrasound.

gene transfer into the skin will be illustrated (Fig. 1) and discussed. The rationale, pros, and cons of each method are summarized (Table 1).

TOPICAL DELIVERY

Topical application of naked plasmid DNA to the skin is particularly attractive to provide a simple approach to deliver genes to large areas of the skin. However, the low permeability of the skin to high-molecular-weight hydrophilic molecules limits the use of this approach. Gene expression after topical delivery of an aqueous solution of DNA on intact skin has been reported to induce gene expression (11), but the expression is rather low. Higher expressions are induced if stratum corneum permeability is increased by mechanical methods, e.g., microabrasion, brushing or tape stripping (11). Formulation of the DNA plasmid can also improve DNA transfection after topical application.

Topical Application of Plasmid Solution

When naked plasmid DNA containing a reporter gene was topically applied to mouse skin submitted to brushing, gene expression was detected in the skin samples as early as four hours after DNA application, reached a plateau after 16 to 72 hours post application, and decreased significantly by seven days post application (11). This expression was confined to the superficial layers of the epidermis and to hair follicles. Topical application of DNA following shaving and brushing was as efficient as intradermal injection.

Quantitative polymerase chain reaction demonstrated that topically applied DNA was capable of penetrating human skin in vitro and keratinocyte layer. In vivo, the levels of plasmid DNA in the serum of mice peaked at four hours. After 24 hours, topically applied DNA existed at higher levels than intravenously administered DNA in almost all tissues and induced a 22-fold higher DNA expression in

TABLE 1 Main Techniques of DNA Delivery in the Skin

	Technique	Principle	Advantages	Disadvantages
Topical delivery	Naked DNA	Topical application of naked DNA solution	Low cost Painless	Low expression level Pretreatment required
	Liposomes	Topical application of DNA–liposome complexes	Easy to use Painless	Liposome preparation Target mainly hair follicles
	Microsized and nanosized formulations	Topical application	Easy to use Painless	Formulation preparation Unknown mechanism
	Hydrogel	Topical application of hydrogel containing plasmid	Easy to use Painless	Hydrogel preparation Only on wounded skin
Intradermal injection		Direct injection of naked DNA into the target tissue	Low cost	Rather low expression level
Mechanical	Microseeding and puncture	Mechanical perforations down to the target tissue before DNA delivery		
	Gene gun	Bombardment of gold particles coated with DNA	Noninvasive Small DNA doses	Particle preparation Device
	Microneedles	Microdisruption of the stratum corneum	Painless	Microneedles manufacture
Physical	Electrotransfer	Application of electric pulses to permeabilize cells and deliver DNA	Very effective Easy to use	Local anesthesia required
	Sonoporation	Enhancement of cell permeability by ultrasound	Painless	Unknown mechanism No in vivo studies with skin
	Laser	Transfer of genetic material by focused laser beam	Painless	Unknown mechanism Expensive, nonportable
Biological	Viruses	Use of transgenic viruses devoid of replication, assembling and infection properties	High efficiency	Immunogenicity Undesired integration in some case

the skin and a sustained expression of the plasmid in the regional lymph node over five days (12).

Topical application of plasmid vectors expressing β-galactosidase (βgal) and hepatitis B surface antigen to intact skin induced antigen-specific immune responses that displayed Th2 features. Topical gene transfer was dependent on the presence of normal hair follicles. In the case of hepatitis B surface antigen, these immune responses approached the magnitude of those produced by the intramuscular injection of the commercially available recombinant polypeptide vaccine (13).

Further studies are required to determine the clinical potential of this simple noninvasive method to transfect large areas of the skin. However, due to the low permeability of the skin to high-molecular-weight hydrophilic molecules, increasing plasmid permeation by using formulations of the DNA plasmid or by enhancing skin permeability must be used for efficient transfection.

Topical Application of Lipid-Based DNA Formulations

Cationic liposomes were described for the first time as gene carriers in 1987 by Felgner et al. (14). Since then, it has been reported that conventional cationic liposomes, nonionic liposomes, transferosomes, and other lipid formulations could be used as gene delivery systems to the skin. In 1995, Alexander et al. reported early gene expression in the epidermis, dermis, and hair follicles after application of plasmid DNA complexed with DOTAP (15). Expression persisted at high levels for 48 hours post treatment but lowered by seven days after application. βgal expression was also observed in hair follicles of mice three days after topical administration of the lacZ gene entrapped in liposomes (PC:Cho:PE 5:3:2), suggesting the feasibility of targeting hair matrix and possibly follicle stem cells (16).

The composition of the lipid-based DNA formulation strongly influences the efficacy of gene expression in the skin. Whereas most studies report an increase in gene expression after the topical application of lipid-based DNA formulations, the benefit from the lipid is not always straightforward. Yu et al. showed that, when the DNA/lipid ratio (μg DNA/nmol lipid) was greater than 1:1, the expression levels observed after topical application of cationic lipids were comparable with those produced by the application of DNA alone (11). With increasing lipid concentrations, reporter gene expression decreased. After topical application of liposomes containing the hemagglutining virus of Japan, a five times lower transfer efficiency was reported than after naked DNA injection (17). Nonionic liposomes were the most efficient vehicle followed by nonionic/cationic and pegylated liposomes, whereas protective interactive noncondensing polymers were relatively inefficient (18). Application (once daily for three consecutive days) of plasmid DNA in various liposomal spray formulations yielded limited gene expression (19). Topical administration of plasmids in biphasic lipid vesicles resulted in gene expression in the lymph node and a Th2 response. However, with intradermal injection, antigen expression was found in the skin and resulted in a Th1 response (20).

Confocal microscopy studies showed that intact liposomes were not able to penetrate into the granular layers of the epidermis (21). This drawback led to the development of highly deformable liposomes (22). In contrast to conventional liposomes, deformable liposomes have been reported to penetrate intact skin. After topical application of a formulation of deformable liposomes (DOTAP-sodium cholate or egg-phosphatidylcholine) loaded with plasmid DNA encoding green fluorescent protein (GFP), the gene was absorbed and transported in several organs in vivo (23,24).

Topical application of DNA encapsulated in liposomes can induce short-term gene expression in the skin. The formulation of the lipid-based complex is a critical factor, which needs to be optimized to enhance gene expression by protecting and condensing the DNA and/or enhancing its cellular penetration.

Topical Application of Other Microsized and Nanosized Formulations

Microcarrier and nanocarrier formulations of plasmid have been shown to enhance DNA penetration and gene expression in the skin. When a water-in-oil nanoemulsion (32 nm) of plasmid was applied to mouse skin, the deposition of the plasmid DNA was primarily in follicular keratinocytes. After a single application of 10 µg in non-hairless mice, expression peaked at 24 hours and was 10 times higher than after aqueous DNA application (25).

Plasmid incorporated in an ethanol-in-fluorocarbon microemulsion also enhanced luciferase expression as well as antibody and Th1 immune response (26). Topical immunization with a topical perfluorocarbon-based microemulsion containing an anthrax protective antigen encoding plasmid led to a significant antibody response (9).

Transcutaneous delivery of a DNA plasmid–dimethylsulfoxide mixture to the untreated skin of chicken resulted in a wide distribution of the plasmid in the body. It induced mucosal and systemic immune response and protection from challenge with the viruses tested. The plasmid persisted until at least 15 weeks post primary vaccination (27).

No general conclusion can be drawn from these studies. In particular, the mechanism(s) by which gene expression is enhanced should be known before a rational design of the formulation can be established.

Topical Application of Hydrogel

Topical delivery of hydrogel containing plasmid could be useful for the treatment of wound healing. Hydrogels can prolong the contact of skin with the plasmid encoding for a growth factor, and they can have a positive effect on wound. Thermosensitive hydrogel made of triblock copolymer PEG–PLGA–PEG containing transforming growth factor-beta1 encoding plasmid significantly increased reepithealization, cell proliferation, and the presence of organized collagen in wound healing in diabetic mice. Maximal gene expression was at 24 hours in the skin wound and dropped by 90% 72 hours later (28,29).

INTRADERMAL INJECTION

One of the simplest ways of gene delivery is injecting naked DNA encoding the therapeutic protein. In 1990, Wolff et al. observed an expression for several months after injection of naked DNA into the muscle (3). Expression following the direct injection of naked plasmid DNA has been established for the skin (30,31). The epidermis and the dermis can take up and transiently express plasmid DNA following direct injection into animal skin.

When pig or human skin (grafted or organ culture) was injected intradermally with naked DNA, the DNA was taken up and expressed in the epidermis. In contrast, DNA injected into mouse skin was expressed in the epidermis, dermis, and underlying tissue (31). Direct local injection of plasmid encoding reporter genes in wounded skin induces gene expression for up to two weeks in fibroblasts, macrophages, and adipocytes in the dermal and subdermal layers. High level of granulocyte-colony-stimulating factor was detected in wounded mouse skin after local delivery of granulocyte-colony-stimulating factor plasmid (32). IL-10 released from transduced keratinocytes can enter the bloodstream and cause biological effects at distant areas of the skin, suggesting that it may be possible to treat systemic disease using naked DNA injection into the skin (33). After intracutaneous injection of a very high dose (2 mg) of naked plasmid DNA, most organs transiently contained the plasmid for several days whereas integration was not detected (34).

Jet injection of DNA in a solution can also be used to transfer DNA into tissues of living animals. A jet of 100 to 300 µL of a DNA solution has sufficient force to travel into and through tissues of adult and juvenile animals. The introduced DNA is found in cells surrounding the path of the jet (35). Jet injection of the naked DNA exhibited a much higher activity than needle injection in human keratinocytes in vivo (36). Cutaneous DNA immunization can be achieved (37).

To prolong gene expression, hydrogel-containing plasmid was investigated. Intradermal injection of agarose hydrogel containing 25 µg plasmid compacted with polylysine was reported to prolong gene expression for aqueous DNA solution from five to seven days to 35 days (38).

MECHANICAL METHODS
Microseeding and Puncture
Mechanical perforation of the skin, e.g., brushing (11), microseeding (39), and puncture (40), can also be used to deliver DNA into the skin. In microseeding, DNA is delivered directly to target cells by multiple perforations with oscillating solid microneedles. Expression of plasmid encoding βgal or human epidermal growth factor in microseeded skin peaked two days after transfection and was higher than after gene transfer by intradermal injection or gene gun. βgal expressing cells were detected in the epidermis and the dermis. The βgal activity corresponded to the localization of the charcoal marker deposits in the epidermis and subepidermal tissue. Pigs microseeded with hemagglutinin encoding plasmid were protected from infection by influenza virus (39). High-frequency puncturing of the skin with fine short needles used for tattooing human skin allowed transfer of reporter genes as well as expression of a transgene leading to the induction of cytolytic T lymphocytes. Expression lasted for at least seven days (40).

Gene Gun
Particle bombardment or biolistic technology provides a useful means for transferring foreign genes into a variety of cells in culture and tissues in vivo. Gene gun consists in accelerating and propelling particles coated with DNA using different kinds of gene devices. It accelerates particles at a sufficient velocity to penetrate into the target cells. Particles are usually composed of gold or tungsten, with a diameter smaller than the target cells (usually between 1 and 5 µm). Devices are based on voltage discharge, helium discharge, or other techniques. Originally, particle-mediated gene transfer was developed to deliver genes to plant cells (41).

In the early 1990s, this approach was extended to mammalian cells and tissues of living animals, including skin. Yang et al. demonstrated a transient expression of marker genes in mouse skin after bombardment with DNA-coated gold microparticles (42). When skin was bombarded with 2–5 μm tungsten or gold particles coated with a plasmid coding luciferase and controlled by a β-actin promoter, ten to twenty percent of the cells in the epidermis expressed the foreign gene. Expression of luciferase in mouse ear was detectable at high level (4000-fold over background) and persisted for up to 10 days. Microprojectiles, which penetrated in the skin, retained the DNA in the tissue and did not induce extensive cell damage or inflammation (43).

    Gene gun is usually applied for gene transfer to external tissues. The application of this technology to other tissues has had limited success. Dileo et al. developed a new design that used helium discharge to propel DNA-coated gold beads that were suspended in liquid, allowing delivery of DNA to deeper tissues, including subcutaneous tumors (44).

    The major application of particle bombardment for gene transfer is DNA immunization. In 1992, Tang et al. detected antibody responses to human growth hormone after genetic inoculation with microprojectiles coated with a plasmid coding human growth hormone gene (8). These initial studies were extended for immunization against various diseases (e.g., influenza, hepatitis B, or HIV). Fynan et al. demonstrated a highly efficient immunization against influenza virus with two to three orders of magnitude less DNA than injection in saline. This could result from the combination of efficient transfection with efficient antigen presentation and recognition (45). Both humoral and cellular immune responses are elicited via gene-gun-mediated nucleic acid immunization. Gene gun vaccination offers the advantages of requiring minimal amounts of DNA and providing a simple means of delivering DNA intracellularly to the epidermis (46). Another application of gene gun is the acceleration of wound healing. Transfer of a human epidermal growth factor by this technique enhanced epidermal repair (47).

    Several clinical trials using gene gun have been carried out. Besides immunization, treatment of melanoma with various cytokines or antigens was investigated (48).

Microneedles

The most direct permeation enhancement relies on physical/mechanical disruption of the stratum corneum. Recently, the ability of microneedles to disrupt the stratum corneum and create microchannels (10 to 20 μm diameter) has been reported (49–53). Microneedles have been widely used to deliver conventional drugs, but only proof of principle of DNA delivery has been reported (49,54). Arrays of micron scale silicon projection (microenhancer arrays) that were dipped into a solution of naked plasmid DNA and scraped across the skin of mice enabled topical gene transfer, resulting in reporter gene activity of up to 2800-fold above topical controls and topical immunization inducing stronger and less variable immune responses than via needle-based injections. In a human clinical study, these devices effectively breached the skin barrier, allowing direct access to the epidermis with minimal associated discomfort and skin irritation (54). Preliminary gene expression studies confirmed that naked DNA plasmid can be locally expressed in excised human skin following disruption of the stratum corneum barrier with longer silicon microneedles (49,55).

    In contrast to solid microneedles, hollow microneedles offer the possibility of transporting drugs by diffusion or by pressure-driven flow. A variety of hollow microneedles have been fabricated, but only limited work has been published on their possible use to deliver nucleic acids into the skin.

PHYSICAL METHODS

Physical methods such as electroporation or sonophoresis developed to enhance transdermal and topical delivery of conventional drugs and to extend their field of application have been reported to enhance DNA transfer into the skin and into cutaneous cells.

Electrotransfer

Electrotransfer has been widely used to introduce DNA into various types of cells in vitro and is one of the most efficient nonviral methods to enhance gene transfer in various tissues in vivo. Electrotransfer involves plasmid injection in the target tissue and application of short high-voltage electric pulses by electrodes. The intensity and the duration of pulses and the more appropriate type of electrodes must be evaluated for each tissue (56). The electric field plays a double part in DNA transfection. Finally, it transiently disturbs membranes and increases cells permeability. Secondly, it promotes electrophoresis of negatively charged DNA (57).

Neumann et al. published the first demonstration of this physical method of gene transfer in 1982. They discovered the possibility to transfer linear or circular DNA plasmid in vitro into cells in suspension by the use of high electric field and showed the simplicity, the easy applicability, and the high efficiency of this technique (58). The confirmation of this result appeared two years later (59).

The earliest published work that used in vivo electrotransfer to deliver genes was conducted by Titomirov et al. (60). A plasmid DNA coding neomycin resistance gene was introduced subcutaneously into newborn mice followed by high-voltage pulses applied to the skin. After electrotransfer, the skin was harvested and skin cells were placed into a selective culture medium. It was demonstrated that plasmid DNA persisted in the cells for at least 30 generations without selection. During the 1990s, electrotransfer using long pulses has been also used for the transfection of other tissues: liver (61), tumors (62), and skeletal muscle (57,63,64).

Electrotransfer may be used to increase transgene expression 10- to 100-fold more than the injection of naked DNA into the skin (65–67). Heller et al. demonstrated that local delivery combined with electrotransfer could result in a significant increase of serum concentrations of a specific protein (68). Neither long-term inflammation nor necroses are generally observed (67,69,70).

After direct intradermal injection of plasmid, the transfected cells are typically restricted to the epidermis and dermis. However, when high-voltage pulses were applied after this intradermal injection, other cells, including adipocytes, fibroblasts, and numerous dendritic-like cells within the dermis and subdermal layers, were transfected (66). After topical application of plasmid on tape-stripped rat skin followed by electrotransfer, GFP expression was also reported but was low and restricted to the epidermis (69).

Duration of expression after electrotransfer depends on the targeted tissue. In contrast to the skeletal muscle where expression lasts for several months, gene expression is limited to only a few weeks into the skin. For example, after intradermal electrotransfer of plasmid coding erythropoietin, the expression persisted for seven weeks at the DNA injection site, and hematocrit levels were increased for 11 weeks (71). With reporter gene, a shorter expression was reported (66,67).

Several authors have tried to increase the effectiveness of the electrotransfer into the skin. By coinjecting the nuclease inhibitor aurintricarboxylic acid with DNA before applying electric pulses, transfection expression was significantly increased (66). The use of a particulate adjuvant (gold particles) enhanced the effectiveness of DNA vaccination by electrotransfer (72). For the skin, combination of one high-voltage pulse and one low-voltage pulse delivered by plate electrodes has been proven to be efficient and well tolerated (67). The design of electrodes can also be optimized (73).

Electrotransfer has no detrimental effect on wound healing and can thus be used in the gene therapy of this pathology (74). A single injection of a plasmid coding keratinocyte growth factor coupled with electrotransfer improved and accelerated wound closure in a wound-healing diabetic mouse model (75). This was recently confirmed in a study in a septic rat model (76).

Vaccination is another interesting application of electrotransfer into the skin. Topical electrotransfer enhances DNA vaccine delivery to the skin and both humoral and cellular immune responses. Hence, it could be developed as a potential alternative for DNA vaccine delivery without inducing any irreversible changes (65,67,77,78). Electrotransfer of DNA in melanoma is currently under investigation in clinical trials.

Sonoporation

Sonoporation is the ultrasound-mediated enhancing of cell permeability. Ultrasound frequencies are in the range of KHz to MHz. Biological effects are mainly due to two mechanisms, cavitation and heating. Acoustic cavitation is the nonthermal interaction between a propagating pressure wave and a gaseous inclusion in aqueous media responsible for mechanical perturbation, collapse, and implosion of gas bubbles (79). The importance of this phenomenon depends on ultrasound intensity and frequency. It might lead to a release of a sufficient energy to permeabilize cell membranes and to enhance drug or gene delivery into cells and tissue. Ultrasound could also generate heat. When a beam is focused down to a small size in target tissue, the thermal energy per area is high. This energy can be absorbed by the tissue, resulting in increased temperature which might perturb biological systems. Thermal effect varies with the exposure time and ultrasound intensity. It has only a minor role in the ultrasound-induced increase in permeability.

The first result of sonoporation gene transfer was obtained in vitro in the mid-1990s (80). Since then, this technique has been used in wide variety of tissues such as muscle (81), tumor, and recently living skin equivalents consisting of keratinocytes seeded upon a fibroblast-populated type I collagen gel and transplanted onto nude mice after the ultrasound-mediated gene transfer (82).

The use of ultrasound contrast microbubbles may improve transfection. These microscopic (1–3 µm) microbubbles contain air or an inert gas with a shell composed of proteins, lipids, or polymers. An example of microbubble that has been proven very effective in sonoporation research is Optison® (perfluoropropane encapsulated in a human albumin sphere, GE Healthcare, Buckinghamshire, U.K.). Gene vectors mixed with microbubbles can be injected locally or systemically before the application of ultrasound on the target area. It is also possible to use polymer-coated microbubbles that can bind and protect the DNA or microbubbles encapsulating DNA (83).

Microchannels
Transient microconduits can be created in human skin by arrays of radiofrequency microelectrodes without impinging underlying blood vessels and nerve endings (84). The transient microconduits of approximately 30 μm diameter and 70 μm depth allow topical DNA delivery and result in gene expression (βgal for example) within the viable epidermal cells surrounding the microchannels. This staining was higher when ViaDerm™ (the radiofrequency-microchannel generator, Taro Pharmaceuticals, Inc., Canada) was applied both prior to and immediately following the topical application of the DNA formulation (50 μg/50 μl) (85).

Laser Irradiation
Laser irradiation is another method to transfer DNA into cells either in vitro or in vivo. The beam is emitted by a laser source, for example, neodymium yttrium–aluminium–garnet or argon ion laser and is focused by a lens. The exact mechanism remains unknown, but the permeability of the cellular membrane is increased, probably by a thermal effect, sufficiently to permit the entry of DNA into the cell. Direct transfer of the neomycin gene by yttrium–aluminium–garnet laser was reported for the first time in 1987 in vitro (86). Laser irradiation was used in vivo to transfer genetic material into the muscle (87) and into the skin (88). Ogura et al. reported levels of luciferase activities after laser irradiation two orders of magnitude higher than those after injection of naked DNA into the skin. No major side effects were observed. Luciferase activity levels were sustained five days after gene transfer. The development of laser gene transfer is limited by the high cost and the size of the laser.

VIRAL METHODS
Historically, viral vectors were the first routes explored to deliver genes into cells. Viruses are obligate intracellular parasites able to deliver genetic material into the infected cell. This innate ability to transfer DNA appeared very useful for gene therapy. The first step of viral vector design is to delete genes allowing replication, assembling, or infection. This step permits to decrease pathogenicity and expression of immunogenic viral antigens. These deleted genes can be replaced by an expression cassette containing promoter and therapeutic gene (the maximal size of the expression cassette depends on the virus considered). This recombinant virus can be replicated only in a cell line which supplies the deleted functions. Production of populations of keratinocytes in which all cells contain the desired therapeutic gene may be important in future genetic therapies. For gene therapy, introduction of a desired gene into keratinocyte stem cells could overcome the problem of achieving persistent gene expression in a significant percentage of keratinocytes.

Transgene can be introduced into fibroblasts or keratinocytes ex vivo and can lead to the expression of gene products with local or systemic effects. The keratinocyte is an attractive target for the purpose of an ex vivo gene therapy. The epidermis can be biopsied to provide the source of keratinocytes, which can be expanded in culture before transfection ex vivo and reimplantation in vivo.

The theoretical advantages of ex vivo therapy, relatively easy delivery and stable integration of the gene, are outbalanced by the expensive, long-lasting procedure and by the risk associated with the procedure. Moreover, the use of viral vectors for gene therapy is limited by immune responses and safety concern. Viruses can cause immunologic reactions and could induce mutagenic or oncogenic effects. These concerns hinder genetic correction of severe inherited skin diseases (10).

Retroviruses

Retroviral vectors to transduce skin cells were initiated in the mid-1990s. Partial and full-thickness wounds made in vitro in a human living skin equivalent were placed in contact with a transduced cell line producing a replication-defective retrovirus containing the βgal gene. Expression of βgal was uniformly present at the wound edge and along the base of the entire partial thickness wound (89).

Human keratinocytes transduced with a retroviral vector for βgal (with 99% efficiency) were grafted onto immunodeficient mice to generate human epidermis. Although integrated vector sequences persisted unchanged in epidermis at 10 weeks post grafting, retroviral long terminal repeat region promoter (LTR)-driven βgal expression ceased in vivo after approximately four weeks (90). While expected in non-integrating viral vectors such as adenovirus, in the case of retrovirus, this loss of gene expression occurred in spite of the retention of vector sequences for several turnover periods. In contrast, LTR defective internal promoter vectors displayed consistently strong levels of sustained marker protein expressions for up to 10 to 12 weeks (90).

Keratinocytes transduced by a retroviral vector have been shown to express the human clotting factor IX, but low levels of human factor were detected for less than a week in the plasma of mice grafted with these cells (91). Factor IX in plasma was twofold to threefold higher with Human Papillomavirus 16 and human keratin 5 elements as promoters than with vector containing the CMV promoter alone (91). Kolodka et al. (92) also showed long-term engraftment and persistence of transgene expression in retrovirus-transduced keratinocytes that could be keratinocyte stem cells. The combined capabilities for efficient retroviral gene transfer and effective pharmacologic selection allow production of entirely engineered populations of human keratinocytes for the use in future efforts to achieve effective cutaneous gene delivery (93). High-level secretion of growth hormone by retrovirally transduced primary human keratinocytes was achieved (94). Retroviral vectors expressing a mutated collagen for gene therapy of recessive dystrophic epidermolysis bullosa in dogs corrected in primary keratinocytes the defect caused by the disease (95). Successful engraftment of retrovirally transduced keratinocytes in pig was demonstrated by the immunohistochemistry of biopsies, showing transgene expression in 40–50% of grafted keratinocytes. After four weeks, keratinocytes expressing a foreign marker gene were lost (96).

Adenoviruses

Gene transfer to the skin using adenovirus has also been demonstrated both ex vivo and in vivo. When murine keratinocytes infected with replication-deficient adenovirus coding for human α1 antitrypsin (hα1AT) were transplanted in mice, hα1AT was detected in the serum for at least 14 days. When Respiratory Syncytial Virus βgal or α1AT adenovirus were administered subcutaneously to mice, expression of βgal was detected after four days in the epidermis and dermis and human α1AT was detectable in the serum for at least 14 days (97). Lu et al. (98,99) showed that the subcutaneous administration of an adenoviral vector containing the luciferase reporter gene induced a strong expression of the transgene in dermal cells, but only a small portion of epidermal cells were transduced.

After topical application of adenovirus CMVlacZ, the entire surface of the treated skin exhibited βgal staining which persisted for seven days, with little or no expression at 10 days. Quantitative analysis showed that the viral-vector-mediated gene transfers were superior to gene gun delivery of plasmid DNA. Epidermal gene transfer by either a gene gun delivery or viral vectors was transient, likely due to the episomal localization of adenoviral vectors as well as terminal differentiation and elimination. Four days after having topically applied an adenoviral vector containing a human TGF-α expression unit, hyperkeratosis and acanthosis were developed by the murine epidermis (99).

Using adenoviruses in which a growth factor inducible element controls the expression of the reporter gene, GFP expression was specifically detected in wound margin keratinocytes from two to 10 days but not in intact skin (100).

After the pioneering studies, adenoviruses have been evaluated for several potential applications. The recombinant adenoviral vector platform is being considered as a cancer vaccine platform because it efficiently induces response to tumor antigen by intradermal immunization (101). Adenoviral vectors carrying the xeroderma pigmentosum complementation group A gene were used to treat xeroderma pigmentosum mutant mice. Subcutaneous injection led to the expression of the xeroderma pigmentosum complementation group A protein in basal keratinocytes and prevented deleterious effect in the skin, including late development of squamous cell carcinoma (102). Tissue-specific expression using the tyrosinase promoter fused to two human tyrosinase enhancers for melanoma-specific expression of genes delivered by adenoviral vectors has been achieved (103).

However, note that first-generation adenoviral vectors are attenuated but not defective viruses that still express several proteins that can lead to immunogenic response, especially in the skin. Consequently, a loss of efficiency of these vectors was observed. Preclinical and clinical studies have demonstrated immunological responses directed toward the adenoviral vectors and inflammation in the target tissues (104). Despite the advantages of adenoviruses over other viral vectors, safety concerns have been raised in clinical trials.

Adeno-Associated Viruses and Lentiviruses

Adeno-associated viruses (AAV) are nonpathogenic, integrating DNA vectors capable of transducing dividing and nondividing cells with the potential of long-term expression. AAV vectors have been transfected successfully in the skin. They function as an autonomous parvovirus in the skin. Following in vivo injection, βgal expression was observed for more than four weeks in keratinocytes as well as hair follicle epithelial cells and exocrine sweat glands. Expression upon readministration was limited (105). AAV expressing vascular endothelial growth factor A administered in wound display tropism for the panniculus carnosus (a part of the subcutaneous tissue) and induce a sustained expression resulting in new vessels formation and reduction of healing time (106,107). In human keloid specimens injected with an AAV vector for four weeks, gene expression was demonstrated by reverse transcriptase polymerase chain reaction and X-gal staining (108). Implantation in nude mice of HeLa keratinocytes transduced by AAV harboring the erythropoietin cDNA induced a high level and long-term (>1 month) increase in hematocrit (109). Injection in the dermis of lentiviral vectors induces transduction of dividing basal and nondividing suprabasal keratinocytes. Ex vivo grafting seemed more efficient (110).

CONCLUSIONS

The delivery of DNA into the skin has many potential applications: treatment of genetic skin diseases but also wound healing, immunotherapy, and vaccination. However, the barrier properties of the skin and the low penetration of the DNA in the skin cells require the development of mechanical, physical, or biological methods to improve gene transfer. Topical delivery of naked DNA to the skin induces a weak expression. Thus, different pretreatments of the skin, like brushing and tape stripping, were designed and proved to be more efficient. DNA formulations enhance expression after topical application, but this expression is often localized to superficial layers of the skin and hair follicles.

Intradermal injection of DNA leads to expression levels higher than those obtained with topical delivery but allows reaching deeper skin structures and so offering the possibility to have a systemic effect through the release of the transgene product to the bloodstream.

Sophisticated methods based on mechanical or physical principles have been developed to improve gene expression with more or less success. Gene gun offers the advantages of a painless, noninvasive delivery at low DNA dose. Therefore, several applications of the gene gun have reached the clinical trials. Solid microneedles have been used to deliver DNA to the skin, particularly for DNA immunization. In vivo electrotransfer is well tolerated and very efficient compared with intradermal injection. This promising technique offers many potential applications into the skin. Sonoporation and microchannels are new methods based on waves of various frequencies to transfer DNA in vivo. The preliminary preclinical data need to be confirmed. Laser irradiation gives also interesting results but the development of this technique is limited by the size and the cost of the laser source.

Comparison of different viral vectors for optimal transduction of primary human keratinocytes indicates that (1) human adenoviral vectors achieve a highly efficient but transient expression; (2) both retroviral and lentiviral can permanently transduce up to 100% cells, but the lentiviral vectors are the most suitable for ex vivo gene therapy because of their ability to transduce clonogenic keratinocytes; and (3) AAV are less suitable (111).

All these technologies offer a large panel of DNA delivery methods into the skin, each with its advantages and disadvantages (Table 1). However, the comparison of techniques is difficult because the DNA doses, the reporter genes, and the expression evaluation methods used are different for each technique and sometimes even for each author. The choice of one technique must take several parameters into consideration, like the therapeutic application, the duration, localization, and intensity of gene expression required, the cost, the accessibility of the material, and the patient comfort.

REFERENCES

1. Spirito F, Meneguzzi G, Danos O, et al. Cutaneous gene transfer and therapy: the present and the future. J Gene Med 2001; 3(1):21–31.
2. Hengge UR. Gene therapy progress and prospects: the skin—easily accessible, but still far away. Gene Ther 2006; 13(22):1555–1563.

3. Wolff JA, Malone RW, Williams P, et al. Direct gene transfer into mouse muscle in vivo. Science 1990; 247(4949 Pt 1):1465–1468.
4. Jeschke MG, Herndon DN, Baer W, et al. Possibilities of non-viral gene transfer to improve cutaneous wound healing. Curr Gene Ther 2001; 1(3):267–278.
5. Branski LK, Pereira CT, Herndon DN et al. Gene therapy in wound healing: present status and future directions. Gene Ther 2007; 14(1):1–10.
6. Meng X, Sawamura D, Ina S, et al. Keratinocyte gene therapy: cytokine gene expression in local keratinocytes and in circulation by introducing cytokine genes into skin. Exp Dermatol 2002; 11(5):456–461.
7. Sawamura D, Akiyama M, Shimizu H. Direct injection of naked DNA and cytokine transgene expression: implications for keratinocyte gene therapy. Clin Exp Dermatol 2002; 27(6):480–484.
8. Tang DC, DeVit M, Johnston SA. Genetic immunization is a simple method for eliciting an immune response. Nature 1992; 356(6365):152–154.
9. Cui Z, Sloat BR. Topical immunization onto mouse skin using a microemulsion incorporated with an anthrax protective antigen protein-encoding plasmid. Int J Pharm 2006; 317(2):187–191.
10. Hengge UR, Bardenheuer W. Gene therapy and the skin. Am J Med Genet C Semin Med Genet 2004; 131C(1):93–100.
11. Yu WH, Kashani-Sabet M, Liggitt D, et al. Topical gene delivery to murine skin. J Invest Dermatol 1999; 112(3):370–375.
12. Kang MJ, Kim CK, Kim MY, et al. Skin permeation, biodistribution, and expression of topically applied plasmid DNA. J Gene Med 2004; 6(11):1238–1246.
13. Fan H, Lin Q, Morrissey GR, et al. Immunization via hair follicles by topical application of naked DNA to normal skin. Nat Biotechnol 1999; 17(9):870–872.
14. Felgner PL. Lipofection: a highly efficient, lipid-mediated DNA-transfection procedure. Proc Natl Acad Sci 1987; 84:7413–7417.
15. Alexander MY, Akhurst RJ. Liposome-medicated gene transfer and expression via the skin. Hum Mol Genet 1995; 4(12):2279–2285.
16. Li L, Hoffman RM. The feasibility of targeted selective gene therapy of the hair follicle. Nat Med 1995; 1(7):705–706.
17. Sawamura D, Meng X, Ina S, et al. In vivo transfer of a foreign gene to keratinocytes using the hemagglutinating virus of Japan-liposome method. J Invest Dermatol 1997; 108(2):195–199.
18. Raghavachari N, Fahl WE. Targeted gene delivery to skin cells in vivo: a comparative study of liposomes and polymers as delivery vehicles. J Pharm Sci 2002; 91(3):615–622.
19. Meykadeh N, Mirmohammadsadegh A, Wang Z, et al. Topical application of plasmid DNA to mouse and human skin. J Mol Med 2005; 83(11):897–903.
20. Babiuk S, Baca-Estrada ME, Pontarollo R et al. Topical delivery of plasmid DNA using biphasic lipid vesicles (Biphasix). J Pharm Pharmacol 2002; 54(12):1609–1614.
21. Kirjavainen M, Urtti A, Valjakka-Koskela R, et al. Liposome-skin interactions and their effects on the skin permeation of drugs. Eur J Pharm Sci 1999; 7(4):279–286.
22. Cevc G. Transfersomes, liposomes and other lipid suspensions on the skin: permeation enhancement, vesicle penetration, and transdermal drug delivery. Crit Rev Ther Drug Carrier Syst 1996; 13(3–4):257–388.
23. Kim A, Lee EH, Choi SH, et al. In vitro and in vivo transfection efficiency of a novel ultradeformable cationic liposome. Biomaterials 2004; 25(2):305–313.
24. Lee EH, Kim A, Oh YK, et al. Effect of edge activators on the formation and transfection efficiency of ultradeformable liposomes. Biomaterials 2005; 26(2):205–210.
25. Wu H, Ramachandran C, Bielinska AU, et al. Topical transfection using plasmid DNA in a water-in-oil nanoemulsion. Int J Pharm 2001; 221(1–2):23–34.
26. Cui Z, Fountain W, Clark M, et al. Novel ethanol-in-fluorocarbon microemulsions for topical genetic immunization. Pharm Res 2003; 20(1):16–23.
27. Heckert RA, Elankumaran S, Oshop GL, et al. A novel transcutaneous plasmid-dimethyl-sulfoxide delivery technique for avian nucleic acid immunization. Vet Immunol Immunopathol 2002; 89(1–2):67–81.
28. Lee PY, Li Z, Huang L. Thermosensitive hydrogel as a TGF-beta1 gene delivery vehicle enhances diabetic wound healing. Pharm Res 2003; 20(12):1995–2000.

29. Li Z, Ning W, Wang J, et al. Controlled gene delivery system based on thermosensitive biodegradable hydrogel. Pharm Res 2003; 20(6):884–888.
30. Hengge UR, Chan EF, Foster RA, et al. Cytokine gene expression in epidermis with biological effects following injection of naked DNA. Nat Genet 1995; 10(2):161–166.
31. Hengge UR, Walker PS, Vogel JC. Expression of naked DNA in human, pig, and mouse skin. J Clin Invest 1996; 97(12):2911–2916.
32. Meuli M, Liu Y, Liggitt D, et al. Efficient gene expression in skin wound sites following local plasmid injection. J Invest Dermatol 2001; 116(1):131–135.
33. Meng X, Sawamura D, Tamai K, et al. Keratinocyte gene therapy for systemic diseases. Circulating interleukin 10 released from gene-transferred keratinocytes inhibits contact hypersensitivity at distant areas of the skin. J Clin Invest 1998; 101(6):1462–1467.
34. Hengge UR, Dexling B, Mirmohammadsadegh A. Safety and pharmacokinetics of naked plasmid DNA in the skin: studies on dissemination and ectopic expression. J Invest Dermatol 2001; 116(6):979–982.
35. Furth PA, Shamay A, Hennighausen L. Gene transfer into mammalian cells by jet injection. Hybridoma 1995; 14(2):149–152.
36. Sawamura D, Ina S, Itai K, et al. In vivo gene introduction into keratinocytes using jet injection. Gene Ther 1999; 6(10):1785–1787.
37. Haensler J, Verdelet C, Sanchez V, et al. Intradermal DNA immunization by using jet-injectors in mice and monkeys. Vaccine 1999; 17(7–8):628–638.
38. Meilander-Lin NJ, Cheung PJ, Wilson DL, et al. Sustained in vivo gene delivery from agarose hydrogel prolongs nonviral gene expression in skin. Tissue Eng 2005; 11(3–4):546–555.
39. Eriksson E, Yao F, Svensjo T, et al. In Vivo Gene Transfer to Skin and Wound by Microseeding. Journal of Surgical Research 1998; 78(2):85–91.
40. Ciernik IF, Krayenbuhl BH, Carbone DP. Puncture-mediated gene transfer to the skin. Hum Gene Ther 1996; 7(8):893–899.
41. Klein RM, Wolf ED, Wu R, et al. High-velocity microprojectiles for delivering nucleic acids into living cells. 1987. Biotechnology 1992; 24:384–386.
42. Yang NS, Burkholder J, Roberts B, et al. In vivo and in vitro gene transfer to mammalian somatic cells by particle bombardment. Proc Natl Acad Sci U S A 1990; 87(24):9568–9572.
43. Williams RS, Johnston SA, Riedy M, et al. Introduction of foreign genes into tissues of living mice by DNA-coated microprojectiles. Proc Natl Acad Sci U S A 1991; 88(7):2726–2730.
44. Dileo J, Miller TE Jr., Chesnoy S, et al. Gene transfer to subdermal tissues via a new gene gun design. Hum Gene Ther 2003; 14(1):79–87.
45. Fynan EF, Webster RG, Fuller DH, et al. DNA vaccines: protective immunizations by parenteral, mucosal, and gene-gun inoculations. Proc Natl Acad Sci U S A 1993; 90(24):11478–11482.
46. Haynes JR, McCabe DE, Swain WF, et al. Particle-mediated nucleic acid immunization. J Biotechnol 1996; 44(1–3):37–42.
47. Andree C, Swain WF, Page CP, et al. In vivo transfer and expression of a human epidermal growth factor gene accelerates wound repair. Proc Natl Acad Sci U S A 1994; 91(25):12188–12192.
48. www.wiley.co.uk/genmed/clinical/. July 2007.
49. Birchall J, Coulman S, Pearton M, et al. Cutaneous DNA delivery and gene expression in ex vivo human skin explants via wet-etch micro-fabricated micro-needles. J Drug Target 2005; 13(7):415–421.
50. Coulman S, Allender C, Birchall J. Microneedles and other physical methods for overcoming the stratum corneum barrier for cutaneous gene therapy. Crit Rev Ther Drug Carrier Syst 2006; 23(3):205–258.
51. Henry S, McAllister DV, Allen MG, et al. Microfabricated microneedles: a novel approach to transdermal drug delivery. J Pharm Sci 1998; 87(8):922–925.
52. Lin W, Cormier M, Samiee A, et al. Transdermal delivery of antisense oligonucleotides with microprojection patch (Macroflux) technology. Pharm Res 2001; 18(12):1789–1793.

53. Matriano JA, Cormier M, Johnson J, et al. Macroflux microprojection array patch technology: a new and efficient approach for intracutaneous immunization. Pharm Res 2002; 19(1):63–70.
54. Mikszta JA, Alarcon JB, Brittingham JM, et al. Improved genetic immunization via micromechanical disruption of skin-barrier function and targeted epidermal delivery. Nat Med 2002; 8(4):415–419.
55. Coulman SA, Barrow D, Anstey A, et al. Minimally invasive cutaneous delivery of macromolecules and plasmid DNA via microneedles. Curr Drug Deliv 2006; 3(1):65–75.
56. Cemazar M, Golzio M, Sersa G, et al. Electrically-assisted nucleic acids delivery to tissues in vivo: where do we stand? Curr Pharm Des 2006; 12(29):3817–3825.
57. Bureau MF, Gehl J, Deleuze V, et al. Importance of association between permeabilization and electrophoretic forces for intramuscular DNA electrotransfer. Biochim Biophys Acta 2000; 1474(3):353–359.
58. Neumann E, Schaefer-Ridder M, Wang Y, et al. Gene transfer into mouse lyoma cells by electroporation in high electric fields. EMBO J 1982; 1(7):841–845.
59. Potter H, Weir L, Leder P. Enhancer-dependent expression of human kappa immunoglobulin genes introduced into mouse pre-B lymphocytes by electroporation. Proc Natl Acad Sci U S A 1984; 81(22):7161–7165.
60. Titomirov AV, Sukharev S, Kistanova E. In vivo electroporation and stable transformation of skin cells of newborn mice by plasmid DNA. Biochim Biophys Acta 1991; 1088(1):131–134.
61. Suzuki T, Shin BC, Fujikura K, et al. Direct gene transfer into rat liver cells by in vivo electroporation. FEBS Lett 1998; 425(3):436–440.
62. Rols MP, Delteil C, Golzio M, et al. In vivo electrically mediated protein and gene transfer in murine melanoma. Nat Biotechnol 1998; 16(2):168–171.
63. Aihara H, Miyazaki J. Gene transfer into muscle by electroporation in vivo. Nat Biotechnol 1998; 16(9):867–870.
64. Mir LM, Bureau MF, Rangara R, et al. Long-term, high level in vivo gene expression after electric pulse-mediated gene transfer into skeletal muscle. C R Acad Sci III 1998; 321(11):893–899.
65. Drabick JJ, Glasspool-Malone J, King A, et al. Cutaneous transfection and immune responses to intradermal nucleic acid vaccination are significantly enhanced by in vivo electropermeabilization. Mol Ther 2001; 3(2):249–255.
66. Glasspool-Malone J, Somiari S, Drabick JJ, et al. Efficient nonviral cutaneous transfection. Mol Ther 2000; 2(2):140–146.
67. Pavselj N, Préat V. DNA electrotransfer into the skin using a combination of one high- and one low-voltage pulse. J Control Release 2005; 106(3):407–415.
68. Heller R, Schultz J, Lucas ML, et al. Intradermal delivery of interleukin-12 plasmid DNA by in vivo electroporation. DNA Cell Biol 2001; 20(1):21–26.
69. Dujardin N, Van Der Smissen P., Préat V. Topical gene transfer into rat skin using electroporation. Pharm Res 2001; 18(1):61–66.
70. Dujardin N, Staes E, Kalia Y, et al. In vivo assessment of skin electroporation using square wave pulses. J Control Release 2002; 79(1–3):219–227.
71. Maruyama H, Ataka K, Higuchi N, et al. Skin-targeted gene transfer using in vivo electroporation. Gene Ther 2001; 8(23):1808–1812.
72. Zhang L, Widera G, Rabussay D. Enhancement of the effectiveness of electroporation-augmented cutaneous DNA vaccination by a particulate adjuvant. Bioelectrochemistry 2004; 63(1–2):369–373.
73. Heller LC, Jaroszeski MJ, Coppola D, et al. Optimization of cutaneous electrically mediated plasmid DNA delivery using novel electrode. Gene Ther 2007; 14(3):275–280.
74. Byrnes CK, Malone RW, Akhter N, et al. Electroporation enhances transfection efficiency in murine cutaneous wounds. Wound Repair Regen 2004; 12(4):397–403.
75. Marti G, Ferguson M, Wang J, et al. Electroporative transfection with KGF-1 DNA improves wound healing in a diabetic mouse model. Gene Ther 2004; 11(24):1780–1785.
76. Lin MP, Marti GP, Dieb R, et al. Delivery of plasmid DNA expression vector for keratinocyte growth factor-1 using electroporation to improve cutaneous wound healing in a septic rat model. Wound Repair Regen 2006; 14(5):618–624.

77. Medi BM, Hoselton S, Marepalli RB, et al. Skin targeted DNA vaccine delivery using electroporation in rabbits: I. Efficacy. Int J Pharm 2005; 294(1–2):53–63.
78. Medi BM, Singh J. Skin targeted DNA vaccine delivery using electroporation in rabbits: II. Safety. Int J Pharm 2006; 308(1–2):61–68.
79. Mitragotri S, Kost J. Low-frequency sonophoresis: a review. Adv Drug Deliv Rev 2004; 56(5):589–601.
80. Kim HJ, Greenleaf JF, Kinnick RR, et al. Ultrasound-mediated transfection of mammalian cells. Hum Gene Ther 1996; 7(11):1339–1346.
81. Taniyama Y, Tachibana K, Hiraoka K, et al. Development of safe and efficient novel nonviral gene transfer using ultrasound: enhancement of transfection efficiency of naked plasmid DNA in skeletal muscle. Gene Ther 2002; 9(6):372–380.
82. Yang L, Shirakata Y, Tamai K, et al. Microbubble-enhanced ultrasound for gene transfer into living skin equivalents. J Dermatol Sci 2005; 40(2):105–114.
83. Lentacker I, De Geest BG, Vandenbroucke RE, et al. Ultrasound-responsive polymer-coated microbubbles that bind and protect DNA. Langmuir 2006; 22(17):7273–7278.
84. Sintov AC, Krymberk I, Daniel D, et al. Radiofrequency-driven skin microchanneling as a new way for electrically assisted transdermal delivery of hydrophilic drugs. J Control Release 2003; 89(2):311–320.
85. Birchall J, Coulman S, Anstey A, et al. Cutaneous gene expression of plasmid DNA in excised human skin following delivery via microchannels created by radio frequency ablation. Int J Pharm 2006; 312(1–2):15–23.
86. Tao W, Wilkinson J, Stanbridge EJ, et al. Direct gene transfer into human cultured cells facilitated by laser micropuncture of the cell membrane. Proc Natl Acad Sci U S A 1987; 84(12):4180–4184.
87. Zeira E, Manevitch A, Khatchatouriants A, et al. Femtosecond infrared laser-an efficient and safe in vivo gene delivery system for prolonged expression. Mol Ther 2003; 8(2):342–350.
88. Ogura M, Sato S, Nakanishi K, et al. In vivo targeted gene transfer in skin by the use of laser-induced stress waves. Lasers Surg Med 2004; 34(3):242–248.
89. Badiavas E, Mehta PP, Falanga V. Retrovirally mediated gene transfer in a skin equivalent model of chronic wounds. J Dermatol Sci 1996; 13(1):56–62.
90. Choate KA, Khavari PA. Sustainability of keratinocyte gene transfer and cell survival in vivo. Hum Gene Ther 1997; 8(8):895–901.
91. Page SM, Brownlee GG. An ex vivo keratinocyte model for gene therapy of hemophilia B. J Invest Dermatol 1997; 109(2):139–145.
92. Kolodka TM, Garlick JA, Taichman LB. Evidence for keratinocyte stem cells in vitro: long term engraftment and persistence of transgene expression from retrovirus-transduced keratinocytes. Proc Natl Acad Sci U S A 1998; 95(8):4356–4361.
93. Deng H, Lin Q, Khavari PA. Sustainable cutaneous gene delivery. Nat Biotechnol 1997; 15(13):1388–1391.
94. Peroni CN, Cecchi CR, Damiani R, et al. High-level secretion of growth hormone by retrovirally transduced primary human keratinocytes: prospects for an animal model of cutaneous gene therapy. Mol Biotechnol 2006; 34(2):239–245.
95. Baldeschi C, Gache Y, Rattenholl A, et al. Genetic correction of canine dystrophic epidermolysis bullosa mediated by retroviral vectors. Hum Mol Genet 2003; 12(15):1897–1905.
96. Pfutzner W, Joari MR, Foster RA, et al. A large preclinical animal model to assess ex vivo skin gene therapy applications. Arch Dermatol Res 2006; 298(1):16–22.
97. Setoguchi Y, Jaffe HA, Danel C, et al. Ex vivo and in vivo gene transfer to the skin using replication-deficient recombinant adenovirus vectors. J Invest Dermatol 1994; 102(4):415–421.
98. Lu B, Scott G, Goldsmith LA. A model for keratinocyte gene therapy: preclinical and therapeutic considerations. Proc Assoc Am Physicians 1996; 108(2):165–172.
99. Lu B, Federoff HJ, Wang Y, et al. Topical application of viral vectors for epidermal gene transfer. J Invest Dermatol 1997; 108(5):803–808.
100. Jaakkola P, Ahonen M, Kahari VM, et al. Transcriptional targeting of adenoviral gene delivery into migrating wound keratinocytes using FiRE, a growth factor-inducible regulatory element. Gene Ther 2000; 7(19):1640–1647.

101. Plog MS, Guyre CA, Roberts BL, et al. Preclinical safety and biodistribution of adenovirus-based cancer vaccines after intradermal delivery. Hum Gene Ther 2006; 17(7):705–716.
102. Marchetto MC, Muotri AR, Burns DK, et al. Gene transduction in skin cells: preventing cancer in xeroderma pigmentosum mice. Proc Natl Acad Sci U S A 2004; 101(51):17759–17764.
103. Lillehammer T, Tveito S, Engesaeter BO, et al. Melanoma-specific expression in first-generation adenoviral vectors in vitro and in vivo—use of the human tyrosinase promoter with human enhancers. Cancer Gene Ther 2005; 12(11):864–872.
104. Rolland AP, Mumper RJ. Plasmid delivery to muscle: Recent advances in polymer delivery systems. Adv Drug Deliv Rev 1998; 30(1–3):151–172.
105. Hengge UR, Mirmohammadsadegh A. Adeno-associated virus expresses transgenes in hair follicles and epidermis. Mol Ther 2000; 2(3):188–194.
106. Deodato B, Arsic N, Zentilin L, et al. Recombinant AAV vector encoding human VEGF165 enhances wound healing. Gene Ther 2002; 9(12):777–785.
107. Galeano M, Deodato B, Altavilla D, et al. Adeno-associated viral vector-mediated human vascular endothelial growth factor gene transfer stimulates angiogenesis and wound healing in the genetically diabetic mouse. Diabetologia 2003; 46(4):546–555.
108. Ma H, Xu R, Cheng H, et al. Gene transfer into human keloid tissue with adeno-associated virus vector. J Trauma 2003; 54(3):569–573.
109. Descamps V, Blumenfeld N, Beuzard Y, et al. Keratinocytes as a target for gene therapy. Sustained production of erythropoietin in mice by human keratinocytes transduced with an adenoassociated virus vector. Arch Dermatol 1996; 132(10):1207–1211.
110. Kuhn U, Terunuma A, Pfutzner W, et al. In vivo assessment of gene delivery to keratinocytes by lentiviral vectors. J Virol 2002; 76(3):1496–1504.
111. Gagnoux-Palacios L, Hervouet C, Spirito F, et al. Assessment of optimal transduction of primary human skin keratinocytes by viral vectors. J Gene Med 2005; 7(9):1178–1186.

34 Pressure Waves for Transdermal Drug Delivery

Apostolos G. Doukas

Wellman Center for Photomedicine, Massachusetts General Hospital, Boston, Massachusetts, U.S.A.

Sumit Paliwal and Samir Mitragotri

Department of Chemical Engineering, University of California, Santa Barbara, Santa Barbara, California, U.S.A.

INTRODUCTION

In clinical therapy, topical application allows localized drug delivery to the site of interest. This enhances the therapeutic effect of the drug while minimizing systemic side effects. Furthermore, topical application of drugs bypasses systemic deactivation or degradation and minimizes gastrointestinal incompatibility and potential toxicological risk. Several physical and chemical methods with varying degrees of effectiveness have been devised. Physical methods have the advantage of decreased skin irritation or allergic responses. Among the physical methods under development or investigation are iontophoresis, electroporation, jet injectors, microneedles, and application of ultrasound and pressure waves (PWs) (see Chapter 1). In this chapter, we review ultrasound and PWs and discuss their applications for drug delivery. Both methods exert mechanical forces on the stratum corneum (SC), the topmost dead layer of skin, which is responsible for the skin's barrier properties. Furthermore, their mechanisms of permeabilization, in terms of effect on skin structure, also appear to be similar.

The primary effect of ultrasound waves is to physically perturb the medium of passage, leading to a variety of effects, such as thermal heating and nonthermal effects caused by acoustic cavitation. These ultrasonic effects have been effectively used to develop a host of medical therapies (1), including lithotripsy (2), hyperthermia (3), thrombolysis (4), lipoplasty (5), wound healing (6), and fracture healing (7). On the other hand, the effects of PWs on biological systems have been studied through laser–tissue interactions (8,9), causing several biological effects induced by short-pulse, high-power lasers. While these phenomena have been traditionally grouped into photochemical, photothermal, and photomechanical effects, the generation of pressure waves and the subsequent interactions with cells, tissue, and organs are chiefly due to the photomechanical effects.

Interestingly, both technologies have been applied to the field of drug delivery in diverse areas of application. Ultrasound has been used to facilitate drug delivery into cells [e.g., sonoporation (10–13), triggered drug release (14–17), and targeted drug delivery (18,19)] and across the skin [e.g., sonophoresis (20–72)]. Similarly, PWs have been shown to permeabilize and enhance delivery of a variety of macromolecules across several biological barriers, including cellular plasma membrane [in vitro (73–75) and in vivo (76,77)] nuclear envelope (78), SC (79), and microbial biofilms (80).

BACKGROUND

Ultrasound is a longitudinal PW operating at a frequency higher than 20 kHz. It is generated by applying an appropriate electrical signal to a piezoelectric transducer that converts the electrical energy into a mechanical wave. The skin's permeability enhancement induced by ultrasound depends on four main parameters: frequency, intensity, duty cycle, and application time. Ultrasound at various frequencies in the range of 20 kHz to 16 MHz has been used to enhance skin permeability. However, transdermal transport enhancement induced by low-frequency ultrasound (f<100 kHz) has been found to be more significant than that induced by high-frequency ultrasound (42,53,81). At each frequency, there exists an intensity below which no detectable enhancement is observed. This intensity is referred to as the threshold intensity. Once the intensity exceeds this threshold, the enhancement increases strongly with the intensity until another threshold intensity, referred to as the decoupling intensity, is reached. Beyond this intensity, the enhancement does not increase with further increase in intensity caused by acoustic decoupling. The threshold intensity for porcine skin increased from approximately 0.11 W/cm² at 19.6 kHz to more than 2 W/cm² at 93.4 kHz (53). At a given intensity, the enhancement decreases with increasing ultrasound frequency.

The dependence of enhancement on intensity, duty cycle, and application time can be combined into a single parameter—the total acoustic energy fluence (E) delivered from the transducer, which is defined as $E=It$, where I is the ultrasound intensity (W/cm²) during each pulse and t is the total "on" time (in seconds). As a general trend, no significant enhancement is observed until a threshold energy fluence dose is reached. The threshold energy fluence doses for various frequencies were found to be 10 J/cm² at 19.6 kHz, 63 J/cm² at 36.9 kHz, 103 J/cm² at 58.9 kHz, 304 J/cm² at 76.6 kHz, and 1305 J/cm² at 93.4 kHz (53). Thus, the threshold energy fluence dose increased by approximately 130-fold as the frequency increased from 19.6 to 93.4 kHz. The dependence of enhancement on energy fluence after the threshold is reached is different for different frequencies. For extremely high-energy doses (e.g., 10⁴ J/cm²), the enhancements induced by all the frequencies are comparable. However, for lower-energy fluence doses, the differences between various frequencies are significant and the choice of frequency may affect the effectiveness of sonophoresis.

In addition to frequency and energy fluence, ultrasonic enhancement also depends on additional parameters, including the distance between the transducer and the skin, gas concentration in the coupling medium, and the transducer geometry. Detailed dependence of enhancement on these parameters has not been studied yet.

As opposed to ultrasound, PWs are finite amplitude waves. The parameters that characterize a PW are peak pressure, rise time (from 10% to 90% of peak value), pulse duration (defined by the full width at half maximum), and decay. However, for drug delivery applications, peak pressure (82), rise time, and pulse duration (83) have been investigated as the critical parameters. The number of pulses applied can also be varied, typically ranging from 1 to 20 pulses. In most cases for transdermal drug delivery, however, 1 pulse has been shown to be sufficient to permeabilize the SC and facilitate drug delivery into the epidermis. The permeabilization of the SC can last, depending on the PW parameters, for several minutes (82,84). Therefore, any additional PW delivered during this time should not affect the efficiency of drug delivery. It is important to notice that the role of PWs in drug delivery is only to permeabilize the SC and that the drug diffuses passively through the SC under its concentration gradient. In addition to the PW parameters, other factors that can influence drug delivery are drug molecular size, skin hydration, and use of chemical enhancers, such as sodium lauryl sulfate (SLS), to pronounce the permeability of the skin by PWs.

Ablation is a reliable method for generating PWs with consistent characteristics. In ablation, the laser radiation causes decomposition of the target material into small fragments that move away from the surface of the target at supersonic speed. Although the amount of material ejected is small, high-amplitude pressure transients can be generated by the imparted recoil momentum that propagates into the material or tissue. The characteristics of the PWs (peak pressure, rise time, and duration) (85) depend on the laser parameters (wavelength, pulse duration, and pulse energy) as well as the optical and mechanical properties of the target material. The peak pressure generated during ablation as a function of irradiance, wavelength, and pulse duration is given by the following equation:

$$P_0 = b \frac{I^{0.7}}{\left(\lambda\sqrt{\tau}\right)^{0.3}} \tag{1}$$

where P_0 is the peak pressure of the wave, b is the proportionality constant that depends on the material properties, I is the laser irradiance, λ is the laser wavelength, and τ is the laser pulse duration. Equation 1 has been shown to hold over a wide range of laser irradiance, wavelength, pulse duration, and pulse energy. In addition, the design of stratified targets and overlays (confined ablation) (86) can produce PWs more efficiently or of higher peak pressure. Although laser-generated PWs have been widely used for drug delivery, other modes of PW generation, such as extracorporeal shock wave lithotripters (87) and a shock wave tube, have been used for the generation of PWs for cytoplasmic (88) and transdermal (89) drug delivery. Figure 1 shows the schematic of the device used for transdermal drug delivery, a typical waveform, and the way the device is applied on the skin, human skin in this particular case.

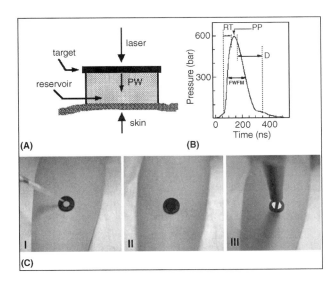

FIGURE 1 (**A**) Schematic of the device used for transdermal drug delivery and (**B**) a typical waveform. (**C**) For the application of PWs for drug delivery in humans, a rubber washer was attached and filled with the drug solution to be delivered into the skin (i). The target material was placed on top of the washer in contact with the solution (ii). The articulating arm of the laser was positioned over the target and the laser was fired once to generate a single PW (iii). *Abbreviations*: PP, peak pressure; RT, rise time; FWHM, full width at half maximum; D, decay.

The nature of PWs as finite amplitude waves can affect the PW parameters because of nonlinear effects. The rise time of a PW propagating through a medium is altered by the linear and nonlinear properties of the medium. The linear attenuation, which increases as a function of frequency, predominantly attenuates the high-frequency components and causes the rise time to increase. On the other hand, the nonlinear properties cause the leading edge of the PW to become steeper as it propagates through the medium. The relative strength of the linear attenuation and nonlinear coefficient of the medium as well as the initial peak pressure, the initial rise time, and the distance traveled in the medium determine the final value of the rise time. It is understood that the large pressure gradients and high-bulk velocity of the molecules within the pressure front account for the unique interactions of the shock waves with matter.

MECHANISM OF ACTION

The skin allows delivery of only a handful of low-molecular-weight (<500 Da) and highly lipophilic molecules, in small quantities as well. This high resistance to molecular transport is a result of the skin's uppermost and dead layer, the SC. The SC possesses a well-packed structure composed of corneocytes, which are filled with keratin and lack nuclei as well as cytoplasmic organelles (90). The intercellular regions are composed of stacks of interdigitating lipid bilayers that provide a robust lipophilic extracellular matrix to the SC. Lipid bilayers chiefly consist of nonpolar and neutral lipids that originate from the membrane-coated granules (lamellar bodies) in the stratum granulosum (91). Three possible pathways, transappendageal, transcellular, and intercellular, have been suggested for molecular transport through the SC (92). The transappendageal pathway represents transport through hair follicles. The transcellular pathway requires the substrates to travel through the corneocytes, whereas the intercellular pathway represents the extracellular matrix between the corneocytes. For intercellular skin transport, hydrophilic substrates are rate limited by the lipid-rich environment of the intercellular matrix of the SC. Alternatively, lipophilic substrates can relatively partition easily into the intercellular lipids of the SC; however, here, the rate-limiting step could be partitioning into the epidermis, which is practically an aqueous environment.

Ultrasound

The transport enhancement induced by ultrasound is mediated by acoustic cavitation, which is characterized by nucleation, growth, and collapse of gaseous pockets. Cavitation is predominantly induced in the coupling medium (the liquid present between the ultrasound transducer and the skin) (60). The size range and maximum radius reached by free cavitating bubbles are related to the frequency and acoustic pressure amplitude. Two types of cavitation, stable and inertial, have been evaluated for their role in sonophoresis. Stable cavitation corresponds to periodic growth and oscillations of bubbles, whereas inertial cavitation corresponds to violent growth and collapse of cavitation bubbles (93). Both types of cavitation have been quantified with the use of acoustic spectroscopy (58,60). The overall dependence of inertial cavitation on ultrasound intensity was found to be similar to that of skin permeability enhancement (58,60). Specifically, ultrasound intensity above the threshold value is required before inception of inertial cavitation is observed. This threshold corresponds to the minimum pressure amplitude required to induce rapid growth and collapse of cavitation nuclei. Beyond this threshold, white noise (indicator of inertial cavitation) increased linearly with ultrasound intensity, although, at any given intensity, inertial cavitation activity decreased rapidly with ultrasound frequency (60). The threshold intensity for the occurrence of inertial cavitation increased with increasing ultrasound frequency. This dependence reflects the fact that growth of cavitation bubbles becomes increasingly difficult with increasing ultrasound frequency. Tezel et al. (60) showed that regardless of the intensity and frequency, skin permeability enhancement correlated universally with a measure proportional to the total acoustic energy fluence. These data suggest a strong role played by inertial cavitation in low-frequency sonophoresis.

Inertial cavitation in the vicinity of a surface is fundamentally different from that away from the surface. Specifically, collapse of spherical cavitation bubbles in the bulk solution is symmetrical and results in the formation of a highly disruptive shock wave with an initial velocity as high as 10^3 m/sec and a pressure amplitude exceeding 10^4 atmospheres (94). However, the amplitude of the shock wave decreases rapidly with distance. Collapse of cavitation bubbles near boundaries (especially rigid ones) has been extensively studied in the literature (95). Specifically, Naude and Ellis (96) showed that cavitation bubbles travel under the influence of the ultrasound field toward the boundary and collapse near the boundary depending on its proximity to the surface. The collapse of cavitation bubbles near the boundary is asymmetrical because of the difference in the surrounding conditions on both sides of the bubbles. Specifically, the asymmetry in the surroundings leads to the generation of pressure gradients, which ultimately leads to the formation of a liquid microjet directed toward the surface. The diameter of the microjet is much smaller than that of the maximum bubble radius. There have been several estimates of the speed of the liquid microjet when it strikes the surface [between 50 and 180 m/sec (97–99)].

Inertial cavitation during sonophoresis occurs in the bulk coupling medium and near the skin surface. Inertial cavitation at both locations may potentially be responsible for permeability enhancement. Tezel and Mitragotri (100) evaluated three mechanisms by which inertial cavitation events might enhance SC permeability. These include bubbles that collapse symmetrically in the bulk medium, emitting shock waves and thereby disrupting the SC lipid bilayers, and acoustic microjets that might impact and disrupt the SC with or without penetrating it. The authors concluded that symmetrical collapses and microjets from asymmetrical collapses are possibly responsible for sonophoresis; however, because histological analysis showed no evidence of surface damage, specific contribution from the SC-penetrating microjets in permeability enhancement was neglected. Regardless of the precise mode of collapse, approximately 10 collapses/sec/cm² in the form of spherical collapses or microjets near the surface of the SC were suggested to explain experimentally observed permeability enhancements. They also reported that bubble collapses only close to the SC surface (~50 µm) contribute to sonophoresis.

Disruption of SC lipid bilayers caused by bubble-induced shock waves or microjet impact may enhance skin permeability by at least two mechanisms. First, a moderate level of disruption decreases the structural order of lipid bilayers and increases the solute diffusion coefficient (101). At a higher level of disruption, lipid bilayers may lose structural integrity and facilitate penetration of the coupling medium into the SC. Because many sonophoresis experiments reported in the literature are performed using coupling media composed of aqueous solutions of surfactants, disruption of SC lipid bilayers enhances incorporation of surfactants into lipid bilayers. Paliwal et al. (102) studied the effect of ultrasound on skin microstructure using electron microscopy. The effects of ultrasound on skin microstructure are similar to those of PWs. Specifically, application of 20 kHz of ultrasound induced heterogeneous and significant distension within the lipid regions of the SC, creating several hundreds of nanometer-wide voids referred to as lacunar domains (Fig. 2C). Incorporation of excessive water and surfactants further promotes bilayer disruption in the SC, thereby opening pathways for solute permeation (103,104). Addition of 1% w/v SLS in the coupling medium yielded pronounced disruption of basic barrier ultrastructures, such as secreted lamellar bodies at the SC–stratum granulosum interface and increased disordering of intercellular lipid bilayers at the SC (Fig. 2D) (102).

Ultrasound has also been shown to induce convective flow across the skin. Morimoto et al. (105) reported that 41 kHz of ultrasound has the potential to induce convective solvent flow to increase the skin permeation of hydrophilic calcein in excised hairless rat skin. Similar conclusions have also been reached by Tang et al. (106). The precise origin of convective flow is not clear, although cavitation is indicated to play a significant role.

PWs

Transdermal delivery can occur when the molecules are either present during the application of the PWs or introduced after the PWs (82,107). Given the short duration of the PWs, a few microseconds at most, the effect of PWs is probably limited to the permeabilization of the SC. The diffusion of the drug occurs under the concentration gradient through the transient channels produced by the PWs in the SC.

Microscopic evaluations of human skin (postfixed with RuO_4) exposed to a PW showed many highly expanded lacunar domains within the SC intercellular lamellae (Fig. 2A and B) (108). The lacunae are defined as electron-lucent areas embedded within the lipid bilayers of the SC's intercellular domains and are consid-

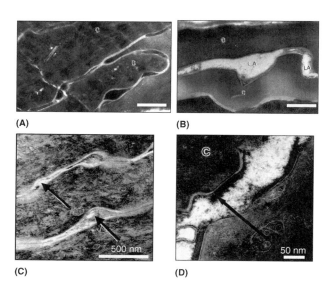

(A)

(B)

(C)

(D)

FIGURE 2 High-magnification electron micrograph of the SC from (**A**) a control site; (**B**) exposed to a single PW with water as the coupling medium, and exposed to ultrasound with (**C**) saline and (**D**) 1% w/v SLS (**D**) as the coupling medium. The expanded lacunar domains within the intercellular lamellae can be seen. "C" depicts corneocytes, and arrows and "LA" depict lacunar domains. Scale bar in (**A**) is 500 nm and in (**B**) is 200 nm.

ered as the putative pores that may facilitate diffusion of drugs through the SC (109). The heterogeneity in lacunae distribution was evident because these domains were not present at every level (i.e., between every corneocyte). Intact lipid bilayer arrangement without any defect could be seen in the extracellular spaces of corneocytes that were present immediately below these domains. However, it should be kept in mind that the lacunae seen in electron micrographs are in essence cross-sections of the three-dimensional trabecular network that may form a continuous, permeable lacunar system. No ultrastructural change was seen in the morphology of individual corneocytes.

The expansion of the lacunar domains could possibly create transient channels that enable drug delivery through the SC and into the epidermis and dermis. We hypothesized that under the action of a PW, the lacunar domains form a continuous pathway that allows the passive diffusion of the drug under the concentration gradient. The actual physical mechanism is not known. The hypothesis is that the free water within the SC is involved in the permeabilization process. Water can be considered incompressible in the time scale of the duration of the PW. The free water has to go somewhere. It is possible that under the pressure gradient generated by the PW, the free water is forced in the constricted domains of the lacunar domains expanding them and thus forming a continuous pathway of transient pores. The observation that the lacunae deep inside the SC, where SC is more hydrated, are dilated more than the surface ones is consistent with this hypothesis.

Electron microscopy of skin postfixed with OsO_4 reveals the cellular ultrastructure details of different strata of the skin. With the use of this technique, human skin biopsies after the application of PWs did not reveal any difference from control sites neither immediately after exposure nor 24 hours after exposure. The nucleated epidermis and the dermis maintained their typical ultrastructural features with no indication of damage either in the extracellular matrix or the cellular components. It is interesting to note that the PWs used in the present experiments could induce extensive changes in the SC without damaging the viable epidermis and dermis. It therefore appears that the threshold for SC permeabilization is lower than the threshold for cell damage. A similar effect has been observed in the application of PWs for drug delivery into the cytoplasm. The peak pressure for the permeabilization of the cell plasma membrane for a number of cell lines was found to be lower than that for cell damage (110).

TRANSDERMAL DELIVERY OF MACROMOLECULES: ANIMAL DATA

Ultrasound and PWs have been used to deliver macromolecules in animal studies. A brief review of the use of these techniques for transdermal macromolecule delivery is presented.

Ultrasound
Proteins
Low-frequency sonophoresis has been shown to deliver several macromolecular drugs. Tachibana and Tachibana (65) demonstrated that a 5-minute exposure to ultrasound (48 kHz, 3000-8000 Pa) induced a significant reduction of blood glucose levels in rats exposed to insulin. Specifically, the glucose level decreased to 34% of the initial value at lower pressures and to 22% of the initial value at higher acoustic pressures. Comparable results were obtained in rabbits at somewhat

higher frequencies (150 kHz). Mitragotri et al. (42) performed in vitro and in vivo evaluations of the effect of low-frequency ultrasound on transdermal delivery of proteins. Application of low-frequency ultrasound (20 kHz, 125 mW/cm^2, 100-ms pulses applied every second) enhanced transdermal transport of proteins, including insulin, γ-interferon, and erythropoietin, across human cadaver skin in vitro (42). Ultrasound under the same conditions delivered therapeutic doses of insulin across hairless rat skin in vivo from a chamber glued on the rat's back and filled with an insulin solution (100 U/ml) (42). A simultaneous application of insulin and ultrasound from outside (20 kHz, 225 mW/cm^2, 100-ms pulses applied every second) reduced the blood glucose level of diabetic hairless rats from approximately 400 to 200 mg/dl in 30 minutes. A corresponding increase in plasma insulin levels was observed during sonophoresis. Boucaud et al. (81) also demonstrated dose-dependent hypoglycemia in hairless rats exposed to ultrasound and insulin. At an energy dose of 900 J/cm^2, a reduction of approximately 75% in glucose levels was reported. Pretreatment of skin by low-frequency ultrasound (20 kHz, ~7 W/cm^2) has also been shown to enhance skin permeability to insulin (111). More recently, Smith et al. (112) demonstrated ultrasonic transdermal insulin delivery in rabbits and rats with a low-profile two-by-two ultrasound array based on the cymbal transducer. In rats, the blood glucose decreased to 233±22 mg/dl in 90 minutes after 5 minutes of pulsed ultrasound exposure. In rabbits, the glucose level was found to decrease to 133±36 mg/dl from the initial baseline in 60 minutes.

Low-Molecular-Weight Heparin

Low-frequency ultrasound has also been shown to deliver low-molecular-weight heparin (LMWH) across the skin (49). Transdermal LMWH delivery was measured by monitoring anti-Factor X activity (aXa) in blood. No significant aXa activity was observed when LMWH was placed on nontreated skin. However, a significant amount of LMWH was transported transdermally after ultrasound pretreatment. aXa in the blood increased slowly for approximately 2 hours, after which it increased rapidly before achieving a steady state after 4 hours at a value of approximately 2 U/ml (49). The effect of transdermally delivered LMWH was observed well beyond 6 hours in contrast to intravenous and subcutaneous injections, which resulted only in transient biological activity.

Oligonucleotides

Low-frequency ultrasound has also been shown to enhance dermal penetration of oligonucleotides (ODNs) (113). A 10-minute application of ultrasound (20 kHz, 2.4 W/cm^2) increased skin ODN permeability to 4.5×10^{-5} cm/hr as compared with nearly undetectable values across nontreated skin. A significant amount of ODNs was also localized in the skin. Greater enhancements of ODN delivery were obtained by simultaneous application of ultrasound and ODNs. Experiments performed with fluorescently-labeled ODNs revealed that ODNs are largely localized in the superficial layers of the skin (Fig. 3A). Estimation of the local concentration of ODNs in the skin was performed. Assuming a depth of penetration of 100 to 1000 μm, the estimated concentration of ODNs in the skin at the end of ultrasound application was approximately 0.53% to 5.3% of the donor concentration. ODN penetration into the skin caused by low-frequency ultrasound was heterogeneous. Heterogeneity of dermal penetration was visualized by monitoring the penetration of a dye, sulforhodamine B, that was incorporated in the coupling medium. Sulforhodamine B penetration clearly indicated four to five intensely stained spots (~1 mm in diameter), which were termed as localized transport pathways. Skin exposed to ISIS 13920 in the presence of ultrasound was assessed using immunohistochemistry to further ensure that ODNs penetrated the skin without losing integrity. No visible staining was observed in the case of passive delivery; however, skin treated with low-frequency ultrasound was heavily stained, suggesting penetration of ODN delivery (Fig. 3C). ODNs were localized in the epidermis and dermis. Furthermore, microscopy studies suggested that ODNs penetrated into epidermal cells (Fig. 3D). This is a particularly appealing feature because viable epidermal cells are an attractive target for ODN delivery.

Vaccines

Recently, low-frequency sonophoresis has also been used to deliver vaccines across the skin (114). Transcutaneous immunization (TCI) promises to be a potent novel vaccination technique because topical immunization elicits both systemic and mucosal immunity (115). The latter form is of great importance because a significant number of pathogens invade the host via mucosal surfaces (116). TCI is based on the premise that systemic and mucosal immune responses can be initiated by the activation of the Langerhans cells (LCs) in the skin. Ultrasonic delivery of tetanus toxoid (TTx) generated a strong systemic immune response in animals. Specifically, ultrasound-assisted transcutaneous delivery of 1.3 µg of TTx generated IgG antibody titers comparable with those induced by 10 µg of subcutaneous injection (Fig. 4A). Studies have shown that an IgG antibody response generated by only 5 µg of subcutaneous injection of TTx is sufficient for protection against a lethal dose of tetanus toxin (117). Ultrasonic delivery of TTx also generated a strong mucosal immune response. A large number of TTx immunoreactive plasma cells were found in the intestine (A Tezel and S Mitragotri, unpublished data). Two possible mechanisms were proposed by the authors to explain why pretreatment of skin

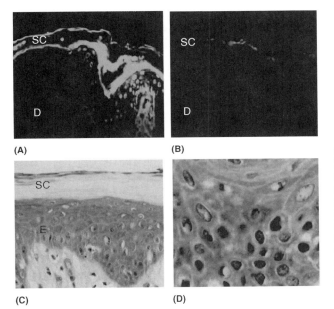

(A) (B) (C) (D)

FIGURE 3 Penetration of fluorescently-labeled oligonucleotides (ODNs) (**A**) after ultrasound treatment of porcine skin and (**B**) through passive diffusion into untreated control skin. Immunohistochemical staining showed extensive penetration of ODNs (**C**) into epidermal tissue and (**D**) into skin cells after ultrasound treatment. *Abbreviations*: SC, stratum corneum; E, epidermis; D, dermis.

with low-frequency ultrasound before contact with the antigen vaccine may enhance the immune response. One possible mechanism is that ultrasound pretreatment results in increased delivery of the vaccine as compared with control, thus enabling a sufficient amount of vaccine to enter the skin to activate the skin's immune response. However, a comparison of the response obtained by TCI with that obtained by subcutaneous immunization shows that the IgG immune response elicited by TCI is almost 10-fold more effective per dose as compared with that elicited by subcutaneous injection. This can possibly be explained by a second mechanism, which pertains to the involvement of LCs and other antigen-presenting cells of the skin that effectively capture the antigen and present it to the immune system. Clear activation of LCs was observed after ultrasonic TTx delivery (Fig. 4B). LC activation is induced partly by the entry of the antigen and partly by the direct effect of ultrasound on skin. Mechanisms responsible for ultrasound-induced activation of LCs are not clear, although barrier disruption and release of pro-inflammatory signals by the keratinocytes are possible candidates.

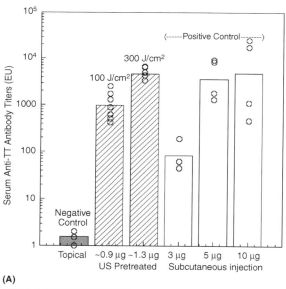

(A)

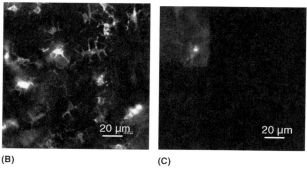

(B)   (C)

FIGURE 4 (A) Tetanus toxin IgG titers in mouse sera after immunization by application of tetanus toxoid on skin with (*shaded bars*) or without (*gray bar*) ultrasound pretreatment. White bars indicate positive controls, obtained by subcutaneous immunization of mice. Assessment of the activation of the skin's Langerhans cells (B) after ultrasound treatment and (C) in untreated control skin samples.

PWs
Insulin
PWs have been used to deliver insulin in streptozotocin-diabetic rats (107). Figure 5 shows the glucose levels of three diabetic rats over time after the procedure. A two-step procedure was used for insulin delivery. For the first step, the reservoir was filled with 2% w/v aqueous solution of SLS, which was allowed to remain in contact with the skin for 2 minutes. This step was intended to enhance the permeabilization of the SC. For the second step, the SLS solution was removed and the reservoirs were filled with a solution of porcine insulin (400 U/ml adjusted to pH 4). The second target was driven by the laser pulse into the reservoir like the plunger of a syringe. Therefore, the first laser pulse in this procedure produced a PW that permeabilized the SC, whereas the second laser pulse drove the target into the reservoir by exerting a hydrodynamic pulse on the insulin solution (118). This treatment reduced the blood glucose of diabetic rats from greater than 350 mg/dl to less than 100 mg/dl (i.e., a reduction of ~80% of the initial glucose level) (107). Overall, the blood glucose levels successfully remained within the normal physiological range for approximately 3 hours. These experiments suggest that therapeutic doses of insulin can be delivered through the SC by PWs. Comparison of glucose kinetics after the application of PWs with the kinetics of intramuscular injection of insulin indicated that the total amount of insulin delivered through the SC was between 0.1 and 0.3 U. With the use of insulin concentration, skin treatment area, and duration for insulin delivery, total insulin solution transported through the skin was estimated to be between 0.3 and 0.9 µl. This corresponds to an average value of skin permeability that is between 4×10^{-4} and 1.2×10^{-3} cm/hr. The application of the PWs did not affect the activity of insulin. This is not surprising because the pressure required to have any effect on molecules or to induce any chemical change is two orders of magnitude higher than that used in these experiments (119).

Allergens
PWs can be applied for rapid delivery of allergens and thus make it possible to differentiate irritants from allergic contact dermatitis. Presently, the suspect allergen is applied at subirritant concentrations to the skin under occlusion (Finn chamber) for a period of up to 48 hours to maximize penetration. Once the patch is removed, the site is clinically examined for morphological evidence of an eczematous response. If

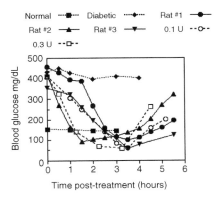

FIGURE 5 Blood glucose kinetics after PW delivery of insulin in diabetic rats. Shown for comparison is the blood glucose kinetics after intramuscular injection of insulin (0.1 and 0.3 U).

the subject develops such a response at a concentration below the irritant threshold concentration, the eczematous lesion is considered to be an allergic response to the tested substance. PWs allowed rapid transdermal delivery of allergens and thus improved the optimal penetration of the allergen across the SC (120). This experiment demonstrated the potential of PWs to reduce the exposure time of allergens for the clinical manifestation of the challenge and improve the accuracy of the procedure.

The allergic skin reaction using PW delivery was compared with 5 minutes and 21 hours of occlusion in a sensitized hairless albino guinea pig model. The pigs were sensitized by intradermal injection of (0.01%) dinitrochlorobenzene and topical administration (0.1%, 1 week later) of the hapten. One month later, testing for the allergic response was performed by the administration of 10 µl of 0.1% dinitrochlorobenzene with a PW. The picture of the back of a pig in Figure 6 shows a skin site treated under occlusion for 21 hours and another treated under occlusion for 5 minutes using the Finn chamber. In addition, a single PW was applied to one site with water as the coupling medium, followed by the application of the allergen for 5 minutes. The skin site treated with the Finn chamber under occlusion for 21 hours showed an erythematous and edematous skin reaction that in some cases resulted in skin maceration and necrosis. These reactions always extended beyond the contact site of the skin with the allergen. On the other hand, skin sites treated with a PW showed a pink, well-demarcated erythematous area confined to the beam diameter at 24 and 48 hours after delivery. The control sites, exposed to the allergen under occlusion for 5 minutes, showed no clinically perceptible reaction.

Nanoparticles and Gene Vectors

Exposure of a single PW was shown to deliver 100-nm microspheres into the epidermis (121), demonstrating the use of PWs for facilitating the transdermal delivery of large particles, such as novel probes (quantum dots, encapsulated probes) and encapsulated drugs. Drugs can be incorporated in time-release microspheres, allowing drug delivery over an extended period. Furthermore, PWs can permeabilize the SC and the cell plasma membrane. This allows use of PWs for gene delivery into keratinocytes and potential gene therapy. Ogura et al. (76) showed recently the de-

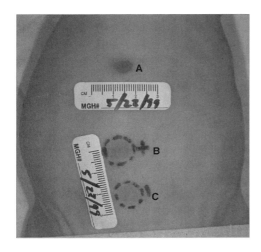

FIGURE 6   The back of a guinea pig treated with the allergen dinitrochlorobenzene with (**A**) the Finn chamber under occlusion for 21 hours, (**B**) a single PW with water as the coupling medium, followed by the application of the allergen for 5 minutes, and (**C**) the Finn chamber under occlusion for 5 minutes as a control.

livery and subsequent expression of luciferace, enhanced green fluorescent protein, and γ-galactosidase genes into the keratinocytes in a rat animal model.

TRANSDERMAL DELIVERY OF MOLECULES: HUMAN DATA
Ultrasound
Several studies on clinical studies of sonophoresis at high frequencies (1–3 MHz) have been reported; however, relatively few clinical studies have been conducted to investigate drug delivery with low-frequency sonophoresis. Recently, Kost (122) reported on the use of low-frequency sonophoresis for topical delivery of the local anesthetic EMLA. This study was sponsored by Sontra Medical (Franklin, Massachusetts, U.S.A.). Rapid onset of topical anesthetics is impeded by low permeability of the SC. Topical anesthesia is required for procedures such as venipuncture, intravenous catheterization, skin biopsy, and other cutaneous procedures. The most prevalent use of EMLA is in pediatrics for alleviating the pain experienced by children during needlestick injections. EMLA cream is indicated for use on normal intact skin to induce adequate local analgesia approximately 60 minutes after application.

The study was a randomized, double blinded, and placebo-controlled crossover trial of the onset and efficacy of cutaneous anesthesia provided by EMLA cream with and that without ultrasound exposure. The anesthetic effect of EMLA cream was compared with that of a placebo cream. The comparison was made on the ventral forearms of 42 healthy human subjects. Two circular sites of approximately 0.8 cm^2 were outlined on both ventral forearms. Each subject had four test sites. Ultrasound skin permeation was accomplished using a device developed by Sontra Medical, the SonoPrep™ skin permeation device. The SonoPrep device delivers ultrasonic energy at 55 kHz to the skin through an aqueous medium. The tip of the device includes a cylindrical ultrasonic horn inside of a housing that positions the horn above the skin. The housing is filled with the coupling buffer, which consists of a phosphate-buffered saline solution and 1% w/v SLS. Ultrasonic skin permeation was controlled by closed-loop feedback measuring an impedance decline during application. Ultrasonic power was delivered to each skin site for an average of 9.0 seconds (n=128, S.E.=0.4 seconds). During ultrasound permeation, the SonoPrep device measures a drop in skin impedance in response to increased skin permeation to control the amount of ultrasonic energy applied and the level of skin permeation achieved.

At the end of ultrasound application, the site was wiped dry and EMLA cream or the placebo cream was placed on the skin. At different times (5, 10, and 15 minutes), anesthesia was examined by pricking the skin site with a 20-G hypodermic needle. The subjects were pricked adjacent to the treated site but not close enough to the site to be affected by ultrasonic permeation of EMLA anesthesia. They were asked to consider the pain of this prick as a reference. The test site was then pricked five times at various positions at each skin site, and the subjects were asked to rate the pain after each prick. *Sharp* was scored as 1.0 and considered as painful as the control prick; *less sharp*, as 0.5; and *painless*, as 0.0. Control experiments were performed by placing EMLA on a nonsonicated site and assessing anesthesia after 60 minutes.

EMLA cream placed on the ultrasound-treated site resulted in statistically significant less pain as compared with the placebo cream at each time point. The onset of cutaneous anesthesia after ultrasound pretreatment was rapid. After only 5 minutes of EMLA application to permeated skin, the level of anesthesia provided was comparable with that of EMLA cream applied to intact skin for 60 minutes. The same effect was observed after 10 and 15 minutes of EMLA application on permeated skin. No significant cutaneous change was observed because of ultrasound application in any patient. A few cases of moderate pallor or moderate needle marks and several cases of mild pallor, redness, piloerection, and needle marks were noted. All resolved without treatment. There was no clinically significant change in vital signs before and after the procedure.

PWs

A very useful probe for human transdermal measurements is δ-aminolevulinic acid (ALA) (82). ALA has been approved by the U.S. Food and Drug Administration and is currently used in photodynamic therapy for skin cancers and in treatment of acne. ALA is a small charged molecule; therefore, the rate of penetration is limited in normal SC. It is the precursor of protoporphyrin IX (PpIX), which is an intermediate in heme biosynthesis. The synthesis of PpIX is the rate-limiting step in the synthesis of heme and is regulated by the inhibition of ALA synthase by the heme. However, application of exogenous ALA enables the cells to bypass this rate-limiting step and produce excess amounts of PpIX because the rate of PpIX production is faster than the rate of conversion of PpIX to heme. Furthermore, because PpIX is produced in viable skin, the presence of ALA in the SC does not interfere with the measurements of PpIX. The peak of PpIX fluorescence is at 634 nm (excitation, 405 nm), whereas ALA does not absorb or fluoresce at this wavelength. Therefore, the transport of ALA through the SC can be followed by monitoring the PpIX fluorescence. The sequence of steps for PW-assisted transdermal delivery was as follows: (1) a rubber washer was attached to the skin with grease, (2) the washer was filled with ALA (5% w/v in water) solution to be delivered into the skin, (3) the target material, black polystyrene, was placed on top of the washer in contact with the solution, and (4) the articulating arm of the laser was positioned over the target and the laser was fired. The laser radiation was totally absorbed by the target and produced a single PW. The PW propagated through the solution, which also acted as the acoustic coupling medium, impinged on the skin, and permeabilized the SC. The permeabilization of the SC was strictly caused by the PW. Molecules diffused into the viable skin under the concentration gradient until the barrier function of the SC was recovered.

Figure 7 shows the fluorescence emission spectrum of PpIX of a site on the forearm of a volunteer exposed to a single PW in the presence of ALA solution. The fluorescence emission of a control site (treated in an identical manner but without exposure to a PW) is also shown for comparison. The permeabilization of the SC and subsequent delivery of ALA depended on the peak pressure. The pressure threshold for the SC permeabilization was observed at approximately 350 bar and increased dramatically at the highest peak pressure (500 bar). It should be pointed out that this pressure threshold value is for a particular site (inner volar forearm) and volunteer. It was observed that the threshold pressure varied among sites, individuals, and skin conditions.

The application of PWs did not cause any pain or discomfort. PWs of 100-ns duration (full width at half maximum) did not produce any sensation whatsoever. On the other hand, PWs of 500-ns duration generated a sensation, but not pain. With respect to skin changes after the application of a PW, the 300-ns PW did not produce any change in the skin, whereas the 500-ns PW produced minor erethyma that disappeared within 10 to 15 minutes.

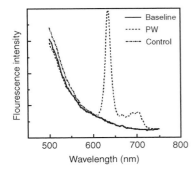

Flourescence intensity

— Baseline
---- PW
----- Control

500   600   700   800
Wavelength (nm)

FIGURE 7 Fluorescence emission spectrum obtained from human skin (the inner volar forearm) exposed to a single PW in the presence of δ-aminolevulinic acid. The fluorescence emission of PpIX peaks at 634 nm (excitation, 405 nm). The fluorescence emission spectra were recorded before the application of PW at baseline and 5 hours after treatment. The fluorescence emission spectra of a control site, a site treated in an identical manner except that no PW was applied at 5 hours, are also shown for comparison. The 5-hour control overlaps with the baseline.

CONCLUSIONS

The skin presents an exciting portal for drug administration into the human body. However, drug delivery through the skin is marred by low drug diffusivity caused by the highly tortuous and poorly permeable pathway provided by the superficial layer of the skin, the SC. Ultrasound and PWs have been proposed as physical methods to transiently open up the skin by exerting high pressure forces onto the SC. Although ultrasound waves induce acoustic cavitation by offering tensile and compressive forces, PWs formed by a laser's target ablation predominantly exert positive pressures through the coupling medium. However, at a mechanistic level, ultrasound and PWs produce similar ultrastructural distensions in the SC's lipid-rich extracellular matrix, causing a transient breach in its barrier properties. Ultrasound has been shown to enhance transport of various macromolecules across the skin, including proteins such as insulin for treating diabetes, ODNs for gene delivery, and immunogens for vaccination. Furthermore, several drugs, including hydrocortisone, salicylic acid, and lidocaine, have been delivered using ultrasound under clinical settings. PWs have also been used to successfully demonstrate the delivery of several protein-based and small-molecule drugs, allergens, and gene vectors across the skin under clinical and preclinical settings. Safety studies on human subjects for ultrasound and PWs have revealed minimal invasiveness for these technologies. Overall, ultrasound and PWs have opened the door to various exciting therapeutic opportunities for safely delivering difficult-to-administer drugs either locally or systemically to the body by physical means.

REFERENCES

1. Mitragotri S., Healing sound: the use of ultrasound in drug delivery and other therapeutic applications. Nat Rev Drug Discov 2005; 4(3):255–60.
2. Coleman AJ, Saunders JE. A review of the physical properties and biological effects of the high amplitude acoustic field used in extracorporeal lithotripsy. Ultrasonics 1993; 31(2):75–89.
3. Diederich CJ, Hynnen K. Ultrasound technology for hyperthemia. Ultrasound Med Biol 1999; 25(6):871–887.
4. Alexandrov AV. Ultrasound-enhanced thrombolysis for stroke: clinical significance. Eur J 2002; 16(1–2):131–140.
5. Goes JC, Landecker A. Ultrasound-Induced Lipoplasty (UAL) in breast surgery. Aesthetic Plast Surg 2002; 26(1):1–9.
6. Speed CA. Therapeutic ultrasound in soft tissue lesions. Rheumatology 2001; 40(12):1331–1336.

7. Hadjiargyrou M, et al. Enhancement of fracture healing by low intensity ultrasound. Clin Orthop 1998; 355 Suppl:S216–S229.
8. Doukas AG, Flotte TJ. Physical characteristics and biological effects of laser-induced stress waves. Ultrasound Med Biol 1996; 22(2):151–164.
9. Doukas AG, McAuliffe DJ, Flotte TJ. Biological effects of laser-induced shock waves: structural and functional cell damage in vitro. Ultrasound Med Biol 1993; 19(2):137–146.
10. Guzman HR, et al. Ultrasound-mediated disruption of cell membranes: I. Quantification of molecular uptake and viability. J Acoustical Soc Am 2001; 110(1):588–596.
11. Sundaram JMB, Mitragotri S. An experimental analysis of ultrasound-induced permeabilization. Biophys J 2003; 84(5):3087-3101.
12. Miller D, Quddus J. Sonoporation of monolayer cells by diagnostic ultrasound activation of contrast-agent gas bodies. Ultrasound Med Biol 2000; 26(4):661–667.
13. Wu J, Ross JP, Chiu J-F. Reparable sonoporation generated by microstreaming. J Acoust Soc Am 2002; 111(3):1460–1464.
14. Nelson JL, et al. Ultrasonically activated chemotherapeutic drug delivery in a rat model. Cancer Res 2002; 62(24):7280–7283.
15. Price RJ, Kaul S. Contrast ultrasound targeted drug and gene delivery: an update on a new therapeutic modality. J Cardiovasc Pharmacol Ther 2002; 7(3):171–180.
16. Kwok CS, et al. Self-assembled molecular structures as ultrasonically-responsive barrier membranes for pulastile delivery. J Biomed Mater Res 2001; 57(2):151–164.
17. Kost J, Leong K, Langer R. Ultrasound-enhanced polymer degradation and release of incorporated substances. Proc Natl Acad Sci 1989; 86:7663–7666.
18. Linder JR. Evolving applications of contrast ultrasound. Am J Cardiol 2002; 90(Suppl. 10A):72J–80J.
19. Unger EC, et al. Local drug and gene delivery through microbubbles. Prog Cardiovasc 2001; 44(1):45–54.
20. Benson HAE, McElnay JC, Harland R. Phonophoresis of lingocaine an prilocaine from Emla cream. Int J Pharm 1988; 44:65–69.
21. Benson HAE, McElnay JC, Harland R. Use of ultrasound to enhance percutaneous absorption of benzydamine. Phys Ther 1989; 69(2):113–118.
22. Benson HAE, McElnay JC, Hadgraft J. Influence of ultrasound on the percutaneous absorption of nicotinate esters. Pharm Res 1991; 9:1279–1283.
23. Bommannan D, et al. Sonophpresis: II. Examination of the mechanism(s) of ultrasound-enhanced transdermal drug delivery. Pharm Res 1992; 9(8):1043–1047.
24. Bommannan D, et al. Sonophoresis: I. The use of high-frequency ultrasound to enhance transdermal drug delivery. Pharm Res 1992; 9(4):559–564.
25. Byl NN, et al, The effects of phonophoresis with corticosteroids: a controlled pilot study. J Orth Sports Phys Ther 1993; 18(5):590–600.
26. Cameroy BM. Ultrasound enhanced local anesthesia. Am J Orthoped 1966; 8:47.
27. Ciccone CD, Leggin BQ, Callamaro JJ. Effects of ultrasound and trolamine salicylate phonophoresis on delayed-onset muscle soreness. Phys Ther 1991; 71(9):666–678.
28. Griffin JE, Touchstone J. Ultrasonic movement of cortisol into pig tissue. Am J Phys Med 1965; 44(1):20–25.
29. Griffin JE, et al. Patients treated with ultrasonic driven hydrocortisone and with ultrasound alone. Phys Ther 1967; 47(7):600–601.
30. Griffin JE, Touchstone JC. Low-intensity phonophoresis of cortisol in swine. Phys Ther 1968; 48(12):1136–1344.
31. Griffin JE, Touchstone JC. Effects of ultrasonic frequency on phonophoresis of cortisol into swine tissues. Am J Phys Med 1972; 51(2):62–78.
32. Johnson ME, et al. Synergistic effect of ultrasound and chemical enhancers on transdermal drug delivery. J Pharm Sci 1996; 85(7):670–679.
33. Kleinkort JA, Wood F. Phonophoresis with 1 percent versus 10 percent hydrocortisone. Phys Ther 1975; 55(12):1320–1324.
34. Kost J, Langer R. Ultrasound-mediated transdermal drug delivery. In: Shah VP, Maibach HI, eds. Topical Drug Bioavailability, Bioequivalence, and Penetration. New York: Plenum, 1993:91–103.
35. Kost J, et al. Enhanced transdermal delivery: synergistic effect of ultrasound and electroporation. Pharm Res 1996; 13(4):633–638.

36. Kost J, Mitragotri S, Langer R. Phonophoresis. In: Bronaugh R, Maibach HI, eds. Percutaneous absorption. New York: Marcel Dekker 1999:615–631.
37. Kost J, et al. Transdermal extraction of glucose and other analytes using ultrasound. Nat Med 2000; 6(3):347–350.
38. Le L, Kost J, Mitragotri S. Combined effect of low-frequency ultrasound and iontophoresis: applications for transdermal heparin delivery. Pharm Res 2000; 17(9):1151–1154.
39. Machluf M, Kost J. Ultrasonically enhanced transdermal drug delivery. Experimental approaches to elucidate the mechanism. J Biomater Sci 1993; 5:147–156.
40. Menon, G, Bommanon D, Elias P. High-frequency sonophoresis: permeation pathways and structural basis for enhanced permeability. Skin Pharmacol 1994; 7(3):130–139.
41. Mitragotri S, et al. A Mechanistic study of ultrasonically enhanced transdermal drug delivery. J Pharm Sci 1995; 84(6):697–706.
42. Mitragotri S, Blankschtein D, Langer R. Ultrasound-mediated transdermal protein delivery. Science 1995; 269:850–853.
43. Mitragotri S, Blankschtein D, Langer R, Sonophoresis: ultrasound mediated transdermal drug delivery. In: Swarbrick J, Boylan J, eds. Encyclopedia of Pharmaceutical Technology. New York: Marcel Dekker, 1995:103-122.
44. Mitragotri S, Blankschtein D, Langer R. Transdermal drug delivery using low-frequency sonophoresis. Pharm Res 1996; 13(3):411–420.
45. Mitragotri S, Blankschtein D, Langer R, Sonophoresis: enhanced transdermal drug delivery by application of ultrasound. In: Swarbrick J, Boylan J, eds. Encyclopedia of Pharmaceutical Technology, 1996:103–122.
46. Mitragotri S, Blankschtein D, Langer R. An explanation for the variation of the sonophoretic transdermal transport enhancement from drug to drug. J Pharm Sci 1997; 86(10):1190–1192.
47. Mitragotri S, et al. Determination of the threshold energy dose for ultrasound-induced transdermal drug delivery. J Control Rel 2000; 63:41–52.
48. Mitragotri S, et al. Synergistic effect of ultrasound and sodium lauryl sulfate on transdermal drug delivery. J Pharm Sci 2000; 89:892–900.
49. Mitragotri S, Kost J. Transdermal delivery of heparin and low-molecular weight heparin using low-frequency ultrasound. Pharm Res 2000; 18(8):1151–1156.
50. Mitragotri S, Kost J. Low-frequency sonophoresis: a non-invasive method for drug delivery and diagnostics. Biotechnol Prog 2000; 16(3):488–492.
51. Mitragotri S. Synergistic effect of enhancers for transdermal drug delivery. Pharm Res 2000; 17(11):1354–1359.
52. Quillen WS. Phonophoresis: a review of the literature and technique. Athl Train 1980; 15:109–110.
53. Tezel A, et al. Frequency dependence of sonophoresis. Pharm Res 2001; 18(12):1694–1700.
54. Tezel A, et al. Synergistic effect of low-frequency ultrasound and surfactant on skin permeability. J Pharm Sci 2001; 91(2):91–100.
55. Terahara TS, Mitragotri S, Langer R. Porous resins as a cavitation enhancer for low-frequency sonophoresis. J Pharm Sci 2002; 91(3):753–759.
56. Terahara T, et al. Dependence of low-frequency sonophoresis on ultrasound parameters; distance of the horn and intensity. Int J Pharm 2002; 235(1–2):35–42.
57. Tang H, Blankschtein D, Langer R. Effects of low-frequency ultrasound on the transdermal penetration of mannitol: comparative studies with in vivo and in vitro studies. J Pharm Sci 2002; 91(8):1776–1794.
58. Tang H, Blankschtein D, Langer R. An investigation of the role of cavitation in low-frequency ultrasound-mediated transdermal drug transport. Pharm Res 2002; 19(8):1160–1169.
59. Tang H, et al. Theoretical description of transdermal transport of hydrophilic permeants: application to low-frequency sonophoresis. J Pharm Sci 2001; 90(5):543–566.
60. Tezel A, Sens A, Mitragotri S. Investigations of the role of cavitation in low-frequency sonophoresis using acoustic spectroscopy. J Pharm Sci 2002; 91(2):444–453.
61. Tezel A, Sens A, Mitragotri S. A theoretical analysis of low-frequency sonophoresis: dependence of transdermal transport pathways on frequency and energy density. Pharm Res 2002; 19(12):1841–1846.

62. Tezel A, Sens A, Mitragotri S. A theoretical description of transdermal transport of hydrophilic solutes induced by low-frequency sonophoresis. J Pharm Sci 2003; 92(1):381–393.
63. Tachibana K. Transdermal delivery of insulin to alloxan-diabetic rabbits by ultrasound exposure. Pharm Res 1992; 9(7):952–954.
64. Tachibana K, Tachibana S. Use of ultrasound to enhance the local anesthetic effect of topically applied aqueous lidocaine. Anesthesiology 1993; 78(6):1091–1096.
65. Tachibana K, Tachibana S. Transdermal delivery of insulin by ultrasonic vibration. J Pharm Pharmacol 1991; 43:270–271.
66. Williams AR. Phonophoresis: an in vivo evaluation using three topical anaesthetic preparations. Ultrasonics 1990; 28(May):137–141.
67. Alvarez-Roman R, et al. Skin permeability enhancement by low-frequency sonophoresis-lipid extraction and transport pathways. J Pharm Sci 2003; 92(6):1138–1146.
68. Merrino G, Kalia YN, Guy RH. Ultrasound-enhanced transdermal transport. J Pharm Sci 2003; 92(6):1125–1137.
69. Merriono G, et al. Frequency and thermal effects on the enhancement of transdermal transport by sonophoresis. J Control Rel 2003; 88(1):85–94.
70. Weimann LJ, Wu J. Transdermal delivery of poly-l-lysine by sonomacroporation. Ultrasound Med. Biol 2002; 28(9):1173–1180.
71. Joshi A, Raje J. Sonicated transdermal drug transport. J Control Release 2002; 83(1):13–22.
72. Machet L, Boucaud A. Phonophoresis: efficiency, mechanisms, and skin tolerance. Int J Pharm 2002; 243(1–2):1–15.
73. Lee S, et al. Alteration of cell membrane by stress waves in vitro. Ultrasound Med Biol 1996; 22(9):1285–1293.
74. Mulholland SE, et al. Cell loading with laser-generated stress waves: the role of the stress gradient. Pharm Res 1999; 16(4):514–518.
75. Terakawa M, et al. Gene transfer into mammalian cells by use of a nanosecond pulsed laser-induced stress wave. Opt Lett 2004; 29(11):1227–1229.
76. Ogura M, et al. In vivo targeted gene transfer in skin by the use of laser-induced stress waves. Lasers Surg Med 2004; 34(3):242–248.
77. Satoh Y, et al. Targeted DNA transfection into the mouse central nervous system using laser-induced stress waves. J Biomed Opt 2005; 10(6)(Article No. 060501)1–3.
78. Lin TY, et al. Nuclear transport by laser-induced pressure transients. Pharm Res 2003; 20(6):879–883.
79. Doukas AG, Kollias N. Transdermal drug delivery with a pressure wave. Adv Drug Deliv Rev 2004; 56(5):559–579.
80. Soukos NS, et al. Photomechanical drug delivery into bacterial biofilms. Pharm Res 2000; 17(4):405–409.
81. Boucaud A, et al. Effect of sonication parameters on transdermal delivery of insulin to hairless rats. J Pharm Sci 2002; 91(3):113–119.
82. Lee S, et al. Topical drug delivery in humans with a single photomechanical wave. Pharm Res 1999; 16(11):1717–1721.
83. Lee S, et al. Photomechanical transdermal delivery: the effect of laser confinement. Lasers Surg Med 2001; 28(4):344–347.
84. Lee S, et al. Photomechanical transcutaneous delivery of macromolecules. J Invest Dermatol 1998; 111(6):925–929.
85. Pirri A. Theory for momentum transfer to a surface with a high-power laser. Phys Fluids 2003; 16(9):1435–1440.
86. Fabbro R, et al. Physical study of laser-produced plasma in confined geometry. J Appl Phys 2006; 68(2):775–784.
87. Gambihler S, Delhis M, Ellwart J. Permeabilization of the plasma membrane of L1210 mouse leukemia cells using lithotripter shock waves. J Membr Biol 1994; 141(3):267–275.
88. Kodama T, Hamblin M, Doukas A. Cytoplasmic molecular delivery with shock waves: importance of impulse. Biophys J 2000; 79(4):1821–1832.
89. Lee S, et al. In vivo transdermal delivery using a shock tube. Shock Waves 2000; 10(5):307–311.
90. SELBY C. An electron microscope study of thin sections of human skin: II. Superficial cell layers of footpad epidermis. J Invest Dermatol 1957; 29(2):131–149.

91. Elias P. Epidermal lipids, barrier function, and desquamation. J Invest Dermatol 1983; 80:44s–49s.
92. Scheuplein RJ. Mechanism of percutaneous adsorption: I. Routes of penetration and the influence of solubility. J Invest Dermatol 1965; 45(5):334–346.
93. Suslick KS. Ultrasound: Its Chemical, Physical and Biological Effects. New York: VCH Publishers, 1989.
94. Pecha R, Gompf B. Microimplosions: cavitation collapse and shock wave emission on a nanosecond time scale. Phys Rev Lett 2000; 84(6):1328–1330.
95. Blake J. Gibson D. Cavitation bubbles near boundaries. In: Lumley J, Van Dyke M, Reed H, eds. Annual Reviews of Fluid Mechanics, 1985:99–123.
96. Naude C, Ellis A. On the mechanisms of cavitation damage by non-hemispherical cavities in contact with solid boundary. Trans ASME J Basic Eng 1961; 83:648–556.
97. Benjamin T, Ellis A. The collapse of cavitation bubbles and the pressures thereby produced against solid boundaries. Philos Trans R Soc Lond Ser A 1966; 260:221–240.
98. Lauterborn W, Bolle H. Experimental Investigations of cavitation bubble collapse in the neighbourhood of a solid boundary. J Fluid Mech 1975; 72:391–399.
99. Plesset M, Chapman R. Collapse of an initially spherical vapour cavity in the neighbourhood of a solid boundary. J Fluid Mech 1971; 47:283–290.
100. Tezel A, Mitragotri S. Interactions of inertial cavitation bubbles with stratum corneum lipid bilayers during low-frequency sonophoresis. Biophys J 2003; 85(6):3502–3512.
101. Mitragotri S. Effect of bilayer disruption on transdermal transport of low-molecular weight hydrophobic solutes. Pharm Res 2001; 18:1022–1028.
102. Paliwal S, Menon GK, Mitragotri S. Low-frequency sonophoresis: ultrastructural basis for stratum corneum permeability assessed using quantum dots. J Invest Dermatol 2006; 126(5):1095–1101.
103. Black G. Interaction between anionic surfactants and skin. In: Walters K, Hadgraft J, eds. Pharmaceutical Skin Penetration Enhancement. New York: Marcel Dekker, 1993:145–174.
104. Walters KA. Surfactants and percutaneous absorption. In: Scott RC, Guy RH, Hadgraft J, eds. Predictions of Percutaneous Penetration. London: IBC Technical Services, 1990:148–162.
105. Morimoto Y, et al. Elucidation of the transport pathway in hairless rat skin enhanced by low-frequency sonophoresis based on the solute-water transport relationship and confocal microscopy. J Control Release 2005; 103(3):587–597.
106. Tang H, et al. Theoretical description of transdermal transport of hydrophilic permeants: application to low-frequency sonophoresis. J Pharm Sci 2001; 90(5):545–568.
107. Lee S, et al. Photomechanical transdermal delivery of insulin in vivo. Lasers Surg Med 2001; 28(3):282–285.
108. Menon G, Kollias N, Doukas A. Ultrastructural evidence of stratum corneum permeabilization induced by photomechanical waves. J Invest Dermatol 2003; 121:104–109.
109. Menon G, Elias P. Morphologic basis for a pore-pathway in mammalian stratum corneum. Skin Pharmacol 1997; 10(5–6):235–246.
110. Lee S, Doukas A. Laser-generated stress waves and their effects on the cell membrane. IEEE J Sel Top Quantum Electron 1999; 5(4):997.
111. Mitragotri S, Kost J. Low-frequency sonophoresis: a review. Adv Drug Deliv Rev 2004: 56(5):589–601.
112. Smith NB. Lee S, Shung KK. Ultrasound-mediated transdermal in vivo transport of insulin with low-profile cymbal arrays. Ultrasound Med Biol 2003; 29(8):1205–1210.
113. Tezel A, et al. Topical delivery of anti-sense oligonucleotides using low-frequency sonophoresis. Pharm Res 2004; 21(12):2219–2225.
114. Tezel A, et al. Low-frequency ultrasound as a transcutaneous immunization adjuvant. Vaccine 2005; 23(29):3800–3807.
115. Gockel CM, Bao S, Beagley KW. Transcutaneous immunization induces mucosal and systemic immunity: a potent method for targeting immunity to the female reproductive tract. Mol Immunol 2000; 37(9):537–544.
116. Kagnoff MF, Eckmann L. Epithelial cells as sensors for microbial infection. J Clinic Inves 1997; 100(1):6–10.
117. Scharton-Kersten T, et al. Transcutaneous immunization with bacterial ADP-ribosylating exotoxins, subunits, and unrelated adjuvants. Infect Immun 2000; 68(9):5306–5313.

118. Lee S, et al. Permeabilization and recovery of the stratum corneum in vivo: The synergy of photomechanical waves and sodium lauryl sulfate. Lasers Surg Med 2001; 29:145–150.
119. Dremin A. Babare L. The shock wave chemistry of organic substances. AIP Conf Proc 2006; 78(1):27–41.
120. Gonzalez S, et al. Rapid allergen delivery with photomechanical waves for inducing allergic skin reactions in the hairless guinea pig animal model. Am J Contact Dermat 2001; 12(3):162–165.
121. Lee S, et al. Photomechanical delivery of 100-nm microspheres through the stratum corneum: implications for transdermal drug delivery. Lasers Surg Med 2002; 31: 207–210.
122. Kost J, Katz N, Shapiro D, et al. Ultrasound skin permeation to accelerate the onset of topical anesthesia. Proceedings of International Symposium on Controlled Release of Bioactive Materials 2003.

35 Microneedle Arrays as Transcutaneous Delivery Devices

James Birchall
Welsh School of Pharmacy, Cardiff University, Cardiff, U.K.

Keith R. Brain
An-eX Analytical Services Ltd. and Cardiff University, Cardiff, U.K.

INTRODUCTION

The barrier properties of the stratum corneum (SC) restrict conventional transdermal delivery to candidates of low molecular weight (<500 Da), but several transcutaneous delivery strategies have been developed to circumvent this restriction (see Chapters 1, 30 and later chapters). This chapter discusses the development as well as advantages and disadvantages of one of these strategies, the microfabricated microneedle array—an innovation with potential to greatly enhance cutaneous delivery of therapeutic agents. Its advantages include adaptability in design, simplicity in use, inexpensive production costs, ease of distribution, and good patient acceptability. It is also anticipated that microneedles would encounter fewer regulatory approval hurdles because of their close analogy with well-characterized hypodermic delivery systems.

Intradermal injection has long been used to provide localized delivery of medicaments to skin compartments. Although this method circumvents the SC barrier, the depth of needle penetration and hence the site of drug delivery are highly variable, dependent on skin properties and operator skill. The typical syringe needle [diameter, >300 μm (1)] creates holes that are too large [diameter, 0.41–0.71 mm (2)] to localize delivery to specific cell types. Intradermal injection also suffers from the disadvantages of inflicting pain at the injection site and presenting risks for phlebitis, hematoma, thrombosis, and infection. Competent personnel and secure disposal procedures are necessary; needlestick injuries and inappropriate needle reuse are further drawbacks. However, because intradermal injection is an assured method for the delivery of significant drug loads, with well-defined pharmacokinetics, it sets the standard with which competitive delivery technologies must be compared.

The original concept of using microneedles for drug administration to skin is almost 30 years old (3). However, it is only relatively recently that microfabrication techniques commonly used in the microelectronics industry have been applied to the manufacture of effective microneedle arrays (4). These comprise an assembly of micron-scale needles (either solid or hollow) that can penetrate the SC and produce micron-scale channels that reach the underlying tissue and provide a direct route for the delivery of a range of therapeutics. Henry et al. (4) were the first to demonstrate enhanced cutaneous penetration of a model compound using a microneedle device consisting of an array of needles etched from silicon on a solid support backing. These short microneedles (~150 μm long) did not reach nerve fibers and blood vessels in the underlying dermis, unlike conventional needles, and therefore facilitated delivery without causing pain or bleeding (5). More recently, collaborations between engineers and drug delivery scientists have resulted in the development of microneedles with a wide range of parameters that are being integrated with formulation science solutions.

Microneedle devices have a number of potential benefits for patients, clinicians, and the pharmaceutical industry as compared with alternative delivery methods, including the following:

1. They can provide direct, controlled delivery of small molecules, macromolecules, vaccines, or nucleic acids into the viable epidermis.
2. They can be mass-produced from a range of materials in a reproducible and cost-effective manner.
3. Array morphology can easily be adjusted by modification of fabrication design and processing.
4. A relatively large surface area can be treated, facilitating access to cellular targets.
5. They are suitable for use with conventional transdermal delivery systems.
6. They are suitable for patient self-administration with minimal clinical input.
7. They can be of single use, easily disposable, and potentially biodegradable.
8. Absence of pain or bleeding makes them more clinically appropriate, particularly in pediatric vaccination or needlephobic patients.

MICRONEEDLE DESIGN AND MANUFACTURE
Silicon Microfabricated Microneedles
The original silicon microfabrication methods of Prausnitz et al. (4) have been adopted and adapted by many research groups (5–13), but the manufacture of silicon microneedles is a complex and expensive process that requires experienced engineers working within established clean-room facilities. Fabrication of such arrays for our own delivery studies, focusing on transcutaneous delivery of plasmid DNA (pDNA), has been performed in collaboration with groups from the Cardiff School of Engineering and Tyndall National Institute (Cork, Ireland). Manufacturing uses an etching process to remove predefined areas from a flat silicon platform to leave needle-shaped islands. Multistep optimization of this procedure creates a desired architecture in a complex, iterative process.

The dry-etch process ("reactive ion etching") uses a lithographically patterned mask and a blend of reactive ion gases. One study (12) combined an isotropic etch with BOSCH Deep Reactive Ion Etching reaction. Silicon wafers are spun coated with a "photoresist" layer, and a high-resolution lithographic mask with an appropriate dot array pattern is used with a UV light exposure step to produce a photoresist etching mask. The surface is etched using a reactive blend of fluorinated gases and oxygen, and regions directly underneath the mask, which are resistant to etching, remain as raised islands. Examples of dry-etch microneedles produced using this process are shown in Figure 1.

Wet-etch fabrication, which relies on the anisotropic behavior of silicon in potassium hydroxide (KOH) solution (13,14), has fewer steps and lower costs as compared with the dry-etch method and is therefore more suitable for mass production. Although this process has not been widely used to fabricate microneedles, Wilke et al. (15) exploited the crystal structure of silicon and its resulting etch characteristics in KOH to develop a reproducible method for the manufacture of microneedle arrays (Fig. 2). Their process relies on precise alignment of the crystal planes within the silicon with the lithographically patterned mask before KOH solution exposure. The difference in resistance between the corners and square planes

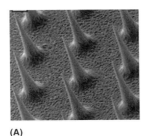

(A)

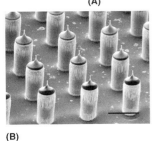

(B)

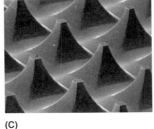

(C)

FIGURE 1 Scanning electron micrographs of silicon microneedles microfabricated using modified deep reactive ion etching processes and microenhancer arrays from (**A**) Georgia Institute of Technology (*Source*: From Ref. 4), (**B**) Cardiff University, and (**C**) BD Technologies (*Source*: From Ref. 42). In each case, the microneedles were between 100 and 200 μm in height.

of the square mask results in underetching of the corners to ultimately create the microneedle structure. The major disadvantage of this process is that, because it relies on the innate etch behavior of silicon, it is difficult to manipulate microneedle geometry and density (13,14), although variant tip morphologies are possible (Fig. 2B and C).

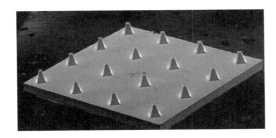

(A)

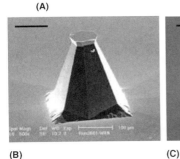

(B)

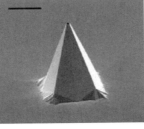

(C)

FIGURE 2 Scanning electron micrographs of (**A**) wet-etch platinum-coated microneedle arrays prepared by Tyndall National Institute, (**B**) sharp-tipped microneedles (bar, 100 μm), and (**C**) frustum-tipped microneedles (bar, 100 μm). *Source*: From Ref. 34.

Use of Alternative Substrates

Because silicon microneedles are generally costly and complex to produce, alternative substrate materials (e.g., metal, glass, and polymers) have been investigated. Many metals and polymers have established biomaterial safety profiles, are more robust, and are less likely to shear upon skin application/removal. As an example, biodegradable polymer microneedles that encapsulate drugs for controlled release in skin have been prepared from molds of silicon master structures (Fig. 3A and B).

Manufacture of titanium and stainless steel microneedles involves laser patterning of a metal surface followed by manipulation to raise the needle structure out of plane (16–18). Alza (Palo Alto, California, U.S.) developed a metal microneedle array incorporated within a patch technology, termed Macroflux® (Fig. 3C). McAllister et al. reported microneedle-mediated delivery of insulin into diabetic hairless rats using a steel microarray, and similar studies have used beveled glass microneedles, created using simple drawn-glass micropipette techniques (19).

Polymer microneedles created by micromolding using silicon microneedles as the primary template (19,20) have had their functionality demonstrated using calcein and bovine serum albumin as model macromolecules (20). Polymer microneedles are robust and biocompatible, and they lend themselves to cost-effective mass production. A further advantage, specific to polymeric material, is their ability to manipulate their composition to produce biodegradable microneedles capable of either in situ biological degradation after application or environmental degradation after use. Multifunctional polymeric microneedles with a multilayer structure have also been prepared and tested (21).

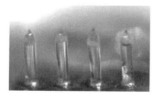

(A)

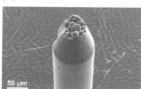

(B)

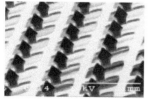

(C)

FIGURE 3   (**A**) Bevel-tipped microneedles made of poly(lactide-*co*-glycolide) (PLGA) and encapsulating calcein within their tips. (**B**) Cutting off the tip of a PLGA microneedle reveals poly(L-lactide) (PLA) microparticles within (imaged by scanning electron micrography). (**C**) Solid microneedles (ALZA Macroflux® Microprojection Array) acid etched from a titanium sheet. *Source*: From Refs. 18, 44.

Hollow Microneedles

Permeation of molecules through microchannels created using a solid microneedle array relies on passive diffusion. Pressurized infusion of a formulation through the bore of a hollow microneedle is a more controllable approach that permits cutaneous delivery of specific volumes at defined rates, allowing fine control over delivery. However, hollow microneedles are inherently structurally weaker than solid microneedles, which is of particular importance for silicon arrays, in which robustness is an issue. Morphological optimization of silicon microneedles can maximize in-use resilience, or more robust materials can be used. Hollow microneedle arrays have now been manufactured using polymer, glass, and silicon to a range of needle heights and geometries (19). Prausnitz et al. have prepared cylindrical hollow composite microneedles by electrodeposition of metals, such as nickel, onto silicon or polymer molds (19,22). These microneedles demonstrated penetration, without breakage or congestion with biological debris, which permitted efficient delivery of liquid formulations (22,23).

A number of commercial companies are developing hollow microneedle devices. For example, the Micropyramid™ (Fig. 4A) is a hollow silicon structure created by NanoPass Technologies (Nes-Ziona, Israel) in conjunction with Silex Microsystems (Järfälla, Sweden) that can be inserted repeatedly with minimal damage to the robust pyramidal structure. The technology is used in conjunction with a sustained delivery device (Nanopump™) and a bolus injection device that combines the array with a jet injection system (MicronJet™). Other commercial devices include 3M's Microstructured Transdermal System™ (3M Company, St. Paul, Minnesota, U.S.) and Becton Dickinson's Microinfusor™ (Becton Dickinson Technologies, Research Triangle, North Carolina, U.S.).

Another advantage of the hollow microneedle is its potential to extract interstitial fluid (ISF) from the skin to monitor levels of drugs or endogenous compounds. Preliminary studies used beveled single glass microneedles (25), but hollow silicon microneedle arrays with multiple tissue sampling points have now been developed (26). Small arrays of beveled solid glass microneedles (27) have been used for collection of ISF for glucose monitoring. Although the insertion of solid glass microneedles followed by vacuum extraction of ISF through the microchannels was successful, extraction of ISF through the bores of a hollow microneedle was not viable. Problems in sampling ISF using hollow arrays may arise from inefficient piercing, which is caused by the elastic nature of the tissue, fracture of the microneedle, and blockage of the needle tip on insertion (26). It may be possible to overcome these problems by modifying the morphology. For example, silicon microneedle arrays with a "snake fang" morphology have successfully sampled ISF using capillary action as the driving force of fluid withdrawal (26).

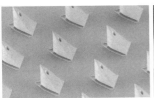

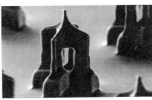

(A) (B)

FIGURE 4 Examples of hollow microneedles. (**A**) Low-cost, disposable, and biocompatible hollow microneedles. *Source*: NanoPass Technologies (Nes-Ziona, Israel) and Silex Microsystems (Järfälla, Sweden). (**B**) Microfluidic transdermal interface microneedles. *Source*: From Ref. 24.

Combination of a micropump with a hollow microneedle array allowed sampling of glucose from ISF and provided controlled continuous infusion of insulin (28). Development of such bioresponsive devices provides the opportunity for feedback-controlled systems in which insulin blood levels are automatically managed in real time in response to the blood glucose levels of individual patients.

Microneedle Mechanics

An appropriate balance is required between miniaturization and maintenance of structural integrity. The length of microneedles used in laboratory and clinical studies varies from 150 μm (4) to 10,000 μm (17), with microneedles from 300 to 600 μm in length routinely used by many research groups. Use of longer microneedles may result in bleeding; any blood loss that occurred after the application of a range of microneedle heights (225, 400, and 600 μm) was found to be minimal and without evidence of infection or scarring (29). The average penetration depths for 50% of the solid titanium microneedles on an array were 165 μm for the 225-μm microneedles and 315 μm for the longer microneedles, which indicated that to circumvent the SC and target viable keratinocytes or Langerhans cells, it is only necessary to use microneedles of approximately 200 μm.

An appropriate application force for the silicon microneedle arrays originally created by Henry et al. was considered to be approximately 10N (4). Application of this force resulted in approximately 95% of microneedles penetrating the skin surface. However, the force required for skin penetration is highly dependent on microneedle diameter, sharpness, length, and interneedle spacing (30) as well as on the elasticity and tension of the tissue. These factors were highlighted in a study (7) in which solid silicon microneedles demonstrated successful, albeit much reduced, calcein permeation in comparison with earlier work (4). A needle will only penetrate the skin when the pressure at the needle tip exceeds the tensile strength of the skin (30), and the reduced efficiency was attributed to the blunt tips of individual microneedles, small interneedle spacing, and the cushioning effect of the underlying subcutaneous fat, resulting in what was termed "the bed of nails effect." Theoretical pressures required to puncture human skin and forces required for effective microneedle penetration have been reported (31). Investigations on the promotion of microneedle insertion, using a piezoelectric actuator (6) and a vibratory (32) actuator, indicated up to 70% reduction in insertion force required.

Precise details on applicator devices are often limited, but these are generally relatively primitive, for example, mounting the array onto metal or wooden rods (4,30) or syringe barrels (7,8). Commercial development of microneedle arrays will presumably result in the production of more effective application devices.

USE OF MICRONEEDLES
In Vitro Studies

Initial studies by Henry et al. showed a 10,000-fold increase in the permeation of calcein (623 Da, 0.6-nm radius) through silicon microneedle–treated human cadaver skin (4). Subsequent studies showed promotion of the delivery of bovine serum albumin (66 kDa, 3.5-nm radius), insulin (6 kDa), and even nanoparticles (25- and 50-nm diameters) (19).

Animal Studies

The Macroflux technology has been used to deliver ovalbumin as a model antigenic protein (16), desmopressin (18), and antisense oligonucleotides (33) into the skin of hairless guinea pigs. Prausnitz et al. recently reported microneedle-mediated delivery of insulin into diabetic hairless rats using a steel microarray. Local microneedle treatment followed by topical insulin application resulted in a reduction of blood glucose levels similar to that observed after subcutaneous insulin injection (17). Similar studies used beveled glass microneedles, created using simple drawn-glass micropipette techniques (19,26).

Human Studies

Most reported microneedle studies have been conducted in animal models (mice, rats, guinea pigs) and/or human cadaver skin. Although these are established experimental models, there are differences in structure between human and animal models, and the mechanical properties of cadaver and freeze-thawed skin are questionable. It is therefore important that studies are conducted on human skin ex vivo or in vivo. In our laboratories, silicon microneedles have been used to deliver pDNA to viable human skin, confirming delivery and expression of reporter plasmid in skin cells proximal to the created microchannels (34,35).

In initial studies of the application of microneedles to human volunteers (4), subjects did not report any pain but occasionally described a mild "wearing" sensation. In subsequent human studies (8,27,36–39), using a variety of microneedle lengths, a sensation of increased pressure, but little associated pain, was reported upon insertion. Indeed, applying needles as long as 2 mm recorded a score of "barely noticeable" (39).

The penetrative efficiency of microneedles in human volunteers has been assessed using skin integrity measurement (4). When a hollow silicon microneedle array mounted on the end of a syringe was used to deliver methyl nicotinate to the arms of 11 human volunteers (8), the lumen position was shown to significantly affect flux.

Delivery of Macromolecules

Early studies were restricted to relatively low-molecular-weight compounds (4,8,19). In many laboratories, the creation of functional microchannels is routinely validated using visual reporter molecules of low molecular weight (e.g., methylene blue). More recently, the use of microneedles has been extended to macromolecular therapeutics, such as proteins, nanoparticles, vaccines, and nucleic acids.

Proteins and Peptides

The in vivo pharmacodynamic response to the therapeutic peptide insulin delivered via microneedles has been demonstrated in a diabetic hairless rat model (17). Stainless steel microneedles were used to enhance the transdermal delivery of insulin, resulting in an 80% reduction in blood glucose levels. It was concluded that microneedles are capable of delivering physiologically relevant amounts of insulin with rapid pharmacodynamic action.

Delivery of desmopressin, a 1.1-kDa synthetic peptide used in the treatment of enuresis, using the Macroflux technology has been assessed (18). Desmopressin was coated onto a microneedle array that was combined with a transdermal patch to hold the array in position for the 15-minute treatment interval. Therapeutically relevant levels were achieved, and, although there was some variability, plasma levels were maintained within the therapeutic window.

Vaccines

The intracutaneous delivery of a model antigen, ovalbumin (45 kDa), using the Macroflux array has been investigated (16,29). This examined the effects of microneedle length, density of microneedles within an array, surface area of treatment, and antigen dose on the systemic immune response within hairless guinea pigs. The results indicated that the immune response obtained was dictated primarily by the antigen dose, although the surface area exposed to the treatment at high antigen doses, at which antigen uptake by Langerhans cells might be saturated, might also play a role. After microneedle treatment, ovalbumin was observed to freely diffuse within skin and was detected throughout the epidermal layer. For soluble vaccines, it may only be necessary to penetrate the SC barrier and rely on subsequent diffusion to facilitate contact of the antigen with cells in the underlying tissue. This would probably not be true for insoluble proteins or more sterically hindered macromolecules, such as nucleic acids. Oligonucleotide delivery using the Macroflux array indicated that lateral diffusion around microchannels was limited (33).

Nucleic Acids

Proof of principle of microneedle-facilitated delivery of nucleic acid to cells within the viable epidermis has been demonstrated. A puncture method similar to a tattooing process (40) and that similar to a microseeding method (41) have been used to transfect skin cells in murine and porcine skin, respectively, with reporter plasmids. Keratinocytes in mice have also been transfected using a "microabrasion" method (42). In our own laboratories, microneedle technology is being exploited to deliver pDNA into and study the subsequent gene expression within excised human skin (12,34,35). Our studies confirmed that delivery of naked pDNA (i.e., pDNA formulated without additional complexing or targeting elements) via microneedle-facilitated microchannels results in considerable levels of reporter gene expression in the viable epidermis. Figure 5 shows a typical result from a human skin transfection study. A solution of pDNA (pCMVβ reporter gene expressing the β-galactosidase enzyme) was applied to the skin surface before the application of an array of microneedles. After incubation, to allow gene uptake into cells and expression to occur, the skin was treated with X-Gal staining solution to identify the gene product. Figure 5 shows microchannels that stained positive for reporter gene expression (dark coloration arising from enzymatic conversion of the X-gal substrate by β-galactosidase). En face imaging of the skin surface showed that a significant proportion of microneedle microchannels were positive for gene expression (Fig. 5A). These studies validated the use of excised skin organ culture where conditions are optimized to maintain cellular viability and provide a realistic assessment of the efficiency of microneedle techniques to facilitate gene transfer. A transverse section photomicrograph of positively expressing microneedle channels is presented in Figure 5B. When microneedles mediate access of pDNA, intense levels of gene expression can be observed in the epidermal layer. Further studies to optimize microneedle morphology as well as application procedures and pDNA formulations to facilitate more reproducible cutaneous gene delivery are ongoing.

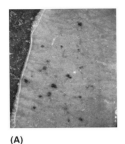

(A)

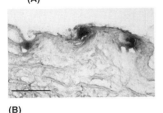

(B)

FIGURE 5   Gene expression in human skin mediated by micro-fabricated microneedles. (**A**) En face image of human skin after the application of solid wet-etch microneedles to skin pretreated topically with pCMVβ reporter plasmid. (**B**) Unstained transverse sections of skin treated with microneedles and pCMVβ (bar, 100 µm).

DNA Vaccines

BD Technologies has used microneedles [termed microenhancer arrays (MEAs)] to deliver genetic vaccines to the skin (42). A solution of pDNA was applied to the surface of mouse skin, and the MEAs laterally scraped across the skin. A 2800-fold increase in reporter gene activity in comparison with conventional topical application to controls was reported. MEAs produced a more proficient and reproducible immune response from a hepatitis B surface antigen–expressing plasmid in comparison with conventional needle injection. Lateral application of the MEAs to human subjects confirmed that the devices breached the skin barrier with negligible to minimal skin irritation, no damage to the array, and no incidence of infection.

NOVEL FORMULATIONS

Optimization of microneedle devices for clinical application will rely on the development of formulations that promote stability and provide controlled cutaneous delivery of a therapeutic entity. Dry coating microneedles not only ensures intimate contact of molecules with cells of the viable epidermis but also offers stability advantages. Materials that are inherently unstable in aqueous formulations, including proteins and nucleic acids, can be dry coated onto an array that is then sealed and stored under nitrogen. This significantly improves shelf life, removes the requirement for costly "cold storage," and allows rapid mass distribution, a particularly important factor in mass immunization schemes. Daddona et al. developed a reproducible method of coating titanium microneedle devices with an ovalbumin formulation (16) and reported that modification of the formulation and refinement of coating methodology permitted precise control over both coating thickness and restriction of coating to the needle extremity (29). Application of coated microneedles resulted in efficient deposition (>50%) of the formulation within the viable epidermis.

The breadth of molecules and particles that can be coated onto microneedle structures using simple, versatile, and controlled methods was recently explored

(43). Using laser cutting and electropolishing, stainless steel microneedles displaying a remarkable range of complex morphologies (Fig. 6A) were prepared and coated under optimized conditions of high viscosity and low surface tension. Successful microneedle coating (Fig. 6B) and decoating in cadaver skin were demonstrated with calcein, vitamin B, bovine serum albumin, pDNA, vaccinia virus, and microparticles.

Surface coating also offers an opportunity to control the release characteristics. The ability to control the release and hence the cutaneous flux of macromolecules from an array by altering the thickness of the coating film was demonstrated using chitosan-coated silicon microneedles (9) The drug was simply dissolved in a hydrophilic chitosan matrix that was cast onto the microneedle surface. This simple process should be suitable for the controlled release of any hydrophilic macromolecule.

Selection of the components of the coating material can control dissolution kinetics, providing an opportunity to administer a bolus dose followed by sustained drug release. Porous calcium phosphate, loaded with trehalose, was coated onto the tips of acupuncture needles (38), which resulted in rapid dissolution of the trehalose reservoir and delivery to the local environment, followed by more prolonged dispersion of the calcium phosphate. Trehalose and calcium phosphate are both candidate vehicles for the delivery of protein- and DNA-based medicines.

As stated previously, biodegradable polymer microneedle arrays provide an exciting alternative approach. Park et al. have investigated biodegradable microneedle arrays formed from biocompatible polylactic acid and polyglycolic acid (20). Use of such materials improves the safety profile because any structural element that may become lodged within the skin will degrade safely. Use of biodegradable materials also provides an opportunity for both dosing and disintegration in situ. Miyano et al. (37) created biodegradable microneedles containing a dispersion of a therapeutic agent within the needle structure. The microneedles in this array were designed to break and be deposited within the upper skin layers so that local release of the therapeutic was controlled by dissolution from individual microneedles. Further recent work published by Park et al. demonstrated

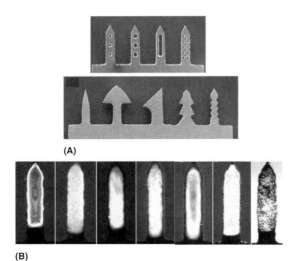

(A)

(B)

FIGURE 6 (**A**) Scanning electron micrographs of microneedles with pockets etched through the microneedle shaft and of microneedles with complex geometries. (**B**) Fluorescent or brightfield micrographs of single microneedles coated with (left to right) calcein, vitamin B, bovine serum albumin conjugated with Texas Red, pDNA conjugated with YOYO-1, modified vaccinia virus—Ankara conjugated with YOYO-1, 1-µm diameter barium sulfate particles, and 10-µm diameter latex particles. *Source*: From Ref. 43.

effective controlled release, from hours to months, from biodegradable polymer microneedles fashioned from drug-loaded polymeric microparticles (44). The use of polymer particle-based micromolding offers further advantages relating to the use of multiple materials, providing microstructures of complex geometries prepared under mild processing conditions (45).

CONCLUSIONS

Although it is possible to deliver a limited range of low-molecular-weight drugs through the defensive skin barrier layers, the challenge of administering larger molecules through the skin is insurmountable unless the skin barrier is significantly disrupted. Use of microfabricated microneedles has been shown to be both effective and painless, and, in comparison with many competing technologies, it provides a realistic opportunity for cost-efficient and potentially disposable patient self-administration of drugs, macromolecules, vaccines, and pDNA. Successful translation of microneedle array technology from the microfabrication clean room, through biological testing, and into clinic practice relies on coordinated, collaborative research to optimize the structure, composition, and mechanical properties of microneedles, develop appropriate methods and devices for microneedle application to skin, and integrate these with effective formulation of the active material.

ACKNOWLEDGEMENTS

The authors acknowledge the significant contributions of Sion Coulman, Chris Allender, Marc Pearton, and Feriel Chabri of the Cardiff University Welsh School of Pharmacy. Noteworthy thanks also go to Dr. Anthony Morrissey of the Tyndall National Institute as well as Professor David Barrow of the Cardiff University Cardiff School of Engineering for their continued microfabrication support and Alexander Anstey, Chris Gateley, and Helen Sweetland (NHS Wales) for their clinical assistance. The financial support provided by the Royal Pharmaceutical Society of Great Britain and BBSRC is gratefully acknowledged.

REFERENCES

1. Zahn JD, Deshmukh AA, Pisano AP, et al. Continuous on-chip micropumping through a microneedle. 4th IEEE International Conference on Micro Electro Mechanical Systems, Interlaken, Switzerland, 2001:503–506.
2. Baxter J, Mitragotri S. Jet-induced skin puncture and its impact on needle-free jet injections: experimental studies and a predictive model. J Control Rel 2005; 106(3): 361–373.
3. Gerstel MS, Place VA. Drug delivery device, U.S. Patent 3,964,482, 1976.
4. Henry S, McAllister DV, Allen M, et al. Microfabricated microneedles: a novel approach to transdermal drug delivery. J Pharm Sci 1998; 87(8):922–925.
5. Henry S, McAllister DV, Allen M, et al. Micromachined microneedles for the transdermal delivery of drugs. 11th IEEE Micro Electro Mech Syst Workshop, Heidelberg, 1998.
6. Newton AM, Lal A, Chen X. Ultrasonically driven microneedle arrays. Adv Drug Delivery Rev 2003; 2003:77–88.
7. Teo MAL, Shearwood C, Ng KC, et al. In vitro and in vivo characterization of MEMS microneedles. Biomed Microdev 2005; 7(1):47–52.
8. Sivamani RK, Stoeber B, Wu GC, et al. Clinical microneedle injection of methyl nicotinate: stratum corneum penetration. Skin Res Technol 2005; 11:152–156.

9.   Xie Y, Xu B, Gao Y. Controlled transdermal delivery of model drug compounds by MEMS microneedle array. Nanomed Nanotechnol Biol Med 2005; 1(2):184–190.

10. Griss P, Tolvanen-Laasko HK, Merilainen P, et al. Characterization of micromachined spiked biopotential electrodes. IEEE Trans Biomed Eng 2002; 49(6):597–603.

11. Prausnitz MR. Microneedles for transdermal drug delivery. Adv Drug Del Rev 2004; 56(5):581–587.

12. Chabri F, Bouris K, Jones T, et al. Microfabricated silicon microneedles for nonviral cutaneous gene delivery. Br J Dermatol 2004; 150(5):869–877.

13. Wilke N, Hibert C, O'Brien J, Morrissey A. Silicon microneedle electrode array with temperature monitoring for electroporation. Sens Actuators A Phys 2005; 123–124:319–25.

14. Wilke N, Mulcahy A, Ye S-R, Morrissey A. Process optimization and characterization of silicon microneedles fabricated by wet etch technology. Microelectronics J 2005; 36(7):650–656.

15. Reed ML, Wu C, Kneller J, et al. Micromechanical devices for intravascular drug delivery. J Pharm Sci 1998; 87(11):1387–1394.

16. Matriano JA, Cormier M, Johnson J, et al. Macroflux microprojection array patch technology: a new and efficient approach for intracutaneous immunization. Pharm Res 2002; 19(1):63–70.

17. Martanto W, Davis SP, Holiday NR, et al. Transdermal delivery of insulin using microneedles *in vivo*. Pharm Res 2004; 21(6):947–952.

18. Cormier M, Johnson B, Ameri M, et al. Transdermal delivery of desmopressin using a coated microneedle array patch system. J Control Rel 2004; 97:503–511.

19. McAllister DV, Wang PM, Davis SP, et al. Microfabricated needles for transdermal delivery of macromolecules and nanoparticles: fabrication methods and transport studies. Proc Nat Acad Sci USA 2003; 100(24):13755–13760.

20. Park J-H, Allen MG, Prausnitz MR. Biodegradable polymer microneedles: fabrication, mechanics and transdermal drug delivery. J Control Rel 2005; 104:51–66.

21. Kuo S, Chou Y. A novel polymer microneedle and PDMS micromolding Technique. Tamkang J Sci Eng 2004; 7(2):95–98.

22. McAllister DV, Cros F, Davis SP, et al. Three-dimensional hollow microneedle and microtube arrays. Transducers 99, International Conference on Solid State Sensors and Actuators, Sendai, June 7–10 1999:1098–1101.

23. Davis SP, Martanto W, Allen MG, et al. Hollow metal microneedles for insulin delivery to diabetic rats. IEEE Trans Biomed Eng 2005; 52(5):909–915.

24. Griss P, Stemme G. Side-opened out-of-plane microneedles for microfluidic transdermal liquid transfer. IEEE J Microelectromech Sys 2003; 12(3):296–301.

25. Wang PM, Cornwell MG, Prausnitz MR. Effects of microneedle tip geometry on injection and extraction in the skin. Joint EMBS BMES 2nd Conference, Houston, Tex, 2002.

26. Mukerjee EV, Collins SD, Isseroff RR, et al. Microneedle array for transdermal biological fluid extraction and *in situ* analysis. Sens Actuators A 2004; 114:267–675.

27. Wang PM, Cornwell M, Prausnitz MR. Minimally invasive extraction of dermal interstitial fluid for glucose monitoring using microneedles. Diabet Technol Ther 2005; 7(1):131–141.

28. Zahn JD, Deshmukh A, Pisano AP, et al. Continuous on-chip micropumping for microneedle enhanced drug delivery. Biomed Microdev 2004; 6(3):183–190.

29. Widera G, Johnson J, Kim L, et al Effect of delivery parameters on immunization to ovalbumin following intracutaneous administration by a coated microneedle array patch system. Vaccine 2006; 24(10):1653–1664.

30. Davis SP, Landis BJ, Adams ZH, et al. Insertion of microneedles into skin: measurement and prediction of insertion force and needle fracture force. J Biomech 2004; 37(8):1155–1163.

31. Aggarwal P, Johnston CR. Geometrical effects in mechanical characterizing of microneedle for biomedical applications. Sens Actuators B 2004; 102:226–234.

32. Yang M, Zahn JD. Microneedle insertion force reduction using vibratory actuation. Biomed Microdev 2004; 6(3):177–182.

33. Lin W, Cormier M, Samiee A, et al. Transdermal delivery of antisense oligonucleotides with microprojection patch (Macroflux) technology. Pharm Res 2001; 18(12):1789–1793.

34. Birchall JC, Coulman S, Pearton M, et al. Cutaneous DNA delivery and gene expression in *ex vivo* human skin explants via wet-etch microfabricated microneedles. J Drug Target 2005; 13(7):415–421.

35. Coulman SA, Barrow D, Anstey A, et al. Minimally invasive cutaneous delivery of macromolecules and plasmid DNA via microneedles. Curr Drug Deliv 2006; 3:65–75.

36. Kaushik S, Hord AH, Denson DD, et al. Lack of pain associated with microfabricated microneedles. Anaesth Analg 2001; 92:502–504.

37. Miyano T, Tobinaga Y, Kanno T, et al. Sugar microneedles as transdermic drug delivery system. Biomed Microdev 2005; 7(3):185–188.

38. Shirkhanzadeh M. Microneedles coated with porous calcium phosphate ceramics: effective vehicles for transdermal delivery of solid trehalose. J Mater Sci Mater Med 2005; 16(1):37–45.

39. Smart WH, Subramanian K. The use of silicon microfabrication technology in painless blood glucose monitoring. Diabet Technol Ther 2000; 2(4):549–559.

40. Ciernik IF, Krayenbuhl BH, Carbone DP. Puncture-mediated gene transfer to the skin. Hum Gene Ther 1996; 7:893–899.

41. Eriksson E, Yao F, Svensjo T, et al. *In vivo* gene transfer to skin and wound by microseeding. J Surg Res 1998; 78(2):85–91.

42. Mikszta JA, Alarcon JB, Brittingham JM, et al. Improved genetic immunization via micromechanical disruption of skin-barrier function and targetted epidermal delivery. Nat Med 2002; 8(4):415–419.

43. Gill HS, Prausnitz MR. Coated microneedles for transdermal delivery. J Control Rel 2007; 117(2):227–237.

44. Park J-H, Allen MG, Prausnitz MR. Polymer microneedles for controlled-release drug delivery. Pharm Res 2006; 23(5):1008–1019.

45. Park J-H, Choi SO, Kamath R, et al. Polymer particle-based micromolding to fabricate novel microstructures. Biomed Microdev 2007; 9(2):223–234.

| **36** | # Needle-Free Ballistic Delivery of Powdered Immunotherapeutics to the Skin Using Supersonic Gas Flow |

Mark A. F. Kendall

Australian Institute for Bioengineering and Nanotechnology (AIBN),
The University of Queensland, Brisbane, Queensland, Australia

ABSTRACT

Millions of people die each year from infectious disease, and many more are affected by allergies. A major stumbling block to the full use of improved immunotherapies (e.g., vaccines) against these problems is our limited ability to deliver genes and drugs to the required sites in the body. Specifically, effective methods to deliver genes and drugs into outer skin and mucosal layers (sites with immunological, physical, and practical advantages that cannot be targeted via traditional delivery methods) are lacking. This chapter investigates this particular challenge for physical delivery approaches. The skin's structural and immunogenic properties are examined in the context of the physical cell targeting requirements of the viable epidermis. Selected current physical cell targeting technologies engineered to meet these needs are examined: needle and syringe, diffusion patches, liquid jet injectors, microneedle arrays/patches, and biolistic particle delivery. The focus then moves to biolistic particle delivery: we first analyze engineering these systems to meet demanding clinical needs. The interaction of biolistic devices with the skin is also examined, focusing on the mechanical interactions of ballistic impact and cell death. Finally, the current clinical outcomes of one key application of engineered delivery devices—DNA vaccines—are discussed.

INTRODUCTION

Immunotherapeutics (e.g., vaccines, allergens) are most commonly administered using a needle and syringe, a method first invented in 1853. The needle and syringe is effective but unpopular and creates a risk of iatrogenic disease from needlestick injury or needle reuse as a consequence of the billions of administrations each year. Further, the needle and syringe does not deliver the vaccine ingredients optimally to the antigen presenting cells, which alone can respond to the combination of antigen and adjuvant (innate immune stimulus) that makes a successful vaccine.

The provision of safe and efficient routes of delivery of immunotherapeutics to the immunologically sensitive dendritic cells in the skin (and mucosa) has the potential to enhance strategies in the treatment of major disease. Examples of these include DNA vaccines and the immunotherapy of allergies. The application of physical methods to achieving this goal presents unique engineering challenges in the physical transport of immunotherapeutic biomolecules (e.g., polynucleotides) to these cells.

In this chapter, the physiology, immunology, and material properties of the skin are examined in the context of the physical cell targeting requirements of the viable epidermis. Selected cell targeting technologies engineered to meet these needs are briefly presented. The operating principles of these approaches are described, together with a discussion of their effectiveness for the noninvasive targeting of viable epidermis cells and the DNA vaccination against major diseases.

The focus then moves to one of these methods, called biolistics, which ballistically delivers millions of microparticles coated with biomolecules to outer skin layers. The engineering of these devices is presented, beginning with earlier prototypes before examining a more advanced system configured for clinical use. Then, follows a theoretical and experimental analysis of the ballistic microparticle impact process, including the examination of induced cell death. Finally, the results of applying this technology to key human clinical trials are presented.

THE IMPORTANCE OF TARGETING SKIN AND MUCOSAL CELLS

Why are outer skin cells important targets in the treatment of disease? The answer is found from a consideration of skin structure, shown schematically in Figures 1 and 3. Human skin can be subdivided into a number of layers: the outer SC (10–20 μm in depth), the viable epidermis (50–100 μm), and the dermis (1–2 mm) (1,2). The SC is the effective physical barrier of dead cells in a "bricks-and-mortar" structure (3,4). The underlying viable epidermis is composed of cells, such as immunologically sensitive Langerhans cells, keratinocytes, stem cells, and melanocytes (2). Unlike the dermis below, the viable epidermis lacks blood vessels and sensory nerve endings—important characteristics of a site for pain-free delivery with minimal damage.

In the viable epidermis, the skin has evolved a highly competent immunological function, with an abundance of Langerhans cells (500–1000 cells mm^{-2}) (5–7), often serving as the first line of defense against many pathogens (8). In particular, Langerhans cells (illustrated in Fig. 3) are extremely effective antigen-presenting cells, responsible for the uptake and processing of foreign materials to generate an effective immune response. Such cells are reported to be up to 1000-fold more effective than keratinocytes, fibroblasts, and myoblasts at eliciting a variety of immune responses (9,10–12). Effective in situ (in vivo) targeting of Langerhans cells and other epidermal cells with polynucleotides or antigens will open up novel applications in disease control (9), including vaccination against major viruses/diseases, such as HIV and cancer.

ENGINEERING OF PHYSICAL APPROACHES FOR THE TARGETING OF SKIN AND MUCOSAL CELLS

Within the viable epidermis, the location of Langerhans cells—as a delivery target for immunotherapeutics—is tightly defined by

- a vertical position at a consistent suprabasal location (13);
- a spatial distribution in the horizontal plane evenly distributed throughout the skin (14); and
- a constitution of 2% of the total epidermal cell population (15) (in human skin).

How can these and other epidermal skin cells be targeted? Despite its recognized potential, the viable epidermis has only recently been viewed as a feasible cellular targeting site with the emergence of new biological and physical technologies. The challenge is the effective penetration of the SC and precise targeting of the cells of interest.

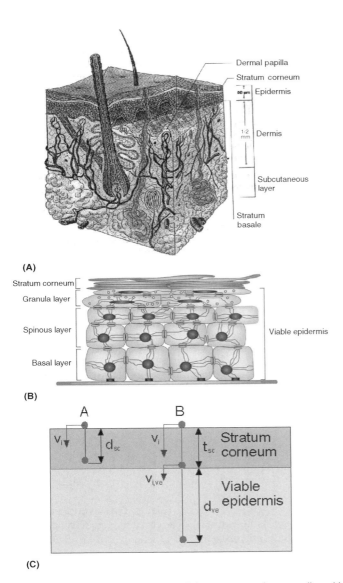

(A)

(B)

(C)

FIGURE 1 A schematic diagram of the structure of mammalian skin (**A**), the epidermis of mammalian skin (**B**), and the corresponding bilayer approximation of the epidermis used for the theoretical penetration model (**C**). Penetration case A denotes particle delivery into the stratum corneum (d_{sc}), whereas in case B, the stratum corneum is fully breached (t_{sc}), and the final particle location is within the viable epidermis (d_{ve}). The impact velocity is v_i, whereas the input velocity for the viable epidermis is $v_{i,ve}$. *Source*: Adapted from Ref. 16.

Mechanical Properties of the SC Barrier

The SC is a semipermeable barrier that—owing to its variable mechanical properties—is challenging to breach, in a minimally invasive manner, to target the viable
epidermal cells below. Mechanically, the SC is classified as a bioviscoelastic solid
and shows highly variable properties. Obvious differences include the huge variation in thickness and composition with the skin site and the age of an individual
(17). However, there are subtler and equally important variations in SC properties
to consider when configuring targeting methods.

As one example, the SC mechanical breaking stress is strongly influenced by
the ambient humidity/moisture content (18–22)—the relative humidity (RH) range
from 0% to 100% results in a decrease in excised human SC breaking stress from 22.5
to 3.2 MPa (23). Similarly, an increase in ambient temperature also results in an SC
breaking stress decrease by an order of magnitude (24).

More recently, with indentation studies using small probes (diameters of 2
and 5 μm) fitted to a NANO-Indenter (25), we have found even more complexity
and variation in key SC—and underlying viable epidermis—mechanical properties.
Specifically,

- the storage modulus and mechanical breaking stress both dramatically decrease
  through the SC (Fig. 2A,B)
- at a given depth within the SC and VE, decreasing the probe size significantly
  increases the storage modulus (Fig. 2A).

These and other sources of variability in the SC mechanical properties present
challenges in configuring approaches to breach, in a minimally invasive manner, the
SC and effectively deliver biomolecules (e.g., polynucleotides, antigens, allergens)
to the underlying cells.

Biological Approaches

Although the focus of this chapter is on physical approaches to target epidermal
cells, it is also important to highlight biological approaches. A powerful biological
approach to the transport of biomolecules to epidermal (and other) cells, in vivo,
exploits the evolved function of viruses in the transport to cells. In gene delivery, researchers have made use of genetically engineered viruses in the DNA vaccination
and gene therapy of major diseases with encouraging results. However, viral gene
delivery is hindered by safety concerns, a limited DNA-carrying capacity, production and packaging problems, and a high cost (26,27).

Physical Cell Targeting Approaches

Alternatively, many physical technologies are being developed. Potentially, they can
overcome some limitations of biological approaches using needle-free mechanisms
to breach the SC barrier to facilitate drug and vaccine administration directly to
epidermal cells. Figure 3 illustrates schematically key physical targeting approaches
relative to the scale of typical skin and the Langerhans cell layer of interest.

Needle and Syringe

For the illustration of the most common physical delivery method, a small-gauge
needle and syringe is shown in half-section in Figure 3A. Although this approach
easily breaches the SC, precise targeting of the Langerhans cell-rich viable epidermis cannot be practically achieved. Hence, the needle and syringe is used for intra-

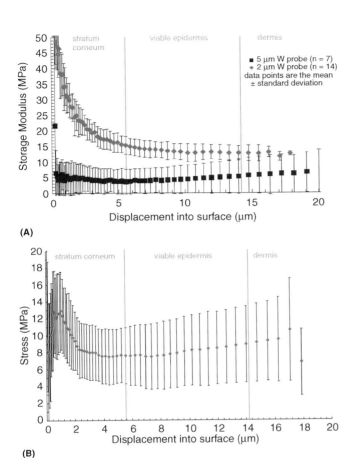

FIGURE 2 Mechanical properties (mean ± standard deviation) as a function of displacement obtained with microprobes indented into murine ears. (**A**) Storage modulus with 5- and 2-μm microprobes. (**B**) Stress with a 2-μm microprobe. *Source*: Adapted from Ref. 25.

dermal or intramuscular injection. This inefficient, indirect targeting of dendritic cells with DNA has resulted in modest immune responses (28). Other disadvantages of the needle and syringe include risks due to needlestick injuries (29) and needle phobia (1).

Diffusion/Permeation Delivery
Perhaps, the least invasive method of breaching the SC is by permeation through it, driven by diffusion from patches applied to the skin (Fig. 3B) (30). However, currently, the general view is that this mode of delivery is best suited to smaller biomolecules [<500 Da (30)]—considerably smaller than oligonucleotides and antigens. This view is being challenged, with a recent study showing that very large recombinant antigens of ~1 MDa can be delivered to elicit systemic responses by diffusion from patches (31). The transport of larger biomolecules through the SC can be further enhanced by simple approaches, including tape stripping with an adhesive tape,

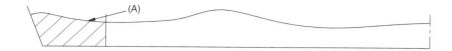

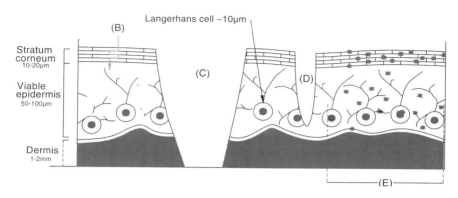

FIGURE 3 A schematic cross-section of the skin showing Langerhans cells. Five physical cell targeting approaches are also shown. (**A**) A half-section of a small gauge needle and syringe; (**B**) route of diffusion from patches; (**C**) penetration from a liquid jet injector; (**D**) a hole from a microinjector; and (**E**) distribution of microparticles after biolistic injection. *Source*: From Ref. 32.

brushing with sandpaper (33,34), or the application of depilatory agents (27,35,36). Among the more advanced technologies are electroporation (37,38), ablation by laser or heat, radiofrequency high-voltage currents (39), iontophoresis (40–42), sonophoresis, and microporation (8). Many of these approaches remain untested for complex entities such as vaccines and immunotherapies. Permeation through the SC can also be enhanced by the coating of plasmid DNA on nanoparticles (~100 nm) for DNA vaccination (43).

Liquid Jet Injectors
Interest in using high-speed liquid jet injectors arose in the mid-20th century because of its needle-free approach (44). This technique has seen a recent resurgence, with liquid delivered around the Langerhans cells in gene transfer and DNA vaccination experiments (44) and the delivery of drugs (45). As shown in Figure 3C, current liquid jet injectors typically disrupt the skin in the epidermal and dermal layer. To target exclusively the viable epidermal cells, such as Langerhans cells, the challenge of more controlled delivery needs to be addressed. With the dermal disruption induced by administration, liquid jet injectors are also reported to cause pain to patients.

Microneedle Arrays/Patches
Researchers have overcome some of the disadvantages described by fabricating arrays of micrometer-scale projections to breach the SC and to deliver naked DNA to several cells in live animals (46). Similar microprojection devices are used to increase the permeability of drugs (47) and "conventional" protein antigen vaccines (47,48). Figure 3D shows that, unlike current liquid jet injectors, these microneedles

can accurately target the viable epidermis. Furthermore, they are as simple to use as patches, while overcoming the SC diffusion barrier to many molecules. Moreover, compared with both the needle and syringe and liquid jet injectors, these microneedle methods are pain-free because of epidermal targeting. By drawing upon a range of manufacturing techniques, McAllister et al. (48) have shown that these microneedle arrays can be made from a range of materials, including silicon, metal, and biodegradable polymers. This advantage makes microneedle patches a promising practical and cost-effective method of delivering oligonucleotides to epidermal cells for DNA vaccination (49).

Biolistics Microparticle Delivery
Currently, the most established physical method of DNA vaccination is biolistic microparticle delivery, otherwise known as gene guns (Fig. 3E). Biolistic delivery is the focus of the remainder of this chapter.

BIOLISTICS MICROPARTICLE DELIVERY
Biolistics Operating Principle
In this needle-free technique, pharmaceutical or immunomodulatory agents, formulated as particles, are accelerated in a supersonic gas jet to sufficient momentum to penetrate the skin (or mucosal) layer and achieve a pharmacological effect.

Sanford and Klein (50) pioneered this innovation with systems designed to deliver DNA-coated metal particles (of diameter of the order of 1 μm) into plant cells for genetic modification, using pistons accelerated along the barrels of adapted guns. The concept was extended to the treatment of humans with particles accelerated by entrainment in a supersonic gas flow (51). Prototype devices embodying this concept have been shown to be effective, painless, and applicable to pharmaceutical therapies ranging from protein delivery (52) to conventional (53) and DNA vaccines (9,54,55).

Different embodiments of the concept (e.g., in Figs. 4 and 6) all have a similar procedure of operation. Consider the prototype shown schematically in Figure 4A as one example.

Before operation, the gas canister is filled with helium or nitrogen to 2–6 MPa, and the vaccine cassette, comprising two 20-μm diaphragms, is loaded with a powdered pharmaceutical payload of 0.5–2 mg. The pharmaceutical material is placed on the lower diaphragm surface. Operation commences when the valve in the gas canister is opened to release gas into the rupture chamber, where the pressure builds up until the two diaphragms retaining the vaccine particles sequentially burst. The rupture of the downstream diaphragm initiates a shock that propagates down the converging–diverging nozzle. The ensuing expansion of stored gas results in a short-duration flow in which the drug particles are entrained and accelerated through the device. After leaving the device, particles impact on the skin and penetrate to the epidermis to deliver a pharmacological effect.

Engineering of Handheld Biolistic Devices for Clinical Use
Biolistic delivery of immunotherapeutics is an application of transonic flow technology that is otherwise applied to aerospace applications. In this section, we introduce prototype devices and discuss the key engineering challenges in applying this aerospace technology to clinical biomedical applications. Key parameters used to guide the engineering of biolistic devices are the following:

1. There is nominally uniform, controlled, and quantified microparticle velocity and spatial distribution impacting the tissue target. Further, the impact momentum is to be within the range needed for delivery to particular locations (e.g., the Langerhans cells for DNA vaccines).
2. There is sufficient "footprint" on the tissue to deliver sufficient payload and target the appropriate number of cells.
3. Noise levels are within the user guidelines, for both the operator and patient.
4. The device should be handheld.
5. For long-term stability, the pharmaceutical is to be stored within a sealed environment.
6. The device is to be produced from biocompatible materials.
7. The devices, manufactured in large numbers, are to be cost-competitive with other relevant technologies.

Earlier Generation Systems

Early attempts to address these parameters were with a prototype device family generated from empirical studies. A schematic of one of these devices, using a convergent-divergent nozzle design is shown in Figure 4A (56). Working with these devices, the challenge was to establish the gas-particle dynamics behavior of the systems. A significant research programme was directed at this goal.

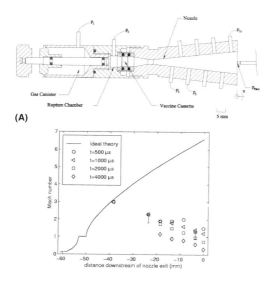

(A)

(B)

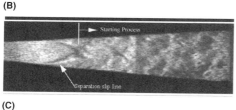

(C)

FIGURE 4 (**A**) Schematic of a simplified prototype vaccine device instrumented for Pitot and static pressure measurements. The static pressure transducers are labeled $p_1–p_{10}$. (**B**) Experimental and ideal axial Mach number within the conical nozzle of investigation. The profiles are provided after the starting process. (**C**) A sample Schlieren image within the nozzle. *Source*: From Ref. 56.

A suite of methods were used to characterize the gas and particle dynamics of these systems. Quinlan et al. (57) performed static pressure measurements to interrogate the gas flow, together with time-integrated Doppler global velocimetry (DGV) measurements of drug particle velocity. These measurements were very useful but gave an incomplete description of the predominantly unsteady flow in the device.

In subsequent, broader studies, the transient gas and particle flow within the device were interrogated with Pitot static pressure measurement (as instrumented in Fig. 4A), together with Schlieren imaging and time-resolved DGV (57) and computational fluid dynamics (CFD) modelling (58). The findings of this study are summarized with measured axial Mach number profiles through the nozzle (Fig. 4B) and a single Schlieren image (Fig. 4C).

The axial profiles of Mach number at various times after termination of the starting process (based on total and Pitot static pressure measurements) are compared with the theoretical Mach number profile for steady isentropic quasi–one-dimensional supersonic flow (with the assumption of a choked throat) in Fig. 4B. Pitot and static pressure measurements (p_2 and p_3, respectively, in Fig. 4A) suggest that 500 μs after diaphragm rupture, the 38.5-mm upstream flow of the nozzle exit is supersonic and close to the isentropic ideal. Further downstream, however, the overexpanded nozzle flow is processed through an oblique shock system that induces flow separation. Consequently, the experimentally determined Mach number (determined from Pitot and static pressure) gradually falls from between 2 and 2.5 (23.5 mm upstream of the exit plane) to 1.5 at the exit plane. The Mach number in the downstream region of the nozzle decays with time as the shock system moves upstream.

Sequences of Schlieren images such as the sample shown in Figure 4C ($t = 132$ μs) reveal the structure of the evolving flow field with greater detail and clarity (56).

The visible oblique shocks have evolved to form at least three oblique shock cells that have interacted with the boundary layer and separated the nozzle flow.

DGV images show particles were entrained in the nozzle starting process and the separated nozzle flow—regimes with large variations in gas density and velocity—giving rise to large variations in particle velocity (200–800 msec^{-1}) and spatial distributions (56). Clearly, the first criterion is not satisfied with this geometry.

Furthermore, the gas flow throughout much of the nozzle (Fig. 4C) is highly sensitive to variations in the nozzle boundary condition imposed by inserting a tissue target and/or a silencer—because the boundary condition information can be communicated upstream. This means that this silenced device applied to the tissue target would have considerably lower and more variable impact velocities. In some cases, it is questionable whether these subsonic nozzle flow–silenced devices would deliver particles with a sufficient momentum to reach the target tissue layer.

Improved Devices for Clinical Use

To overcome the large variations in particle impact conditions in described earlier devices—and meet the other important criteria of a practical clinical system (outlined above)—a next-generation biolistic device, called the contoured shock tube (CST), was conceived and developed (59–62). The devices operate with the principle of delivering a payload of microparticles to the skin with a narrow range of velocities, by entraining the drug payload in a quasi–one-dimensional, steady supersonic flow field.

In experiments with simple prototype CST devices, it was shown that the desired gas flow was achieved repeatedly (59). Importantly, further work with

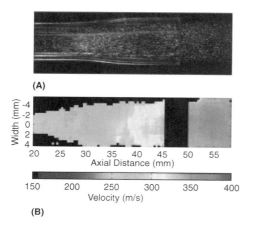

(A)

(B)

FIGURE 5 A raw image (**A**) and derived particle image velocimetry (PIV) velocity map (**B**) of the instantaneous particle flow field of a contoured shock tube (CST) prototype, taken 225 μs after diaphragm rupture. The payload was 2.2 mg of 39-μm-diameter polystyrene spheres. *Source*: From Ref. 59.

particle payloads measured a variation in free-jet particle velocity of ±4% (59). In this research, measurements were made with particle image velocimetry (PIV). A sample PIV result is shown in Figure 5. Similar PIV images at a range of times after diaphragm rupture were processed to extract the mean centerline axial particle velocity profiles. Importantly, these PIV measurements show particle payloads do achieve near uniform exit-plane velocities at the device exit over the time interval studied. This CST device prototype was a bench-top prototype, not addressing the key criteria for a practical, handheld clinical immunotherapeutic system.

An embodiment of the CST configured to meet these clinical needs is shown in Figure 6, with the key components labeled. The device was fabricated from biocompatible materials, and the device wall thickness was kept relatively constant to meet autoclave sterilization requirements.

To reduce the overall system length, the bottle reservoir (which operates by an actuation pin) is located within the driver annulus. A challenge of this coaxial arrangement was to maintain integrity of transonic gas flow within the driver-initiated after diaphragm rupture. This challenge was met by carefully contouring the driver and obstacle of the mounting arrangement (62). Possible fragments from opening of the aluminium gas bottle are contained by a sealed filter at the bottle head.

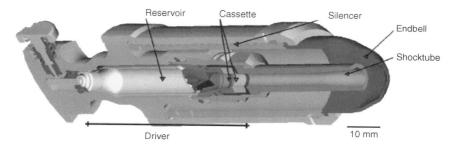

FIGURE 6 A contoured shock tube (CST) prototype configured for clinical biolistic delivery. *Source*: From Ref. 59.

The powdered pharmaceutical is enclosed and sealed by a cassette created by the inclusion of additional diaphragms upstream of the particle payload. In this case, the cassette houses two jets designed to mix the particles into a cloud, hence reducing the dependence on the initial particle location (59,61). Therefore, a nominally uniform spatial distribution of particles is released within the quasi-steady flow through the shock tube and nozzle. Repeated in vitro and in vivo experiments show that polycarbonate diaphragm fragments do not damage the target.

Elements of the silencing system are also shown in Figure 6. The primary shock initiated by diaphragm rupture, reflected from the target, is identified as the main source of sound to be attenuated. This shock is collapsed into compression waves by a series of compressions–expansions induced by an array of orifices and sawtooth baffles, resulting in appropriate sound levels for the operator and patient.

The device lift-off force is also to be well within user constraints. A peak lift-off force of 13 N is achieved by the careful selection of end-bell contact diameter, silencer volume, flow rates through the reservoir, and silencer geometry. This peak was for only a very short time within a gas flow, lasting only ~200 μs (with a helium driver gas). The point of contact between the device and skin target was selected to maintain a target seal and minimize the lift-off force, while not adversely affecting the impact velocities of the particles The effect of silencing was also minimized by maintaining a supersonic gas flow transporting particles through the nozzle—so changes in the nozzle boundary condition were not fed upstream.

The range of impact conditions for the CST platform was achieved by the selection of appropriate helium/nitrogen mixtures within the gas bottle driver/driven area ratios.

Ballistics Microparticle Delivery to Skin

We now examine delivery of microparticles from these quantified and highly controlled biolistics devices that are impacting the skin. Shown in Figure 1, this skin is a highly variable, bioviscoelastic material.

The described biolistic devices have been applied to a range of tissue targets for immunotherapeutic applications, including the skin of rodents (63), pigs (16), dogs (64), and humans (65). Typically, two classes of particles are delivered to the tissue. In the powder delivery of conventional vaccines and allergens for allergy immunotherapy, particles of 10–20 μm in radius are delivered to the epidermis of the skin to achieve a therapeutic effect (63). DNA vaccination, however, is an application in which smaller (radius 0.5–2 μm) gold particles coated with a DNA construct are targeted at the nuclei of key immunologically sensitive cells within the epidermis (55).

Theoretical Model for Ballistic Impact Into Skin

In these particle impact studies, the mechanisms of particle impact were explored with a theoretical model, based on a representation first proposed by Dehn (66). The model attributes the particle resistive force (D) to plastic deformation and target inertia,

$$D = \frac{1}{2}\rho_t A v^2 + 3A\sigma_y, \tag{1}$$

where ρ_t and σ_y are the density and yield stress of the target, A is the particle cross-sectional area, and v is the particle velocity. The yield stress (sometimes known as

TABLE 1 Parameters and Assigned Values Used in Theoretical Calculations of Particle Penetration Depth as a Function of Relative Humidity

Skin region	Parameter	Value	Source
SC	σ_{sc} (MPa)	22.5–3.2 (0–100% RH)	Wildnauer et al. (1971)
	ρ_{sc} (kg m^{-3})	1500	Duck (1990)
	t_{sc} (μm)	10–15.6 (0–93% RH)	Blank et al. (1984) and measurement
Viable epidermis	σ_{ve} (MPa)	2.2	Actin tensile: Kishino and Yanagida (1988)
		10	Epithelium: Mitchell et al. (2003)
	ρ_{ve} (kg m^{-3})	1150	Duck (1990)

Abbreviations: RH, relative humidity; SC, stratum corneum. *Source*: From Ref. 16.

the breaking stress) is the stress at which the tissue begins to exhibit plastic behavior. Equation (1) may be integrated to obtain the penetration depth as a function of particle impact and target parameters. The key parameters of the skin used in the model are summarized in Table 1. Note that these parameters have all been obtained at low, quasi-static strain rates and not the high ballistic strain rates.

The theoretical model of particle penetration into the epidermis using expression (1) in a two layer model is shown in Figure 1C. Expression (1) shows that the yield stress and density of the SC and viable epidermis are important in the ballistic delivery of particles to the epidermis.

In the case of particle delivery only to the SC (labeled "A" in Fig. 1C), the particle depth into the SC (d_{sc}) is obtained by the integration of expression (1),

$$d_{sc} = \frac{4\rho_p r_p}{3\rho_{sc}} \left\{ \ln\left(\frac{1}{2} \rho_{sc} v_i^2 + 3\sigma_{sc} \right) - \ln\left(3\sigma_{sc} \right) \right\}, \tag{2}$$

where the subscripts sc and p denote the SC and particle properties, respectively. Also, v_i and σ_{sc}, respectively, are the particle impact velocity and SC yield stress.

If the particle impact momentum is sufficient to breach the SC (labeled "B" in Fig. 1C), expression (2) is rearranged to obtain the velocity of the particle at the SC–viable epidermis boundary ($v_{i,ve}$), that is,

$$v_i = \left\{ \left(v_i^2 + \frac{6\sigma_{sc}}{\rho_{sc}} \right) e^{\frac{-3\rho_{sc} t_{sc}}{4\rho_p r_p}} - \frac{6\sigma_{sc}}{\rho_{sc}} \right\}^{\frac{1}{2}} \tag{3}$$

where t_{sc} is the thickness of the SC.

The subsequent particle penetration in the viable epidermis (d_{ve}) is then calculated using expression (2), using instead the material properties of the viable epidermis and $v_{i,ve}$. The total particle penetration depth (d_t) is, thus,

$$d_t = t_{sc} + d_{ve} \tag{4}$$

An alternative fully numerical discrete element model approach has also been applied (70) but will not be discussed here.

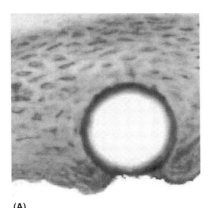

(A)

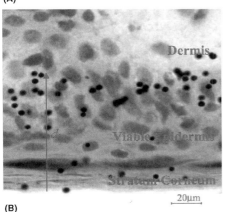

(B)

FIGURE 7   Photomicrographs of particles delivered to human skin. A 20-μm-radius glass sphere delivered at 260 m/sec (**A**) and gold particles (1.0 ± 0.2 μm radius) delivered at 580 ±50 m/sec (**B**) are shown. *Source*: From Ref. 65.

Locations of Microparticles Into Skin

As one example, particle delivery to excised human skin is shown for both classes of particles (Fig. 7) (65). In Figure 7A, a glass particle with a radius of 20 μm delivered to the skin at a nominal entry velocity of 260 m/sec is shown. Note the variation in both the SC and epidermal thicknesses. Histological sampling of the three skin sites from the backs of cadavers. Measured SC and epidermal thickness compared very well with previous reports from the literature. More than 1800 readings of the deepest particle edge and size of the particles were made on similar histological sections with polystyrene, stainless steel, and glass particles, selected for different density and size ranges.

In Figure 7B, a histological section is shown after the impact of gold particles with a measured mean radius of 1 ± 0.2 μm on the skin with a mean calculated impact velocity of 580 ± 50 m/sec. A sample particle depth measurement is labeled as d_i. More than 1200 readings of the deepest edge and size of the gold particles were made on similar histological sections. All the raw data collected from the histology sections (such as in Fig. 7) are plotted as a function of the particle impact parameter, $\rho v r$, where ρ is the density, v is the velocity, and r is the radius (Fig. 8). The variability of penetration as shown in Figure 8 is typical of results obtained with other tissues.

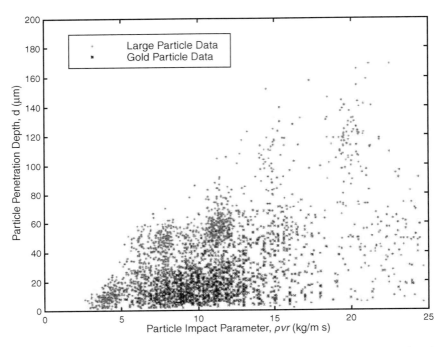

FIGURE 8 Raw gold and larger particle penetration into excised human skin as a function of the particle radius, density, and impact velocity. *Source*: From Ref. 65.

Some insights into the sources of scatter in the penetration data of Figure 8 can be gained when the data are grouped and processed. Consider, for instance, the gold data shown in Fig. 7 grouped by particle radius as shown in Figure 9. The error bars correspond to one standard deviation in collapsed particle penetration depth and ρvr. Note the trend indicating that for a given value of ρvr, an increase in radius (and hence, a decrease in impact velocity) corresponds to a decrease in penetration depth. These data, together with other (unpublished) work, show the different particle sizes and the cell matrix results in different penetration depths. For instance, the gold particles are smaller than the average cell size and, during deceleration through the skin tissue, are more likely to penetrate through individual cell membranes. For the larger particles, however, the tissue would primarily fail between the cell boundaries. Indeed, these ballistic penetration data are qualitatively consistent with findings from microprobe indentation studies (25), albeit at considerably higher strain rates.

Corresponding calculated penetration profiles using the theoretical model are also shown in Figure 8 and illustrate a similar trend with good agreement. Importantly, in this case, the yield stress was held constant at 40 MPa to achieve the closest fit with the data. This is considerably higher than the quasi-static yield stresses reported in the literature (summarized in Table 1 and Fig. 2). This discrepancy is attributed to a huge strain rate effect: the ballistic impact of the microparticle has a peak strain rate of ~10^6 sec^{-1}. In a subsequent, more refined study (16), these strain rate effects are further elucidated.

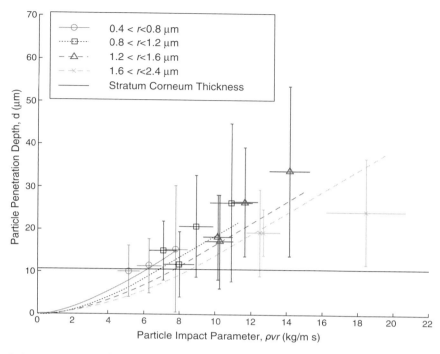

FIGURE 9 Impact parameters and penetration depth of gold particles within excised human skin. *Source*: From 65.

In addition to the described scale and strain rate effects, another source of variability stems from the high sensitivity in SC mechanical properties to hydration and temperature, deriving from variation in ambient conditions [detailed in Ref. 16]. Increasing the RH from 15% to 95% (temperature at 25°C) led to a particle penetration increase by a factor of 1.8. Temperature increases from 20°C to 40°C (RH at 15%) enhanced particle penetration 2-fold. In both cases, these increases were sufficient to move the target layer from the SC to the viable epidermis. In immunotherapeutic applications, this is the difference between the ineffectual delivery of particles to the SC and the targeted delivery of specific cells in the viable epidermis.

These collective data show the momentum range obtained from the described biolistic devices primarily translate into delivery within targeted viable epidermis and SC. With the precise delivery conditions achieved from these devices, we have obtained new insights into the important biological variability in microparticle impact. This variability, together with more obvious differences in tissue thicknesses (with the tissue site of target, age, and sex), must be considered when selecting device conditions for clinical biolistic immunotherapeutic delivery.

Skin Cell Death From Ballistic Impact

Of great importance in biolistics applications is the biological responses induced by biolistic impact. When delivered to the tissue surface, the microparticles undergo a tremendous deceleration—peaking at ~10^{10} g—and coming to rest within ~100–200 ns. Such deceleration induces shock and stress waves within the tissue, and it is important to determine under which conditions skin cells are killed. This was investigated in mice, where following the delivery of gold microparticles, the cell death was assayed with mixtures of ethidium bromide and acridine orange and images noninvasively with multiphoton microscopy (71). It was found that each direct impact of a gold microparticle resulted in cell death. Further, even in cases where microparticles passed within ~10 μm of the cell surface—but not touching the cell—cell death resulted. A sufficiently high number density in the tissue can result in complete cell death within the viable epidermis. Clearly, this is important when considering the biological responses induced by microparticle impact.

Clinical Results and Commercial Application
Commercial Application
Biolistics is a platform technology for delivering a broad range of drugs and immunotherapeutics. Currently, the technology is progressing commercially in two streams:

- Delivery of local lidocaine anesthetic to the skin (the larger class of particles shown in Figure 8), approved by the FDA for market application (Zingo™; Anesiva, San Francisco, California, U.S.)
- Delivery of DNA vaccines on gold microparticles (PowderMed™; Pfizer, New York, New York, U.S.; undergoing phase III clinical trials).

Clinical Results
Although strong results are achieved in other immunotherapeutics such as allergy immunotherapy of the animal model (63) and lidocaine for anesthesia, the key clinical progress with DNA vaccines is discussed here.

The DNA plasmid that forms the active component DNA vaccines is precipitated onto microscopic gold particles (typically 2 μg DNA on 1 mg of gold). Microscopic elemental gold particles (mean particle diameter ~2 μm) are used as the plasmid DNA carrier, because it is inert and has the appropriate density needed to deliver the vaccine directly into the target epidermal immunologically sensitive cells, including Langerhans cells.

Following delivery into the antigen-presenting cell, the DNA elutes off the gold particle and is transcribed into RNA. The RNA, in turn, is translated into the relevant antigen, which is then processed and presented on the cell surface as if it were an intracellular viral protein. An efficient cellular and humoral immune response is thus induced.

A series of clinical trials have been conducted to assess the immunogenicity and safety of a prophylactic hepatitis B virus DNA vaccine (54,72,73). These studies have demonstrated that biolistic DNA vaccination can elicit antigen-specific humoral and T cell responses. In the study by Roy et al. (54), DNA vaccination with 1 to 4 μg of hepatitis B surface antigen elicited measurable cytotoxic T cell responses and T_H cell responses in all 12 healthy adults who had not previously been immunized with a hepatitis B vaccine (54). Furthermore, all 12 previously nonvaccinated subjects also seroconverted with levels of hepatitis B–specific antibody ranging from 10 to >5000 mIU/mL. This is of particular significance as intramuscular delivery of DNA—using the needle and syringe—with up to 1000-fold more DNA has generated only low or no antibody responses (74,75). The same biolistic hepatitis B DNA

TABLE 2 Serum Antibody Responses, Seroconversion, and Seroprotection Rate

Group	Day	GMT (range)	Seroconversion[a] (%)	Seroprotection[b] (%)	Mean GMT increase (fold)
1	0	16 (5–40)	–	17 (2/12)	–
	14	23 (5–160)	8 (1/12)	42 (5/12)	1.4
	21	28 (10–240)	17 (2/12)	33 (4/12)	1.7
	56	44 (10–320)	33 (4/12)	58 (7/12)	**2.8**
2	0	17 (5–40)	–	33 (4/12)	–
	14	29 (10–60)	17 (2/12)	50 (6/12)	1.7
	21	36 (20–80)	8 (1/12)	58 (7/12)	2.1
	56	65 (20–320)	**67 (8/12)**	**92 (11/12)**	3.9
3	0	12 (5–40)	–	8 (1/12)	–
	14	21 (5–80)	17 (2/12)	25 (3/12)	1.8
	21	40 (10–160)	33 (4/12)	67 (8/12)	3.4
	56	97 (40–640)	**64 (7/11)**	**100 (11/11)**	8.1

Note: Values meeting CPMP criteria are in bold.
[a]Seroconversion is defined as either a negative prevaccination titer (≤ 10) to a postvaccination titer ≥ 40 or a significant increase in antibody titer (i.e., at least a fourfold increase between prevaccination and postvaccination titers where the prevaccination titer is ≥ 10).
[b]Seroprotection rate is defined as the proportion of subjects achieving a titer ≥ 40.
Source: From Ref. 76.

vaccine was also shown to increase serum antibody titers in 7 of 11 subjects who had previously failed to seroconvert after three or more doses of conventional vaccination with licensed recombinant protein vaccine (72). Finally this plasmid DNA construct has been used to successfully bridge between the earlier bulky experimental device and the simple, handheld disposable device that will be used for product commercialization (73).

A phase I study (76) has been carried out to investigate the safety and immunogenicity of biolistic administration of an influenza prophylactic plasmid, which encodes a single hemagglutination (HA) antigen of influenza A/Panama/2007/99 (H3N2). A total of 36 healthy subjects with low preexisting serological responses to this strain received a vaccination of 1, 2, or 4 µg of DNA at a single administration session. The antibody response was then assessed according to the Committee for Medicinal Products for Human Use criteria for the approval of annual flu vaccines in the European Union. Table 2 summarizes these humoral responses, determined as a hemagglutination inhibition titer elicited on days 0 (predose), 14, 21, and 56. Time points, where responses met the levels required by the CHMP guidelines for licensing of annual influenza vaccine, are shown in bold.

The 4-µg-dose group met the CHMP criteria at day 21, demonstrating the ability of biolistic DNA vaccination to stimulate serological responses equivalent to those seen in protein based approaches. Furthermore, the responses in all groups continued to increase up to day 56 (the last day monitored) indicating that responses to biolistic vaccination may show a more sustained increase than is typically seen with protein vaccines. By day 56 100% of those subjects vaccinated with the 4 µg dose were seroprotected.

Overall vaccination was well tolerated, and local reactogenicity results were typical of those seen in other biolistics studies.

CONCLUSION

Many immunotherapeutics (e.g., vaccines) can be radically improved by targeted delivery to particular immunologically sensitive cells within the outer skin layers. The push is on to develop a range of technologies to meet this need, either using physical or biological targeting approaches. One of these methods, called biolistics, ballistically delivers biomolecule-coated gold microparticles to the outer layers of the skin. The method of particle acceleration relies heavily on approaches usually applied to the aerospace industry. Consequently, many unique challenges had to be overcome in engineering biolistic devices for clinical use. Research with the resultant devices has yielded unique insights into the skin at microscale dynamic loading—both from mechanical and biological perspectives. Important progress is also being made in clinical trials using biolistic devices to deliver DNA vaccines in the following fields: hepatitis B, influenza, genital herpes, human papillomavirus, HIV/AIDS, Hantaan virus, melanoma, and a variety of other cancers.

REFERENCES

1. Givens B, Oberle S, Lander J. Taking the jab out of needles. Can Nurs J 1993;89:37–40.
2. Fuchs E, Raghavan S. Getting under the skin of epidermal morphogenesis. Nat Rev Genet 2002; 3:199–209.
3. Menton DN, Eisen AZ. Structure and organization of mammalian stratum corneum. J Ultrastruct Res 1971; 35(3):247–264.
4. Nemes Z, Steinert PM. Bricks and mortar of the epidermal barrier. Exp Mol Med 1999; 31:5–19.
5. Stenn KS, Goldenhersh MA, Trepeta RW. Structure and Functions of the Skin. The Skin. Vol. 9. London: Churchill Livingstone, 1992.
6. Chen H, Yuan J, Wang Y, Silvers WK. Distribution of ATPase-positive Langerhans cells in normal adult human skin. Br J Dermatol 1985; 113(6):707–711.
7. Berman B, Chen VL, France DS, Dotz WI, Petroni G. Anatomical mapping of epidermal Langerhans cell densities in adults. Br J Dermatol 1983; 109(5): 553–558.
8. Babiuk S, Baca-Estrada M, Babiuk LA, Ewen C, Foldvari M. Cutaneous vaccination: the skin as an immunologically active tissue and the challenge of antigen delivery. J Control Release 2000; 66:199–214.
9. Chen D, Maa Y, Haynes JR. Needle-free epidermal powder immunization. Expert Rev Vaccines 2002; 1(3):89–100.
10. Banchereau J, Steinman RM. Dendritic cells and the control of immunity. Nature 1998; 19(392):245–252.
11. McKinney EC, Streilein JW. On the extraordinary capacity of allogeneic epidermal Langerhans cells to prime cytotoxic T cells *in vivo*. J Immunol 1989; 143:1560–1564.
12. Timares L, Takashima A, Johnston SA. Quantitative analysis of the immunopotency of genetically transfected dendritic cells. Proc Natl Acad Sci USA 1998; 95:13147–13152.
13. Hoath SB, Leahy DG. Formation and function of the stratum corneum. In: Marks R, Levenge J, Voegli R, eds. The Essential Stratum Corneum. London, U.K.: Martin Dunitz, 2002.
14. Numahara T, Tanemura M, Nakagawa T, Takaiwa T. Spatial data analysis by epidermal Langerhans cells reveals an elegant system. J Dermatol Sci 2001; 25:219–228.
15. Bauer J, Bahmer FA, Worl J, Neuhuber W, Schuler G, Fartasch M. A strikingly constant ratio exists between Langerhans cells and other epidermal cells in human skin. A stereologic study using the optical dissector method and the confocal laser-scanning microscope. J Invest Dermatol 2001; 116:313–318.
16. Kendall MAF, Rishworth S, Carter FV, Mitchell TJ. The effects of relative humidity and ambient temperature on the ballistic delivery of micro-particles into excised porcine skin. J Invest Dermatol 2004; 122(3):739–746.
17. Hopewell JW. The skin: its structure and response to ionizing radiation. Int J Radiat Biol 1990; 57(4):751–773.

18. Wildnauer RH, Bothwell JW, Douglas AB. Stratum corneum properties. I. Influence of relative humidity on normal and extracted stratum corneum. J Invest Dermatol 1971; 56:72–78.
19. Christensen MS, Hargens CW, Nacht S, Gans EH. Viscoelastic properties of intact human skin: instrumentation, hydration effects and the contribution of the stratum corneum. J Invest Dermatol 1977; 69:282–286.
20. Rawlings A, Harding C, Watkinson A, Banks J, Ackerman O, Sabin R. The effect of glycerol and humidity on desmosome degradation in the stratum corneum. Arch Dermatol Res 1995; 287:457–464.
21. Dobrev H. In vivo non-invasive study of the mechanical properties of the human skin after single application of topical corticosteroids. Folia Med (Plovdiv) 1996; 38: 7–11.
22. Nicolopoulos CS, Giannoudis PV, Glaros KD, Barbanel JC. In vitro study of the failure of skin surface after influence of hydration and reconditioning. Arch Dermatol Res 1998; 290:638–640.
23. Kendall MAF, Rishworth S, Carter FV, Mitchell TJ. The effects of relative humidity and ambient temperature on the ballistic delivery of micro-particles into excised porcine skin. J Invest Dermatol 2004; 122(3):739–746.
24. Papir YS, Hsu, K-H, Wildnauer RH. The mechanical properties of stratum corneum I. The effect of water and ambient temperature on the tensile properties of newborn rat stratum corneum. Biochim Biophys Acta 1975; 399:170–180.
25. Kendall MAF, Chong Y, Cock A. The mechanical properties of the skin epidermis in relation to targeted gene and drug delivery. Biomaterials 2007; 28:4968–4977.
26. Lu B, Federoff HJ, Wang Y, Goldsmith LA, Scott G. Topical application of viral vectors for epidermal gene transfer. J Invest Dermatol 1997; 108, 803–808.
27. Tang D-C, Shi Z, Curiael DT. Vaccination onto bare skin. Nature 1997; 388:729–730.
28. Mumper RJ, Ledebur HC. Dendritic cell delivery of plasmid DNA: application for controlled nucleic acid-based vaccines. Mol Biotech 2001; 19, 79–95.
29. World Health Organisation. Safety of Injections, Facts, Figures Fact Sheet No. 232. Geneva, Switzerland: World Health Organisation, 1999.
30. Glenn GM, Kenney RT, Ellingsworth LR, Frech SA, Hammond SA, Zoeteweweij JP. Transcutaneous immunization and immunostimulant strategies: capitalizing on the immunocompetence of the skin. Expert Rev Vaccines 2003; 2(2):253–267.
31. Guerena-Burgueno F, Hall ER, Taylor DN. Safety and immunogenicity of a prototype enterotoxigenic *Escherichia coli* vaccine administered transcutaneously. Infect Immun 2002; 70(4):1874–1880.
32. Kendall MAF Engineering of needle-free physical methods to target epidermal cells for DNA vaccination. Vaccine 2006; 24(21):4651–4656.
33. Liu LJ, Watabe S, Yang J, et al. Topical application of HIV DNA vaccine with cytokine-expression plasmids induces strong antigen-specific immune responses. Vaccine 2001; 20(1–2):42–48.
34. Watabe S, Xin KQ, Ihata A, et al. Protection against influenza virus challenge by topical application of influenza DNA vaccine. Vaccine 2001; 19(31):4434–4444.
35. Shi Z, Zeng M, Yang G, et al. Protection against tetanus by needle-free inoculation of adenovirus-vectored nasal and epicutaneous vaccines. J Virol 2001; 75(23): 11474–11482.
36. Shi Z, Curiel DT, Tang DC. DNA-based non-invasive vaccination onto the skin. Vaccine 1999; 17(17):2136–2141.
37. Widera G, Austin M, Rabussay D, et al. Increased DNA vaccine delivery and immunogenicity by electroporation in vivo. J Immunol 2000; 164:4635–4640.
38. Zucchelli S, Capone S, Fattori E, et al. Enhancing B- and T-cell immune response to a hepatitis C virus E2 DNA vaccine by intramuscular electrical gene transfer. J Virol 2000; 74:11598–11607.
39. Sintov AC, Krymberk I, Daniel D, Hannan T, Sohn Z, Levin G. Radiofrequency-driven skin microchanneling as a new way for electrically assisted transdermal delivery of hydrophilic drugs. J Control Release 2003; 89(2):311–320.
40. Alexander MY, Akhurst RJ. Liposome-mediated gene transfer and expression via the skin. Hum Molec Genet 1995; 4:2279–2285.

41. Li L, Hoffman RM. The feasibility of targeted selective gene therapy of the hair follicle. Nat Med 1995; 1:705–706.
42. Domashenko A, Gupta S, Cotsarelis G. Efficient delivery of transgenes to human hair follicle progenitor cells using topical lipoplex. Nat Biotechnol 2000; 18:420–423.
43. Cui Z, Mumper RJ. Dendritic cell-targeted genetic vaccines engineered from novel microemulsion precursors. Mol Ther 2001; 3:S352.
44. Furth PA, Shamay A, Henninghausen L. Gene transfer into mammalian cells by jet injection. Hybridoma 1995; 14:149–152.
45. Bremseth DL, Pass F. Delivery of insulin by jet injection: recent observations. Diabetes Technol Ther 2001; 3:225–232.
46. Mikszta JA, Alarcon JB, Brittingham JM, Sutter DE, Pettis RJ, Harvery NG. Improved genetic immunization via micromechanical disruption of skin-barrier function and targeted epidermal delivery. Nature 2002; 8(4):415–419.
47. Matriano JA, Cormier M, Johnson J, et al. Macroflux microprojection array patch technology: a new and efficient approach for intracutaneous immunization. Pharm Res 2002; 19(1):63–70.
48. McAllister DV, Wang PM, Davis SP, et al. Microfabricated needles for transdermal delivery of macromolecules and nanoparticles: fabrication methods and transport studies. Proc Natl Acad Sci USA 2003; 25(100):13755–13760.
49. Kendall MAF. Device for Delivery of Bioactive Materials and Other Stimuli. U.S. Patent Application, U.S. 11/496,053, filed August 2006.
50. Sanford JC, Klein MC. Delivery of substances into cells and tissues using a particle bombardment process. J Part Sci Technol 1987; 5:27–37.
51. Bellhouse BJ, Sarphie DF, Greenford JC. Needleless syringe using supersonic gas flow for particle delivery. International Patent WO94/24263, 1994.
52. Burkoth TL, Bellhouse BJ, Hewson G, Longridge DJ, Muddle AG, Sarphie DF. Transdermal and transmucosal powdered drug delivery. Crit Rev Ther Drug Carrier Syst 1999; 16(4):331–384.
53. Chen DX, Endres RL, Erickson CA, et al. Epidermal immunization by a needle-free powder delivery technology: immunogenicity of influenza vaccine and protection in mice. Nat Med 2000; 6:1187–1190.
54. Roy MJ, Wu MS, Barr LJ, et al. Induction of antigen-specific CD8+ T cells, T helper cells, and protective levels of antibody in humans by particle mediated administration of a hepatitis B virus DNA vaccine. Vaccine 2000; 19:764–778.
55. Lesinski GB, Smithson SL, Srivastava N, Chen DX, Widera G, Westerink JA. DNA vaccine encoding a peptide mimic of *Streptococcus pneumoniae* serotype 4 capsular polysaccharide induces specific anti-carbohydrate antibodies in Balb/c mice. Vaccine 2001;19:1717–1726.
56. Kendall MAF, Quinlan NJ, Thorpe SJ, Ainsworth RW, Bellhouse BJ. Measurements of the gas and particle flow within a converging–diverging nozzle for high speed powdered vaccine and drug delivery. Exp Fluids 2004; 37:128–136.
57. Quinlan NJ, Kendall MAF, Bellhouse BJ, Ainsworth RW. Investigations of gas and particle dynamics in first generation needle-free drug delivery devices. Int J Shock Waves 2001; 10(6):395–404.
58. Liu Y, Kendall MAF. Numerical study of a transient gas and particle flow in a high-speed needle-free ballistic particulate vaccine delivery system. J Mech Med Biol 2004; 4(4):1–20.
59. Kendall MAF. The delivery of particulate vaccines and drugs to human skin with a practical, hand-held shock tube-based system. Shock Waves J 2002; 12(1):22–30.
60. Liu Y, Kendall MAF. Numerical simulation of heat transfer from a transonic jet impinging on skin for needle-free powdered drug and vaccine delivery. J Mech Eng Sci Proc Inst Mech Eng 2004; 218(C):1373–1383.
61. Truong NK, Liu Y, Kendall MAF. Gas-particle dynamics characterisation of a pre-clinical contoured shock tube for vaccine and drug delivery. *Shock Waves* 2007; 15:149–154.
62. Marrion M, Kendall MAF, Liu Y. The gas-dynamic effects of a hemisphere-cylinder obstacle in a shock-tube driver. Exp Fluids 2005; 38:319–327.

63. Kendall MAF, Mitchell TJ, Costigan G, et al. Down regulation of IgE allergic responses in the lung by epidermal biolistic micro-particle delivery. Allergy Clin Immunol J 2006; 117(2):275–282.

64. Mitchell TJ, Kendall MAF, Bellhouse BJ. A ballistic study of micro-particle penetration to the oral mucosa. Int J Impact Eng 2003; 28:581–599.

65. Kendall MAF, Mitchell TJ, Wrighton-Smith P. Intradermal ballistic delivery of micro-particles into excised human skin for drug and vaccine applications. J Biomechanics 2004; 37(11):1733–1741.

66. Dehn J. A unified theory of penetration. Int J Impact Eng 1976; 5:239–248.

67. Duck FA. Physical Properties of Tissue: A Comprehensive Reference Book. London: Academic Press, 1990.

68. Blank IH, Ernslie AG, Simon I, Apt C. The diffusion of water across the stratum corneum as a function of its water content. J Invest Dermatol 1984; 82:188–94.

69. Kishino A, Yanagida T. Force measurements by micromanipulation of a single actin filament by glass needles. Nature 1988; 334:74–76.

70. Mitchell TM. The ballistics of micro-particles into the mucosa and skin. DPhil thesis, Engineering Science, University of Oxford, 2003.

71. Raju PA, Truong NK, Kendall MAF. Assessment of epidermal cell viability by near infra-red two-photon microscopy following ballistic delivery of gold micro-particles. Vaccine 2006; 24(21):4644–4647.

72. Rottinghaus ST, Poland GA, Jacobson RM, Barr LJ, Roy MJ. Hepatitis B DNA vaccine induces protective antibody responses in human non-responders to conventional vaccination. Vaccine 2003; 21(31):4604–4608.

73. Roberts LK, Barr LJ, Fuller DH, McMahon CW, Leese PT, Jones S. Clinical safety and efficacy of a powdered hepatitis B nucleic acid vaccine delivered to the epidermis by a commercial prototype device. Vaccine 2005; 23(40):4867–4878.

74. MacGregor RR, Boyer JD, Ugen KE, et al. First human trial of a DNA-based vaccine for treatment of human immunodeficiency virus type 1 infection: safety and host response. J Infect Dis 1998; 178(1):92–100.

75. MacGregor RR, Ginsberg R, Ugen KE, et al. T-cell responses induced in normal volunteers immunized with a DNA-based vaccine containing HIV-1 env and rev. AIDS 2002; 16(16):2137–2143.

76. Drape RJ. Macklin MD, Barr LJ, Jones S, Haynes JR, Dean HJ. Epidermal DNA vaccine for influenza is immunogenic in humans. Vaccine 2006; 24(21):4475–4481.

Index